Handbuch der Urologie · Encyclopedia of Urology

Founded by C. E. Alken, V. W. Dix, H. M. Weyrauch, E. Wildbolz
Edited by L. Andersson, R. F. Gittes, W. E. Goodwin
W. Lutzeyer, E. Zingg

Disturbances in Male Fertility

By

K. Bandhauer   G. Bartsch   D. M. de Kretser
A. Eshkol   J. Frick   M. Glezerman   J. B. Kerr
B. Lunenfeld   W. Pöldinger   H. P. Rohr
F. Scharfetter   P. D. Temple-Smith

Edited by

K. Bandhauer · J. Frick

With 153 Figures

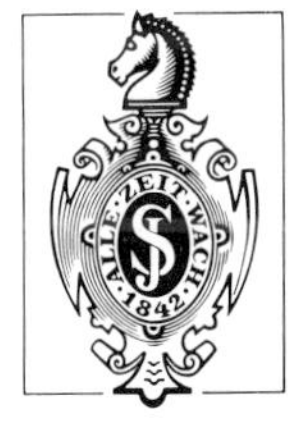

Springer-Verlag Berlin Heidelberg New York 1982

Handbuch der Urologie · Encyclopedia of Urology · Band XVI

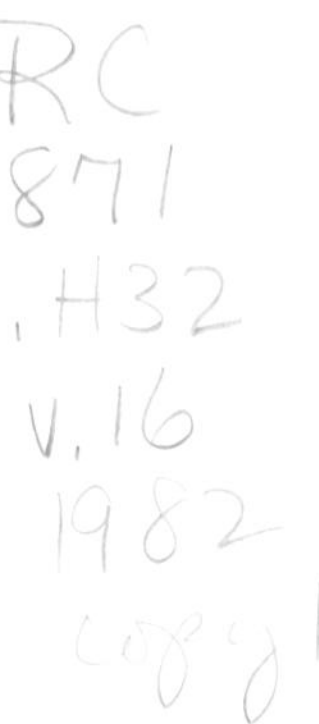

ISBN 3-540-05279-8 Springer-Verlag Berlin Heidelberg New York
ISBN 0-387-05279-8 Springer-Verlag New York Heidelberg Berlin

Library of Congress Cataloging in Publication Data (Revised)
Main entry under title: Handbuch der Urologie. Vols. published after 1964 have imprint:
Berlin, New York, Springer Verlag.
Includes bibliographies.
CONTENTS: 1. Anatomie und Embryologie, von K. CONRAD et al. 1969. – 2. Physiologie und pathologische
Physiologie, von B. FEY et al. 1965. – . –
16 Disturbances in male fertility, by K. Bandhauer [et al.] 1981.
1. Urology – Collected works. I. ALKEN, CARL ERICH, 1912– ed. II. Title: Encyclopedia of urology. [DNLM:
1. Sterility, Male. WJ 100 H237] RC871.H28   616.6   58-4788   AACR1
ISBN 3-540-05279-8 ISBN 0-387-05279-8

Typesetting, printing and bookbinding: Universitätsdruckerei H. Stürtz AG, Würzburg
2122/3130-543210

List of Contributors

K. BANDHAUER, Klinik für Urologie, Kantonsspital St. Gallen, CH-9007 St. Gallen

J. FRICK, Urologische Abteilung, Landeskrankenanstalten Salzburg, A-5020 Salzburg

G. BARTSCH, Universitätsklinik für Urologie, Anichstraße 35, A-6020 Innsbruck

D.M. DE KRETSER, Department of Anatomy, Monash University, Clayton Victoria Australia 3168

A. ESHKOL, Institut of Endocrinology, Sackler School of Medicine, The Chaim Sheba Medical Center, Tel-Aviv University, The State of Israel Ministry of Health, Tel-Hashomer, Israel 52621

M. GLEZERMAN, Department of Obstetrics and Gynecology, Soroka Medical Center and Ben Gurion University, Assa Street 3, Beer Sheva, Israel

J.B. KERR, Department of Anatomy, Monash University, Clayton Victoria Australia 3168

B. LUNENFELD, Institut of Endocrinology, Sackler School of Medicine, The Chaim Sheba Medical Center, Tel-Aviv University, The State of Israel Ministry of Health, Tel-Hashomer, Israel 52621

W. PÖLDINGER, Kantonale Psychiatrische Klinik Wil, Zürcherstraße 30, CH-9500 Wil/SG

H.P. ROHR, Pathologisches Institut, Universität Basel, Schönbeinstraße 40, CH-4031 Basel

F. SCHARFETTER, Klinik für Neurochirurgie, Kantonsspital St. Gallen, CH-9007 St. Gallen

P.D. TEMPLE-SMITH, Department of Anatomy, Monash University, Clayton Victoria Australia 3168

Preface

Impending famine and a terrifying rate of consumption of natural resources are vital issues which have focussed public interest in the ecologic, social and political problems of ever increasing overpopulation in many countries of the world. As well as the vast material and intellectual expenditure lavished on family planning and birth control, the past decade has seen an immense research effort in the elaboration of improved methods of fertility control, both for men and for women. During the same period, however, research into the causes of male fertility disorders has proceeded with equal intensity, and a number of promising therapeutic approaches have become the subject of clinical trials. The wish of an individual or of a couple to have offspring is an absolute which requires no further justification, and there can be few challenges to a physician as essential as the spouses' predicament in a childless marriage. Only with a special knowledge of the function, pathology and pathophysiology of the reproductive system is he properly equipped to meet that challenge.

Even today it is frequently considered that the wife in such a childless marriage is "at fault", and although in the light of our present knowledge the cause is almost equally likely to be found in either partner, it has for many years been traditional first and foremost to investigate the wife. At the root of these so widely held attitudes lies not only the historical and social development of the world's major cultures nor indeed merely the image of woman, the conceiver and seat of fertility, but also the erroneous concept that the coital potency and fertility of a man are one and the same. This prejudice, in addition to the evident and apparently more easily assessed cyclic events of ovulation, has for many years placed female sterility in the limelight of diagnostic and therapeutic endeavour. Nevertheless it would be quite wrong to believe that understanding of fertility disorders in men is purely an achievement of recent decade. LESKY[1] (1950) and MÜLLER[2] (1957) have reviewed an almost unbroken historical record of efforts to understand male fertility problems, reaching from antiquity to the present day. Their monographs reveal that fertility and sterility in men have occupied medical and scientific minds to an exceptional degree ever since classical time. Anyone interested in these fascinating problems should refer to their publications, the principal features

---

[1] LESKY, E.: Die Zeugungs- und Vererbungslehre der Antike und ihre Nachwirken. Akademie der Wissenschaften und der Literatur. 1950, 19, 1226.

[2] MÜLLER, W.: Über die Bedeutung der Infertilität des Mannes in der Medizingeschichte mit Beispielen aus der Weltgeschichte. Diss. Würzburg 1957.

of which HEINKE and DÖPFMER [3] have summarised in their Handbook of Dermatology and Venereology (Volume VI/3). However long this preoccupation may have existed, it cannot be denied that, until the past decade, the management of male fertility disorders has never achieved the same standard as is the case for female sterility. Although Johann Ham "discovered" spermatoza as early as 1677, and despite the great advances made in our knowledge of intracellular hormone metabolism ever since the basic descriptions of testicular morphology by LEYDIG [4] (1850) and SERTOLI [5] (1878), there are still a remarkable number of unsolved problems in understanding spermatogenesis. The most intense research efforts in the fields of endocrinology and biochemistry have so far failed to answer the ultimate questions as to the hormonal control of spermatogenesis, the influence of seminal fluid on the fertility of semen or the mechanisms of maturation, transport and motility of the individual fertilising sperm. The investigation of male fertility disorders remains dependent on rather crude empirical parameters of the quality and quantity of semen. Therapeutic successes are sparse, corresponding to this dubious state of knowledge, and there remain few precisely defined causes of impaired fertility accessible to specific treatment. Whereas female sterility has for a long time been the domain of a single medical speciality – gynecology – the problems of male sterility have been, and remain, contrastingly divided between a multitude of disciplines. This fact alone must surely go a long way towards explaining the discrepancy in the results obtained when investigating and treating fertility disorders in men and women. Urologists, gynecologists, dermatologists and endocrinologists are all involved in the problems of male fertility, with one or another speciality taking the lead, according to regional preferences. Repeated attempts to establish a specialist field of Andrology have so far failed to produce concrete results although in many countries urologists have come to show an increasing interest in the various aspects of male fertility disorders and have thus moved towards Andrologic practice. One should not however conclude from these developments that any one of the present specialist fields is so situated as to be able to encompass all the complexities of reproductive problems and do justice to them either in clinical practice or in co-ordinated research. Only the closest interdisciplinary co-operation and recognition that anatomical, endocrine, biochemical, genetic and immune disorders all represent important causes of impaired male fertility is likely to lead to further advances in the management of male sterility. In particular, further research into the physiology and pathophysiology of the male reproductive tract demands such co-operation.

This volume is intended for those among our colleagues whose principal interest lies in the clinical problems of male infertility. Appearing as it does in the "Encyclopedia of Urology" series it is obviously primarily directed at

---

[3] HEINKE, E. und R. DÖPFMER: Entwurf einer Medizingeschichte der Fertilitätsstörungen beim Manne. In: Handbuch der Haut- und Geschlechtskrankheiten, Ergänzungswerk, Band VI/3, 1960. Springer-Verlag Berlin-Göttingen-Heidelberg 1960.

[4] LEYDIG, A.: Untersuchungen zur Anatomie und Histologie der Tiere, Z. Wiss. Zool. 2, 47 (1850).

[5] SERTOLI, E.: Sulla struttura dei canalicoli semeniferi dei testicoli studiata in rapport allo sviluppe dei nemaspermi, Torino 1878.

the urologist. It is the latter, after all, whose field brings him into the closest contact with these issues, whether he is principally concerned with clinical investigation and treatment or whether his opinion has been sought on a specific issue by a specialist in another field. It has already been pointed out that numerous problems of male fertility and sterility spill over into adjacent medical and scientific fields, such as biochemistry, genetics, immunology, etc., and therefore our treatment of the subject is necessarily incomplete and lays no claim to being encyclopedic or exhaustive. We have rather attempted to guide the clinician in his encounter with male sterility, illuminating various problems by reference to their physiologic and pathophysiologic basis.

We owe our gratitude to all those who have contributed to this volume and take this opportunity of thanking them for their great efforts and for their help in its completion. Every one of them has exerted a decisive influence on the shape of the final product.

K. BANDHAUER   J. FRICK

Contents

Contents

Quantitative Morphology of the Prostate and Epididymis
G. Bartsch and H.P. Rohr
With 32 Figures

Etiology of Fertility Disturbances in Man
M. GLEZERMAN
With 2 Figures

Male Fertility Disorders – History and Clinical Examination
K. BANDHAUER
With 1 Figure

Semen Analysis
M. GLEZERMAN
With 3 Figures

Testicular Biopsy
M. GLEZERMAN
With 7 Figures

Radiologic Investigation of Male Fertility Disorders
K. BANDHAUER
With 6 Figures

Endocrine Evalution of Male Fertility Disorders
B. Lunenfeld and M. Glezerman
With 2 Figures

Neurology of Male Fertility Disorders
F. Scharfetter
With 1 Figure

Immunologic Causes of Male Fertility Disorders

K. Bandhauer

Treatment of Male Infertility
M. GLEZERMAN and B. LUNENFELD

Operative Therapy of Male Infertility
J. Frick
With 11 Figures

Artificial Insemination and Semen Preservation
M. Glezerman
With 3 Figures

Male Contraception
J. Frick
With 17 Figures

Impotence

K. BANDHAUER

Functional Sexual Disorders in the Male
W. Pöldinger

Male Climacteric?
B. Lunenfeld, A. Eshkol, and M. Glezerman
With 2 Figures

Anatomical and Functional Aspects of the Male Reproductive Organs

D.M. de Kretser, P.D. Temple-Smith, and J.B. Kerr

With 66 Figures

A. Testis

I. Development

The testis develops on the dorsal wall of the embryo within a condensation of mesoderm termed the gonadal ridge derived from the intermediate cell mass. The gonadal ridge in man first becomes a discernible structure by the 5th–6th week of gestation and provides the precursors for Sertoli and Leydig cells and for the connective tissue stroma of the testis (Witschi, 1951). The germ cell component is provided by the migration of primordial germ cells from the yolk sac to the developing gonad at approximately the 6th week of gestation. The arrival of the primordial germ cells is followed by a period of mitotic cell division and a general reorganization of the gonad into a series of seminiferous cords and intercordal tissue. This stage of testicular differentiation is clearly dependent on a Y chromosome that contains the genome for testis differentiation and results in the production of a specific protein on the surface of cells in the male. This substance is recognizable by immunological techniques such as the H-Y antigen and is thought to determine the formation of seminiferous cords (Ohno, 1977).

The seminiferous cords are composed of primordial germ cells which are centrally placed and supporting cells which are essentially immature or undifferentiated Sertoli cells (Pelliniemi and Niemi, 1969; Jost et al. 1974). The intercordal tissue contains mesenchymal precursors that by the 8th–10th week of gestation give rise to the fetal generation of Leydig cells presumably due to stimulation by the high levels of human chorionic gonadotrophin (HCG) for which receptors have been demonstrated on the fetal Leydig cells (Catt et al. 1975). The secretion of testosterone by the fetal generation of interstitial cells is responsible for the masculization of the genital tract but is not responsible for regression of the Müllerian duct. The latter is dependent on the secretion of a large protein termed antiMüllerian hormone, produced by the testis, most likely from the immature Sertoli cells (Josso et al., 1977).

Centrally, the seminiferous cords link with an anastomosing system of ducts to form the rete testis, which in turn link with tubules of the mesonephric system, these forming the definitive ductule efferentes. These ducts become aggregated to form the head of the epidymis linking with the mesonephric duct, which in turn forms the duct of the epididymis and vas deferens (Jost, 1973).

The initial stages of testicular development take place on the dorsal abdominal wall in the upper lumbar region, and hence the testis derives vascular connections at that level. With subsequent growth of the embryo, the testis effectively descends to reach the inguinal region by the 7th month of gestation, and in 90% of full-term infants the testes are scrotally placed. In a further 7%–8%, descent later takes place within the 1st year of life, but in the remaining boys with cryptorchidism (1.7%–3.0%) the testes are arrested in the line of normal descent or are found in ectopic sites such as the superficial inguinal pouch, superficial abdominal region, the perineum and the thigh (PAULSEN, 1974). The exact role played by the gubernaculum in descent of the testis is controversial, but recent studies in the rat indicate that transsection of this structure during development will cause cryptorchidism (BERGH et al., 1978).

Descent into the scrotum is preceded by a peritoneal sac, the process vaginalis. The testis invaginates the posterior aspect of this sac, which definitively remains as the tunica vaginalis, while in normal development the cranial part of the peritoneal sac becomes obliterated. In some individuals, frequently in association with maldescent of the testis, the processus vaginalis remains patent.

II. General Anatomy

The testis lies within the scrotum surrounded on its anterior and lateral sides by the tunica vaginalis, which does not extend onto the posterior aspects covered by the epididymis. The nerve supply to the testis arises from the renal and aortic plexuses, reaching the testis by running with the testicular artery (MITCHELL, 1935). Afferent fibers enter the spinal cord at the level of the T10–12 spinal segments.

The principal arterial supply is derived from the testicular artery arising directly from the aorta. The testicular artery descends within the coverings of the spermatic cord and is surrounded by the pampiniform plexus of veins. This intimate relationship of the plexus of veins with the testicular artery is thought to be a countercurrent mechanism capable of acting is a heat exchanger, thus lowering the temperature of blood reaching the testis by way of the testicular artery (WAITES and MOULE, 1961). Evidence also exists that testosterone may diffuse from the high concentrations in the venous drainage of the testis into the testicular artery, thus providing a countercurrent mechanism to aid the maintenance of a high testosterone concentration within the testis (FREE et al., 1973).

An additional arterial supply to the testis arises from the deferential artery, and it has been claimed that this supply alone is sufficient to maintain the testis. Based on the above data, the testicular artery has been divided during surgery for cryptorchidism or ligated together with the testicular veins in surgery for varicocele (PALOMO 1949). The long-term results of surgery for cryptorchidism involving disruption of the testicular artery are only now being assessed in terms of fertility, and certainly in some cases no germ cells are found in the testis. Until more extensive data can be provided, the testicular artery should be preserved if at all possible though the results of high ligation of veins for varicocele show no difference if the artery is included in the ligature.

The venous drainage of the testis is of some importance with reference to surgery for varicocele. The pampiniform plexus runs with the spermatic cord to the internal inguinal ring by which stage it is in the form of one or two trunks which run with the testicular artery to drain on the left into the left renal vein and on the right to the inferior vena cava. The use of venography in the diagnosis of varicocele has led to the discovery of a number of sites of anomalous drainage. These include: (1) drainage of the right testicular vein into the right renal vein, (2) venous connections with the distal branches of the renal veins on both sides, (3) divergence of a major venous channel away from the testicular artery and testicular vein beyond the internal inguinal ring, and (4) connections of the pampiniform plexus with veins draining into the external iliac vein. The most likely site of locating the entire venous drainage of the testis thus appears to be within 1 or 2 cm of the internal inguinal ring (COMHAIRE and KUNNEN, 1976).

The major lymphatic channels follow the course of the vascular supply. At their origin, extensive lymphatic sinusoids have been demonstrated in the intertubular tissue of the testis in a number of species carefully fixed by arterial perfusion. However, no extensive network has been demonstrated in man by perfusion techniques. Because of their close proximity to the Leydig cells, the lymph draining the testis has concentrations of testosterone equal to the venous outflow from the testis.

III. Cytological Features

A well-defined fibrous capsule, the tunica albuginea, surrounds the testis and sends septa which incompletely divide the testis into lobules. Posteriorly, extensions of this capsule form the mediastinum of the testis and contains the anastomotic duct system forming the rete testis. Within the lobules lie the coiled seminiferous tubules surrounded by a lamina propria. Between the tubules, the intertubular tissue contains the interstitial cells, lymphatics and the vascular and nerve supply.

1. Seminiferous Tubules

Within the seminiferous tubules, the germ cells undergo the process of spermatogenesis, a complex sequence of changes which can be subdivided into phases (a) replication of stem cells, (b) meiosis, (c) spermiogenesis and (d) Sertoli cells.

a) Replication of Stem Cells

For spermatogenesis to continue to produce a large number of spermatozoa, replication of the stem cells termed spermatogonia (Fig. 1) must continue to provide a pool of cells which can commence the process of meiosis. Several different types of spermatogonia have been identified by CLERMONT (1963), who considered that the type A dark (Ad) constituted the most primitive form. These cells can be recognized by their deeply staining granular chromatin and central nuclear vacuole. They divide to produce pale type A spermatogonia

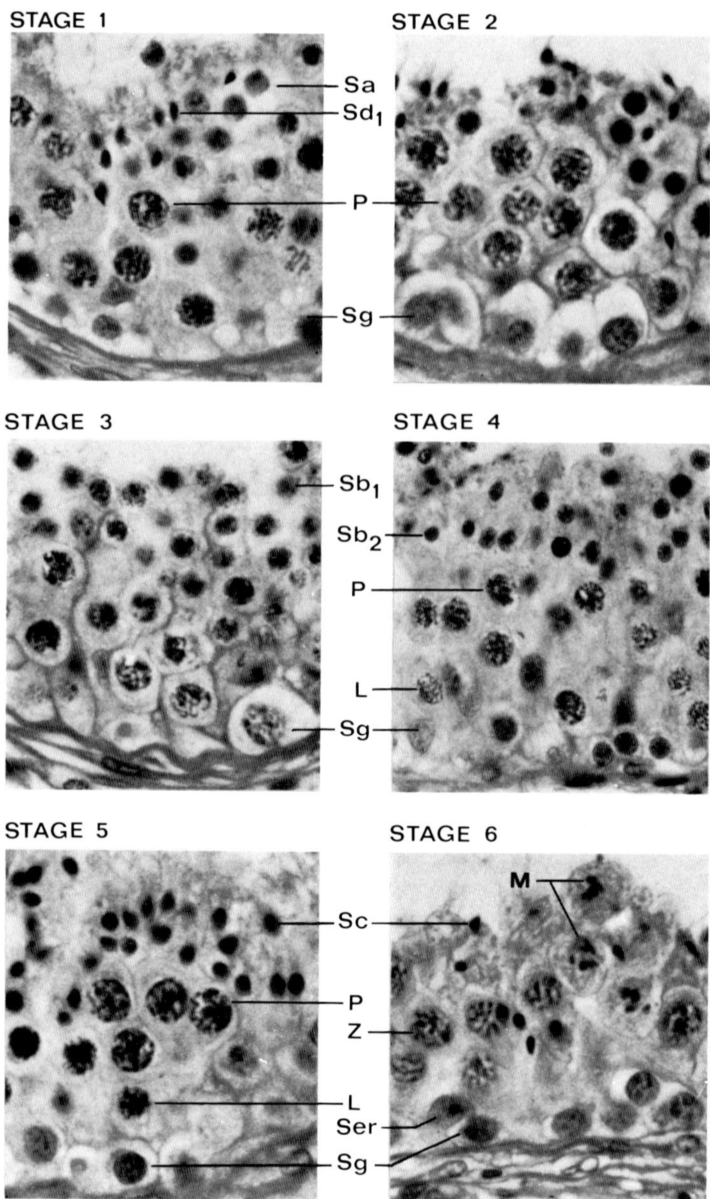

Fig. 1. Photomicrographs illustrate the six stages of the seminiferous cycle in the human testis. *Sg*, spermatogonia; *L*, leptotene; *Z*, zygotene; *P*, pachytene primary spermatocytes; *Sa, Sb$_1$, Sb$_2$, Sc, Sd$_1$* indicate spermatids during spermiogenesis; *Ser*, Sertoli cell nuclei. (After CLERMONT, 1963)

(Ap), which have a nucleus containing finely granular chromatin and one or more nucleoli. Their division results in the emergence of type B spermatogonia, recognized by the presence of peripheral aggregations of chromatin adjacent to the nuclear membrane. Furthermore, their cytoplasm is only partly in contact with the basement membrane of the tubule in contrast to types Ad and Ap. Destruction of the spermatogonial complement of the testis results in irreversible sterility.

b) Meiosis

The reduction of the chromosomal number from the diploid to the haploid state occurs by the process of meiosis, which involves two separate cell divisions. The type B spermatogonia lose their contact with the basement membrane and divide to form the primary spermatocytes which commence the first meiotic division. This division is characterized by a long prophase during which homologous chromosomes pair to form bivalents which may exchange chromosomal material between the pairs by the process of crossing-over. The appearance and behaviour of the chromosomes during this prophase enables classification of primary spermatocytes into several categories: (1) leptotene, (2) zygotene; (3) pachytene, (4) diplotene and (5) diakinesis (Fig. 1). During the prophase, growth occurs in these cells, which become the largest germ cells within the epithelium.

Ultrastructurally, the cytoplasm is characterized by a Golgi complex which increases in size throughout the prophase of meiosis and mitochondria which in the leptotene and zygotene stages form groups surrounded by a granular intermitochondrial material. The cristae of the mitochondria dilate such that the intracristal space frequently forms a central electron-lucid area. The nuclear features characterize many of the phases of the meiotic prophase. In the leptotene stage, single electron-dense threads appear, being representative of the condensing chromosomes. Later in zygotene these threads pair and correspond to the bivalents formed by homologous chromosomes. In zygotene, between the paired threads a central linear electron-dense component develops, forming a tripartite structure, being termed a synaptinemal complex, which persists through pachytene and disappears during diplotene and diakinesis (SOLARI and TRES, 1970). By serial reconstruction, WETTSTEIN and SOTELO (1967) demonstrated that the number of synaptinemal complexes correspond to the number of bivalents.

The division of primary spermatocytes results in the formation of the secondary spermatocytes, which have an extremely short life span before they divide to form the spermatids. Because of their short life span, profiles of secondary spermatocytes are infrequently seen but can be recognized by their position close to the lumen of the seminiferous tubule, their spherical nucleus with large globular chromatin masses and their size of 10–12 µm in diameter (CLERMONT, 1963).

c) Spermiogenesis

No further cell division occurs after the division of secondary spermatocytes to form spermatids. The sequence of changes which result in the transformation

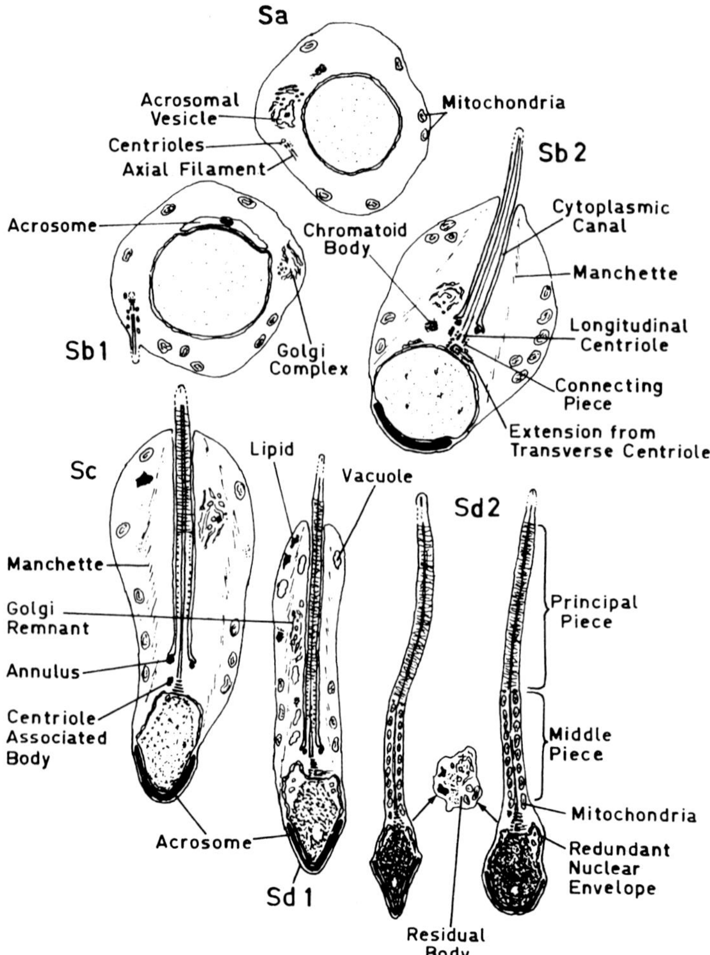

Fig. 2. The ultrastructural features of the stages of spermiogenesis are shown at each phase of spermatid development defined by CLERMONT (1963). [DE KRETSER, Z. Zellforsch *98*, 477–505 (1969)]

of the early spermatid, a conventionally shaped cell, into the highly organized spermatozoon is termed spermiogenesis, but some authors use the term spermateleosis. The cytological changes can be grouped into several areas: (1) formation of the acrosome, (2) development of the flagellum or tail, (3) nuclear changes, (4) reorganization of cell organelles and cytoplasm and (5) release of spermatozoon from epithelium (Fig. 2). Though partially visible by light microscopy, many of the changes can only be observed by electron microscopy (DE KRETSER, 1969; HOLSTEIN, 1976).

α) Formation of the Acrosome

This structure develops by the formation of a large vacuole in the Golgi complex (Fig. 3A). The vacuole is applied to the nuclear membrane on the

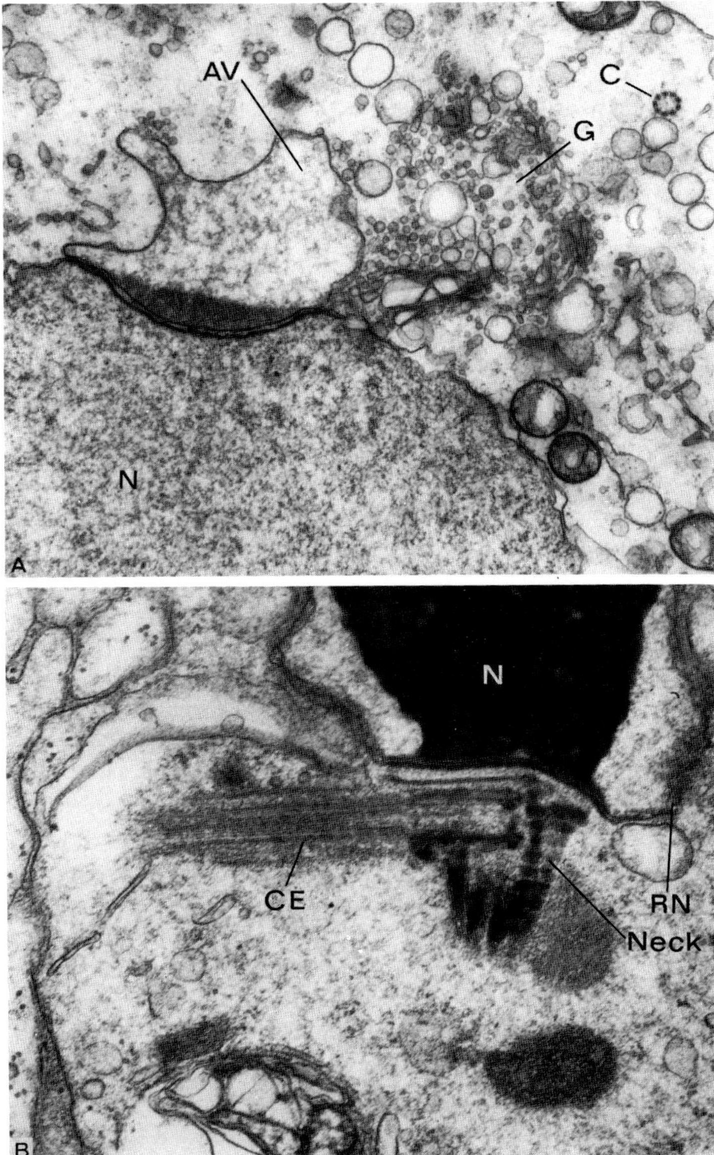

Fig. 3. A The Golgi complex (*G*) giving rise to the acrosomal vesicle (*AV*) lodged against the spermatid nucleus (*N*); note adjacent centriole (*C*). **B** A late phase of spermatid development illustrates the condensed nucleus (*N*), redundant nuclear membrane (*RN*), and the *neck* of sperm; note the extension of microtubule (*CE*) from the proximal centriole lodged in the neck of the sperm

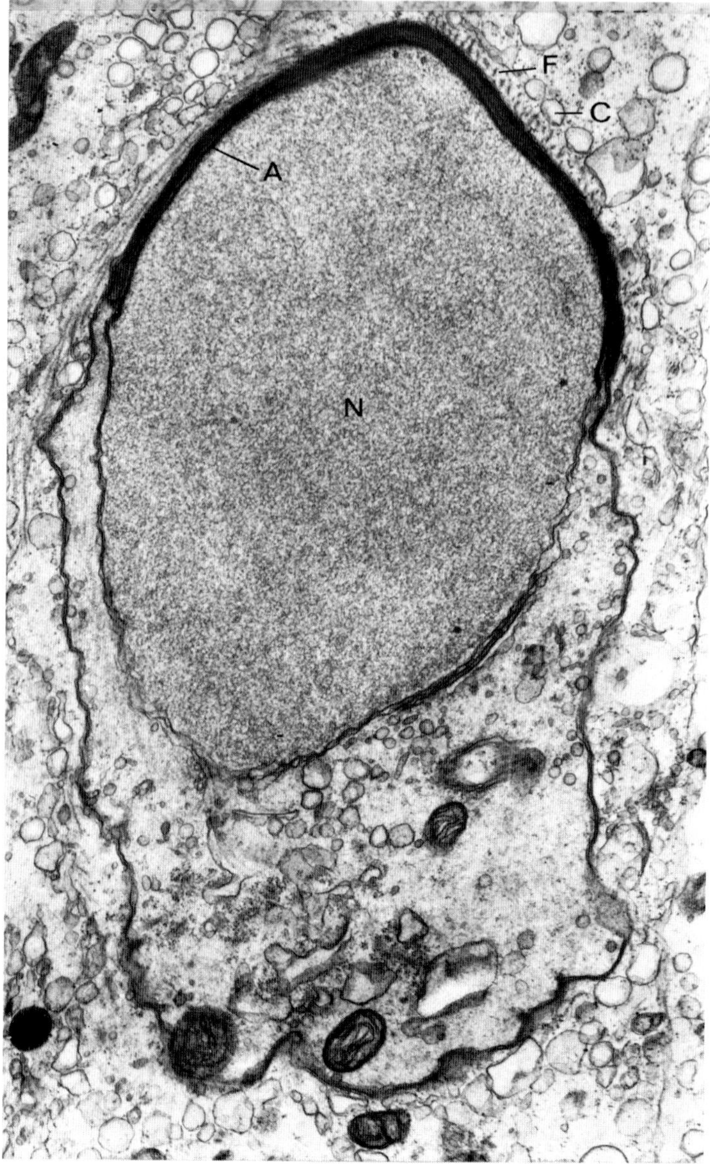

Fig. 4. The Sb stage of spermiogenesis is illustrated and shows the nucleus (*N*), acrosome (*A*), and specialized cell function at the Sertoli cell spermatid interface with cisternae (*C*) and fibrils (*F*)

opposite side of the nucleus to the developing tail or axial filament. Some enlargement of the acrosome occurs by aggregation of vacuoles from the adjacent Golgi complex, and it finally forms a cap-like structure covering the cranial half of the head of the sperm (Figs. 4, 6A). With the change in position of the nucleus, the acrosome separates the nucleus from the cell membrane. It contains glycoprotein material, which includes the specific protein acrosin and enzymes necessary for penetration of the zona pellucida of the ovum (see review by CHANG and HUNTER, 1975).

β) Development of the Flagellum

This structure is formed from one of the pair of centrioles which can be found adjacent to the Golgi complex (Fig. 3 A). Initial development proceeds while the centriole lies free in the cytoplasm and a substantial length of the flagellum has already been formed before it lodges in a depression in the nucleus at the abacrosomal plane. The early development of the flagellum consists of the elaboration of the axial filament which is formed by an outer circle of nine equally spaced doubled microtubules surrounding two centrally placed microtubules (Fig. 7). The proximal portion of the axial filament becomes modified to form the complex structure of the neck of the sperm, which will articulate with the base of the nucleus (Fig. 3 B). In this region of the axial filament, a series of electron-dense columns surround its origin from the distal centriole and also form a fossa in which the proximal centriole is housed at right angles to the plane of the tail. Extending from these columns in the neck, a circular arrangement of nine electron-dense fibers surround the axial filament forming part of the middle piece and principal piece of the sperm tail (Figs. 6, 7). In the latter area, the outer dense fibers become attenuated except for a single pair on opposite sides of the tail, which remain substantial and are joined together by a circumferentially disposed series of ribs. In the terminal segment of the tail, the central core of nine doublets is covered only by the cell membrane.

γ) Nuclear Changes

The central nucleus of the early spermatid becomes displaced to the periphery of the cell and that portion covered by the acrosome comes into contact with the cell membrane (Figs. 4, 5). Associated with this change in position, the chromatin of the spermatid begins to form granules which increase in electron density and eventually coalesce. During these changes there is a progressive reduction in nuclear volume, which is associated with an ill-defined stabilization of the DNA such that it is resistant to digestion by the enzyme DNA-ase (GLEDHILL et al., 1966).

δ) Reorganization of Cell Organelles and Cytoplasm

Having given rise to the acrosome, the Golgi complex migrates to the caudal end of the spermatid. The mitochondria, which early in spermiogenesis are peripherally placed in the cytoplasm, later form a helical sheath surrounding the region of the sperm called the middle piece. This event occurs late in spermiogenesis just prior to loss of the cytoplasm in the form of residual body. The latter process involves the invagination of processes of Sertoli cell cytoplasm into spermatid cytoplasm, which is thereby "pulled off" the developing tail. Little is known about the mechanisms by which the cytoplasm reorganization occurs, but it is likely that the early positional changes of the nucleus may be caused by a palisade of microtubules, termed the manchette (Figs. 5, 6 B), which appear to surround the nucleus.

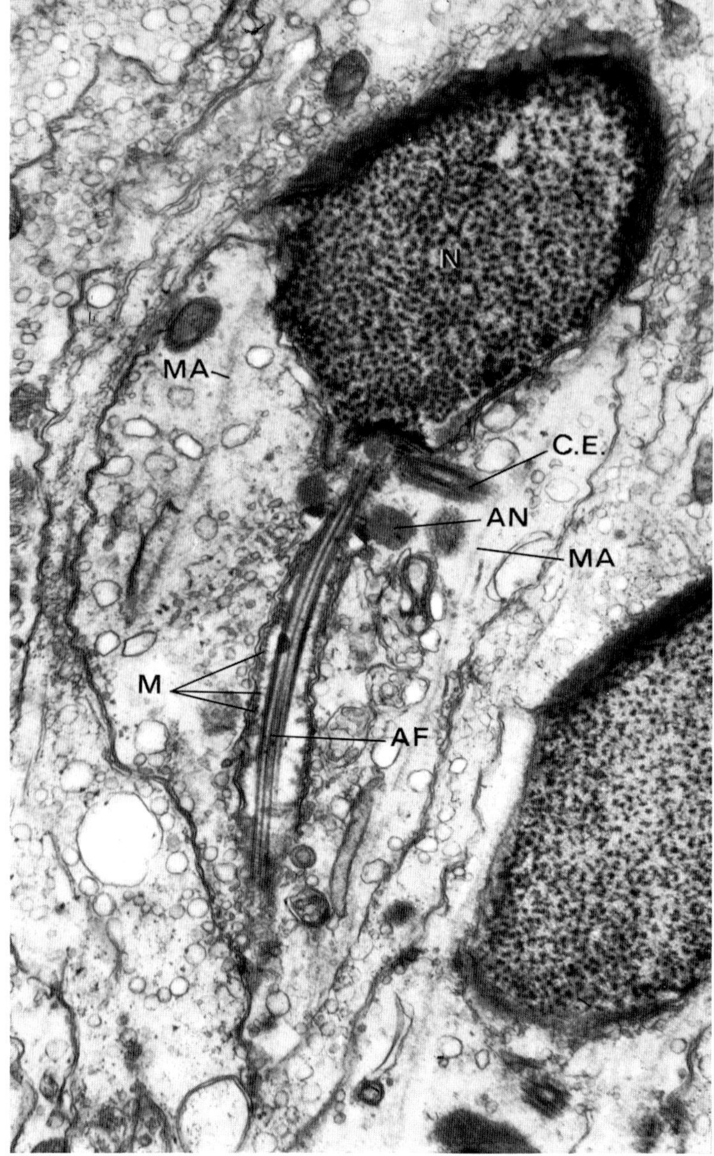

Fig. 5. A spermatid at the Sc stage shows the more heavily condensed nucleus (*N*), axial filament (*AF*), centriolar extension (*CE*) from the proximal centriole, manchette of microtubules (*MA*) and microtubules (*M*), which probably form the precursors of the ribs of the principal piece whose cranial limit is marked by the annulus (*AN*)

ε) Spermiation

The process by which sperm are finally shed from the epithelium is called spermiation. It partly involves the removal of the residual cytoplasm by processes of adjacent Sertoli cells, which appear to invaginate the spermatid cytoplasm. Little else is known about the exact mechanisms.

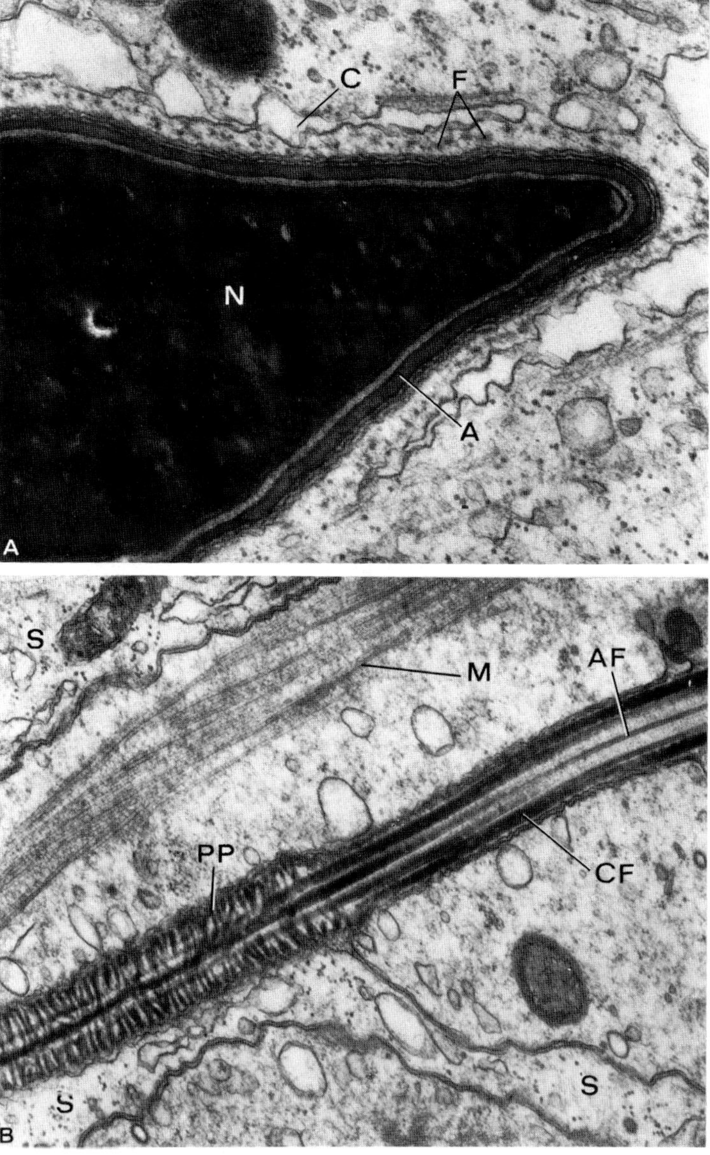

Fig. 6. A The heavily condensed nucleus (N) of an Sd$_2$ spermatid is shown, also illustrating the acrosome (A) and specialized Sertoli cell-spermatid interface with cisternae (C) and microfibrils (F). **B** Portion of an Sd$_1$ spermatid tail and cytoplasm shows the axial filament (AF), outer coarse fibers (CF), principal piece (PP), and manchette (M). Adjacent Sertoli cell cytoplasmic processes (S) surround the spermatid

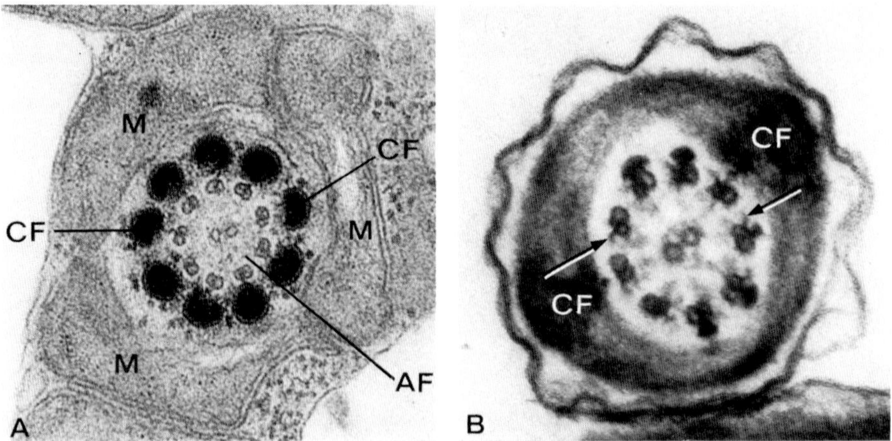

Fig. 7A, B. Cross sections of the sperm tail at middle piece (**A**) and principal piece (**B**) levels illustrate the axial filament complex (*AF*), outer coarse fibers (*CF*), and mitochondria (*M*). The sperm in **B** are obtained from a normal male and illustrate the presence of dyenin arms (*arrow*) that are absent in the sperm from a man with the immotile cilia syndrome (**A**)

d) Sertoli Cells

The supporting or Sertoli cells extend from the basement membrane of the tubule to the lumen and send an arborizing network of cytoplasmic processes between the adjacent germ cells. Many of these processes are so small that they can only be visualized by use of the electron microscope and the outlines of the Sertoli cell are extremely difficult to discern by light microscopy (Fig. 8). Each Sertoli cell forms an individual unit, and where the cell membrane of adjacent Sertoli cells abut, specialized cell junctions are formed (Fig. 9). At these points, the intercellular space is markedly reduced and in some places obliterated and recent freeze-fracture studies indicate that at these sites parallel arrays of intramembranous particles interdigitate (FAWCETT, 1975). By the use of tracer techniques employing lanthanum, it has been shown that intercellular transport is prevented at these special junctions (DYM and FAWCETT, 1970) and that they constitute the major component of the blood-testis barrier (see page 21). Adjacent to the cell membrane in this region, parallel cisternae of endoplasmic reticulum delineate a narrow band of cytoplasm, which contains bundles of microfibrils (Fig. 9). The location of these specialized inter-Sertoli cell junctions subdivide the tubule into a basal and adluminal compartment, the latter containing all the germ cells beyond the preleptotene stage of meiosis (DYM and FAWCETT, 1970). The special cell junctions are absent in the prepubertal testis and appear just prior to the onset of meiosis within the testis (FLICK-INGER, 1967; DE KRETSER and BURGER, 1972).

No special cell junctions exist between the Sertoli cells and the spermatogonia and spermatocytes. However, adjacent to the cell membrane of spermatids, the Sertoli cell again demonstrates parallel cisternae of endoplasmic reticulum,

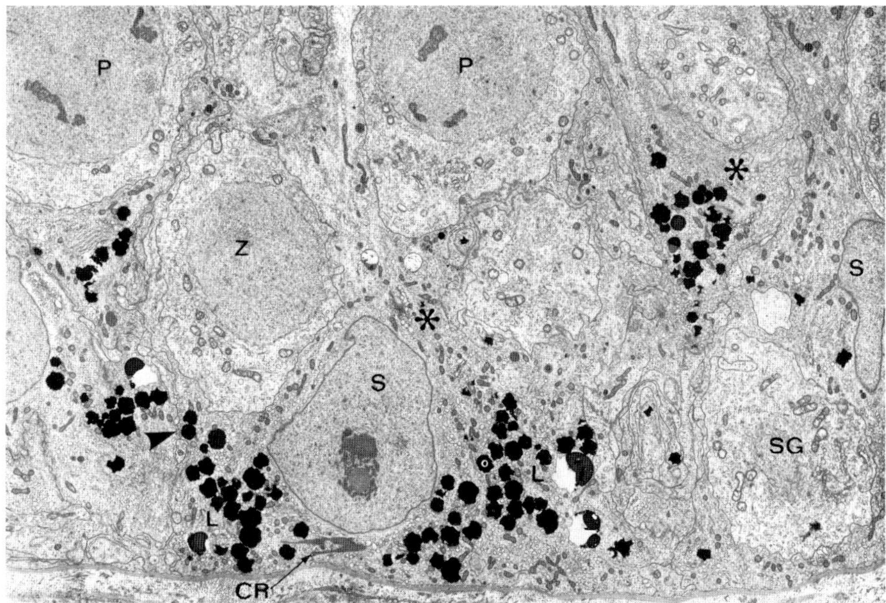

Fig. 8. Basal aspect of seminiferous tubule illustrates the Sertoli cell nucleus (*S*), lipid inclusions (*L*), cytoplasmic extensions (*), and specialized cell junctions (*arrowheads*). Adjacent spermatogonia (*SG*) and primary spermatocytes at the zygotene (*Z*) and pachytene phase (*P*), as well as crystals of Charcot-Böttcher (*CR*) are indicated

which delineate a narrow band of cytoplasm containing bundles of fibrils (Figs. 4, 6).

The nucleus of the Sertoli cell is partly lobulated and basally placed, containing a large centrally placed nucleolus (Fig. 8). The latter is poorly developed in the prepubertal testis and appears to result from the gonadotrophic stimulation at puberty. The mitochondria of the Sertoli cell are ovoid to rod shaped and are found throughout the cytoplasm, but frequently collections of mitochondria are found adjacent to the basement membrane of the tubule where pinocytotic vesicles and coated vesicles are seen. The cristae of mitochondria are both plate-like and tubular.

Profiles of smooth endoplasmic reticulum are plentiful in the mature Sertoli cell but less so in the prepubertal testis. In the perinuclear area, parallel arrays of interconnecting cisternae of smooth endoplasmic reticulum are found concentrically distributed around a cytoplasmic core which frequently contains a lipid inclusion. These collections have been termed lamellar bodies, and the cytoplasm between the parallel arrays of cisternae sometimes contain membrane-bound granules. A network of microfibrils extends throughout the Sertoli cell cytoplasm but is particularly noticeable around the perinuclear area. Among the other organelles found in the perinuclear area are the Golgi complex, lipid inclusions of variable dimensions, lysosomes and the crystalloids of Charcot-Böttcher. Profiles of rough endoplasmic reticulum are scattered throughout

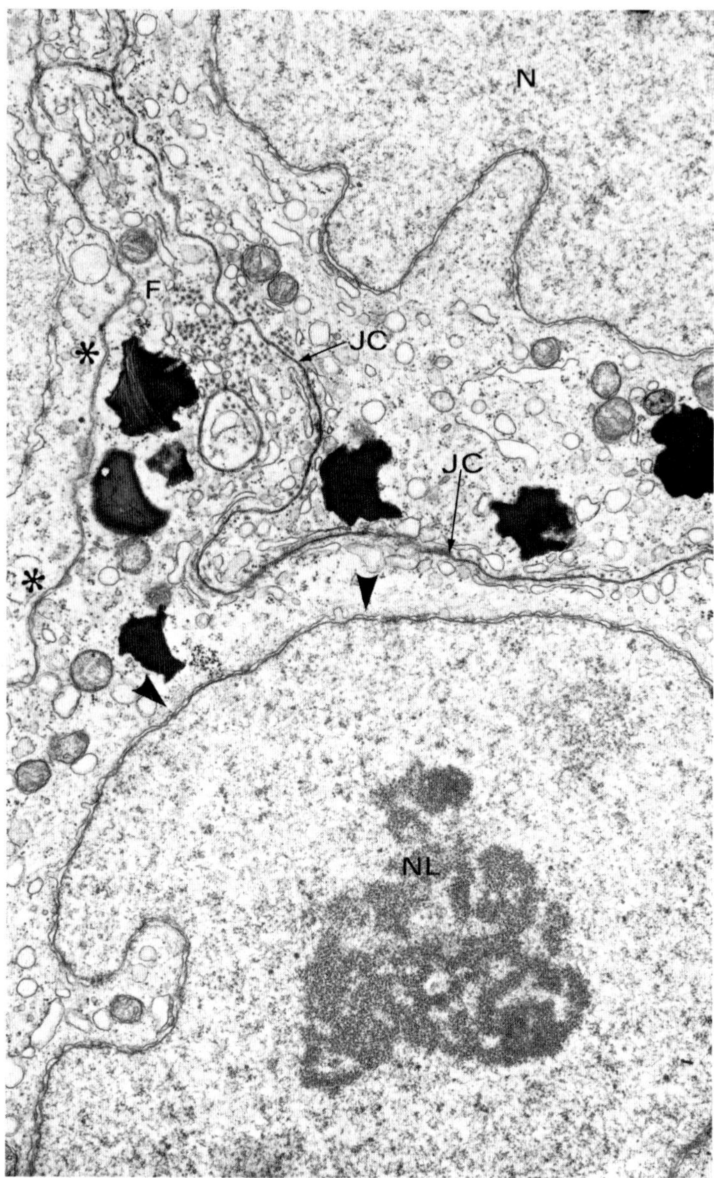

Fig. 9. The nucleus and (*N*) nucleolus (*NL*) of Sertoli cells are shown together with the perinuclear network of microfilaments (*arrowheads*). Specialized inter-Sertoli cell junctions (*JC*) and associated bundles of microfibrils (*F*) and nonspecialized Sertoli cell-germ cell interface (*) can be seen

the basal cytoplasm but are not associated with any secretory granules. Ribosomes and polysomes are also frequently seen.

It has been shown that in the rat testis, the structure of the Sertoli cell varies cyclically with the stages of the spermatogenic cycle (LACY, 1960; KERR and DE KRETSER, 1975). This is most evident in the form and numbers of lipid inclusions present at the basal aspects of the Sertoli cell but also involves the form and quantity of smooth endoplasmic reticulum. In addition, at stages 10–14 of the cycle, certain views suggested transfer of lipid inclusions from the Sertoli cell to the diplotene and diakinetic primary spermatocytes (KERR and DE KRETSER, 1975). No such cyclic variation was noted in studies of the monkey testis by DYM (1973), and to date no detailed electron-microscopic analysis of the Sertoli cell structure has been attempted at the various stages of the human seminiferous cycle.

e) Seminiferous Cycle

In many mammals, spermatogenesis is a highly organized and coordinated process such that long segments of tubules can be occupied by the same phase of spermatogenesis. By careful histological analysis, CLERMONT (1972) has established a seminiferous cycle for many species and has determined the length of time taken for spermatogenesis from the spermatogonial stage to the release of spermatozoa from the epithelium. The length of time taken for the process is a biological constant for each species and cannot be altered, namely, it is not possible to stimulate the germ cells to rush through the spermatogenic process. In man, the length of time required for spermatogenesis is 70 ± 4 days (HELLER and CLERMONT 1964) and the phases of the process are illustrated in Fig. 1.

2. Intertubular Tissue

a) Lamina Propria of the Seminiferous Tubules

The seminiferous tubules are surrounded by a basement membrane which usually consists of a thin relatively amorphous single layer of moderately electron-dense material (Fig. 10). Around some tubules from normal biopsies, the basement membrane consists of one or more lamellae, an appearance more commonly seen in biopsies from men with testicular damage (DE KRETSER et al., 1975). Immediately external to the basement membrane is a thin layer of collagen up to 2 μm wide, external to which the tubule is surrounded by a layer of fusiform, elongated cells which form a circumferential sheath. These cells, termed myoid cells because of their contractile properties, are characterized by a spindle-shaped nucleus, and the perinuclear cytoplasm contains many pinocytotic vesicles and plexiform arrays of intracellular microfibrils 40–60 Å in width, which exhibit areas of increased electron density similar to those seen in smooth muscle cells (ROSS and LONG, 1966). Studies using immunofluorescent methods have shown that the fibrils consist of an actin-like protein. Closely apposed to both surfaces of the myoid cells is a thin layer of moderately electron-dense material similar in appearance to the basement membrane, but in other areas plexiform bundles of fine filaments lie in association to the myoid cells.

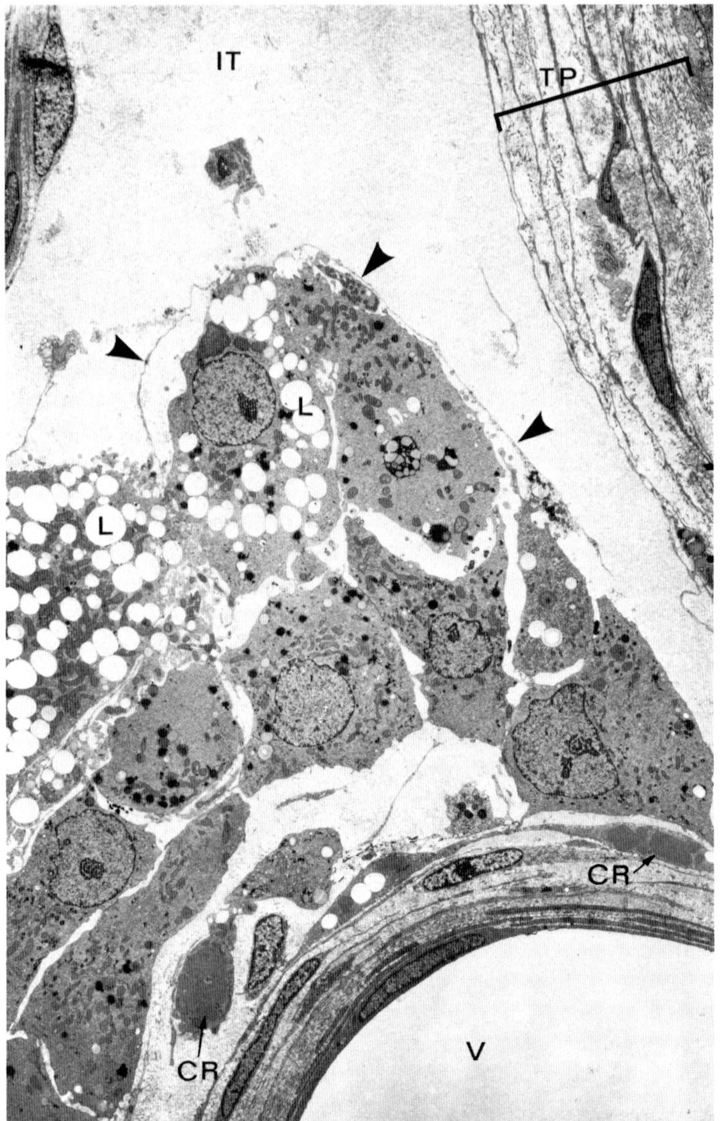

Fig. 10. A low power electron micrograph demonstrates a venule (*V*) surrounded by Leydig cells some of which contain lipid inclusions (*L*) and crystals of Reinke (*CR*). The endothelium of lymphatic vesicles (*arrowheads*), the intertubular tissue (*IT*), and tunica propria (*TP*) are also shown

One or more layers of myoid cells surround the human seminiferous tubule, and interspersed between them are layers of collagen fibres. In states of seminiferous tubule damage, the thickness of the layer of collagen fibres increases constituting the condition of peritubular fibrosis. Around severely damaged tubules there is also a proliferation of the layers of fine fibrillar material apposed to each surface of the myoid cells, most likely representing the "hyaline" material described by light microscopy (DE KRETSER et al., 1975). No blood vessels are seen within the layers of myoid cells though occasionally a small nerve fibre penetrates into the lamina propria.

b) Interstitial Cells

Surrounding the capillaries within the intertubular area, irregular collections of cells form groups which appear to be randomly distributed amongst the seminiferous tubules (Fig. 10). These cells are termed interstitial cells and consist of a heterogenous group of cells of two major types described originally in the human testis by FAWCETT and BURGOS (1960). The first consist of a group of fusiform cells representing the immature interstitial cells (SNIFFEN, 1950; FAWCETT and BURGOS, 1960) and are characterized by an elliptical nucleus, cytoplasmic fibrils, a small Golgi complex and variable small amounts of granular and agranular endoplasmic reticulum. These cells comprise the principal feature of the intertubular tissue in the immature testis and in early pubertal maturation.

The second type can be termed mature interstitial cells and correspond to the cells originally described by Leydig consisting of large polyhedral epitheloid cells varying in diameter from 10–25 µm with an oval nucleus and prominent nucleolus. Considerable variation occurs in their light-microscopic appearance, some cells contain eosinophilic granules which can be aggregated to one pole of the cell leaving relatively pale agranular areas (SNIFFEN, 1950; TILLINGER, 1957). Variable amounts of lipid and lipofuscin pigment are also seen. To date it has not been possible to associate specific light-microscopic features with degrees of steroidogenic activity.

Ultrastructurally, the mature interstitial or Leydig cells contain large quantities of agranular endoplasmic reticulum consisting of vesicles and tubular profiles (DE KRETSER, 1967a; CHRISTENSEN, 1975). The mitochondria demonstrate tubular cristae similar to other steroid-producing cells and are variable in size and shape (Fig. 11). The cells contain a well-developed Golgi complex, some lipid inclusions and lysosomes, as well as aggregates of lipofuscin pigment. Crystals of Reinke are frequently found (Fig. 12) and in some planes demonstrate a striking hexagonal lattice arrangement (DE KRETSER, 1967a). In some cells smaller crystalline tubular inclusions can be found, and it has been suggested that these represent precursors of the larger crystals (DE KRETSER, 1967a). No functional significance has been ascribed to these crystals. Comparative data covering the interstitial cells of different species have recently been reviewed by CHRISTENSEN (1975) and demonstrated certain features in common, namely, agranular endoplasmic reticulum, mitochondria with tubular cristae and lipid inclusions – all features of steroid-secreting cells. Stimulation with human chorionic gonadotrophin results in an increased plasma testosterone and in the above cytological components together with enlargement of the Golgi complex (DE KRETSER, 1967b).

c) Vasculature

The arrangement of the blood vessels and lymphatics in relation to the Leydig cells varies between species, and these features have been reviewed by

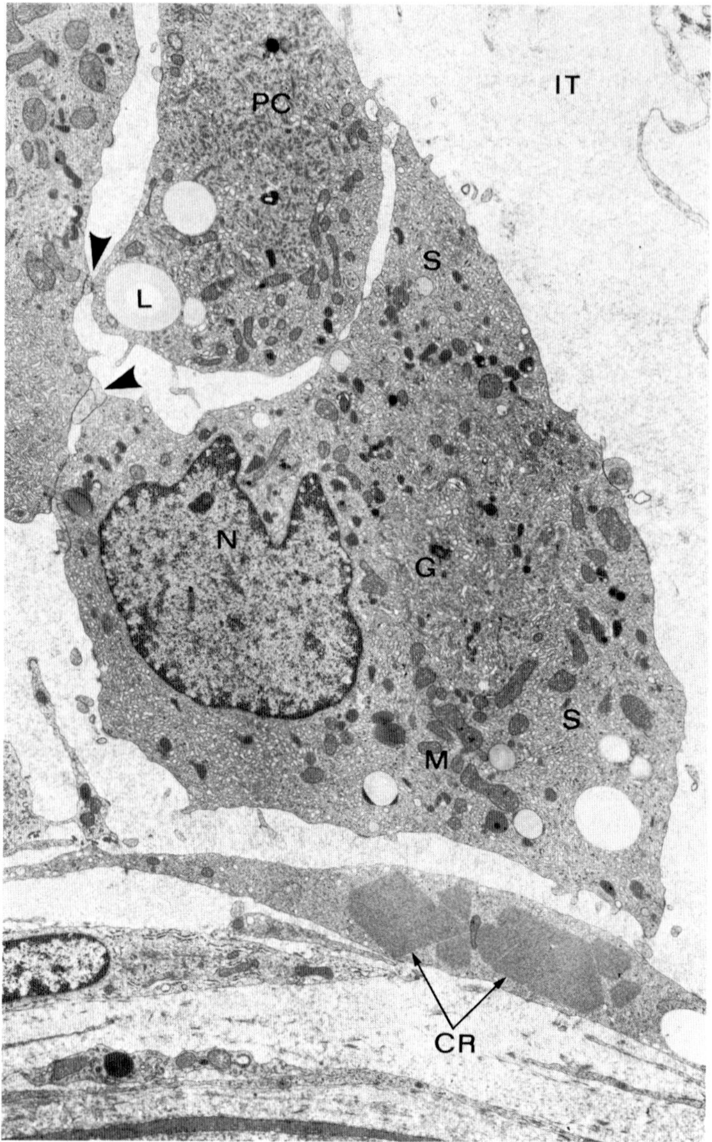

Fig. 11. A higher magnification of Leydig cells demonstrates the nucleus (*N*), Golgi complex (*G*), the intertubular tissue (*IT*), mitochondria (*M*), smooth endoplasmic reticulum (*S*), lipid inclusions (*L*), crystals of Reinke (*CR*) and their probable precursors, and the paracrystalline inclusions (*PC*). Where adjacent Leydig cells are closely apposed, the intercellular space (*arrow*) is sometimes narrowed to 20 Å, forming gap junctions

FAWCETT et al. (1973). In some species such as the rat, large lymphatic sinusoids dominate the intertubular area, but in the human testis the lymphatics are more limited in extent forming single centrally placed vessels. The Leydig cells surround the capillaries, which are not fenestrated in type.

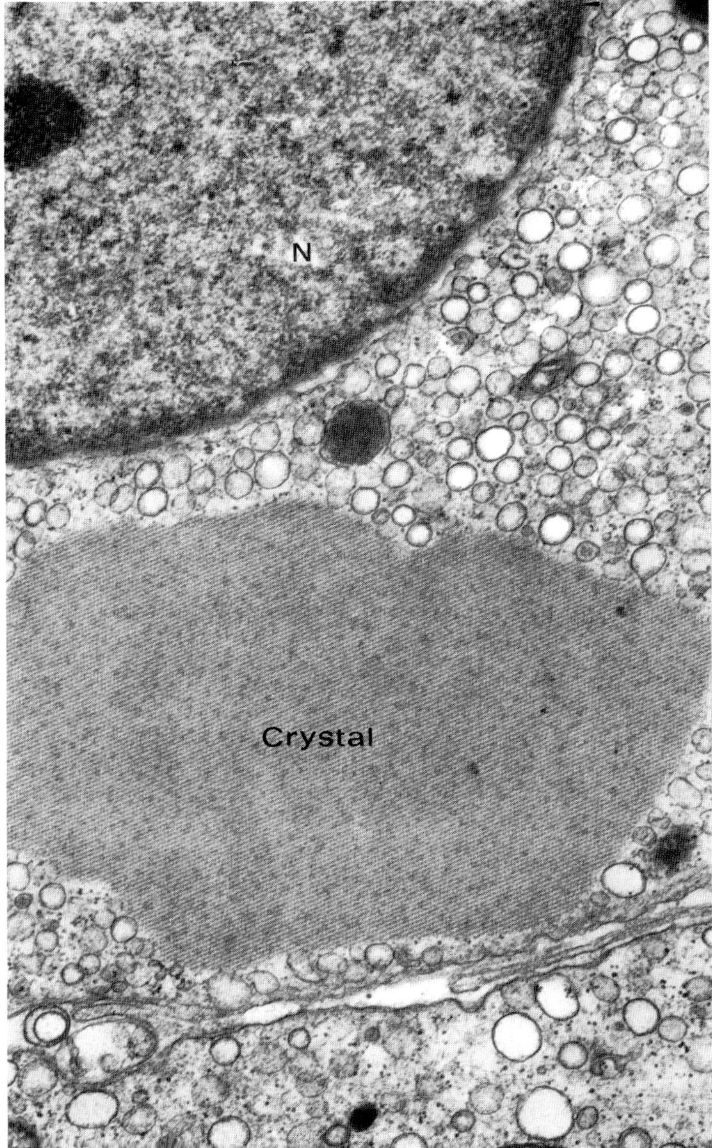

Fig. 12. A *crystal* of Reinke in this cytoplasm of a Leydig cell is shown; *N*, nucleus

IV. Function

1. Control of Testicular Function

Adequate spermatogenic and androgenic function of the testis is dependent on the secretion of the gonadotropic hormones by the pituitary gland, which in turn requires stimulation by the gonadotropin-releasing hormone (GNRH) produced by the hypothalamus. GNRH is a decapeptide which has been isolated and synthesized (AMOSS et al., 1971; SCHALLY et al., 1971) and is secreted into the pituitary portal system in episodic bursts (CARMEL et al., 1976). In adult men, it rapidly induces the secretion of the two gonadotropic hormones, luteinizing hormone (LH) and follicle-stimulating hormone (FSH). The ratio of LH released is greater than FSH and increases in a dose-response relationship (WOLLESEN et al., 1976). Recent studies indicate that in addition to stimulating secretion, GNRH also induces production of the LH and FSH by the gonadotropes of the pituitary (BREMNER and PAULSEN, 1974; EDWARDSON and GILBERT, 1975; PICKERING and FINK, 1976).

FSH and LH are secreted in episodic bursts; the spikes of secretion are more easily discernible in the profiles of LH levels (ALFORD et al., 1973). In view of the episodic secretion, care should be taken in the interpretation of single levels of these hormones, especially LH (SANTEN and BARDIN, 1973). The levels of FSH and LH increase during puberty and are responsible for stimulating testicular growth (BAKER et al., 1976). Receptors for each hormone have been demonstrated; those for LH are restricted to the interstitial cell (DE KRETSER et al., 1971) and those for FSH to the seminiferous tubules (MEANS and VAITUKAITIS, 1972), in particular to the Sertoli cells and spermatogonia (ORTH and CHRISTENSEN, 1978). Though the sites of these receptors appear to compartmentalize the actions of LH and FSH on the testis, there is evidence that FSH can influence interstitial cell function (ODELL et al., 1973) and that LH, through the stimulation of testosterone secretion, is vital for spermatogenesis, probably exerting its action through the androgen receptors found in Sertoli cells (TINDALL et al., 1977).

As with any endocrine secretion, feedback mechanisms enable the target tissue to exert a controlling influence over the hormones stimulating its function. It is well established that the interstitial cells, through the secretion of testosterone and estradiol, control the secretion of LH (SANTEN, 1975). However, controversy exists as to the nature of the physiological feedback signal for FSH. Testosterone and estradiol do exert a suppressive influence on FSH secretion, but recent studies have provided evidence for the existence of a nonsteroid substance in the testis termed inhibin, which can exert a suppressive action on FSH secretion (see review DE KRETSER et al., 1977). Since the feedback signal for FSH emanates principally from the seminiferous tubules, correlations have been established between the function of the tubules and the level of FSH in serum (DE KRETSER et al., 1974a; RICH and DE KRETSER, 1977) which enable the FSH level to be used as an index of the state of the seminiferous epithelium in the evaluation of the infertile male (DE KRETSER, 1974b).

2. Spermatogenic Function

The production of spermatozoa by the seminiferous epithelium requires the combined action of FSH and LH, the latter through testosterone secretion by the Leydig cells. Some data in other species suggest that FSH may not be required for the maintenance of spermatogenesis (see review by STEINBERGER, 1971), but the results of investigations in man indicate the need for both gonadotropic hormones (PAULSEN, 1966; MACLEOD et al., 1966; MANCINI et al., 1971).

Though FSH and LH are necessary for spermatogenesis, they are unable to increase the rate of germ cell development, which is constant for each species. Studies in man indicate that the time necessary for development from spermatogonia to spermatozoa is 70 ± 4 days (HELLER and CLERMONT, 1964). From evidence presented by MEANS and HUCKINS (1974), it is likely that FSH may increase sperm production by decreasing the number of germ cells that degenerate during spermatogenesis.

The action of both FSH and testosterone on the seminiferous epithelium appears to be exerted by their action on the Sertoli cell. In response to FSH and testosterone secretion during pubertal maturation, the Sertoli cells develop their specialized cell junctions, which constitute the blood-testis barrier (DE KRETSER and BURGER 1972; SETCHELL and WAITES, 1975). The effect of the barrier is to create two compartments in the tubule: an adluminal compartment that contains the bases of the Sertoli cells and spermatogonia has access to the extratubular environment, whereas access to germ cells of the luminal compartment must be through the Sertoli cell cytoplasm since the specialized cell junctions prevent intercellular transport of metabolites (DYM and FAWCETT, 1970). Consequently, the metabolic and hormonal requirements for the germ cells undergoing meiosis and spermiogenesis must be met by adequate Sertoli cell function.

It is presumed that the nature of the blood-testis barrier is determined by the Sertoli cells. The data reviewed by SETCHELL and WAITES (1975) indicate that different substances have variable rates of penetration from the extratubular to the intratubular environment and that this selective permeability appears coincidentally with the appearance of the specialized inter-Sertoli cell junctions.

The physiology of the Sertoli cell has therefore been the subject of intensive study over the past 5 years, and many advances have been made in our understanding of this cell. The action of FSH on the testis is now thought to be expressed principally by its action on the Sertoli cell. MEANS et al. (1976) have reviewed data indicating that FSH stimulates RNA and protein synthesis in the testes of rats that had been depleted of germ cells. Furthermore, cultures of Sertoli cells have been shown to respond to FSH by increasing cyclic AMP levels (DORRINGTON et al., 1975), the secretion of androgen-binding protein (ABP) and their mitotic activity (GRISWOLD et al., 1977). STEINBERGER and STEINBERGER (1976) have demonstrated that in culture Sertoli cells produce an nonsteroid factor which is capable of suppressing FSH secretion by pituitary cell cultures.

The ability of the Sertoli cell to produce ABP was first detected in the rat and subsequently confirmed in a number of species (see review HANSSON et al., 1975a). Although some investigators have claimed they could demonstrate ABP in cytosols from human testes, the identification of this product in man is difficult because of the similarity of ABP to sex steroid-binding globulin (SSBG), which circulates in human plasma (BURKE et al., 1977; HSU et al., 1977). In the rabbit, where parallel purification of ABP and SSBG has been attempted, the only significant difference appeared to be one of charge; these data suggest that two very similar proteins are produced by the liver (SSBG) and the testes (ABP) (HANSSON et al., 1975b). In the rat, ABP production is stimulated by both FSH and testosterone (Hansson et al., 1975a; Means et al., 1976) and is secreted into seminiferous tubule fluid in which it reaches the caput epididymis where a portion is reabsorbed (French and Ritzen, 1973; Pelliniemi et al., 1979). The high concentrations of testosterone carried bound to ABP are probably of significance in maintaining the androgen-dependent cells in the caput epididymis. Lower ABP levels have been detected in the remainder of the epididymis and also in semen (Hansson et al., 1975a), but their significance at these sites remains to be identified.

Attempts to purify and concentrate ABP in the rat have led to the development of a radio-immunoassay for ABP (Gunsalus et al., 1978). The increased sensitivity of this technique has made it possible to detect this protein in the blood of male rats, whereas previous studies had been unable to do so. One of the major benefits of the discovery that the Sertoli cell produces ABP is that the function of these cells can now be assessed by a biochemical marker, both in the testis and in blood. A number of investigators have now demonstrated that in states of seminiferous tubule damage induced by a host of factors (e.g. cryptorchidism, vitamin A deficiency, hydroxyurea, fetal irradiation), the ability of the Sertoli cell to produce ABP is impaired, which indicates that germ cells are not the only type whose function is disrupted by these agents (Hagenäs and Ritzén, 1976; Rich and de Kretser, 1977). Thus, the measurement of ABP production provides a useful tool for investigating the function of the Sertoli cell in various physiological and pathological states.

It is well recognized that spermatogenesis is a coordinated sequence of development, a feature that is especially evident in certain species such as the rat (Clermont, 1972). The method by which this coordination is achieved is of some interest and may involve two mechanisms. First, the dividing germ cells have been shown to remain connected by intercellular cytoplasmic bridges so that large numbers of germ cells at the spermatogonial, spermatocyte and spermatid stages are joined (Dym and Fawcett, 1971). The second possibility may involve the Sertoli cell since, due to the arborizing nature of its cytoplasmic processes, a single Sertoli cell may be in contact with large numbers of germ cells, especially in a radial direction within the epithelium. It is therefore of interest that the cytology of the Sertoli cells shows cyclic variation governed by the stage of the seminiferous cycle (Kerr and de Kretser, 1975). Furthermore, Parvinen et al. (1979) have demonstrated that functional parameters such as the capacity for FSH binding, the amount of FSH-generated cyclic AMP production and the secretion of ABP vary in concert with the stage of the cycle.

3. Steroidogenic Function

The early experiments of Berthold (1849) demonstrated that the presence of a testis governed the appearance of secondary sexual characteristics. This concept was further developed by Bouin and Ancel (1903), who implicated the interstitial cells of the testis in the establishment of the secondary sex characteristics. The isolation of testosterone from the testis (David et al., 1935) was followed by studies to establish the biochemical pathways by which testosterone was synthesized from precursors such as acetate (BRADY, 1951; SAVARD et al., 1952; SLAUNWHITE and SAMUELS, 1956; DORFMAN et al., 1968). However, it was not until 1965 that the interstitial cells were conclusively established as the major source of testosterone production by the testis (CHRISTENSEN and MASON, 1965). The human testis produces approximately 7 mg of testosterone per day (LIPSETT et al., 1966), which leaves the testis via the spermatic vein and testicular lymphatics.

In recent years, a number of studies have evaluated the events involved in the secretion of testosterone by interstitial cells following the binding of LH to receptors on their surface (DE KRETSER et al., 1971). These studies reviewed by DUFAU et al. (1978) have established that binding of LH to receptors initiates an increase in cyclic AMP, which in turn is responsible for changes in the metabolism of the cells resulting in the secretion of testosterone. The rise in cyclic AMP in turn activates protein kinase, which is involved in the phosphorylation of protein substrates. The specific role of these phosphorylated proteins in the activation of the early steps in the steroidogenic pathway still remains to be determined, but it is known that LH probably stimulates an increase in free cholesterol and the conversion of this material to 22-α-hydroxycholesterol prior to the side chain cleavage step involved in the formation of pregnenolone. The use of human chorionic gonadotropin (HCG) as a source of LH has demonstrated that chronic stimulation will elevate plasma testosterone levels (LIPSETT et al., 1966) and will result in an increase in the organelles in steroid biosynthesis, namely, smooth endoplasmic reticulum, mitochondria and the Golgi complex (DE KRETSER, 1967). The specific role of each organelle in steroid biosynthesis and the cytological location of the necessary enzymes have been reviewed by CHRISTENSEN (1975). The measurement of plasma testosterone following administration of HCG for 4 days has been used as a test of Leydig cell function in man and has demonstrated abnormalities in the function of these cells in testicular disorders (PAULSEN et al., 1968; DE KRETSER et al., 1975). It is also of use in determining whether testicular tissue is present in boys with intra-abdominal cryptorchidism.

The function of the Leydig cells varies with age. The secretion of testosterone by the fetal generation is important in the differentiation of the male genitalia. This generation of Leydig cells degenerates late in fetal life or shortly after birth, depending on the species (LORDING and DE KRETSER, 1972; CATT et al., 1975). In boys, a short-lived increase in testosterone occurs shortly after birth, but the significance of this observation remains unknown (FOREST and CATHIARD, 1975). In man, the Leydig cells remain quiescent, as judged by their ability to secrete testosterone, until the commencement of puberty when incremental increases of testosterone can be associated with the stages of pubertal maturation (KELCH et al., 1972b; BAKER et al., 1976). However, in the rat, a number of investigators have suggested that the Leydig cells secrete other products before the pubertal rise of testosterone occurs (FICHER and STEINBERGER, 1968; PODESTA and RIVAROLA, 1974). Some of these substances represent 5α-reduced products of testosterone, such as 5α-androstan-3α-17β-diol, which may be important in the initiation of spermatogenesis (RIVAROLA et al., 1972). No comparable data are available in man.

The site of production of estradiol in the male remains controversial. In man, studies of estradiol concentrations in spermatic vein blood have led to the conclusion that 30%–50% of estradiol is produced in the testes, the remainder by peripheral conversion of testosterone (KELCH et al., 1972a). It has been claimed that the Leydig cells are the source of oestrogen production in the testis (MADDOCK and NELSON, 1952) and this claim has received support by the demonstration that cultures of Leydig cells can respond to HCG by converting testosterone to oestradiol (VALLADARES and PAYNE, 1979). However, DORRINGTON and ARMSTRONG (1975) have demonstrated that Sertoli cells from immature rats can also convert testosterone to oestradiol under the influence of FSH, and this observation suggests that the Sertoli cell may be the source of oestradiol production. The latter hypothesis would be in keeping with the observations that the seminiferous tubules have the capacity to utilize precursors such as pregnenolone by converting them to testosterone (CHRISTENSEN and MASON, 1965; HALL et al., 1969). The actual site of oestradiol production by the adult testis remains undefined, but the concept that both compartments of the testis may have a cooperative role in total testicular steroidogenesis must be borne in mind since data are available to indicate that the seminiferous tubules are unable to utilize early precursors of steroids such as cholesterol (HALL et al., 1969). Evidence from studies of a number of different functions of the testis make it likely that the activities of the two compartments are very closely interrelated, and both should always be evaluated (AOKI and FAWCETT, 1978; RICH et al., 1979; KERR et al., 1979). Both studies indicate the possibility that the two compartments of the testis influence each other since Leydig cell hypertrophy is commonly observed around damaged seminiferous tubules. Furthermore, in the areas of normal testicular tissue surrounding the areas of focal damage, the Leydig cells were normal (AOKI and FAWCETT, 1978).

B. Anatomy of the Male Reproductive Tract and Accessory Glands

I. Introduction

The human ejaculate is a complex association of cells and secretions derived from a series of interconnected, androgen-dependent ducts and glands which together comprise the male genital tract. In the preceding section, the structural organization and contribution to the seminal plasma of one component of this system, the testis, has been described and the remaining sections of this chapter discuss the development, anatomy and cytology of the other structures forming the male tract; the intratesticular ducts, ductuli efferentes, epididymis, ductus deferens, ampullae, seminal vesicles, ejaculatory ducts, prostate, bulbourethral glands and urethral glands.

II. Embryogenesis of the Male Reproductive Tract

Whereas there is a common origin for the gonad in both sexes, the male and female genital tracts develop from two distinct transitional duct systems, the mesonephric (or Wolffian) ducts and the adjacent paramesonephric (or Müllerian) ducts, which are both present in the embryo before sexual differentiation.

In lower vertebrates the mesonephros forms both the excretory and reproductive systems but in mammals the metanephros has supplanted the mesonephros as progenitor of the excretory system in both sexes and the mesonephros is retained only in male embryos to form part of the genital tract.

The mesonephros consists of mesonephric tubules which begin to differentiate in the embryo during the 4th week of fetal development. These tubules are the main components of the urogenital ridges, which are well defined by the end of the 5th week. During subsequent development, the mesonephric tubules grow laterally until they contact and fuse with the mesonephric duct, which in turn opens on each side into the urogenital sinus.

In the male, during the period of sexual differentiation, when the gonad is organized into a testis (see Sect. A), the mesonephric tubules and duct persist and develop into epididymis, ductus deferens, seminal vesicles and ejaculatory duct. The paramesonephric ducts regress in the male and are obliterated during the 3rd month (JIRASEK, 1967). Steroid and protein hormones secreted by the testis influence both the differentiation and development of the male duct system and the regression of the paramesonephric ducts (JOST et al., 1973; see also Sect. A).

In contrast to the mesonephric derivation of the proximal region of the male tract, the structures situated more distally in the male reproductive system, the prostate, bulbourethral gland and urethra, are derived from the urogenital sinus (NARBAITZ, 1974).

Segments of both the mesonephric and paramesonephric ducts are retained as vestigial structures in the male. The blind cranial end of the mesonephric duct persists as an appendix of the epididymis which is usually associated with the caput epididymidis, and some caudal remnants of the mesonephric tubules may be retained below the ductuli efferentes as the paradidymis. The cranial end of the paramesonephric ducts may be retained attached to the superior pole of the testis as the vesicular appendix of the testis.

III. Intratesticular Ducts

Spermatozoa and fluids produced by the seminiferous tubules of the testis are transported to the extra-testicular ductuli efferentes along an anastomosing system of channels in the mediastinum of the testis (Fig. 13). Two structurally different ducts take part in this anastomosis: the transitional distal segment of the seminiferous tubules and the channels of the rete testis (ROOSEN-RUNGE and HOLSTEIN, 1978).

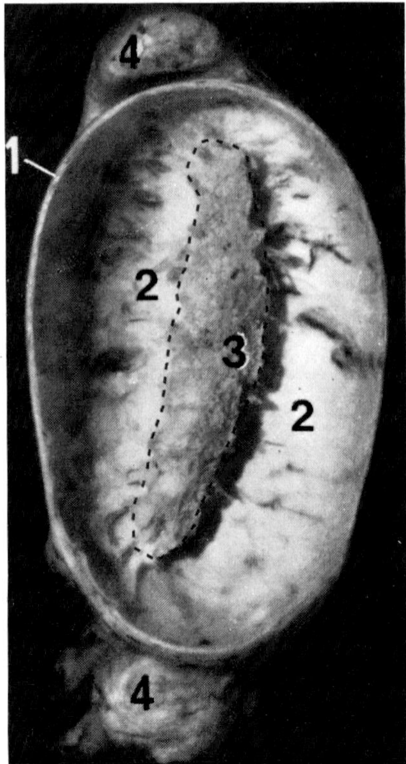

Fig. 13. Coronal bisection of an adult human testis showing the location of the intratesticular ducts in relation to the tunica albuginea and the long axis of the epididymis. All testicular tissue except the mediastinum (*inside broken line*) has been removed to demonstrate the curved axis of the rete testis. *1,* tunica albuginea; *2,* inner wall of tunica albuginea with testicular parenchyma removed; *3,* mediastinum containing anastomosing channels of the rete testis and mediastinal connective tissue; *4,* head and tail of epididymis. (E.C. Roosen-Runge, A.F. Holstein, 1978) × 1.5

1. Transitional Distal Segment of Seminiferous Tubule

The terminal segment of each seminiferous tubule consists of a transitional zone comprising a simple columnar epithelium of Sertoli cells without germ cells. The lumen at the distal extremity of these tubules narrows and a plug-like arrangement of epithelial cells projects into the wider lumen of the tubuli recti (Fig. 14). The ultrastructure of these cells has not been examined in detail in man but Dym (1974) has shown in the monkey that they differ in several ways from the germ cell associated Sertoli cells in the seminiferous epithelium; they contain less smooth endoplasmic reticulum but more lipid droplets, a more extensive rough endoplasmic reticulum and a profusion of cytoplasmic filaments. Intra-epithelial lymphocytes were also present amongst the Sertoli cells in this region, an observation not recorded within the normal seminiferous epithelium.

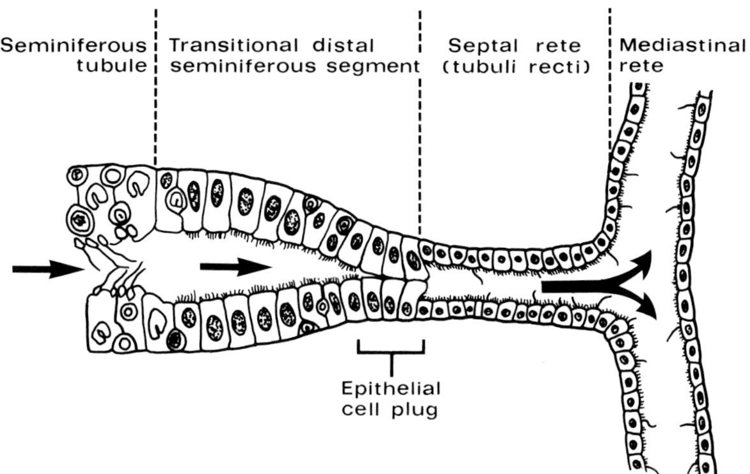

Fig. 14. Transitional region between the seminiferous tubule and rete testis. This diagram shows the change in epithelial structure between the seminiferous tubule and its distal segment, which is lined by columnar cells without germ cells, and the tubules of the septal rete testis, which are lined by a low cuboidal or squamous epithelium. A plug of columnar epithelial cells partially occludes the lumen of the tubule at the site of transition between the two epithelial types. *Arrows* indicate direction of flow of fluids in the tubule. Redrawn from DYM, 1974

The lamina propria around the transitional segments is intermediate between those characteristic of the seminiferous tubules and the tubuli recti and rete testis. It consists of a thick basal lamina supported by loose bundles of collagen fibres, and enclosed by several layers of circularly oriented myoid cells and a peripheral layer of fibrocytes and collagen fibres.

Prominent bundles of filaments within these modified Sertoli cells resemble tonofilaments rather than contractile filaments and may therefore function as cytoskeletal elements which confer structural rigidity on the epithelial cells in this region. Why these cells need more structural reinforcement than cell types on either side of the transition zone has not yet been determined. ROOSEN-RUNGE (1961) has suggested that the function of this plug of cells is to provide a valve which allows movement of fluid and cells from the seminiferous tubules into the rete testis but which prevents reflux of this fluid into these tubules when contractions of the *tunica albuginea* increase the intratesticular pressure. DYM (1974) has observed that when Sertoli cells of the transitional segment appear to occlude the lumen, their apices always point towards the rete testis. He concluded that the shape and narrowness of the lumen make it difficult to envision a reflux from the rete testis into the seminiferous tubules but suggests that the lumen is always patent in vivo.

2. Rete Testis

The rete testis is a collecting reservoir for testicular fluids in the mediastinum of the testis. It extends along the longitudinal axis of the testis, parallel to the axis of the epididymis, and opens into the ductuli efferentes at the cranial

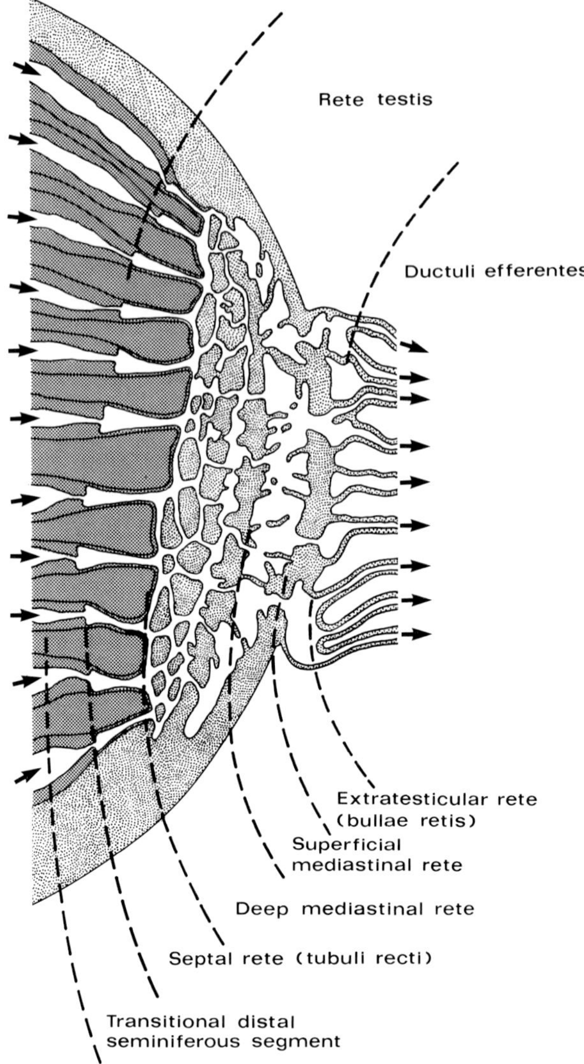

Fig. 15. Structural divisions within the rete testis. *Arrows* indicate the direction of flow of fluids and cells from the seminiferous tubules to the ductuli efferentes

pole of the testis (Fig. 13). The epithelium lining the ducts and channels of the rete testis is essentially the same in composition and ultrastructural features throughout; however, differences in the size and configuration of the ducts and passages in different regions of the rete have been used to subdivide it into distinct regions (Fig. 15). Three major subdivisions have been described (ROOSEN-RUNGE and HOLSTEIN, 1978): a septal (intralobular) portion which is formed by the tubuli recti, a mediastinal (tunical) region which includes the true network of interconnecting channels – this is the most extensive part of the rete testis – and an extratesticular zone consisting of a series of terminal dilatations which have been termed bullae retes. In the connective tissue which encloses the rete channels are blood vessels, various types of nerve fibres and numerous, irregular lymphatic channels.

a) Septal Rete

The septal rete is derived entirely from the tubuli recti which are short, straight tubules connecting the distal seminiferous segments to the mediastinal rete (Figs. 14, 15). These emerge from the connective tissue partitions which separate the lobules of the testis and empty into the cavities of the mediastinal rete.

b) Mediastinal Rete

This part of the rete testis consists of an extensive network of channels which extend into the tunica albuginea. Based on differences in structure, ROOSEN-RUNGE and HOLSTEIN (1978) have subdivided the mediastinal rete into deep and superficial regions. The deep mediastinal rete is formed by a dense maze of anastomosing passages which drain the straight tubules of the septal rete and empty, via numerous openings, into a series of relatively wide longitudinal channels which comprise the superficial mediastinal rete. Using scanning electron microscopy, ROOSEN-RUNGE and HOLSTEIN (1978) have examined the three-dimensional structure of the rete testis channels. From these observations, they not only confirmed the general complexity of the network of passages but also found that these anastomosing channels contain an irregular meshwork of cylindrical tissue strands, the chordae retis, of widely varying morphologies which traverse the rete channels in many directions (Fig. 16A). The diameters of the chordae retis vary from 5 to 40 µm and an excellent account of their various forms and morphological relationships in the human rete testis is given by ROOSEN-RUNGE and HOLSTEIN (1978). Chordae retis are covered by a simple, microvillous epithelium consisting of squamous or cuboidal cells, with similar structural features to those lining the channels of the rete testis (Fig. 16B). Thicker chordae are vascularized but those with diameters less than 20 µm are usually avascular.

The subepithelial tissue core of each chorda contains myofibroblastic cellular elements closely associated with a fibro-elastic matrix. The myoid cell component consists of elongated cells with elongate, ovoid nuclei, extensively branching cytoplasmic processes, and intracellular aggregates of 60 Å microfilaments inserted into thickenings of the plasma membrane (Fig. 17). These cellular processes are intimately associated with bundles of connective tissue fibres comprising small aggregates of collagen fibrils, interspersed with bundles of microfilaments which resemble elastin fibres. The function of the chordae retis has not been determined but their structural associations suggest two possibilities. First, it seems likely that their strut-like arrangement controls the degree of distension of the thin-walled rete channels by exocrine fluid secretions of the testis; and secondly, and perhaps of even greater functional significance, contraction of the myoid elements in the tissue core of the chordae may provide a sensitive and effective mechanism within the testis for raising intrarete pressures and forcing rete testis fluid into the excurrent ducts and ductus epididymidis.

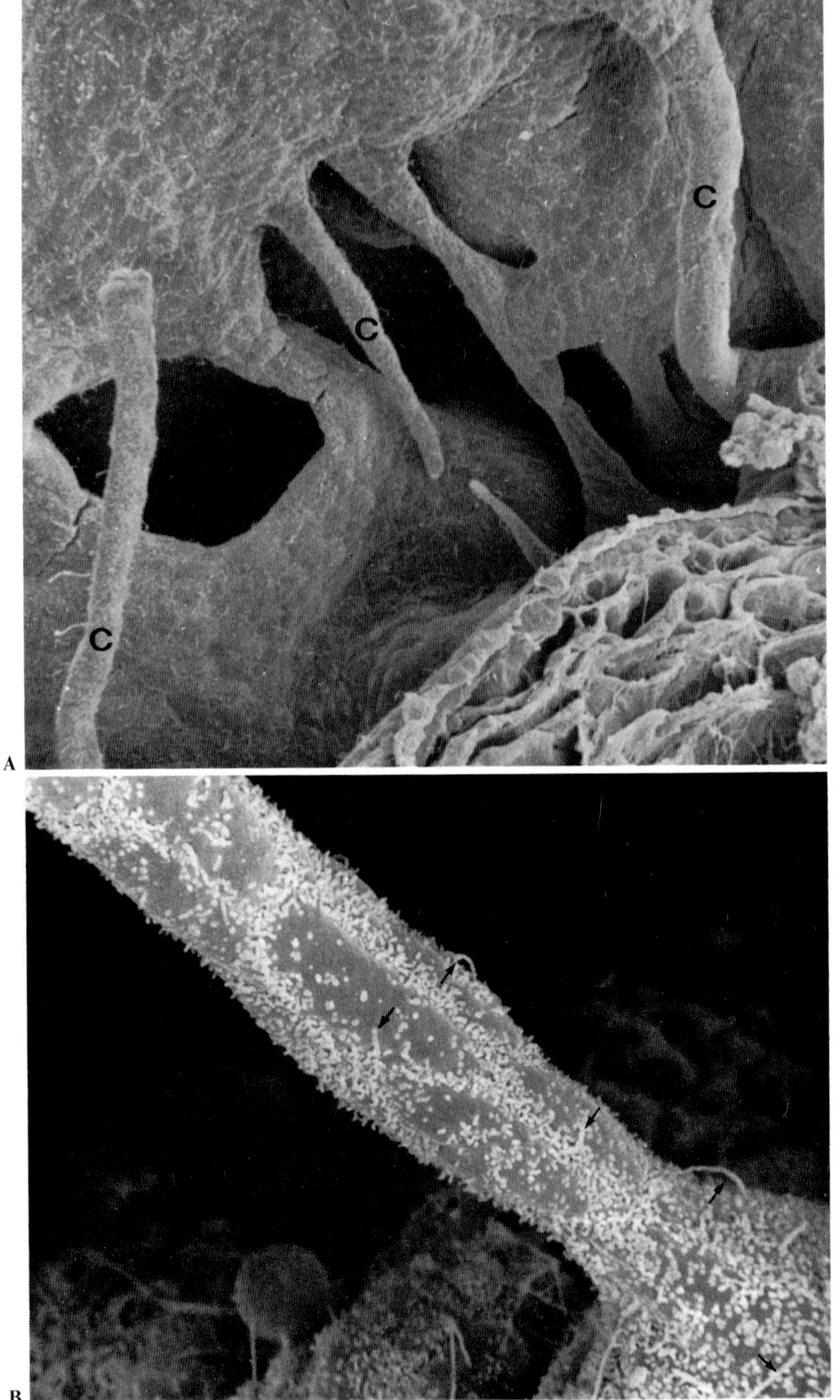

Fig. 16

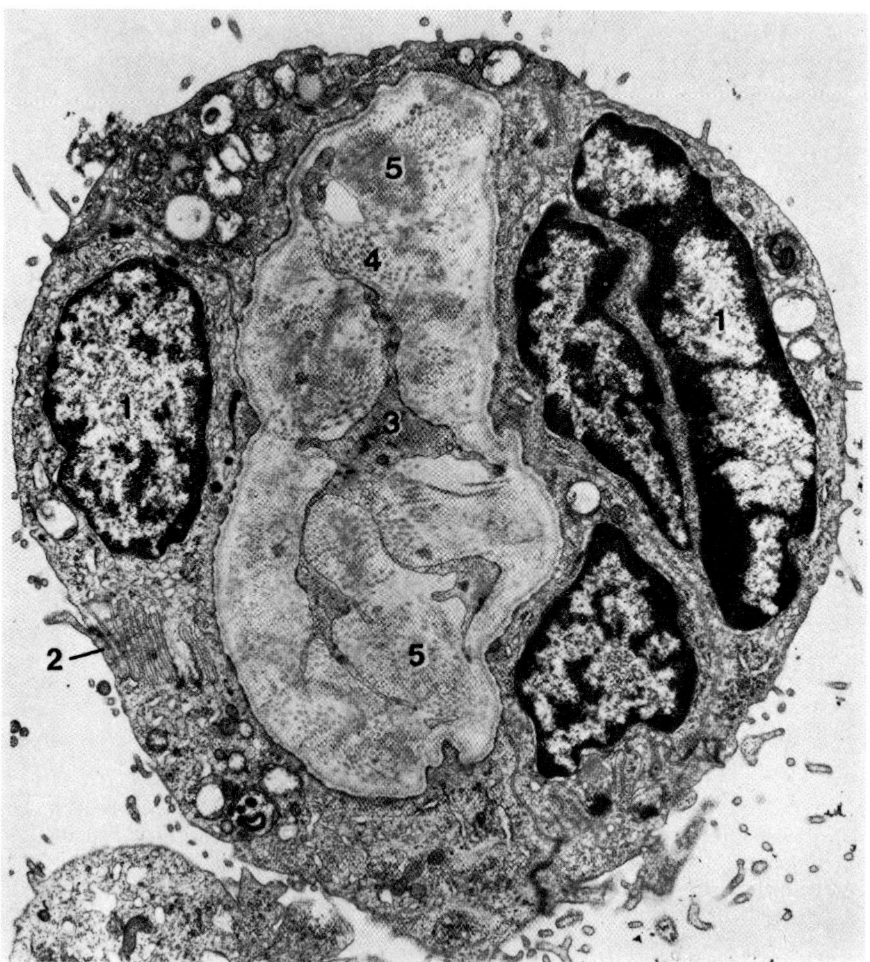

Fig. 17. Transverse section through a non-vascular chorda retis, showing peripheral squamous cells (*1*) and lateral cell membrane interdigitations (*2*) between them. The central core contains a myofibroblast (*3*) with branching processes surrounded by collagen fibres (*4*) and bundles of microfilaments (*5*). (Courtesy of E.C. ROOSEN-RUNGE and A.F. HOLSTEIN.) ×14000

Fig. 16A, B. Scanning electron micrographs showing the internal structure of the rete testis. (Courtesy of E.C. ROOSEN-RUNGE and A.F. HOLSTEIN.) **A** Low-power view of the mediastinal rete testis showing the irregular arrangement of anastomosing channels and chordae retis (*C*) and the lining of squamous epithelial cells. ×750. **B** Higher magnification of a mediastinal chorda retis showing the arrangement of squamous epithelial cells and surface microvilli. *Arrows* indicate long single cilia commonly present on these cells. ×2000

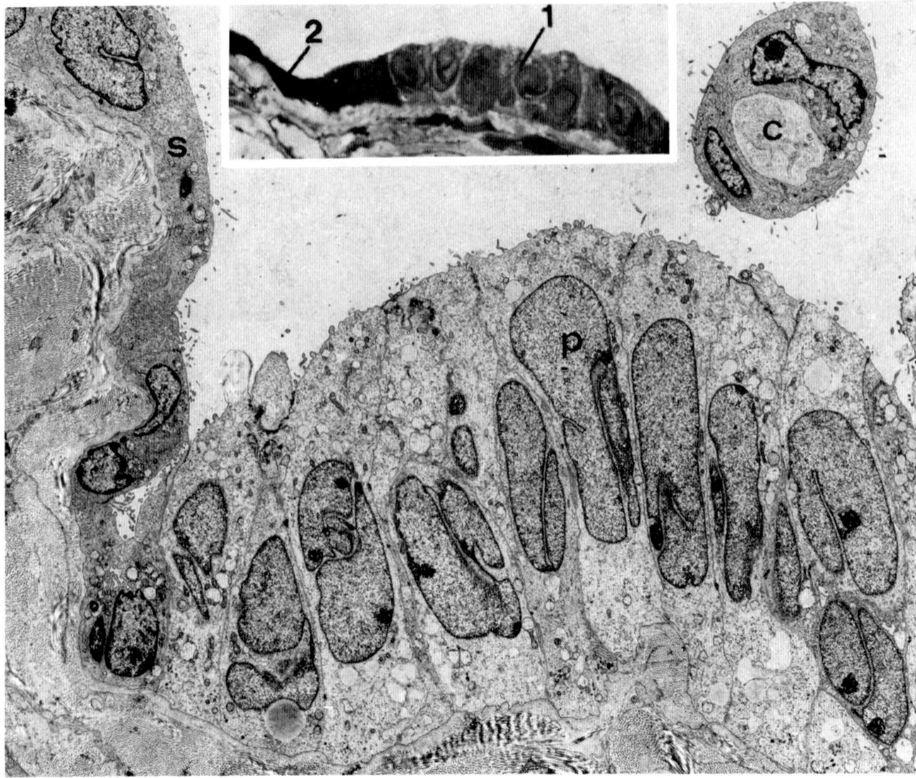

Fig. 18. Epithelial cell lining of the mediastinal rete testis showing epithelial cells, a dense subepithelial layer of connective tissue fibres and thin basal lamina. The squamous (*s*) and prismatic (*p*) cells are shown and a chorda retis (*c*) appears in transverse section. (Courtesy of E. BUSTOS-OBREGON and A.F. HOLSTEIN.) ×3000. *Inset:* light micrograph of the epithelium showing squamous cells (*2*) interspersed by a small island of prismatic cells (*1*). (Courtesy of E.C. ROOSEN-RUNGE and A.F. HOLSTEIN.) ×450

c) Extratesticular Rete

From the wide channels of the superficial mediastinal rete, fluids empty into the extratesticular rete – the bullae retis – which is characterised by vesicular dilatations often exceeding 3 mm in diameter and visible macroscopically. These dilatations are lined by a squamous epithelium and traversed by chords and pillars similar to those found in the mediastinal rete testis. The bullae are regarded by ROOSEN-RUNGE and HOLSTEIN (1978) as vestibules or antichambers to the excurrent duct system.

d) Cytological Features

Although the epithelium shows considerable variability, two distinct cell types (Fig. 18), squamous and prismatic cells, have been described (BUSTOS-OBREGON and HOLSTEIN, 1975). Most of the rete testis, including the chordae retis, is lined by squamous cells (Figs. 19, 20). These are flat, osmophilic and

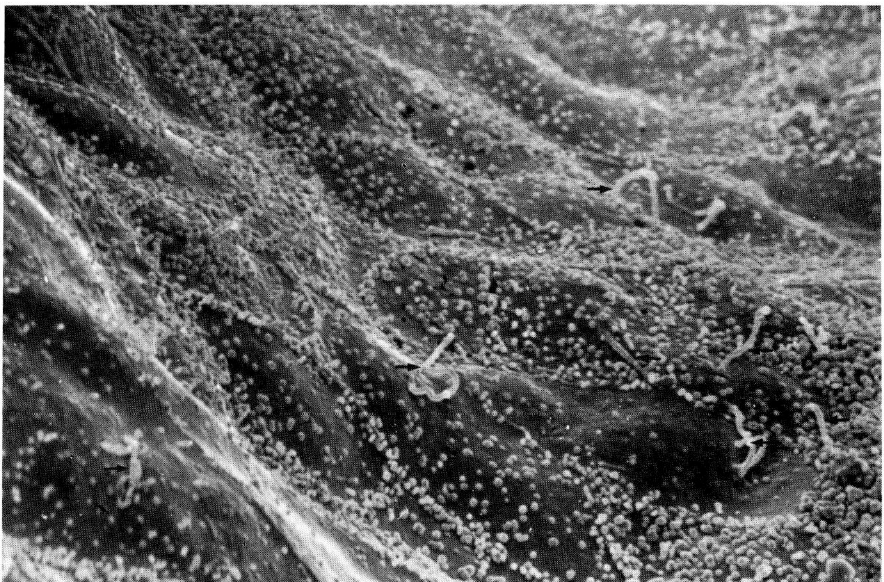

Fig. 19. Low-paper scanning electron micrograph of the undulating squamous epithelium lining the mediastinal rete testis. Short microvilli and isolated single cilia (*arrows*) cover the surface of these cells. (Courtesy of E.C. ROOSEN-RUNGE and A.F. HOLSTEIN.) ×2500

basophilic cells containing a few fat droplets, glycogen particles in the cytoplasm, dense areas of chromatin associated with the nuclear envelope and isolated areas of compacted smooth endoplasmic reticulum. The apical surfaces of these cells are sparsely studded with short microvilli which are usually more densely aggregated around the apical borders of each cell (Figs. 16 B, 19 and 20). An additional structural characteristic is the long single cilium which develops in the central region of the apical surface of each cell (Figs. 19, 20).

The lateral surfaces of adjacent cells are attached by short tight junctions at their apices and by discrete apical and basal desmosomes. The lateral cell membranes also show complex interdigitations which are often lined by rows of microvesicles.

Prismatic cells occur in isolated clusters amongst the squamous cells and can be seen bulging into lumen at bends and corners in the channels (Figs. 18, 22). These cells are light staining and contain irregular nuclei with fine, granular chromatin and prominent nucleoli. Like the squamous cells, they possess a single central cilium (Fig. 21) and variable concentrations of short microvilli over the apical surface (Fig. 21). The cytoplasmic organelles are polarized in their distribution with basally located fat droplets, few glycogen particles and supranuclear aggregations of Golgi and mitochondria (Fig. 22). The apical cytoplasm lacks microvesicles, and microvilli are fewer, thicker and shorter than in the squamous cells.

The rete epithelium rests on a 300–400 Å thick basal lamina, which is in turn enclosed in a connective tissue sheath, consisting of fibrocytes, smooth

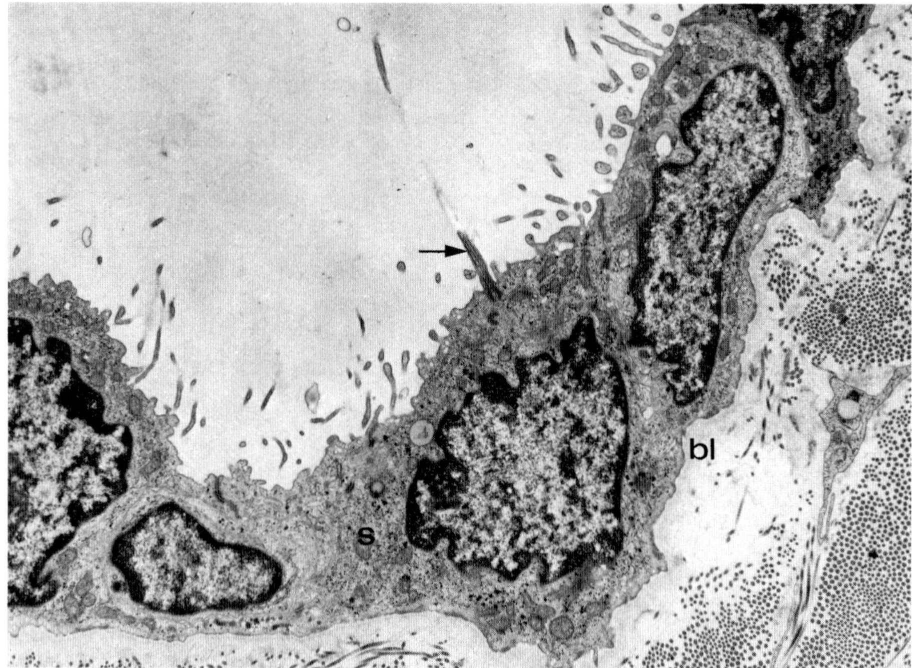

Fig. 20. Ultrastructural features of mediastinal squamous cells. Cytoplasmic organelles are sparse; a thin, amorphous basal lamina (*bl*) separates the squamous epithelial cells (*s*) from dense peritubular bundles of collagen and elastin fibres. Part of a cilium (*arrow*) is shown in longitudinal section. (Courtesy of E.C. ROOSEN-RUNGE and A.F. HOLSTEIN.) × 8700

muscle cells and an intercellular ground substance containing conspicuous bundles of collagen fibres and more dispersed elastin fibres (Figs. 18, 20 and 22).

IV. Epididymis

1. Derivation and Development

The epididymis is derived from the tubules and duct of the mesonephric system, which give rise to two structurally different regions, the ductuli efferentes and the ductus epididymidis. In mammals, including man, the mesonephros consists of an aggregation of tubules which begin their development during the 4th week of fetal life and increase in mass during the 5th week to form the bulk of the urogenital crests. At this time the mesonephros functions as a primitive excretory organ, with each mesonephric tubule being proximally associated with a vascular glomerulus and the excretory filtrates voided into the mesonephric (Wolffian) duct. The excretory function of the mesonephros is transient in mammals. Later in development the excretory role of the mesonephric duct is usurped by the metanephric system, which forms the definitive kidney, and the mesonephric duct and tubules become intimately associated

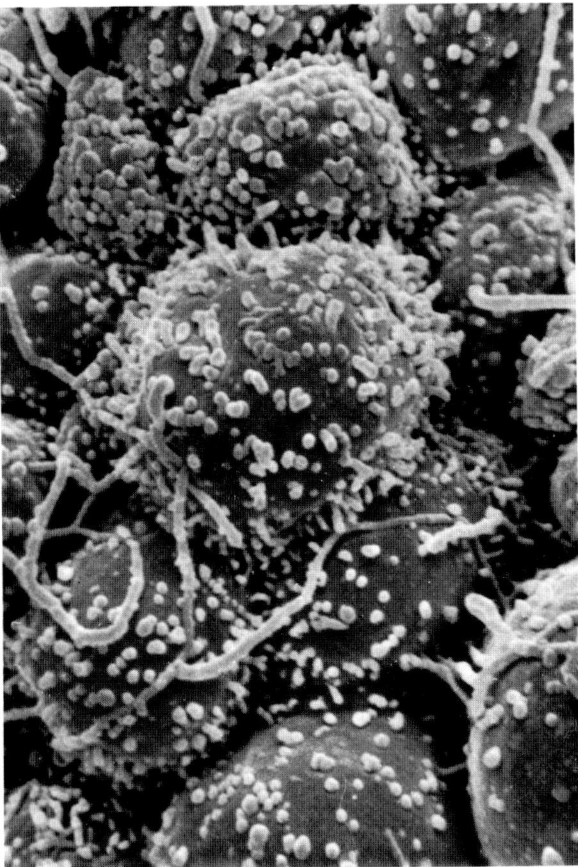

Fig. 21. Topographical features of an enclave of prismatic cells in the mediastinal rete testis. (Courtesy of E.C. ROOSEN-RUNGE and A.F. HOLSTEIN.) ×4500

with the developing gonad to form the excurrent ducts of the male reproductive system (Fig. 23).

This association is formed during the 3rd month of embryonic development after the developing seminiferous cords connect at their distal ends to form the rete testis, which then lies in direct contact with the central portion of mesonephric tubules. During the 3rd–4th month, the rete testis makes connections with between 6 and 12 adjacent mesonephric tubules and in the ensuing few months the gonadal rete acquires a lumen which provides direct continuity between the developing seminiferous tubules and these mesonephric tubules. The mesonephric tubules above and below the central connecting group do not develop a direct communication with the developing testis but gradually atrophy along with the cranial portion of the mesonephric duct associated with these tubules. As described previously (see Sect. B.II) parts of the degenerating mesonephric system persist in the definitive male reproductive tract as the rudimentary appendix of the epididymis and the paradidymis. The mesonephric

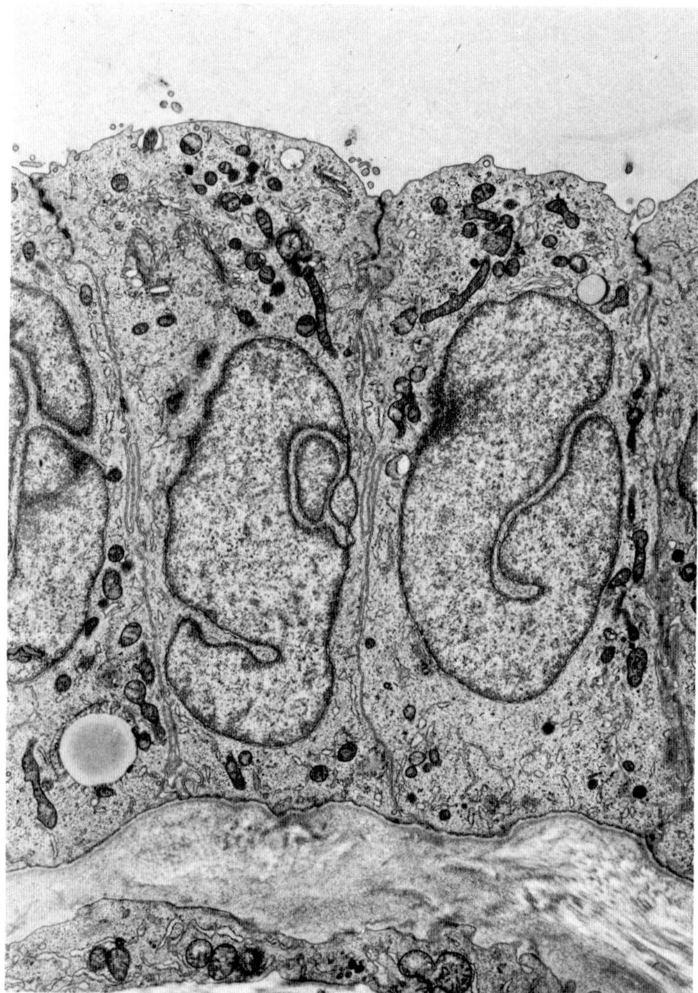

Fig. 22. Ultrastructural features of prismatic cells of the rete testis. Nuclei are large and irregular with fine granular chromatin; mitochondria, Golgi system and other organelles are sparse and concentrated in the apical region of the cell; microvesicles are absent from the apical cytoplasm. (Courtesy of E. BUSTOS-OBREGON and A.F. HOLSTEIN.) × 5000

duct associated with the captured mesonephric tubules persists, enlarges and convolutes to form, with the convoluted, vascularized cone-like aggregates of mesonephric tubules, the coni vasculosi, in the head of the epididymis. The body and tail regions of the epididymis are derived from enlarged, aggregated convolutions of the mesonephric duct below the tubule-associated portion. The mesonephric duct continues caudally into the ductus deferens which, as described in detail in Sect. B.V.1, is derived from the distal segment of the mesonephric duct.

The epididymis is well developed at the time of testicular descent in man. Because of its close relationship with the testis, the epididymis is also directed

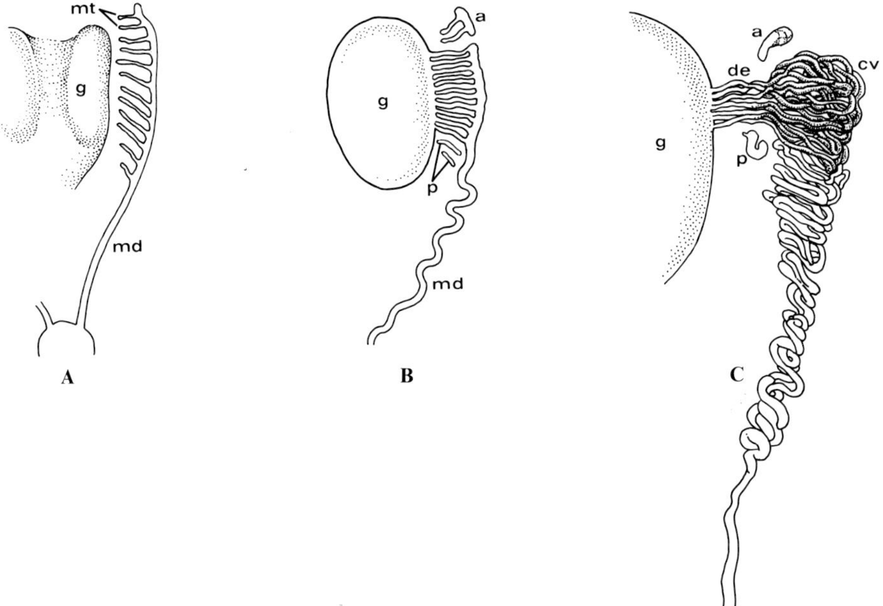

Fig. 23 A–C. Early stages in the development of the epididymis. **A** 6–8 weeks: The mesonephric tubules (*mt*) and duct (*md*) have differentiated but are not yet connected to the developing gonad (*g*). At this stage the mesonephric duct is still functioning as a primitive excretory system. **B** 12–16 weeks: The mesonephric duct and tubules become connected to the developing gonad to form the excurrent system. The tubules above and below the central tubules atrophy to form the appendix of the epididymis (*a*) and the paradidymis (*p*). **C** 20–28 weeks: The mesonephric tubules enlarge to form the ductuli efferentes (*de*) and the coni vasculosi (*cv*) of the head of the epididymis (*stippled*). The distal region of the head of the epididymis and its body and tail develop from the mesonephric duct which also forms the ductus deferens

through the inguinal canal to a definitive position in the scrotum by the same forces responsible for the descent of the testis.

2. General Anatomy

a) Anatomical Relationships

The epididymis is normally contained within the scrotal sac along the posterolateral surface of the testis (Fig. 24). It is closely related to the ductus deferens, which lies along the medial surface of the body and head of the epididymis as it passes upward into the inguinal canal. Superiorly the epididymis is connected to the testis by the ductuli efferentes (vasa efferentia) and by a layer of mesorchium, and inferiorly the tail of the epididymis is attached posterolaterally to the inferior pole of the testis by a narrow band of fibrous connective tissue. This band, in addition to providing a point of attachment of the epididymis to the testis also functions to transmit intratesticular branches of the testicular artery which provide an important collateral blood supply to the tail of the epididymis (see Sect. B.IV.2.6). The gubernaculum provides an additional

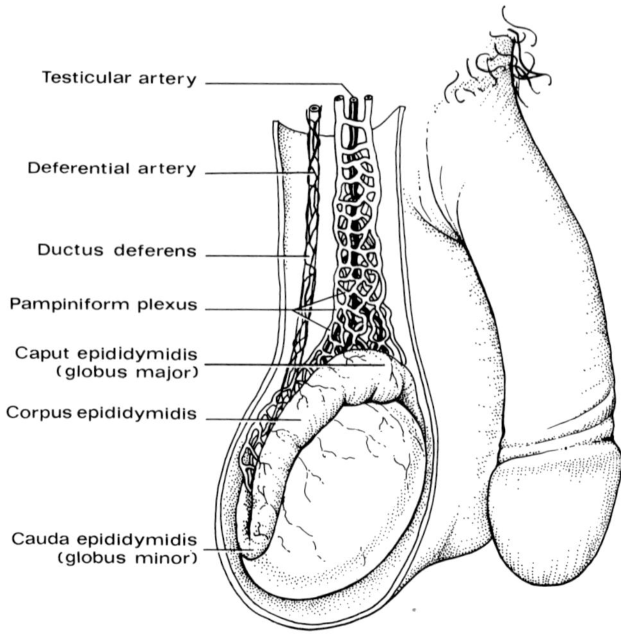

Fig. 24. Scrotal contents in situ. For simplicity the tunica vaginalis and the coverings of the spermatic cord have been omitted from this diagram

zone of attachment between the tail of the epididymis and the wall of the scrotal sac. In man, as in most other scrotal mammals, the epididymis and testis descend into the scrotal sac from the fetal intraabdominal position behind a diverticulum of parietal peritoneum, the *processus vaginalis*. Testiculo-epididymal descent usually occurs during the 7th and 8th months of fetal life and is thought to be influenced by the gubernaculum, which at this stage consists of a thin, longitudinal band of retroperitoneal mesenchyme extending from the inferior pole of the testis and caudal region of the epididymis through the presumptive inguinal canal to the labioscrotal swelling. Although the role of the gubernaculum in testicular descent is still disputed it is widely accepted that it acts to guide the testis and epididymis into the scrotum and, in the definitive position, helps to maintain these structures within the scrotal sac. This idea is supported by experiments which have demonstrated that transection of the gubernaculum before testicular descent results in maldescent of the testis and epididymis. Traditionally it has been held that the primary reason for testicular descent is to provide a cooler environment for sustained testicular function. Recently, however, BEDFORD (1978) has produced compelling evidence to support an alternative suggestion that the need for a cool position for the caudal sperm storage region of the epididymis was in fact the primary selective factor which led to the descent of the epididymis and its associated testis into the cooler environment of the scrotum.

The epididymis is a firm, elongated, crescent-shaped structure, about 4–5 cm long, with an enlarged flattened superior pole, the caput epididymidis or globus

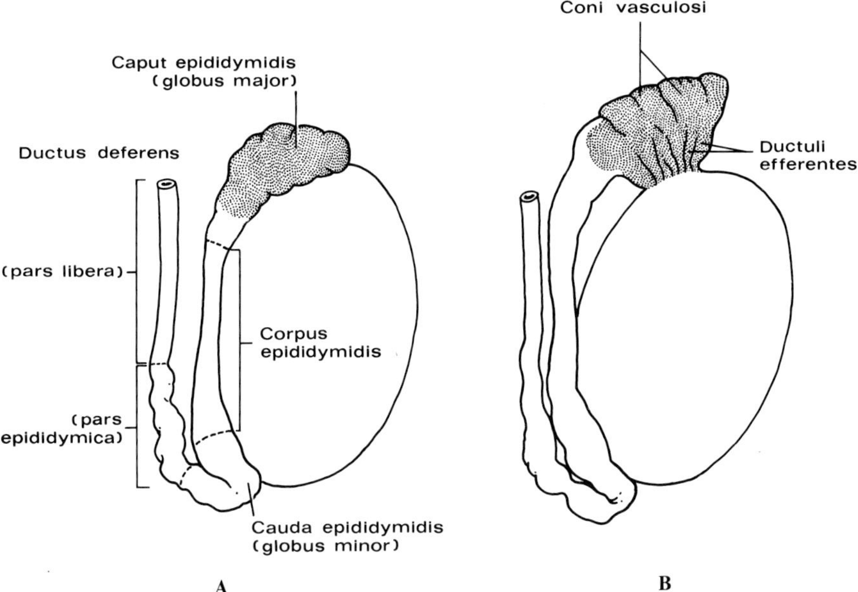

Fig. 25 A, B. The regional organisation of the human epididymis and its relationship to the testis. **A** In situ, the ductus deferens has been subdivided into convoluted and straight portions, the *pars epididymica* and the *pars libera*. **B** The caput epididymidis has been reflected from the testis to show the ductuli efferentes and coni vasculosi. The *stippled region* in the head of the epididymis corresponds to that part derived from the ciliated tubules of the ductuli efferentes

major, and a bulbous inferior pole, the cauda epididymidis or globus minor, which are connected by a narrower isthmus, the body or corpus epididymidis (Fig. 25). The epididymis consists of extensive convolutions of the ductuli efferenti and the ductus epididymidis set in a thin connective tissue stroma and enclosed by a thick outer connective tissue capsule. The organization and structure of the epididymis is described in more detail in Sect. B.IV.3.

The anterolateral surfaces of the epididymis are covered by visceral tunica vaginalis. This is a scrotal remnant of the fetal peritoneal sac, the processus vaginalis, which extends into the scrotum prior to the scrotal descent of the testis and epididymis. The visceral layer is reflected posterolaterally from the epididymis to become the parietal layer of the tunica vaginalis. The posteromedial surface of the epididymis in direct contact with the testis is not covered by the visceral layer (Fig. 26). Similarly the ductus deferens, the posterior surface of the testis and the associated vasculature have no contact with the visceral layer of the tunica. Along the medial surface of the corpus epididymidis, where there is no attachment or fusion of the epididymis to the testis, a shallow pocket of visceral tunica vaginalis separates the adjacent surfaces of the testis and epididymis forming the sinus epididymidis (Fig. 26 B).

b) Vasculature

α) Arterial

The epididymis receives a dual blood supply from branches of the testicular (internal spermatic) and the deferential arteries (Hollinshead, 1966). In general, the principal blood supply to the head of the epididymis is from the testicular artery whereas that to the epididymal tail is from the deferential artery (Fig. 24). However, this simplified scheme is complicated by extensive anastomoses between the two blood supplies and by minor additional supplies to the cauda epididymidis from extra and intratesticular branches of the testicular artery.

In man, and most other mammals, the testicular artery provides an extensive blood supply to the caput epididymidis via a series of branches, up to 0.25 mm in diameter, which originate from the distal part of the artery close to the superior pole of the testis. The caput epididymidis receives a small additional blood supply from small terminal intratesticular branches of the testicular artery and there is also commonly an anastomosis near the superior pole of the testis between the arterial supply of the caput epididymidis and terminal intratesticular branches of the testicular artery.

The corpus epididymidis is poorly supplied by the testicular artery, receiving only a few small branches from it close to the testis. A more extensive blood supply to this region is derived from terminal branches of the deferential artery.

The cauda epididymidis receives its blood supply from three sources. The principal blood supply is from branches of the deferential artery which extends along the ductus deferens to the tail, and subsequently to the body, of the epididymis. Alternative blood supplies to the cauda epididymidis arise from extra- and intratesticular branches of the testicular artery. The cauda is usually supplied by one or a few extra testicular branches which arise either from the main arterial stem, a secondary branch of the main stem or from an arterial branch to the caput epididymidis.

Intratesticular branches of the testicular artery provide an important supplementary blood supply to the tail of the epididymis. These blood vessels leave the testis close to the inferior pole where the epididymis is not separated from the testis by tunica vaginalis and reach the cauda epididymidis by piercing areolar tissue which attaches it to the testis. These branches either directly supply the cauda epididymidis or anastomose with branches of the deferential artery to establish important pathways of collateral circulation to the testis and epididymis. The importance of this and other collateral circulations to the testis after surgical disruption of the testicular artery has already been discussed in Sect. A.

β) Venous

Venous blood from the epididymis drains into the pampiniform plexus, which is formed from three main drainage systems: (1) internal spermatic veins (anterior group) which, as described in Sect. A, leave the testis and accompany the internal spermatic artery to the inferior vena cava; (2) deferential veins (central group), which run back along the ductus deferens in association with the deferential artery and (3) the cremasteric or external spermatic veins (posterior group), which empty into branches of the inferior epigastric and pudendal veins. These three groups anastomose freely with each other in the spermatic cord and therefore provide alternative collateral circulations for testicular and epididymal venous blood. These alternative routes are of great clinical significance in the treatment of varicocele since ligation of the internal testicular vessels above the exit point of the deferential and cremasteric vessels from the spermatic cord ensures adequate circulation from these vessels to maintain testicular function (HOLLINSHEAD, 1966). Although some variations exist, venous blood from the head of the epididymis commonly drains into the internal spermatic venous plexus whereas venous drainage from the body and tail regions of the epididymis is to the deferential veins.

γ) Lymphatics

The pattern of lymphatic drainage of the epididymis is similar to the venous drainage. Major lymphatic channels from the epididymis usually drain into the lymphatic vessels accompanying the testicular (internal spermatic) vessels or into those which follow the course of the deferential vessels. In general, lymphatic drainage from the head of the epididymis accompanies lymph from the testis in lymph vessels which follow the testicular vessels and drain to pre-aortic nodes, whereas lymph from the body and tail of the epididymis drains to the internal group of external iliac nodes in lymph channels which accompany the deferential artery.

c) Innervation

Two groups of sympathetic nerve fibres, the middle and inferior spermatic nerves, provide efferent innervation to the epididymis (MITCHELL, 1935, 1938; NETTER, 1954). The middle spermatic nerves carry fibres from the superior hypogastric plexus which join the ductus deferens at the internal inguinal ring. These fibres provide the principal nerve supply to the ductus deferens and a lesser innervation to the epididymis. The epididymis receives its innervation mostly from the inferior spermatic nerves. These nerves carry sympathetic fibres from the lower end of the inferior hypogastric plexus or the upper end of the pelvic plexus along the ductus deferens to the epididymis. As well as supplying the epididymis they provide a minor innervation to the ductus deferens as they pass along it.

Although not yet demonstrated in man, it seems possible from the close relationship of the head of the epididymis with the testis and similarities in the origin of their blood supplies and lymphatic drainage, that the superior spermatic nerve which innervates the testis and its associated structures may also provide a nerve supply to the caput epididymidis.

While there is some evidence for parasympathetic innervation of the epididymis in other mammals there is, as yet, none to suggest this in man. It is generally accepted that the smooth muscle associated with the epididymis and vas deferens is innervated by adrenergic sympathetic fibres (BAUMGARTEN et al., 1968, 1971).

Afferent innervation from the epididymis is carried by fibres which pass to the superior hypogastric (presacral) plexus and then ascend through the aortic plexus or lumbar chains. These fibres are thought to enter the spinal cord from the sympathetic chain at spinal segments T11, 12 and L1, but variations to this pattern presumably exist. HOLLINSHEAD (1966) has suggested that, because of the similarity in the pathways of afferent fibres from the epididymis and testis, pain derived from the epididymis is not usually distinguishable from testicular pain.

3. Cytological Features

As indicated previously, the superior pole of the epididymis is connected to the testis by a series of 8–15 excurrent ducts, the ductuli efferentes, which receive the accumulated testicular fluids and spermatozoa from the rete testis (see Sect. B.III.2). The ductuli efferentes form tightly packed conical coils, known as the lobules of the head of the epididymis or coni vasculosi (HOLLINS-HEAD, 1966; MORITA, 1966; HOLSTEIN, 1976), which comprise the bulk of the caput epididymidis (Fig. 25). This arrangement in man is unusual since in most other mammals the ductuli efferentes unite to form a single excurrent duct before entering the head of the epididymis (DYM, 1976; GLOVER and NICANDER, 1971; HAMILTON, 1972, 1975; HOFFER and GREENBERG, 1978) and do not therefore contribute directly to the main structure of the epididymis. In these mammals the epididymis is formed solely by aggregations of convoluted coils of the ductus epididymidis. Exceptions to this are found in the dog, horse and bull where the organization of the head of the epididymis is apparently similar to that described in man (BENOIT, 1926; MANEELY, 1959; HEMEIDA et al., 1978).

In man the ductuli efferentes gradually coalesce in the distal region of the head of the epididymis to form the ductus epididymidis, a single, highly convoluted duct which forms the remainder of the caput epididymidis and all of the corpus and cauda epididymidis. As it extends distally the ductus epididymidis gradually increases in diameter and its convolutions become less tortuous. At its distal end it merges into the proximal convoluted portion of the ductus deferens, the pars epididymica (Fig. 25). Several structural features mark the transition from ductus epididymidis to ductus deferens (see Sect. B.V.2.a).

The traditional approach to the structure of the epididymis has been to subdivide it into sequential zones which represent morphological and/or functional regions within the epididymis. The most commonly used system of nomenclature is that already described in Sect. B.IV.2.a, in which the epididymis is subdivided into three regions, the caput, corpus and cauda epididymidis, representing morphological regions of the epididymis which can be recognized macroscopically (Fig. 25). Alternative systems are the zonal nomenclature of REID and CLELAND (1957), which was used to subdivide the rat epididymis into a series of histologically recognizable zones, and the functionally oriented nomenclature of GLOVER and NICANDER (1971), in which the traditional regions of the epididymis were replaced by a zonal system representing regions of the epididymis with particular functional attributes. The terms initial, middle and terminal segments have been used in this system to signify regions of the epididymis in which fluid absorption, sperm maturation and sperm storage, respectively, occur. In this section we have retained the traditional nomenclature to describe the epididymis. The caput epididymidis, which contains the ductuli

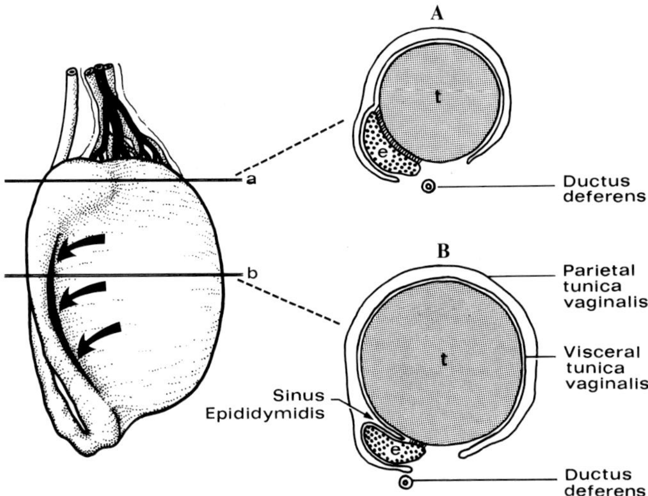

Fig. 26. The relationships of the tunica vaginalis to the testis and epididymis. A lateral surface view of the testis and epididymis covered by visceral tunica vaginalis (the parietal layer has been removed) shows the position of the sinus epididymis (*arrows*) and the planes of sections *a* and *b* which correspond to the levels of transverse sections (*a*) and (*b*). Sections (*a*) and (*b*) demonstrate the relationships between parietal and visceral tunica vaginalis and the testis (*t*), epididymis (*e*) and sinus epididymidis

efferentes and the initial part of the ductus epididymidis, represents the principal zone of fluid resorption and the initiation of sperm maturation. The corpus epididymidis is the principal region for completion of sperm maturation (BED-FORD et al., 1973) and the cauda epididymidis functions as a region for sperm storage.

Few studies have been made of the structure or ultrastructure of the human epididymis. The details included in this section are drawn from the observations of MORITA (1966), HOLSTEIN (1969, 1976), BAUMGARTEN et al. (1968, 1971) and BRANDES (1974) and are augmented by unpublished observations from this department. As with other parts of the human male reproductive system the paucity of information on the morphology of the human epididymis results from the difficulties usually encountered in obtaining fresh normal biopsy and necropsy specimens.

The ductuli efferentes differ considerably in structure from the ductus epididymis. As a result in this section the histological characteristics of these two components of the excurrent duct are considered separately.

a) Ductuli efferentes

The shape of the ductuli efferentes changes with increasing distance from the testis; the tubules become narrower and the populations of non-ciliated cells in the epithelium lining the tubules change from being predominantly secretory in function in the proximal segments of the tubules to predominantly absorptive in the distal segments (MORITA, 1966; HOLSTEIN, 1969, 1976b). The morphological correlates of these functions will be described later in this section.

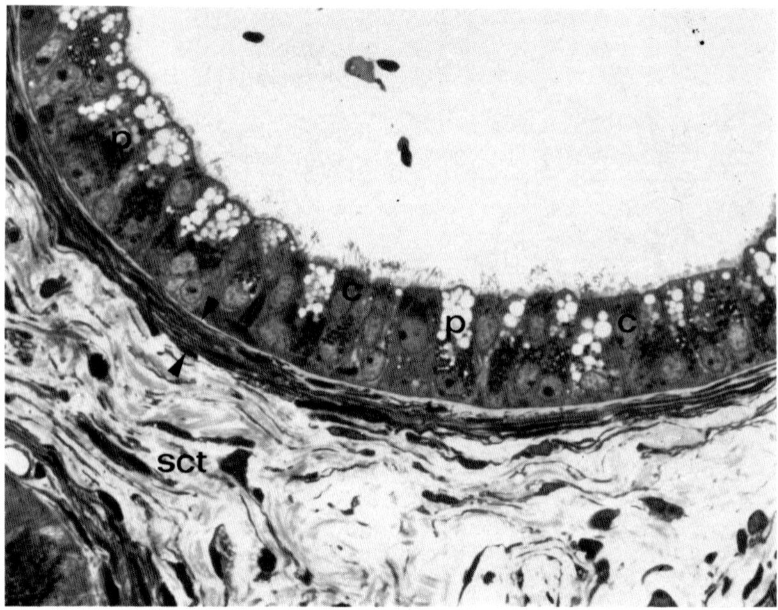

Fig. 27. High-power light micrograph of the epithelium of a human ductulus efferentis, showing principal cells (*p*) interspersed by ciliated cells (*c*). Each tubule is set in stromal connective tissue (*sct*), which contains fibroblasts, and collagen and elastin fibres, and is surrounded by 4–6 layers of thin contractile cells (*between arrowheads*). × 520

While there is some variation, there is a general trend to reduction in epithelial height towards the distal extremities of the ductuli efferentes. The epithelium of the proximal segments measures approximately 35–40 µm in height whereas distal epithelial heights are reduced to 20–30 µm.

α) Epithelium

A simple columnar epithelium consisting mostly of ciliated and non-ciliated principal cells lines the ductuli efferentes (Fig. 27). Small, rounded intra-epithelial cells which resemble lymphocytes are also present, sparsely distributed amongst the epithelial cells. These cells appear to correspond to the "halo" cells described by REID and CLELAND (1957) in the epithelium of the rat epididymis.

Ciliated cells occur only in the ductuli efferentes. By definition the commencement of the ductus epididymidis is regarded as the zone of transition from a ciliated to a non-ciliated epithelium.

Ciliated cells in the ductuli efferentes of man are morphologically similar to ciliated cells found in ductuli efferentes of other mammals (LADMAN and YOUNG, 1958; LADMAN, 1967; HAMILTON, 1975; RAMOS and DYM, 1977; HEMEIDA et al., 1978; HOFFER and GREENBERG, 1978). The most prominent feature of these cells is the dense aggregation of cilia which protude from their apical surface into the lumen of the duct (Figs. 27, 28). The cells are columnar and

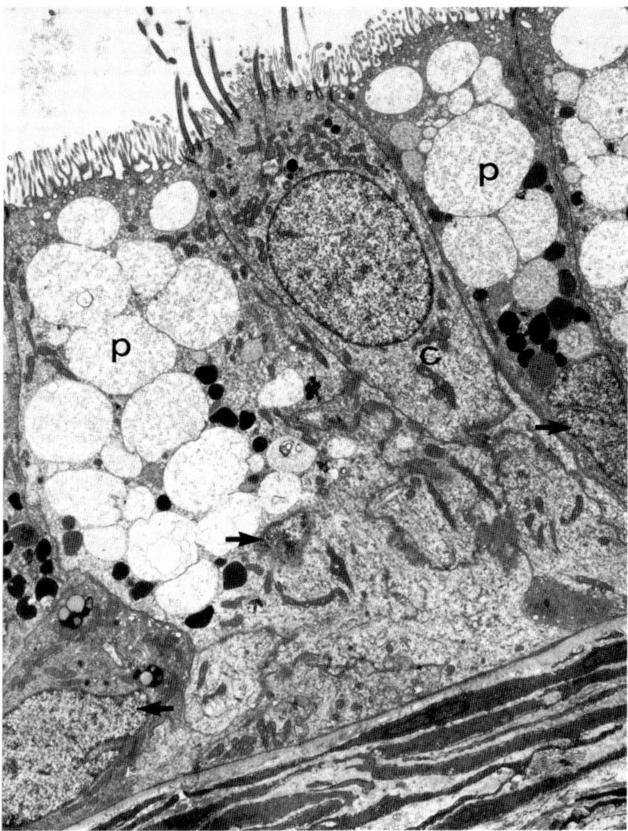

Fig. 28. Low-power electron micrograph of the ciliated epithelium lining the proximal segment of a human ductulus efferentis, showing a ciliated cell (*c*) flanked by principal cells (*p*). The ciliated cell features cilia, dense apical aggregations of mitochondria and a large, spherical, apically situated nucleus. The principal cells are distinguished by irregular, basally situated nuclei (*arrows*), short microvilli, supranuclear aggregates of large, round vesicles containing a floccular matrix and small, dense granules. × 3100

vary in height, depending on their position along the ductuli efferentes, from 40 to 25 μm. In cross-section they usually appear goblet shaped, increasing from a basal width of 3–6 μm to a width of 7–10 μm in the expanded apical region. Ciliated cell nuclei are usually located in the central or expanded apical region of the cell, and are large, spherical and euchromatic with one or more prominent nucleoli (Figs. 27, 28).

Dense aggregations of mitochondria occur in the apical region of these cells. These are found clustered around the ciliary rootlets, which extend obliquely in a basal direction towards the nucleus as lateral extensions of the basal body of each cilium (Fig. 29), suggesting an energy-related association with these structures. The ciliary rootlets are similar to those seen in the ciliated cells of the rhesus monkey ductuli efferentes (RAMOS and DYM, 1977) and comprise tightly packed aggregates of microfilaments with prominent cross striations.

The cilia, which display a standard 9+2 arrangement of axial filaments, are much longer than either the small fine apical microvilli, which are sparsely dispersed between them over the apical surface of the ciliated cells, or those protruding from the luminal surface of non-ciliated cells. Each cilium is 0.25–0.4 µm in diameter and terminates proximally in a prominent basal body. The function of cilia in the ductuli efferentes has not been clearly defined. It has been suggested that they aid the movement of fluid along the tubules from the rete testis to the ductus epididymidis, a concept which is to some extent confirmed by the observations of a high incidence of obstructive azoospermia in men with a history of bronchiectasis. However, any conclusions of cilia dysfunction drawn from these observations need to take into consideration the observations of PEDERSON and REBBE (1975), AFZELIUS (1976) and ELIASSON et al. (1977) that some men exhibiting the "immotile cilia syndrome" are still able to produce ejaculates containing normal concentrations of immotile spermatozoa.

Apart from dense aggregations of mitochondria, ciliated cells possess few cytoplasmic organelles, and those present are mostly confined to the apical cytoplasm (Fig. 28). Profiles of smooth and rough endoplasmic reticulum and Golgi bodies are sparse, suggesting little capacity in these cells for synthesis and secretion, and few pinocytotic vacuoles are evident in the apical region, indicating a low rate of absorption of material from the lumen. This conclusion is supported by observations in the hamster using intraluminal colloid injection techniques (MONTORZI and BURGOS, 1967).

Dark and light membrane-bound vesicles are the only other abundant organelles. These occur in the supranuclear and apical cytoplasm, often closely associated with mitochondria, and are of various sizes and shapes (Fig. 30). The more homogeneous electron-translucent vesicles resemble lipid droplets, and may provide a potential energy source for the associated mitochondria, while the darker heterogeneous structures are more akin to primary and secondary lysosomes, which may function to degrade the contents of the lighter vesicles.

A few free ribosomes and polyribosomes occur scattered through the cytoplasm of ciliated cells. The small fine microvilli which extended between the cilia on the luminal surface of these cells appear to differ ultrastructurally from the microvilli on adjacent non-ciliated principal cells. They are shorter and narrower and appear more electron translucent.

Non-ciliated Principal Cells. Principal cells are easily distinguished from ciliated cells by three morphological characteristics (Figs. 27, 28, 31): the absence of cilia, basally positioned nuclei and a more basophilic and electron-dense cytoplasm (HOLSTEIN, 1976b). A gradual change in function of the principal cells from secretion in the proximal regions to absorption in the distal regions of the ductuli efferentes is reflected in the ultrastructural features of cells from each region (MORITA, 1966; HOLSTEIN, 1969; BRANDES, 1974). In contrast to this view, however, BLOOM and FAWCETT (1975) have suggested that ultrastructural and histochemical studies indicate that "secretory vacuoles" are, in fact, lysosomes and that there is no direct evidence to support the suggestion that the non-ciliated cells of the ductuli efferentes have a secretory function. More

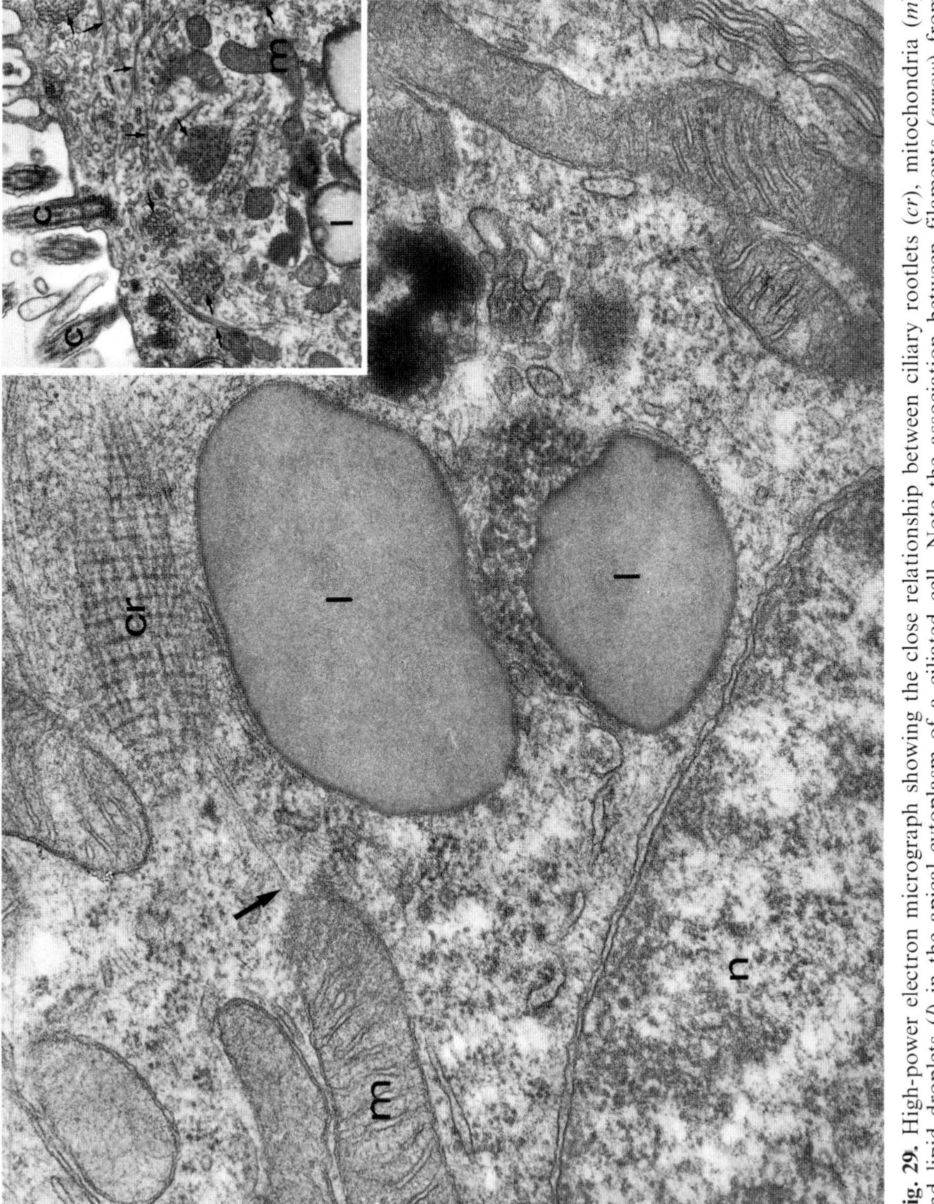

Fig. 29. High-power electron micrograph showing the close relationship between ciliary rootlets (*cr*), mitochondria (*m*) and lipid droplets (*l*) in the apical cytoplasm of a ciliated cell. Note the association between filaments (*arrow*) from the ciliary rootlets and the outer mitochondrial membrane. *n*, nucleus. ×51 500 *Inset*: the apical region of a ciliated cell at low magnification showing mitochondria (*m*), lipid droplets (*l*), cilia (*c*), ciliary rootlets (*arrows*) and microvilli. ×13 500

detailed observations are required to resolve this contention. Both MORITA (1966) and HOLSTEIN (1969) have described a number of non-ciliated cell types based on morphological features of the luminal surface of the cell. Principal cells lining the proximal ductuli efferentes have smoothly contoured free surfaces which protrude slightly into the lumen in a manner which MORITA (1966) suggests

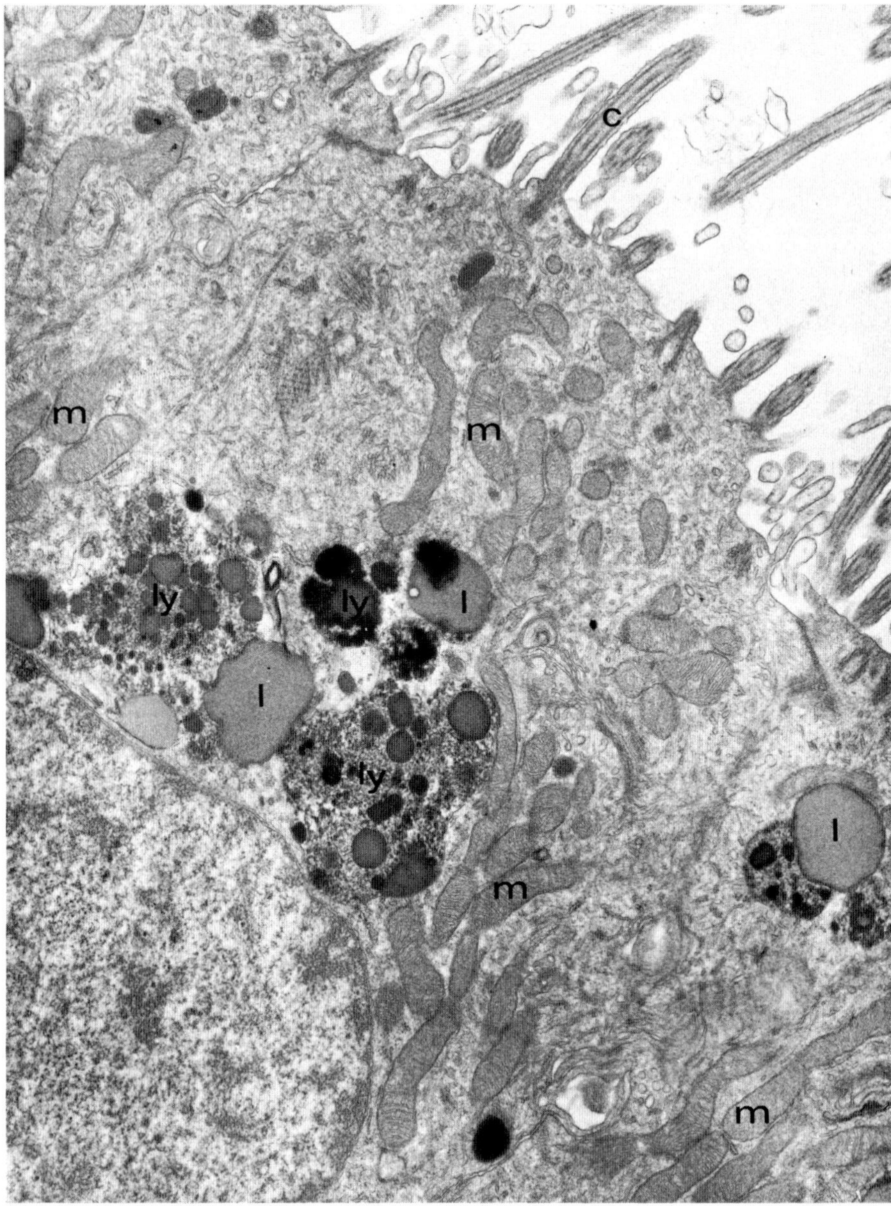

Fig. 30. Supranuclear and apical regions of the ciliated cell. The intimate association between lysosomes (*ly*), lipid droplets (*l*), mitochondria (*m*) and cilia (*c*) suggests an energy-related function which may sustain ciliary movement. × 16000

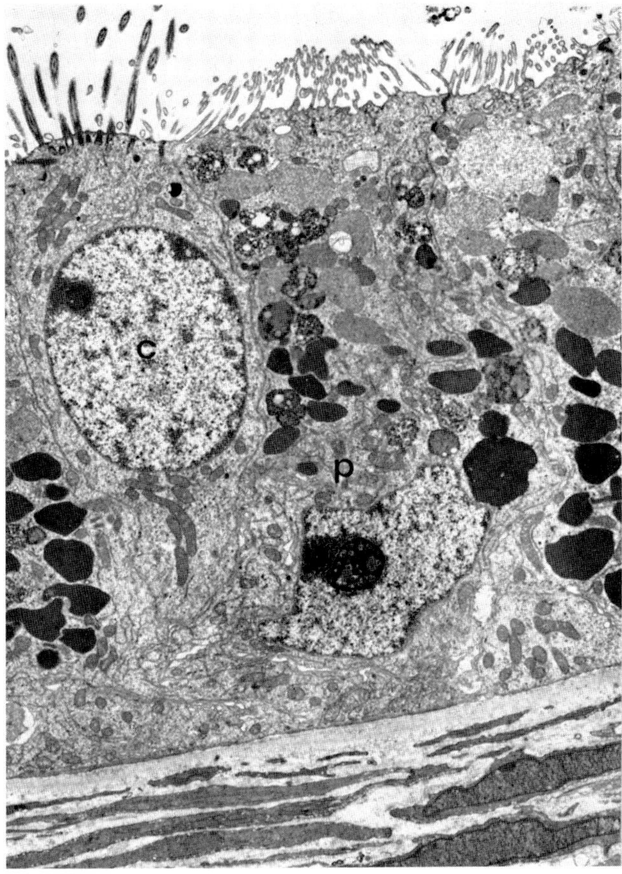

Fig. 31. Low-power electron micrograph of the ciliated epithelium lining the distal ductuli efferentes. The structure of the ciliated cell (*c*) is similar to those seen in the proximal segment. Principal cells (*p*) contain irregular basal nuclei, a dense brush border of microvilli and supranuclear aggregations heteromorphiic dense bodies and mitochondria. ×4750

is characteristic of apocrine or microapocrine secretory activity. Short microvilli protrude in an irregular fashion from the luminal surface of the principal cells but are often concentrated around the periphery of the free surface of the cell. The nuclei of non-ciliated principal cells contrast in shape and position with those of the adjacent ciliated cells. The ovoid principal cell nuclei are positioned in the basal region of the cell with their long axes aligned towards the lumen of the ductule. Nuclear shape is often irregular due to infolding and invagination of the nuclear membrane into the nucleoplasm. Micropinocytotic vesicles and canalicular invaginations, which are characteristic of the absorptive principal cells in the distal ductuli efferentes are rarely seen in proximal principal cells, but aggregations of granules and vesicles are common (compare Figs. 28, 31). These vary in morphology from 2–4 μm apical granules containing a heterogeneous matrix to smaller vesicles containing aggregates of dense parti-

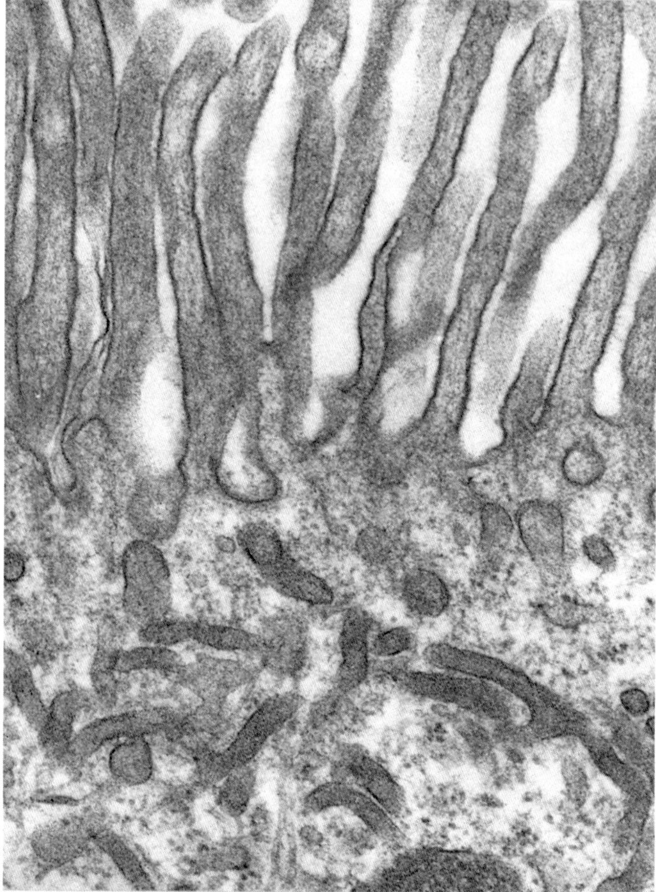

Fig. 32. High magnification of the apical region and luminal surface of a principal cell from the distal ductuli efferentes showing coiled canaliculi and coated micropinocytic vesicles between the dense aggregates of surface microvilli. × 55000

cles within a fine granular matrix. Small irregular dense bodies containing granules of various sizes and density are also observed (MORITA, 1966).

Round or spherical vacuoles, up to 2.5 µm in diameter are common in the apical cytoplasm. These increase in diameter close to the apical surface of the cell and are often surrounded by smaller granules containing a heterogeneous matrix. In many cells, aggregations of osmophilic structures resembling residual bodies or lipofuscin granules are present in the supranuclear cytoplasm. A poorly to moderately developed Golgi complex is also situated in this region of the cell. Terminal dilations of the Golgi cisternae suggest an active secretory function, but the large accumulations of secretory granules in the cytoplasm do not appear to correspond to the observed secretory activity of the Golgi system. Rough and smooth endoplasmic reticulum are sparsely distributed in the cytoplasm. Rough endoplasmic reticulum is abundant in the apical region of the cell, often in close association with cytoplasmic vesicles and mitochondria. A prominent single cilium is often observed extending from the luminal surface of ductuli principal cells (MORITA, 1966).

In more distal regions of the ductuli efferentes the secretory cells are gradually replaced by absorptive principal cells (Fig. 31). In these, the luminal free surface is covered by a dense brush border of microvilli of uniform shape and size. Between adjacent microvilli the plasma membrane penetrates into the apical cytoplasm to form coiled tubular canaliculi and coated micropinocytotic vesicles which are commonly related to an absorptive function (Fig. 32). Flocculent material is often present in the vesicles and invaginations deep within the apical cytoplasm and the proximal ends of the canaliculi are often dilated and associated with small vesicles. Cisternae of rough endoplasmic reticulum are evenly distributed throughout the cytoplasm and are often observed in close association with mitochondria. Multivesicular bodies are commonly observed in the apical and supranuclear cytoplasm. Lysosome-like bodies, 0.8–1.2 μm in diameter and containing a heterogeneous matrix with membrane vesicles and lamellae, are also present in the supranuclear region.

Fluid absorption has been demonstrated in the ductuli efferentes and proximal caput epididymidis of mammals using a variety of experimental techniques and it has been calculated that more than 90% of the fluid secreted by the testis is absorbed into and across epithelial cells in these regions (CRABO, 1965).

β) Lamina Propria and Muscularis

Unlike more distal regions of the reproductive tract, the thin layers of the lamina propria and muscularis externa of the ductuli efferentes blend into each other and are not easily distinguished (Figs. 27, 28, 33).

The epithelium lining the efferentes is set on a thin basal lamina (600 Å–900 Å), which increases in thickness in the distal regions of the ductuli efferentes. Immediately beneath the basal lamina is a dense network of connective tissue fibres which are often separated by zones of amorphous extracellular matrix resembling the matrix of the basal lamina. Peripheral to this layer, and often making minor incursions into it, is a thin layer of circularly or spirally arranged contractile cells interspersed by occasional differentiated cells which resemble fibrocytes (BAUMGARTEN et al., 1971). The thickness of this muscle coat varies with the diameter and degree of contraction of the tubules. In the proximal regions of the ductuli efferentes the muscle coat comprises two layers of thin contractile cells but in more distal regions of the ductules, near their junction with the ductus epididymidis, the muscle coat increases in thickness and the number of contractile cell layers may double or treble (BAUMGARTEN et al., 1971).

Ultrastructural studies of the fibromuscular sheath of the ductuli efferentes by BAUMGARTEN et al. (1971) provide an extremely detailed account of the structure both of contractile cells and the connective tissue matrix which separates them.

The contractile cells are intermediate in morphology between the myoid contractile cells associated with the seminiferous tubules and the ordinary

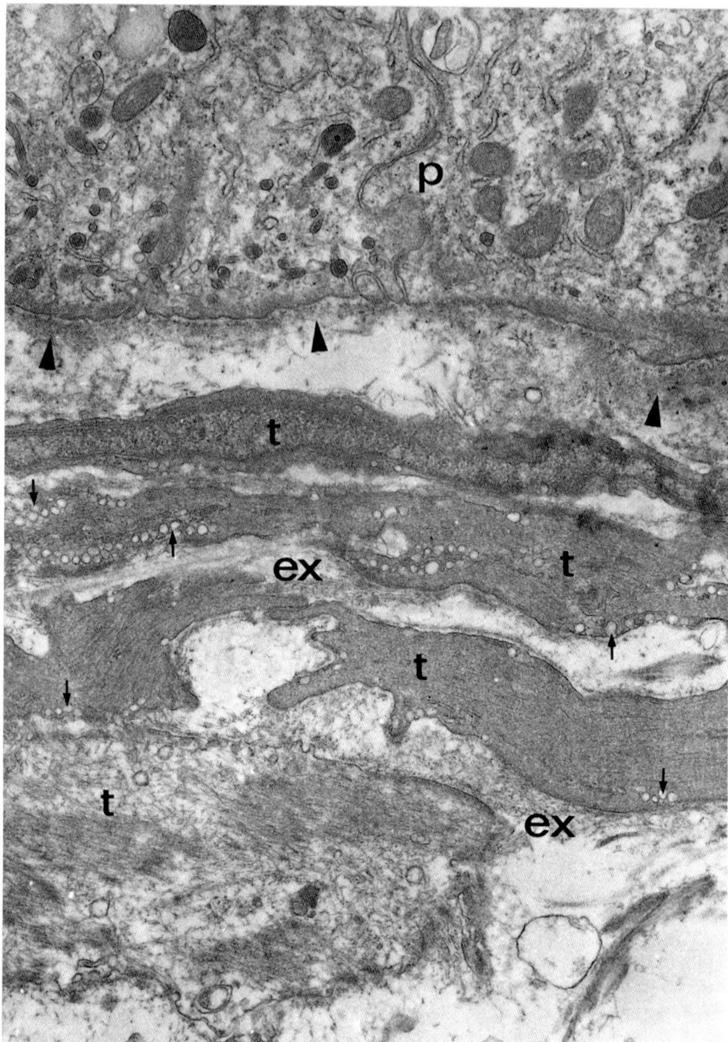

Fig. 33. Low magnification electron micrograph showing a longitudinal section through the peritubular fibromuscular sheath of a ductulus efferentis. The basal regions of two principal cells (*p*) can be seen in association with an indistinct basal lamina (*arrowheads*). The thin contractile cells (*t*) of the muscularis are separated by wide tracts of extracellular matrix (*ex*) containing loosely organized collagen and elastin fibres. Note the densely packed bundles of intracellular myofilaments and numerous membrane calveoli (*arrows*) characteristic of the contractile cells. × 16 000

smooth muscle cells which form the muscle sheath around the ductus deferens and the distal cauda epididymidis. These cells are not epithelial derivatives, as are the myoid "basket" cells associated with various secretory epithelia (BLOOM and FAWCETT, 1975), but are thought to represent an intermediate stage in evolutionary development between the undifferentiated mesenchymal stem cells and differentiated ordinary smooth muscle cells (BAUMGARTEN et al., 1971).

The identification of contractile elements in the wall of the ductuli efferentes and ductus epididymidis has proved extremely difficult by conventional microscopic techniques (EBNER, 1902; HEIDENHAIN and WERNER, 1924; BAUMGARTEN et al., 1971). However, this difficulty has been resolved by the use of semi-thin sections of plastic-embedded tissues correlated with ultrastructural observations and has enabled identification and description of contractile cells of varying morphologies in the fibromuscular sheath around the excurrent ducts.

Contractile cells associated with the ductuli efferentes are more akin in morphology to those which surround the seminiferous epithelium than the ordinary smooth muscle cells associated with the distal cauda epididymidis and ductus deferens. They differ, however, from the contractile cells of the seminiferous tubules in having a more elaborate arrangement of cytoplasmic myofilaments and more dense aggregations of cytoplasmic organelles which BAUMGARTEN et al. (1971) have suggested are special adaptations for rhythmic autocontractility.

The thin contractile cells contain an elongated, centrally positioned nucleus surrounded by a thin veil of cytoplasm containing bundles of myofilaments, either 60 Å or 140 Å in diameter, arranged longitudinally in tightly packed layers which usually enclose the nucleus and extend to the tapering ends of the cell (Fig. 33). Dense patches representing sites of attachment and fusion of diverging and converging myofilaments are rarely seen but, as in ordinary smooth muscle cells, the contractile filaments are attached at specific sites to the inner surface of the plasma membrane. These sites are characterized by membrane-associated plaques of electron-dense material and are separated by segments of plasma membrane containing high densities of micropinocytotic vesicles or calveoli. Aggregations of cytoplasmic organelles, including mitochondria, smooth and rough endoplasmic reticulum, glycogen granules and occasional large lipid droplets, occur in small filament-free areas of cytoplasm at each pole of the nucleus. While contractile cells of different morphology are present in the peritubular fibromuscular sheath of the ductuli efferentes, they are not easily classified into the three different structural categories described by BAUMGARTEN et al. (1971). This may indicate that the dark and translucent cell types of BAUMGARTEN et al. (1971) do not develop in this region or that a continuum of cell types exist in the fibromuscular sheath of both the ductuli efferentes and ductus epididymidis but that the dark and translucent cells, which represent morphological extremes, only appear in the more distal regions.

The fibroblast-like cells present in the peritubular sheath differ from the contractile cells in having a more irregular nuclear shape and cell outline, few or no intracellular filament bundles and large aggregations of rough endoplasmic reticulum. Dense submembrane plaques and adjacent regions of calveolated plasma membrane, which are distinguishing features of contractile cells, are not found in these cells.

Characteristically in the peritubular sheath of the ductuli efferentes, and also in the segments of the ductus epididymidis containing thin contractile cell elements, the cellular elements are separated by wide tracts of intercellular matrix (Fig. 33). These tracts contain loosely intertwining bundles of collagen fibres interspersed by aggregates of smaller 100 Å diameter electron-dense elastin-like fibres. The latter are attached to the plasma membrane of adjacent contractile cells in the regions of the dense, submembrane plaques and are particularly concentrated at each pole of the cell (BAUMGARTEN et al., 1971). These provide a complex system of intercellular connections which may aid coordination and synchronization of the contractile elements in this layer.

The pattern of adrenergic innervation of the contractile cells of the ductuli efferentes with low densities of single adrenergic terminal fibres penetrating the muscle coat, medium noradrenaline content adrenergic terminals and a mostly distant (more then 1000 Å) association of adrenergic synapses with the contractile cells, correlates closely with the observed peristaltic-like autocontractility of the ductuli efferentes (BAUMGARTEN et al., 1971).

b) Ductus Epididymidis

As indicated in the previous section, the ductus epididymidis is a single, highly convoluted duct which commences from below the final confluence of the distal convolutions of the coni vasculosi of the ductuli efferentes (BLOOM and FAWCETT, 1975; HOLSTEIN, 1976b). The general structure and function of the ductus epididymidis in man is similar to that described for other mammals (NICANDER, 1957a, b; REID and CLELAND, 1957; MANEELY, 1959; HAMILTON, 1972, 1975). The prime function of the epithelium is to maintain a suitable luminal environment for the maturation and storage of spermatozoa (YOUNG, 1931; BEDFORD, 1963, 1975; GLOVER, 1969; HAMILTON, 1972; TURNER, 1979) and the peritubular sheath of smooth muscle provides the appropriate contractile forces which transport maturing spermatozoa to the caudal storage region and eventually into the ejaculate (BAUMGARTEN et al., 1971). In the distal region of the coni vasculosi the ductuli efferentes are reduced in diameter to half that of the proximal ductuli efferentes but below the zone of transition of the ductus epididymidis there is an obvious enlargement of the ductus to a diameter similar to that seen in the proximal ductuli efferentes (HOLSTEIN, 1969, 1976). An initial segment, similar to that described in other mammalian species (REID and CLELAND, 1957; HAMILTON, 1975) has not yet been identified in the human epididymis. Along the ductus epididymidis there is a gradual proximodistal reduction in tubule diameter to the transition zone between the distal corpus and proximal cauda epididymidis, where tubule and luminal diameters reach a minimum. Below this, there is a rapid increase again in tubule diameter, particularly in the distal cauda epididymidis, where most of the sperm storage capacity of the epididymis resides. Concomitant with the distal enlargement of the ductus deferens in this region is a reduction in the height of the epithelium and an increase in the luminal concentration of spermatozoa.

Distal to the caudal flexure of the epididymis the duct starts to acquire the morphological characteristics of the ductus deferens. The mucosa is arranged into a series of folds which correspond to the longitudinal ridges of the ductus deferens mucosa partially obliterating the lumen of the duct. There is an increase in epithelial height, when compared with that of more proximal regions of the cauda epididymidis, an increase in the thickness of the connective tissue

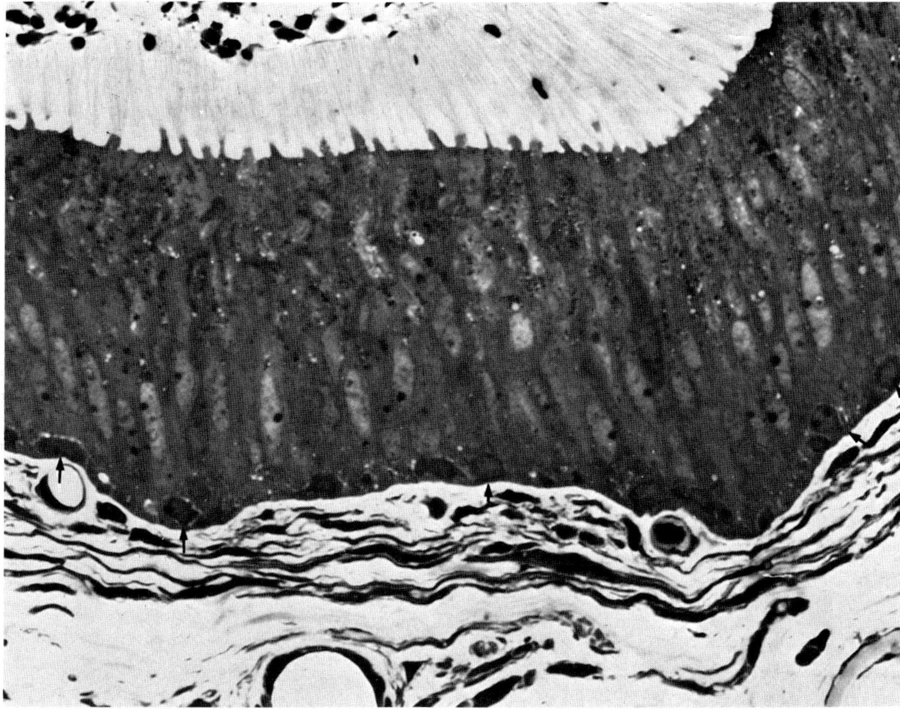

Fig. 34. High-power light micrograph of the pseudostratified columnar epithelium lining the proximal ductus epididymidis showing principal cells, with long, dense apical stereocilia and large ovoid nuclei, and basal cells (*arrows*). Spermatozoa, in various planes of section, can be seen in the lumen of the duct. ×440

component of the lamina propria and an absence of spermatozoa from the lumen.

α) Epithelium

The transition from ductuli efferentes to ductus epididymidis is marked by the loss of ciliated cells from the epithelium and the development of a pseudostratified epithelium consisting of principal cells and basal cells, interspersed by occasional intra-epithelial lymphocytes (HORSTMANN, 1962; HOLSTEIN, 1976b).

The microscopic appearance of the epithelium varies due to changes in its height and cross-sectional outline along the ductus epididymidis. There is a gradual proximodistal reduction in epithelial height (MANEELY, 1959; HOLSTEIN, 1969; BLOOM and FAWCETT, 1975) from a tall, pseudostratified columnar epithelium 45–60 μm in height in the proximal ductus epididymidis (Fig. 34) to a low columnar or cuboidal pseudostratified epithelium 10–20 μm in height in the distal cauda region (Fig. 35). In the distal caput and proximal corpus epididymidis the epithelium forms a smooth inner lining around the duct. As tubule diameter decreases and the lumen gradually narrows in the distal corpus epididymidis, the epithelium gradually acquires a ruffled cross-sectional appear-

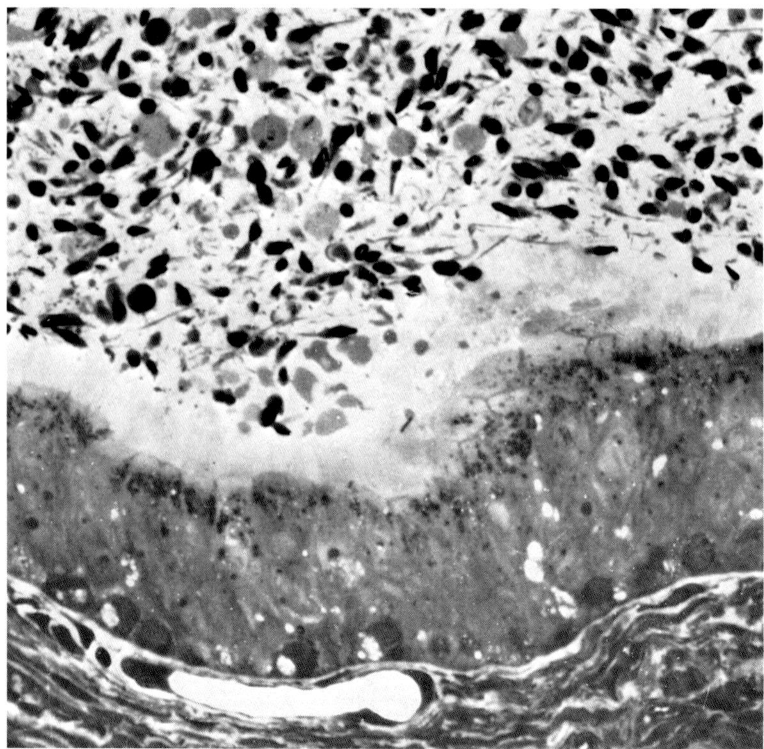

Fig. 35. High-power light electron micrograph showing the pseudostratified epithelium of the distal ductus epididymidis. The principal cells in this region of the epididymis show a decreased cell height and a reduction in the length of the apical stereocilia, when compared to proximal principal cells. Basal cells can be seen interspersed between the principal cells. × 390

ance as it becomes pushed up into irregular longitudinal folds. These folds are lost abruptly as tubule diameter increases in more distal regions of the duct and the epithelium again assumes a smooth outline (HOLSTEIN, 1976b).

As with other epithelia in the glands or ducts of the male reproductive tract, the epithelium of the ductus epididymidis is androgen-dependent. Androgen deficiency causes structural and functional changes in the epididymal epithelial cells which result in a large decrease in epididymal weight due to regression of the epithelial cells and subsequent reduction in tubule and luminal diameter. These changes can be reversed by androgen therapy.

Principal Cells. The gradual decrease in epithelial height along the ductus epididymidis reflects morphological changes in the principal cells. In the initial portion of the ductus epididymidis (distal caput) the principal cells (Fig. 34) are tall, narrow columnar cells, 50–60 μm in height and 6–10 μm wide, with large lenticulate nuclei and prominent apical brush borders of fine stereocilia, 15–20 μm long, which project deep into the lumen of the duct (HORSTMANN, 1962; HOLSTEIN, 1969, 1976b).

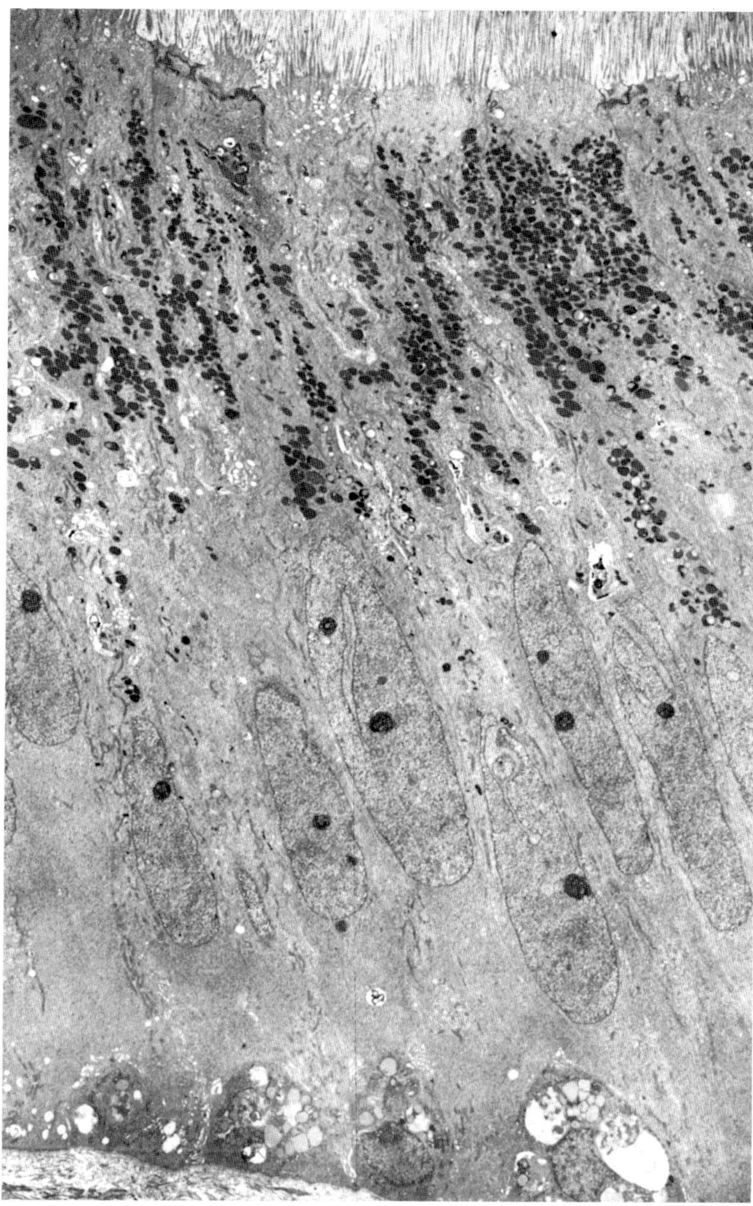

Fig. 36. Low-power electron micrograph showing ultrastructural features of the epithelium of the proximal ductus epididymidis. The principal cells are tall, narrow columnar cells with smooth, elongated nuclei, an extensive supranuclear Golgi complex and long stereocilia. Basal cells occur along the basal lamina lodged between the bases of adjacent principal cells. × 2 500

Principal cell nuclei have a smooth, regular outline with only occasional indentations (Fig. 36). The nucleoplasm shows little affinity for standard histological and ultrastructural stains and is usually pale and electron translucent, with little or no condensed chromatin along the nuclear membrane. Principal cell nuclei are elongated and commonly situated in the basal region of the cell with the long axis oriented radially towards the lumen. Variations in the positions of nuclei in adjacent cells give rise, with the basal cells, to the pseudo-stratified appearance of the epithelium. Each nucleus contains one to three prominent nucleoli, and aggregates of small, round, dense intranuclear granules are sometimes observed. The composition and function of these granules remains unknown.

Basal, perinuclear, supranuclear and apical regions have been described (HORSTMANN, 1962), with each region containing a characteristic array of organelles. In toluidine blue stained Epon sections of human epididymis the basal and perinuclear cytoplasm stains slightly more than the supranuclear and apical cytoplasm, reflecting differences in cytoplasmic organelles in these regions, which have subsequently been confirmed by ultrastructural observations (HORSTMANN, 1962; HOLSTEIN, 1969).

Cisternae of endoplasmic reticulum are widely distributed through the principal cell cytoplasm but are more concentrated, in association with free ribosomes and polyribosomes, in the basal and perinuclear regions of the cell (Fig. 37). Profiles of smooth endoplasmic reticulum are also present, but less numerous, in these regions. Mitochondria occur in all cytoplasmic compartments but appear to be more numerous in the apical and perinuclear compartments, where they are often in close association with profiles of rough endoplasmic reticulum.

The supranuclear compartment is characterized by an extensive Golgi complex which can be identified by light microscopy as an area of low density (Fig. 36). At higher magnification the Golgi complex appears as a series of fenestrated cisternae of smooth reticular membranes arranged in extensive parallel stacks. These stacks are often closely associated with mitochondria, small coated and smooth vesicles, and numerous dense lysosome-like bodies of various dimensions. Lysosomes and small vesicles are known to be derived from the Golgi system, which is recognized as the source of various lytic enzymes (FRIEND and FARQUAR, 1967). As in the rat (HAMILTON, 1975), smooth endoplasmic reticulum forms a comparatively small component of the reticular system in human principal cells, and the dense whorls of smooth endoplasmic reticulum observed in mouse and rabbit principal cells (HAMILTON, 1975) have not been observed in man.

Apart from dense bodies and small vesicles, there is no evidence of synthesis and packaging of secretory granules from the extensive Golgi apparatus of the principal cell. It appears that production of lytic enzymes to assist in the degradation of luminal material absorbed by the principal cells is the most important, if not the sole, activity of the Golgi system in these cells.

The apical region is characterized by a dense brush border of stereocilia and by numerous pinocytotic vesicles, multivesicular bodies and dense, membrane-bound primary and secondary lysosomes in the cytoplasm (Fig. 38).

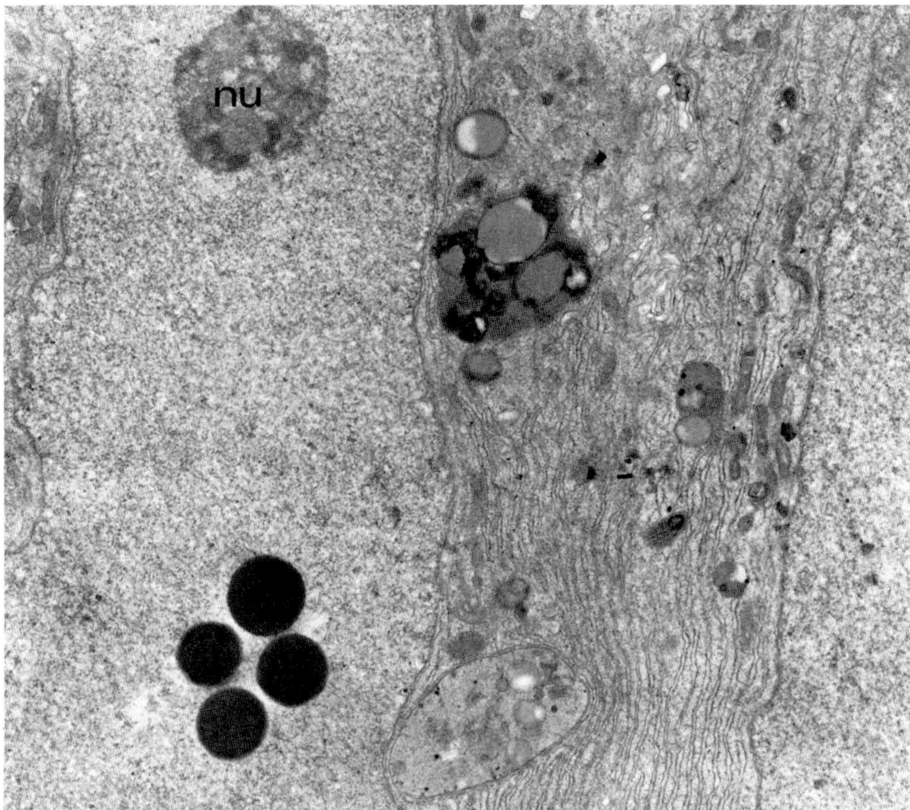

Fig. 37. Perinuclear region of a principal cell from the proximal ductus epididymidis. Dense, parallel stacks of rough endoplasmic reticulum are common in the cytoplasm of this region. A few lipid droplets, dense lysosome-like bodies and mitochondria are also present, and a prominent nucleolus (*nu*) and four dense intranuclear inclusions can be seen in one of the nuclei. × 10 500

Contrary to their name, the stereocilia are non-motile structures which bear a closer morphological resemblance to elongated microvilli than cilia. They lack the 9+2 axonemal complex, basal bodies and striated rootlets of cilia but possess a dense core of microfilaments which extend into the apical cytoplasm and probably provide a structural support for the stereocilia. Like microvilli, they provide an extensive surface area for absorption and their extreme length in proximal principal cells corresponds with functional observations made in laboratory animals (HOWARDS et al., 1975; JOHNSON and HOWARDS, 1977; TURNER, 1979) that fluid absorption is greatest in the initial portion of the duct. The functional relationship between length of stereocilia and fluid absorption has not been examined in the human epididymis.

Other morphological indicators of fluid absorption in these cells are the elaborate spiral canaliculi, which extend between adjacent stereocilia into the

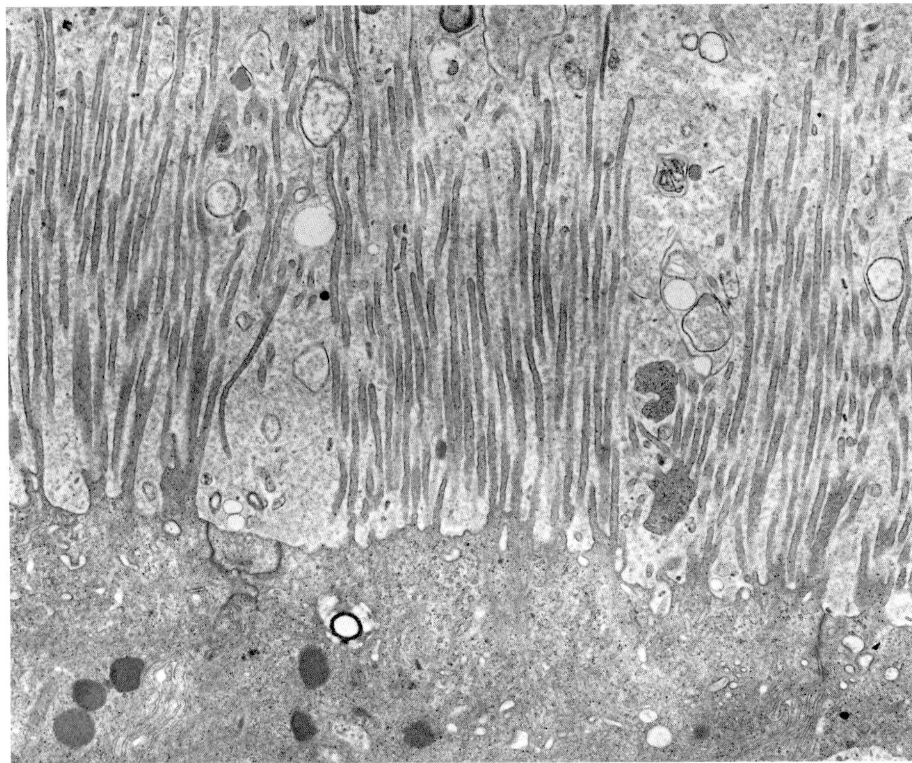

Fig. 38. Apical region of a proximal principal cell showing dense aggregations of long, fine stereocilia, numerous pinocytotic vesicles and profiles of spiral canaliculi, and some dense lysosome-like bodies. Dense apical tight junctions can be clearly seen between adjacent cells. × 12 300

apical cytoplasm, and numerous pinocytotic vesicles. Multivesicular bodies, coated vesicles and various lysosomes and dense bodies are numerous in the apical cytoplasm and can be regarded as additional evidence of absorptive activity by the principal cells. The multivesicular bodies, which appear as large vesicles containing variable amounts of flocculent material and internalized vesicles, are particularly numerous in the apical cytoplasm of principal cells in the proximal region of the duct (Fig. 38).

The lateral plasma membranes of adjacent principal cells show no interesting specializations. Extensive interdigitations are sometimes observed in the basal region of adjacent cells but towards the lumen the lateral plasma membranes become smooth and are attached only at infrequent intervals by desmosomes. Around the apex of each cell the lateral membranes are attached by an apical junctional complex, which isolates the luminal compartment and restricts the passage of substances into and out of the lumen. SUZUKI and NAGANO (1978) have recently shown an increase in the width and complexity of the apical tight junctions between principal cells along the ductus epididymidis of the rat and have suggested that this indicates a decrease in leakiness of the epithelium in the caudal regions of the duct.

In more distal regions of the epididymis the principal cells show a decrease in height and an increased width, and their nuclei appear slightly larger and more spherical in shape (Figs. 35, 39). Associated with decreased cell height is a reduction in the density of intracellular organelles, especially endoplasmic reticulum and Golgi system. The length and density of stereocilia are also reduced and the decrease in numbers of multivesicular bodies, pinocytotic vesicles and lysosomal granules in the apical cytoplasm (Fig. 40) suggests a decrease in absorptive activity of the caudal principal cells.

In addition to absorptive function, principal cells in other mammals have been shown to have the capacity for de novo steroidogenesis (HAMILTON et al., 1969; HAMILTON and FAWCETT, 1970; HAMILTON, 1971) and for secretion of various substances into the lumen of the ductus epididymidis. These substances include specific epididymal proteins (BLAQUIER, 1975; CAMEO and BLAQUIER, 1976), carnitine (MARQUIS and FRITZ, 1965; BROOKS et al., 1974), glycerylphosphorylcholine (DAWSON and ROWLANDS, 1959; SCOTT et al., 1963; BROOKS et al., 1974) and sialic acids (FOURNIER, 1966). None of these secretory functions have yet been demonstrated in principal cells of the human epididymis although high concentrations of carnitine, thought to be derived from the epididymis, have been identified in human seminal plasma (FRENKEL et al., 1974; KOHENG-KUL et al., 1977). While the smooth endoplasmic reticulum observed in principal cells of man is likely to be able to participate in steroidogenesis, as it has been shown to in epididymal cells of other mammals, there is no structural evidence in principal cells of the human epididymis which would indicate the traditional synthesis and elaboration of secretory products into the lumen of the duct. This paradox has also been described in principal cells of other mammals which are known to synthesize and release secretory materials into the lumen (HAMILTON, 1975).

Basal Cells. These cells are similar in structure to basal cells found in epithelium lining the ductus deferens (Sect. B.V.3.a), seminal vesicle (Sect. B.VI.3.a) and prostate (Sect. B.VII.3.a). They are 5–8 µm in diameter and vary in shape from spherical to pyramidal. In the proximal ductus epididymidis spherical basal cells predominate whereas in the caudal regions, where the epithelial height is reduced, pyramidally shaped basal cells are more common. Epididymal basal cells occur randomly over the basal lamina interspersed between the bases of adjacent principal cells. Each basal cell contains an ovoid nucleus surrounded by a thin layer of essentially featureless cytoplasm (Fig. 41). The cytoplasm contains few organelles – occasional mitochondria and lipid droplets, a few profiles of endoplasmic reticulum and free ribosomes – and lacks the dense bundles of filaments, which are a feature of the basal cells of the ductus deferens (HOFFER, 1976).

The function of basal cells in epithelia of the male reproductive system is obscure. A commonly held view is that they form a stem cell population from which degenerating principal cells are replaced. If this is so, recent studies in the rat, at least, suggest that the rate of replacement of principal cells in

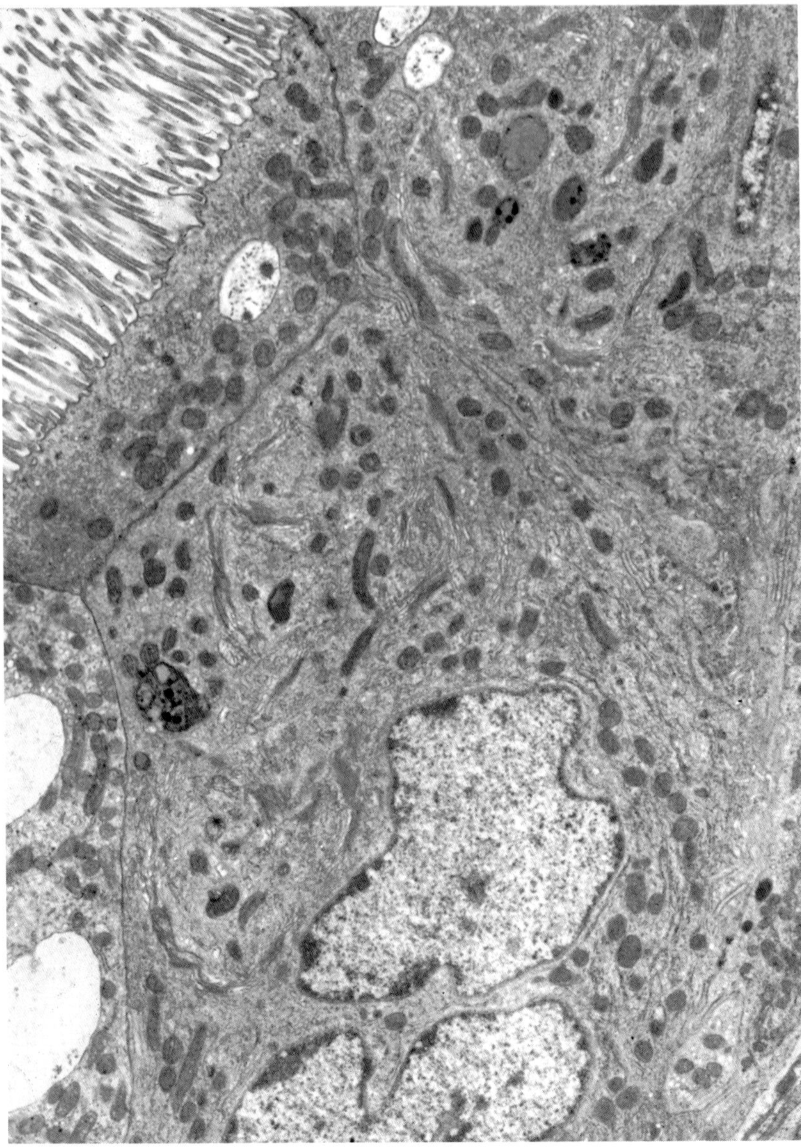

Fig. 39. Oblique section through principal cells of the distal ductus epididymidis showing larger, rounded nuclei, decreased stereocilial length, dispersed profiles of Golgi cisternae in the supranuclear region, some multivesicular bodies and apical aggregations of mitochondria. Reduced absorptive activity by these cells is suggested by decreased numbers of apical pinocytotic vesicles and lysosomal granules. ×4200

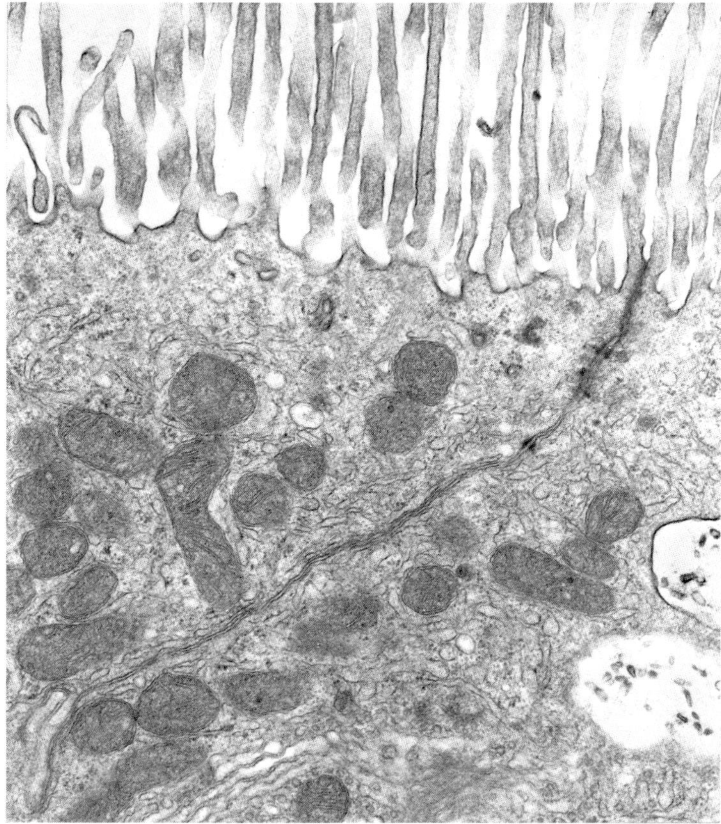

Fig. 40. High-magnification electron micrograph of the apical region of distal ductus principal cells. ×16800

the mature epididymis must be very slow since few mitotically active basal cells were observed (NAGY and EDMONDS, 1975).

Intra-epithelial lymphocytes. REID and CLELAND (1957) originally described these cells as halo cells but subsequent ultrastructural observations show that they have a close similarity in structure to lymphocytes (HAMILTON, 1972; HOFFER et al., 1973; DYM and ROMRELL, 1975). These cells are sparsely and randomly distributed in the epithelium between principal cells and are found throughout the epididymis, although they appear to be more common in the proximal regions of the duct. Like lymphocytes, they consist of a dark spherical nucleus invested by a thin peripheral sheath of pale cytoplasm, containing few organelles. They are lodged at various levels between adjacent principal cells. Some cells remain in contact with the basal lamina whereas others are found in the apical region of the epithelium just below the apical junctional complex, which connects neighbouring principal cells. As with basal cells, the function of intra-epithelial lymphocytes is still unknown. DYM and ROMRELL (1975) have suggested that, since intra-epithelial lymphocytes are located in segments of the duct where

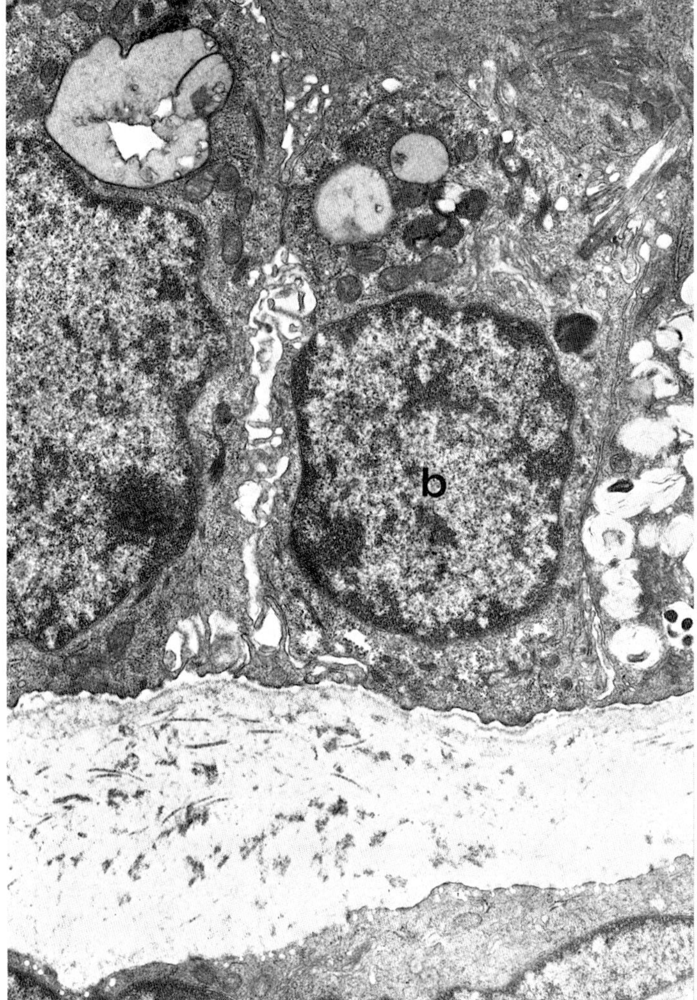

Fig. 41. Basal cell (*b*) from the epithelium of the ductus epididymidis showing the characteristic rounded, heterochromatic nucleus and thin peripheral layer of cytoplasm containing a few apical lipid droplets, mitochondria and profiles of endoplasmic reticulum. × 8800

luminal material is absorbed, they may form a resident population of immunocompetent cells which function to sequester sperm and epididymal antigens and prevent them from reaching the general circulation.

β) Lamina Propria

The lamina propria of the ductus epididymidis is unremarkable. It shows a gradual transition in structure along its length from a narrow subepithelial layer in the proximal regions of the epididymis (Figs. 34, 42), which resembles

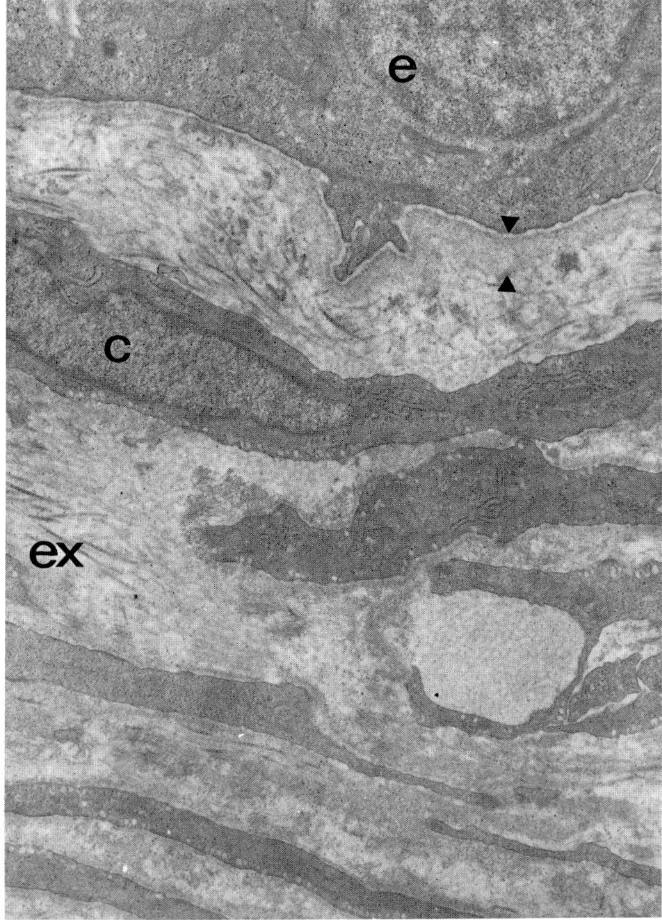

Fig. 42. The basal lamina (*between arrow heads*) and associated elements of the lamina propria of the proximal ductus epididymidis. *c,* thin contractile cell; *e,* epithelium; *ex,* extracellular matrix. × 12000

the lamina propria of the distal ductuli efferentes (see Sect. B.IV.3.a), to a thicker layer in the distal cauda epididymidis (Fig. 35), which is similar in structure to the lamina propria of the ductus deferens (Sect. B.V.3.b). While the basal lamina, which provides a supporting layer of glycoprotein matrix for the epithelial cells, shows an increase in thickness from caput to cauda epididymidis, most of the increase in thickness of the lamina propria is due to increases in outer layers of connective tissue elements. Throughout the length of the ductus epididymidis small capillary loops can be observed penetrating across the lamina propria and making contact with the basal membrane of principal cells across the thin expanse of the basal lamina. These contacts appear to be more common in the distal corpus and cauda regions of the epididymis but their function is unknown.

γ) Muscularis

The muscle coat which surrounds the ductus epididymidis shows a gradual transition along its length from a thin myoid sheath similar in its proximal extremity to that described for the ductuli efferentes (Sect. B.IV.3.a)γ) to a thick muscular sheath which blends into the trilaminar sheath of ordinary smooth muscle cells which form the muscularis externa of the ductus deferens (BAUMGARTEN et al., 1971).

The tubules of the caput epididymidis are surrounded by up to six layers of predominantly circularly arranged contractile cells (Fig. 43 A). In the corpus epididymidis the muscle coat gradually increases in thickness and, in addition to circularly and obliquely arranged contractile myoid cells, strips of longitudinally oriented muscle strands appear peripherally. The muscle cells are separated from each other by wide bands of connective tissue. The transition zone between corpus and cauda epididymidis is marked by a further increase in the thickness of the muscle coat due to the appearance of large ordinary smooth muscle cells at the periphery of the peritubular muscle coat (Fig. 43 B). The thin contractile cells which characterize the more proximal parts of the epididymis are gradually reduced in numbers in the cauda epididymidis and replaced by large smooth muscle cells. These become organized into three interconnected layers and eventually merge with the trilaminar muscle coat of the ductus deferens (BAUMGARTEN et al., 1971). Concomitant with these changes is a reduction in the size of the connective tissue interspaces between the smooth muscle cells to the narrow zones found in the trilaminar peritubular sheath of the ductus deferens. The ultrastructural features of the thin contractile cells, connective tissue elements and the large ordinary smooth muscle cells of the ductus epididymidis are similar to those described for the ductuli efferentes (see Sect. B.IV.3.a)γ) and the ductus deferens (see Sect. B.V.3.γ).

The thin contractile cells are easily distinguished from adjacent connective tissue cells by the presence of myofilaments. Based on cytological features three different types of contractile cells have been described (BAUMGARTEN et al., 1971). The most common contractile cell type resembles that already described in the peritubular sheath of the ductuli efferentes. It contains elongated nuclei with polar aggregations of cytoplasmic organelles and dense bundles of myofilaments which span the length of each cell and attach to dense fibrous plaques along the inside of the cell membrane. Dark contractile cells can be distinguished by an electron-dense cytoplasm containing large accumulations of endoplasmic reticulum which are often associated with aggregations of glycogen granules. These cells contain interweaving bundles of myofilaments which have an average diameter of 60 Å. Coarser single tubular myofilaments with an approximate cross-sectional diameter of 140 Å are also found in the cytoplasm of these cells. The third type of contractile cell can be distinguished by its translucent cytoplasm and irregular, loosely arranged myofilaments which often run parallel to the long axis of the cell and interweave obliquely with parallel fibre bundles. As with the single myofilaments of the dark cells, these myofilaments are tubular in cross-section with an average diameter of 140 Å (BAUMGARTEN et al., 1971). Thin 100 Å extracellular elastin filaments form a loose fibre network about

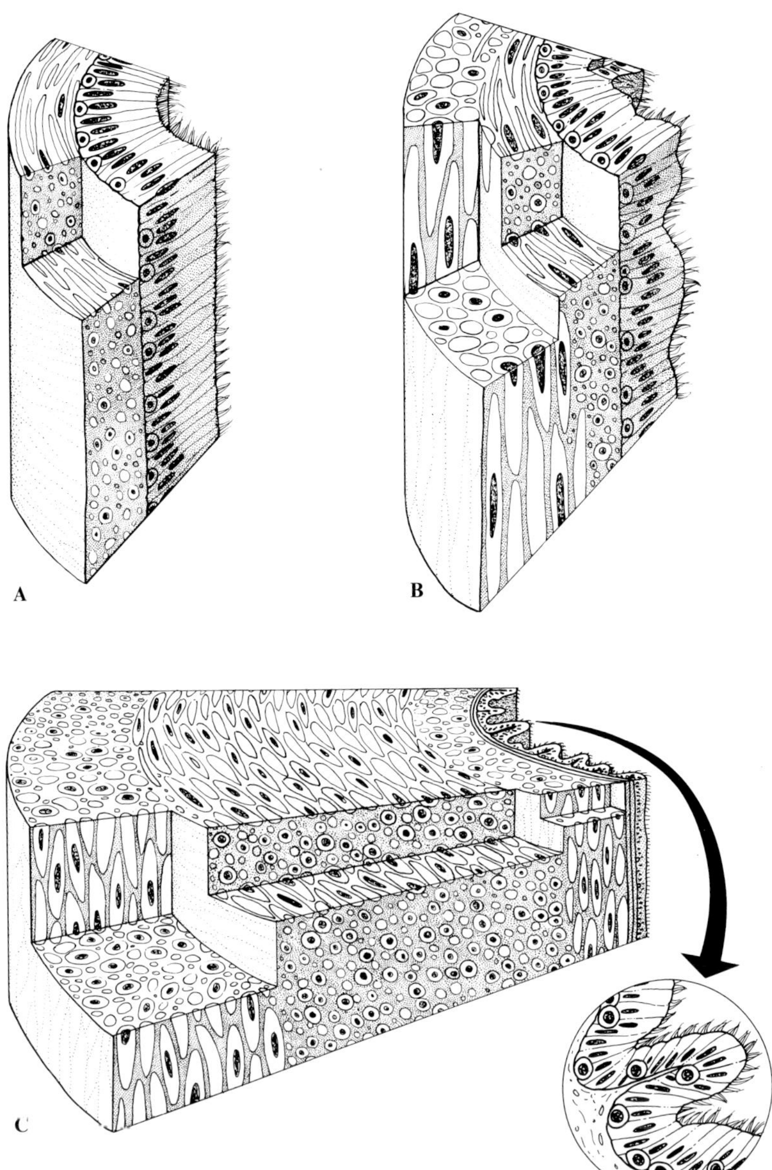

Fig. 43 A–C. Differences in the morphology and arrangement of contractile cells around the male reproductive tract at three levels. **A** Proximal caput epididymidis: this region is surrounded by about six layers of thin contractile cells arranged in circular layers. **B** Proximal cauda epididymidis: the epithelium in this region is surrounded by circularly arranged layers of thin contractile cells, which are in turn enclosed by an outer longitudinal layer of large ordinary smooth muscle cells. In the distal cauda the inner layer of thin contractile cells are gradually lost and replaced by a layer of circularly oriented ordinary smooth muscle cells. **C** Ductus deferens: in this region the muscle coat comprises three distinct layers of large ordinary smooth muscle cells. The inner and outer layers are arranged longitudinally and the middle layer is oriented in a circular fashion around the duct (scale of c is ×10 that of a. and b.). (**A** and **B** redrawn from Baumgarten et al., 1971)

0.3 μm thick around each contractile cell. Bundles of these filaments extend from the tapering ends of each contractile cell and gradually diverge into small strand-like aggregations which penetrate large adjacent aggregates of collagen fibres.

The large "ordinary" smooth muscle cells of the cauda ductus epididymidis are easily distinguished from the associated thin contractile cells. As indicated previously, large smooth muscle cells are characteristic of the cauda epididymidis. They contain numerous 60-Å-diameter myofilaments and their structural features are similar to those of ordinary smooth muscle cells from other parts of the reproductive tract. The cell organelles and glycogen granules are scattered irregularly throughout the cytoplasm between bundles of myofilaments. The myofilaments are inserted into dense zones on the inner surface of the cell membrane which are separated by adjacent areas of calveolated plasma membrane. The narrow extracellular spaces between adjacent cells are filled with a more or less continuous layer of granular extracellular matrix containing bundles of 100 Å elastin fibres, which appear to extend between and are attached to adjacent cells. Aggregates of collagen fibres and fibrocytes occur in wider intercellular spaces. Nexus-like junctions occur infrequently between smooth muscle cells and are commonly observed between narrow cellular processes which extend towards neighbouring cells, often interdigitating with their surface processes.

As with the arrangement of the peritubular muscle coat, there is a transition in the innervation of the muscle sheath along the ductus epididymidis. The proximal portions of the epididymis, from the caput to the distal corpus, are innervated by a few single terminal adrenergic fibres. These do not usually penetrate the wide intercellular spaces but form a loose plexus at the periphery of the layer of thin contractile cells (BAUMGARTEN et al., 1971). In more distal parts of the epididymis, in association with the large smooth muscle cells, adrenergic terminals with numerous varicosities are found in close proximity to the smooth muscle cells and within the narrow extracellular spaces. The density of these fibres gradually increases in the distal cauda epididymidis as the number of ordinary smooth muscle cells increases. Innervation of these cells is mainly by adrenergic terminals, but a few cholinergic terminals can also be identified.

The morphological differences in distribution and arrangement of peritubular smooth muscle in the ductus epididymidis correspond to differences in the motor activity of the epididymis along its length. In the ductuli efferentes and proximal regions of the ductus epididymidis, where the peritubular sheath is composed mostly of thin, contractile cells, the duct undergoes spontaneous rhythmic contractions, both in vivo and in vitro (BATTAGLIA, 1956; RISLEY, 1958), which resemble peristaltic movements. These contractions are reduced in magnitude and frequency with increasing distance from the testis. In the more distal regions of the ductus epididymidis, which are enclosed in a thick bilaminar or trilaminar coat of large, ordinary smooth muscle cells, the motor activity of the tubule resembles that of the ductus deferens (see Sect. B.V.3.γ). This usually shows little spontaneous muscular activity but is capable, at ejaculation, of highly coordinated muscular contractions initiated by stimulation of adrenergic sympathetic fibres from the middle and inferior spermatic nerves.

These motor activities correspond closely with the functions ascribed to the proximal and distal regions of the epididymis. The proximal region is responsible for the continuous transport of maturing spermatozoa to the site of storage. The more inactive distal segment of the duct is well suited to its generally accepted function as a storage site for matured spermatozoa. The flow rate of spermatozoa is considerably reduced in the cauda epididymidis and they gradually become concentrated into dense aggregations by further absorption of epididymal fluids by the cauda epithelial cells. The average capacity of this caudal sperm reservoir in man has not been established. In some mammals, in particular marsupials and rodents, overflow of spermatozoa into the urine (spermatorrhea) is commonly observed in celibate males, indicating that, once full, the continual inflow of spermatozoa into the reservoir is balanced by an equivalent overflow into the ductus deferens, and eventually the urethra.

4. Function

The complex of ducts constituting the epididymis serves as a transport mechanism by which sperm are conveyed from the testis to the vas deferens. The transit time for sperm through the epididymis in man is approximately 12 days (ROWLEY et al., 1970), and a remarkable interspecies similarity exists (BEDFORD, 1975). However, not all sperm traverse the epididymis at the same rate, and consequently, at any one point in the duct system, the spermatozoal population is heterogeneous in terms of its time in contact with the epididymal duct systems. The passage of sperm is facilitated by the peristaltic activity of the smooth muscle surrounding the duct, and the coordination of contraction is particularly evident in the caudal region. This peristaltic activity results in sperm being moved from the epididymis to the vas deferens during the ejaculatory process, but it should be noted that frequent ejaculation can only reduce the total transit time by 10%–20% (BEDFORD, 1975).

In addition to its role in the transport of sperm, it is clear that the epididymis has a number of other functions which result in the maturation of sperm. When they are released from the epithelium, spermatozoa differ considerably from ejaculated sperm in their morphology, motility, metabolism and fertilizing ability (see reviews by BEDFORD, 1975; HAMILTON, 1975). Many of these parameters alter during their passage through the epididymis, and the changes appear to be dependent on the epididymal environment. The changes that occur in spermatozoa during maturation are associated with the development of the capacity to fertilize ova. Studies in many species have indicated that sperm collected in the caput epididymis are unable to fertilize ova but that they have acquired this ability by the time they reach the cauda (ORGEBIN-CRIST, 1969). Part of the maturational changes appear to be intrinsic to spermatozoa, but others require the epididymal environment since the interruption of the passage of sperm through the proximal part of the epididymis does not halt the maturational change many of the ova fertilized by such sperm do not develop normally

(GADDUM and GLOVER, 1965; ORGEBIN-CHRIST, 1967; PAUFLER and FOOTE, 1968; BEDFORD, 1975).

Many of the changes associated with sperm maturation remain unknown, but a number of differences have been noted, though no single change can be associated with the acquisition of fertilizing ability (BEDFORD, 1975). During passage through the epididymis, sperm acquire the ability for purposeful, forward motility, though no structural change has been associated with this change (BLANDAU and RUMERY, 1964; BEDFORD, 1966; ORGEBIN-CRIST, 1967). The changes in sperm motility can be induced by treating epididymal sperm in vitro with dibutyryl cyclic AMP and by phosphodiesterase inhibitors (HOSKINS and CASILLAS, 1975). Other morphological changes do occur but the nature and type vary between species. Migration and loss of the cytoplasmic droplet occur in most species, while acrosomal changes are frequently prominent, resulting in significant changes in shape (FAWCETT and HOLLENBERG, 1963; BEDFORD, 1963, 1965). Subtle changes in the plasmalemma also occur as seen in their electrophoretic mobility, surface charge patterns, swelling of the membrane and alterations in the patterns of agglutination of sperm (BEDFORD, 1975). Changes also occur in the nucleus, rendering the chromatin stable against the action of agents capable of disrupting S–S bonds (GLEDHILL et al., 1966; CALVIN and BEDFORD, 1971). Significant metabolic changes also occur in sperm during their passage through the epididymis, and these involve changes in oxygen uptake, gluconeogenesis, lipid metabolism and inositol synthesis (see review BEDFORD, 1975; HAMILTON, 1975). The relationship of these changes to the acquisition of motility and fertilizing ability still remains unclear.

Regional differences in the epididymis have been noted in different species by a number of investigators. Consequently, interspecies comparison in terms of function can be difficult and designation of specific functions to any one cell type has proved difficult.

a) Absorption

The results of a number of studies support the conclusion that over 90% of the fluid produced in the testis is absorbed in the proximal portion of the epididymis. It seems clear that the microvilli present on the cells of the epididymis throughout its length aid in the reabsorption of fluid, and it seems likely that the principal cells play a major role in this respect (HAMILTON, 1972). The recent demonstration that androgen-binding protein (ABP) can be localized by immunofluorescent techniques to the principal cells of a very limited segment of the epididymis makes it likely that the function of these cells may vary in different segments (PELLINIEMI et al., 1979). In addition to fluid, particulate matter introduced into the lumen is rapidly phagocytosed by the epithelium throughout its length (BURGOS, 1964; NICANDER, 1965).

b) Secretion

The epididymis is known to secrete several substances, though the specific cellular source of each remains obscure. The micropuncture studies of LEVINE and Marsh (1971) have demonstrated a progressive decrease in the sodium concentration during progression down the epididymal duct, and studies of osmotic pressures suggest the development of an anion gap indicating epididymal secretion. Glycerophosphorylcholine (GPC) is synthesized by the epididymis and may be responsible for maintaining osmotic pressure as sodium is reabsorbed (Hamilton, 1975). High concentrations of carnitine are also found in the epididymis, but its source and role are unknown. However, since the levels are dependent on androgen secretion, there is little doubt that it is an epididymal secretion (Marquis and Fritz, 1965; Pearson and Tubbs, 1967). A number of glycoproteins and sialic acid are also secreted by the epididymis, the sialic acid possibly functioning as a lubricant, a sperm-coating substance, or a mechanism of altering change on the surfaces of sperm (Hamilton, 1975). Recently, a glycoprotein found in fluid from the caput epididymis, was shown to have the capacity to stimulate forward motility in immotile epididymal sperm (Brandt et al., 1978).

c) Androgen Dependence

The structure and function of the epididymis is clearly dependent on the secretion of testosterone. Sperm-fertilizing ability is rapidly lost following hypophysectomy or castration but regained with androgen replacement (Dyson and Orgebin-Crist, 1973). The uptake of androgens is facilitated by the presence of androgen receptors within the epididymis (Blaquier, 1971; Danzo et al., 1973). The high concentration of testosterone in the caput epididymis is maintained by the binding of testosterone to ABP. The specific role of ABP and its importance in maintaining the epididymis still remains to be established. It has also been demonstrated that the epididymis can also produce testosterone by metabolism from a number of precursors, but the exact role of this metabolic capability remains unknown (Hamilton et al., 1969; Frankel and Eik-Nes, 1970). It seems surprising that a tissue with a synthetic capability for testosterone should be dependent on the capacity of the testis to secrete testosterone since the steroid synthetic activity is lost following castration (Frankel and Eik-Nes, 1970; Inano et al., 1969).

Much work still remains to be done to establish the specific role of different cells and segments of the epididymis in the acquisition of fertilizing ability of sperm. It is also evident that for adequate function the epididymis is dependent on mechanisms designed to maintain its temperature below that of body temperature (Bedford, 1975). In fact, Bedford (1977) postulates that the temperature dependence of the epididymis is the prime mover in the development of the scrotum.

V. Ductus Deferens

1. Development

The ductus deferens is derived from the caudal portion of the mesonephric duct. At about 3 months in man an outpouching, the presumptive seminal vesicle, arises in the distal region of the mesonephric duct (Fig. 50 A), which divides the developing duct into ductus deferens and ejaculatory duct (MOORE, 1973). The thick muscular coat which surrounds the mucosa of the definitive ductus is derived from condensations of mesenchymal cells which subsequently differentiate into myoblasts and, eventually, large mature smooth muscle cells.

A spindle-shaped enlargement of the ductus deferens develops just proximal to the seminal vesicle forming the ampulla (Fig. 50 B). The function of this part of the ductus deferens is not known in man, although similar glandular enlargements in rodents have recently been shown to have a spermiophagic capacity (COOPER and HAMILTON, 1977). There is considerable controversy, based on the similarities in organization and cytological features, as to whether the ampulla should be regarded as a distal portion of the ductus deferens or a proximal extension of the seminal vesicles. Recently AUMÜLLER and BRUHL (1977) have put forward a persuasive argument for the latter.

2. General Anatomy

a) Anatomical Relationships

The ductus deferens (vas deferens) is a distal extension of the ductus epididymidis, which carries spermatozoa and seminal fluids from the cauda epididymidis (Fig. 26) to the ejaculatory duct (Fig. 51), where it joins with the excretory duct of the seminal vesicle. It is commonly divided into four segments – testicular (scrotal), inguinal, abdominal and pelvic – which correspond to the anatomical positions of various parts of the ductus deferens. In man there is no evidence to suggest any structural or functional differences between these regional segments, but recent studies in the rat (FLICKINGER, 1973; HAMILTON and COOPER, 1978) have described variation in both structure and function along the ductus deferens.

The testicular portion of the ductus deferens extends from the terminal convolutions of the cauda epididymidis at the distal pole of the testis to the distal end of the spermatic cord. The ductus deferens extends as a continuation of the ductus epididymidis from a region distal to the caudal flexure of the epididymis. BAUMGARTEN et al. (1971) have described an initial convoluted portion, the *pars epididymica,* which extends from the ductus epididymidis to the straight portion of the testicular ductus deferens, the *pars libera* (Fig. 25). There is no distinct morphological transition zone between epididymis and ductus deferens but three structural differences have been described. First, the epithelium lining the cauda epididymidis gradually changes from shorter columnar or cuboidal cells with short stereocilia and basally situated nuclei to tall columnar, pseudostratified epithelium with longer stereocilia. Secondly, the epithelium and lamina propia are arranged in a series of longitudinal ridges which extend deep into the lumen of the ductus deferens and, thirdly, the remaining bundles of subepithelial thin smooth muscle cells, characteristic of the ductus epididymidis, are replaced by stratae of ordinary thick smooth muscle cells to form the three distinct layers characteristic of the ductus deferens. As will be discussed later in this chapter these different arrangements of smooth muscle seem to be important in determining the muscular activity of each region of the duct.

From the distal pole of the testis the ductus deferens ascends posteromedially along the epididymis, initially enclosed in mesorchium derived from the *processus vaginalis,* to join with the vascular, lymphatic and neural structures supplying the testis and epididymis. These structures, together with the ductus deferens, form the spermatic cord immediately above the superior pole of the testis.

In the inguinal region the vas extends superiorly as the posterior component of the spermatic cord. Because of its thick muscular wall and narrow lumen, it is easily distinguished by palpation from adjacent structures in the cord.

After passing through the inguinal canal and deep inguinal ring the ductus deferens parts company with the other components of the spermatic cord and continues beneath the parietal peritoneum, passing the lateral margin of the inferior epigastric artery around the iliac fossa. Here it ascends for about 2.5 cm anterosuperior to the external iliac artery to cross the external iliac vessels at the junction of the anterior and middle thirds of the pelvic brim to enter the pelvic cavity.

The pelvic ductus deferens then continues beneath the peritoneum passing inferiorly, posteriorly and medially along the lateral wall of the pelvis, where it crosses above the ureter at the upper pole of the seminal vesicle. It then changes direction to pass anteromedially along the medial aspect of the seminal vesicle and then courses down the posterior surface of the bladder to join with the duct of the seminal vesicle to form the ejaculatory duct (Fig. 51). Proximal to this junction the ductus deferens widens to form the bulb-shaped dilatation of the ampulla.

The ejaculatory duct is a tube about 2 cm in length which pierces the prostate and opens into the prostatic urethra just lateral to the "orifice" of the utriculus of the prostate (Fig. 51).

External and luminal diameters of the human ductus deferens have been measured by BRUESCHKE et al. (1974) in segments of the scrotal vas removed during vasectomy. The average external diameter ($\eta=23$) was 2.85 ± 0.43 mm and the internal diameter measured 0.85 ± 0.07 mm with "no resistance" to the measuring gauge and 1.06 ± 0.72 mm with "significant" resistance. No measurements are available for other regions of the ductus deferens.

b) Vasculature

Arterial. The ductus deferens receives its blood supply from the deferential artery. This is a branch of the vesiculodeferential artery, which usually arises in the angle between the umbilical derivative of the superior vesical artery and the terminal portion of the anterior division of the internal iliac artery (Fig. 44a). The deferential artery joins the ductus deferens at its distal end, close to the ampulla, and runs proximally within the adventitial sheath of the duct to provide blood supply to the entire length of the ductus deferens and, as described in the previous section, to the cauda and corpus epididymidis. It terminates in an extensive anastomosis with the epididymal branches of the

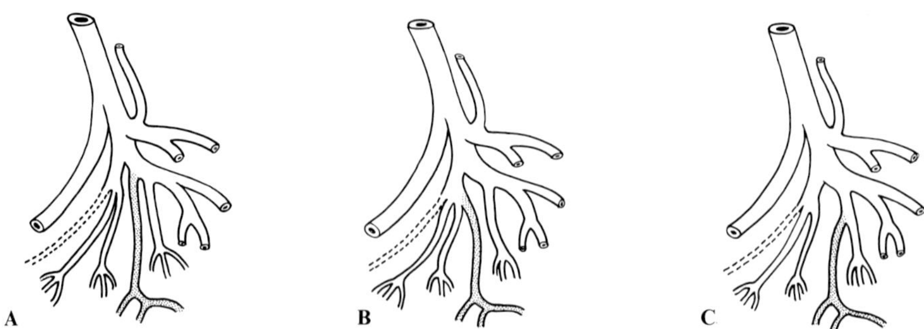

Fig. 44 A–C. Variations in the origin of the vesiculo-deferential artery to the ductus deferens. **A** Common origin in the angle between the superior vesicle artery and the anterior division of the internal iliac (94.3%). **B** Origin as a branch of the umbilical segment of the superior vesicle artery. **C** Origin from the inferior vesicle artery. (Redrawn from BRAITHWAITE, 1952)

testicular artery (HARRISON and BARCLAY, 1948). In the inguinal canal the deferential artery is a component of the spermatic cord.

Some confusion exists, even within reputable texts on pelvic anatomy, as to the origin of the blood supply to the ductus deferens. The inferior vesical artery is often described as giving off a branch to the ductus deferens, as well as supplying the seminal vesicles in man, but this is now regarded as a failure to distinguished between the inferior vesical and vesiculodeferential arteries (HOLLINSHEAD, 1966). Although the larger arterial branches to the ductus deferens, and also the seminal vesicles, are commonly derived from the vesiculo-deferential artery some variations to this arrangement have been described (BRAITHWAITE, 1952). In the two most common variations the vesiculodeferential artery arises as a branch of either the superior vesical (Fig. 44 B), in its umbilical remnant, or the inferior vesical artery (Fig. 44 C).

Venous. Venous blood from the ductus deferens drains along the deferential veins into the prostatic (pudendal) plexus, which also receives venous drainage from the other male accessory glands. From the prostatic plexus venous blood drains to the internal iliac veins and the inferior vena cava.

In the rat an extensive venous plexus has been described around the distal ductus deferens (HAMILTON and COOPER, 1978). This plexus is supplied directly by the deferential artery, drains into the deferential vein and is connected to the erectile tissue of the corpus spongiosum, suggesting an erectile function. The presence of a similar venous plexus in man has yet to be described.

Lymphatics. Lymphatic vessels of the ductus deferens join those of the cauda epididymidis and drain mostly into the internal group of external iliac lymph nodes. A variable collateral drainage of lymph also occurs into the internal iliac (hypogastric) nodes.

c) Innervation

As described in Sect. C.IV.2.c, innervation to the ductus deferens is carried by the middle and inferior spermatic nerves, which also supply the epididymis. Sympathetic fibres from the middle spermatic nerve provide the principal supply to the ductus deferens but this is augmented by a few fibres from the inferior spermatic nerve as it passes along the ductus deferens to the epididymis. As with the epididymis, there is no evidence of parasympathetic innervation to the ductus deferens.

Afferent innervation of the ductus deferens has not yet been clearly defined (HOLLINSHEAD, 1966). It has been suggested that the proximal end of the ductus deferens is innervated by afferent fibres accompanying sympathetic fibres from spinal segments T11, T12 and L1, which reach the spinal cord via the superior hypogastric and aortic plexuses. The distal (or pelvic) portion of the ductus deferens is thought to be supplied by afferent fibres associated with the pelvic splanchnic nerves from sacral segments S2, S3 and S4, as for the prostate and seminal vesicles.

3. Cytological Features

The structural organization of the ductus deferens is similar to that of the caudal ductus epididymidis. It comprises a mucous membrane, lining the lumen of the duct, which is surrounded by a thick coat of smooth muscle and a thin outer adventitial layer of connective tissue in which the major vessels and nerves of the duct are located. The mucous membrane is formed by an inner epithelial lining enclosed by a lamina propria. The epithelium and its adjacent lamina propria are thrown up into a series of longitudinal folds (Fig. 45), a feature which distinguishes the vas from the adjacent duct of the cauda epididymidis.

a) Epithelium

The structure of the scrotal vas epithelium has been described in detail by HOFFER (1976). It comprises a pseudostratified epithelium containing a discontinuous layer of basal cells along the basal lamina and thin, tall columnar cells from which three types can be distinguished (Fig. 45): (1) principal cells, (2) mitochondrion-rich cells and (3) pencil cells. In addition to these, a few agranular leucocytes, which resemble the intra-epithelial lymphocytes found in the rhesus monkey and rat epididymis (DYM and ROMRELL, 1975), are present interspersed amongst the epithelial cells.

Principal Cells. These tall columnar cells contain large irregularly shaped nuclei and dense aggregations of cytoplasmic organelles (Figs. 45, 46). The nuclei have deeply convoluted surfaces and contain prominent nucleoli and a high euchromatin-heterochromatin ratio, an indication of high metabolic activity. Large aggregates of tubular and vesicular rough endoplasmic reticulum occur in the basal and perinuclear cytoplasm in association with polysomes and free ribosomes but only small isolated profiles of typical agranular endoplasmic reticulum are present. This contrasts with the extensive whorls of agranular

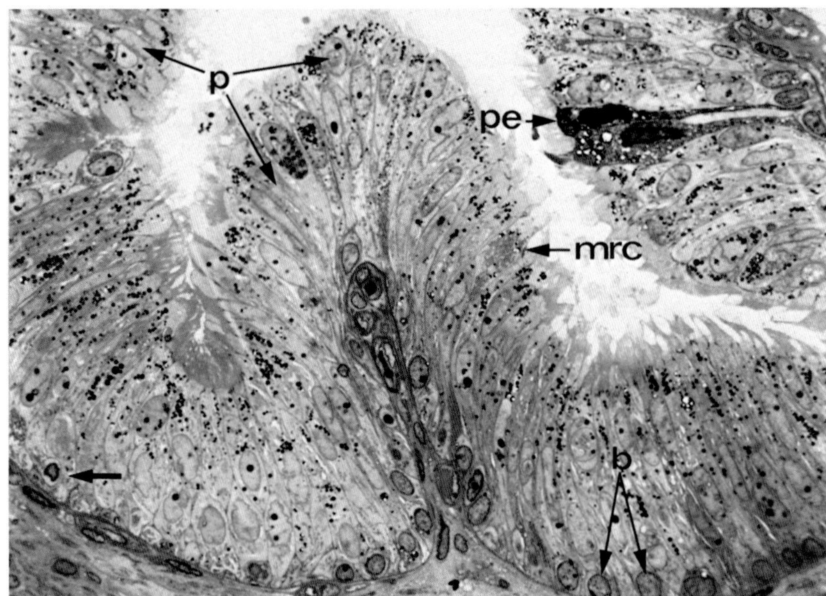

Fig. 45. High-magnification light micrograph of the pseudostratified, columnar epithelium of the human ductus deferens showing the five epithelial cell types: principal (*p*), basal (*b*), mitochondrion-rich (*mrc*) and pencil cells (*pe*), and an intra-epithelial leucocyte (*arrow*). The epithelium and peritubular connective tissue of the ductus deferens is characteristically pushed up into distinctive longitudinal folds. (Courtesy of ANITA P. HOFFER)

endoplasmic reticulum which have been described in vas principal cells of some rodents (HAMILTON et al., 1969; FLICKINGER, 1973) but does not exclude the possibility that, as in the rat (FLICKINGER, 1973), principal cells containing large quantities of agranular endoplasmic reticulum are restricted to more distal regions of the ductus deferens which have not yet been examined at the ultra-structural level in man. Numerous mitochondria, prominent apical and/or para-nuclear Golgi complexes, and multivesicular bodies and lysosomes in the apical and supranuclear cytoplasm, are also present within the principal cells.

Typical junctional complexes hold the principal cells together near their luminal surfaces and desmosomes are present at intervals along the lateral membranes of adjacent cells. Long stereocilia extend into the lumen from the apical surface of each principal cell and coated invaginations occur between the stereocilia, suggesting active endocytotic activity similar to principal cells in the ductus epididymidis (Fig. 47).

These structural features suggest that principal cells have the capacity for steroidogenesis (agranular endoplasmic reticulum), absorption and degradation (coated vesicles, multivesicular bodies and lysosomes), and protein and glycopro-tein synthesis (granular endoplasmic reticulum and Golgi complex). Each of these functions have been demonstrated in vas principal cells of rodents (FRIEND and FARQUAR, 1967; HAMILTON, 1975; BENNETT et al., 1974) but their occurrence

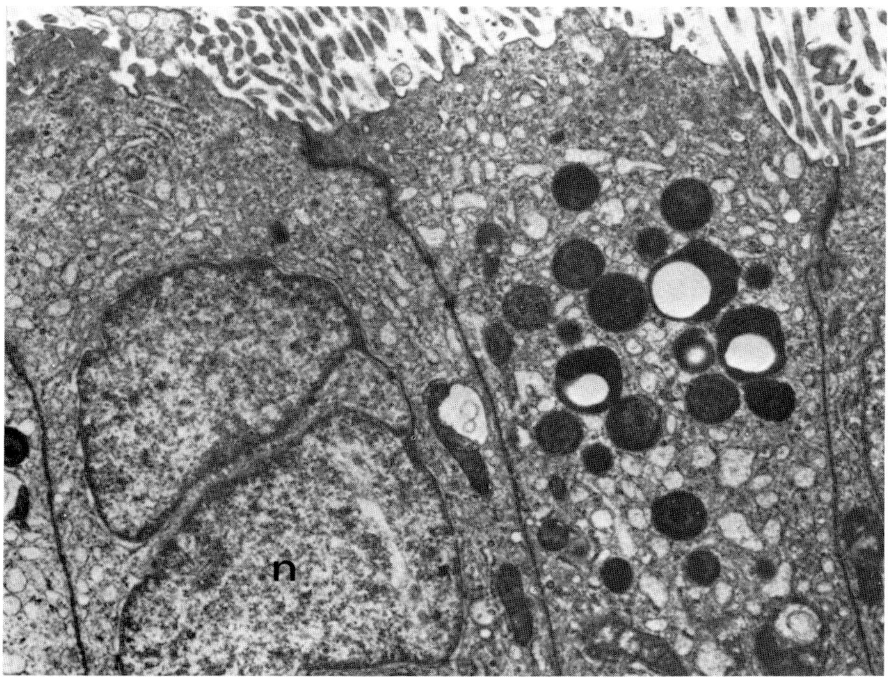

Fig. 46. Ultrastructural features of the apical region of two principal cells in the human ductus deferens. (Courtesy of ANITA P. HOFFER)

in and significance to the function of the ductus deferens in man awaits further investigation.

Basal Cells. These cells lie along the basement membrane (Fig. 35) and have simple ultrastructural features which are similar to those of basal cells in the epididymis (Fig. 41).

Each contains an ovoid nucleus enclosed in a thin peripheral layer of cytoplasm. The nucleus contains little nucleolar material or heterochromatin and the cytoplasm has only a few organelles, including small amounts of rough and agranular endoplasmic reticulum, Golgi complex and mitochondria scattered through it. The only remarkable cytoplasmic inclusions in these cells are dense aggregations of 100-Å-diameter filaments similar to those seen in various cell types, including muscle cells. HOFFER (1976) has speculated that this dense network of filaments may act as a cytoskeleton to provide stability to the epithelium when the duct is at maximum distension.

Mitochondrion-Rich Cells. Mitochondrion-rich cells are infrequent but constant elements in the human ductus deferens which are easily distinguished from principal cells by their densely-packed aggregates of mitochondria (Figs. 45, 48). These cells are cylindrical or tapered with long apical stereocilia and nuclei which are similar in morphology to those of principal cells. Endoplasmic reticu-

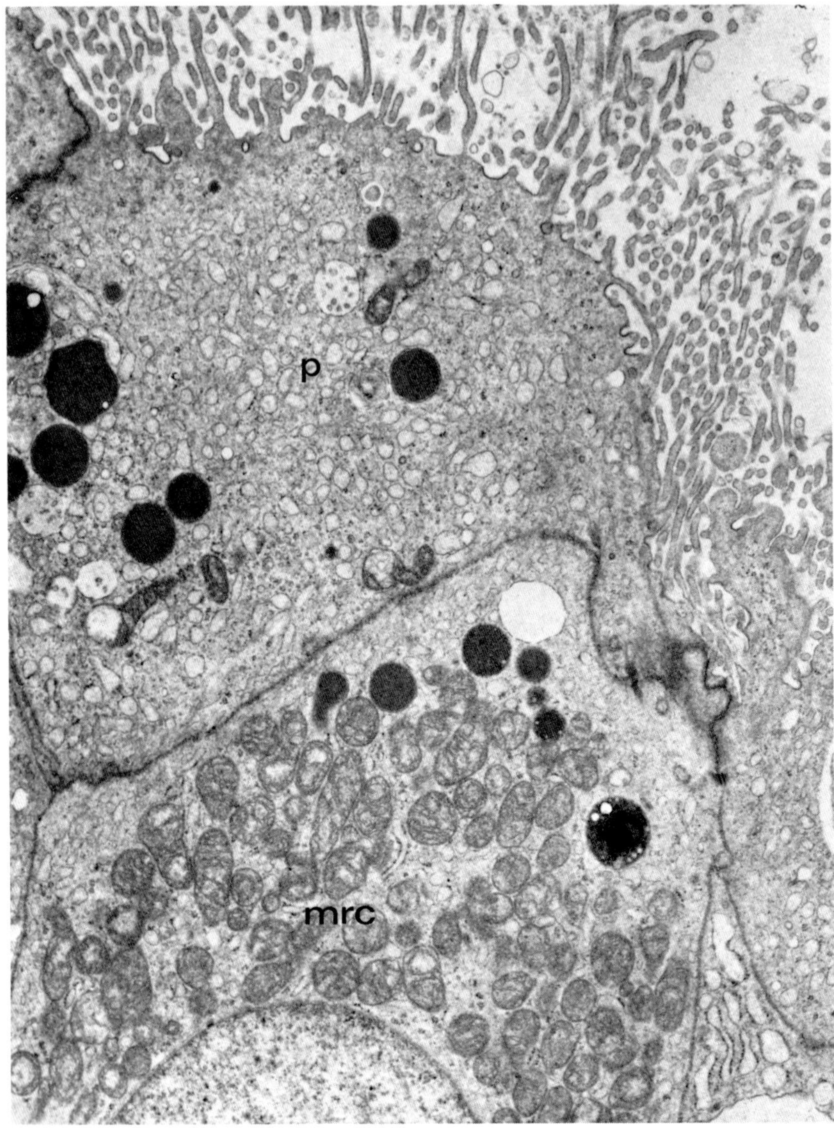

Fig. 47. Oblique section through the apical regions of a principal cell (*p*) and an adjacent mitochondrion-rich cell (*mrc*). Long stereocilia can be seen extending from the luminal surface of the principal cell with coated membrane invaginations between them. Multivesicular bodies, profiles of agranular endoplasmic reticulum and dense bodies are also present. (Courtesy of ANITA P. HOFFER)

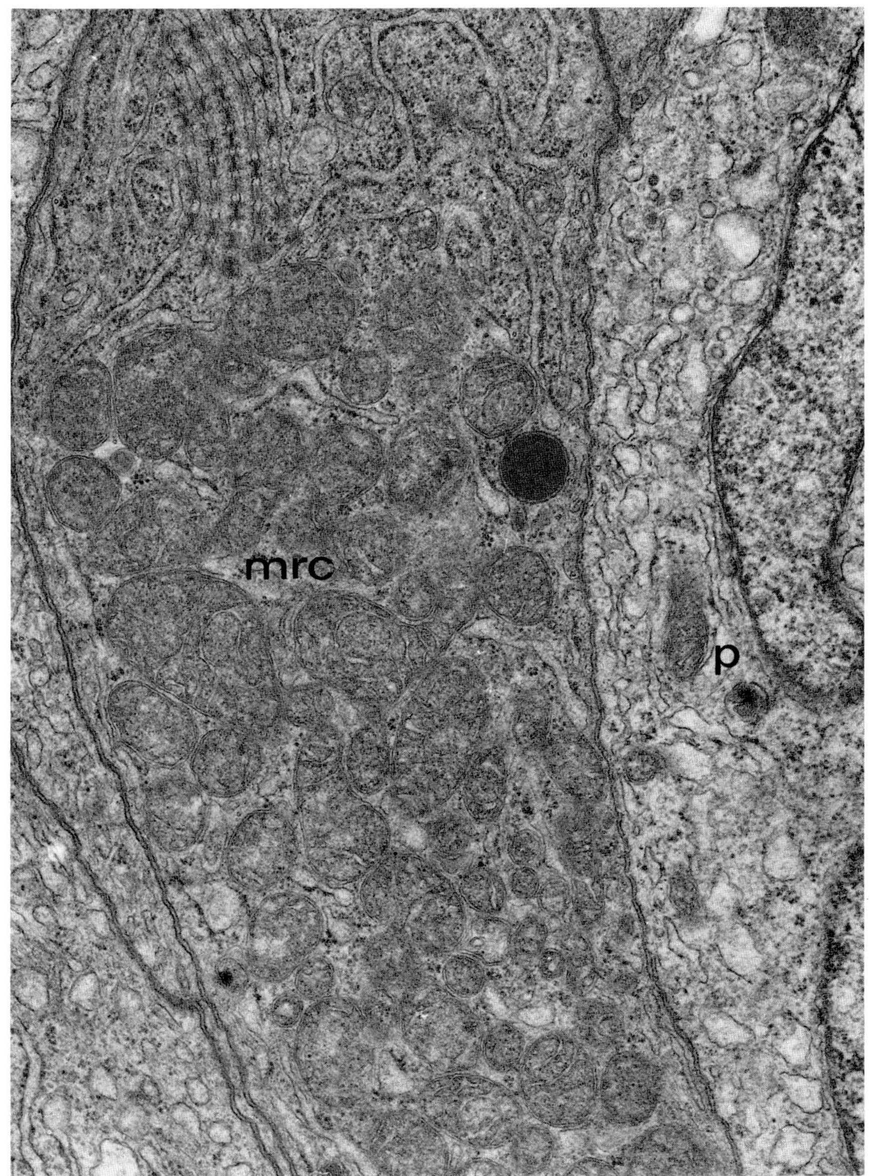

Fig. 48. A mitochondrion-rich cell (*mrc*) flanked by principal cells (*p*). The cell is easily recognized by the presence of densely packed aggregates of mitochondria. Profiles of granular and agranular endoplasmic reticulum and groups of ribosomes are also apparent. (Courtesy of ANITA P. HOFFER)

lum and Golgi complexes are poorly developed and other organelles are few and sparsely distributed through cytoplasm. The function of these cells is unknown, but they may be involved in acidification of the luminal fluid or in transport of electrolytes and water across the mucosa (HOFFER, 1976), as has been demonstrated for mitochondrion-rich cells in the gastric mucosa and the nephron.

Pencil Cells. These are goblet-shaped cells with pyknotic nuclei and intensely osmophilic cytoplasm (Fig. 45). The cytoplasm contains numerous vacuoles and debris, few mitochondria and dilated fragments of endoplasmic reticulum (Fig. 49). Their function has been variously described as absorptive (POPOVIC et al., 1973) or secretory (MARTAN et al., 1964), but HOFFER (1976) has suggested from her observations that they are simply dead or dying columnar epithelial cells.

b) Lamina Propria

The lamina propria enclosing the epithelium of the ductus deferens consists of two layers: (1) a basal lamina, an amorphous glycoprotein matrix of relatively uniform width, and (2) an outer layer of connective tissue elements of variable thickness.

The outer connective tissue layer contains fibroblasts, collagen fibres and a dense irregular network of elastin fibres set in a matrix of extracellular ground substance. Smooth muscle cells, and their associated intercellular elastin fibres, from the inner longitudinal smooth muscle layer are often observed in direct contact with the basal lamina. The dense aggregates of elastin fibres in the lamina propria and the muscularis (Sect. B.V.3.c) are thought to provide elastic recoil of the duct following contraction and dilation at ejaculation.

c) Muscularis

The main structural component of the ductus deferens is the extensive coat of smooth muscle which forms a layer approximately 1 mm thick around the mucous membrane (BENOIT, 1926; BAUMGARTEN et al., 1971). A very detailed description of the components, ultrastructure and innervation of this layer is given in BAUMGARTEN et al. (1971). As in the distal cauda epididymidis, the muscularis is trilaminate consisting of inner and outer layers of longitudinally oriented smooth muscle cells and a thicker intermediate layer of circumferentially arranged muscle fibres (Fig. 43 C). In contrast to the small contractile cells which form the thin muscularis of the proximal regions of the ductus epididymidis, the muscular layers around the vas are formed exclusively by "ordinary" smooth muscle cells similar to those described in the cauda epididymidis. These large smooth muscle cells contain dense aggregations of myofilaments of uniform size and about 60 Å diameter, which form a regular pattern of dense patches in the cytoplasm as a result of the frequent intermeshing of small bundles of myofilaments. Cytoplasmic organelles and glycogen granules are irregularly dispersed throughout the cytoplasm between myofilament bundles. Electron-dense regions along the inner surface of each cell mark the zones of attachment of myofilaments to the inner leaflet of the cell membrane. These regions alternate

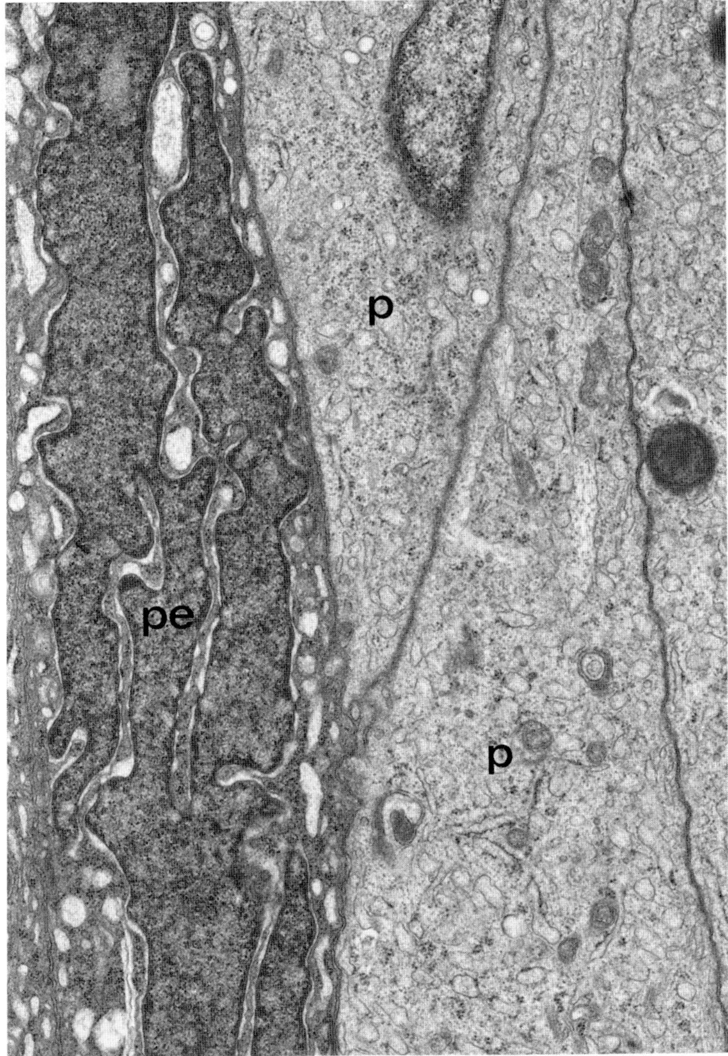

Fig. 49. Electron micrograph showing the perinuclear region of a pencil cell (*pe*) adjacent to two principal cells (*p*). The nucleus is extremely irregular in shape and is enclosed by darkly staining cytoplasm containing profiles of dilated endoplasmic reticulum, vacuoles and aggregates of ribosomes. (Courtesy of ANITA P. HOFFER)

with zones of micropinocytotic invaginations of the cell membrane; a characteristic feature of smooth muscle cells (MUGGLI and BAUMGARTNER, 1972; ORCINI and PERRELET, 1973). Smooth muscle cells in the three layers of the muscle coat are closely associated, separated only by narrow intercellular spaces which are filled with an amorphous mucoprotein matrix containing scattered aggregates of elastin filaments (100 Å), and occasional fibroblasts and collagen fibres.

Finger-like processes extend from each cell and interdigitate with those from adjacent cells. Occasionally nexus-like junctions are established between these processes.

As with the large "ordinary" smooth muscle cells of the cauda epididymidis (Sect. B.IV.3.b), those of the ductus deferens are innervated by adrenergic terminal nerve fibres which are endowed with many small but distinct varicosities. These nerve fibres pass along small connective tissue spaces adjacent to smooth muscle elements and there is a continuous gradual increase in density of such fibres in the distal cauda epididymidis and ductus deferens (BAUMGARTEN et al., 1971). Similar observations have been made in the distal region of the reproduction tract of the monkey and rat (NORBERG et al., 1967). The main nerve supply to the ductus deferens, and the cauda epididymidis, is adrenergic; only a few cholinergic terminals have been observed close to the effector cells. The importance of an intact adrenergic system in the human ductus deferens for normal ejaculation is substantiated by impotence due to emission failure in patients treated with prejunctional adrenergic blocking agents (NICKERSON, 1970).

Unlike the more proximal regions of the ductus epididymidis, which have been shown to undergo spontaneous, slow rhythmic, migrating contractions reminiscent of peristaltic movements (see Sect. B.IV.3.b), the ductus deferens, like the adjacent caudal segment of the ductus epididymidis, is usually inactive unless involved in neurally controlled reflex contractions associated with ejaculation.

Adrenergic and cholinergic stimulation of the ductus deferens are excitatory but BAUMGARTEN et al. (1971) have suggested that the highly differentiated smooth muscle cells can endogenously suppress spontaneous contractility. They discuss in detail the influence of an observed unequal distribution of functionally heterogeneous receptor sites on the outer cell membrane of these smooth muscle cells in providing a selective effect of neurotransmitter release. This is associated with the predominance of inhibitory β-adrenoreceptors at sites facing the synapses and the distribution of α-adrenoreceptors over the remainder of the cell membrane. BAUMGARTEN et al. (1971) suggest that this receptor distribution pattern favours a selective inhibitory effect of small releases of transmitter on restricted areas of membrane close to the synapse while facilitating excitation of the more widely dispersed α-receptors when enhanced stimulation resulted in hypersecretion of neurotransmitter from the nerve endings.

BAUMGARTEN et al., (1971) have concluded that the structure and innervation of smooth muscle in the ductus deferens and distal cauda epididymidis permit both the storage of large concentrations of mature spermatozoa in the lower regions of the reproductive tract and the expulsion of part or all of these stored products at ejaculation by strong adrenergically mediated contractions of the distal ductus epididymidis and ductus deferens.

VI. Seminal Vesicles

1. Development

As described previously (Sect. B.I, B.V.1), the seminal vesicles are derived from the mesonephric duct and first appear as swellings at the distal end of

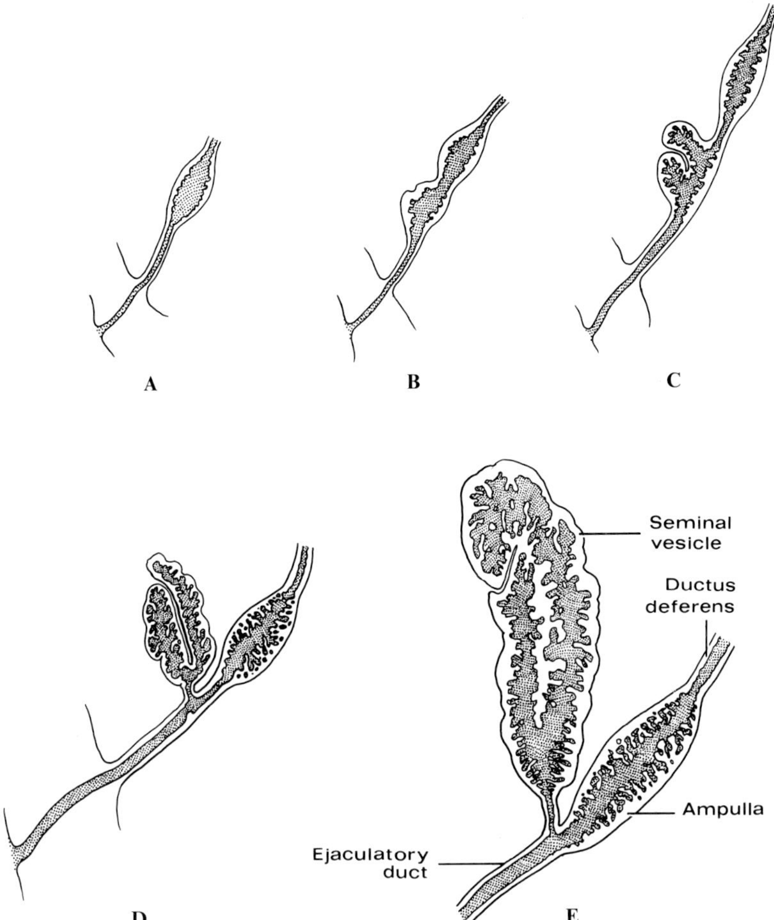

Fig. 50 A–E. Development of the seminal vesicle and ampulla of the ductus deferens. **A** 10–12 weeks: a spindle-shaped swelling appears in the mesonephric duct close to the bladder. **B** 12–14 weeks: the primordial seminal vesicle develops as a lateral diverticulum distal to the presumptive ampulla. **C** 16–20 weeks: latral and dorsolateral components of the developing seminal vesicle are apparent and secondary sacculations appear along the main tubular duct and also in the developing ampulla. **D** Neonatal: the seminal vesicle consists of a sacculate diverticulum connected to the ductus deferens by a narrow main duct. **E** Adult: below the confluence of the ampulla and the main duct of the seminal vesicle the ejaculatory duct is formed

the mesonephric duct during the third fetal month (Fig. 50 A). Early embryogenesis of the human seminal vesicles has been described by Lowsley (1912), and more recently by Nilsson and Bengmark (1962). The studies show that at 10–12 weeks of age a spindle-shaped enlargement develops in the mesonephric duct close to the bladder neck (Fig. 50 B). Subsequently the primordial seminal vesicle appears as lateral diverticulum which can be subdivided into dorsolateral and lateral components. These enlarge in different directions producing a tubular structure folded back on itself. During the period from 16 to 20 weeks secondary sacculations develop from this main tubular duct (Fig. 50C). These appear initially in the lower regions of the developing seminal vesicle but gradually increase in number towards the apex of the gland. At birth each seminal vesicle consists of a sacculate diverticulum a few millimetres long which communicates by a narrow main duct with the ductus deferens (Fig. 50D). The gland at this stage is invested in a thick layer of smooth muscle and the epithelium, which consists of a pseudostratified layer of columnar principal cells interspersed with basal cuboidal cells (LANGERHANS, 1875; VITALI-MAZZA, 1956), is attached to a well-defined basement membrane and supported on numerous primary and secondary folds of fibrous stromal connective tissue.

As with the prostate (Sect. B.VII.1), postnatal growth and differentiation of the seminal vesicles is gradual until the increasing levels of androgen at puberty facilitate a rapid phase of growth, development and maturation (Fig. 50C). A comprehensive review of the embryogenesis, growth and development of the seminal vesicles is given by AUMÜLLER (1979).

2. General Anatomy

a) Anatomical Relationships

As described in the previous section, the seminal vesicle originates from a diverticulum of the developing vas deferens to form a tubular structure with a "blind end". During development this tube increases in length and folds back on itself so that the fundus of the tube, which is only visible at dissection, becomes situated laterally at approximately one-third of the distance from the apex of the mature gland (Fig. 50E). When dissected from the connective tissue stroma the tube has an overall length of 10–15 cm (NILSSON and BENGMARK, 1962; GRAY, 1973) and diameter of 0.3–0.5 cm. At its proximal end the main central duct narrows to form a straight excretory duct which usually enters the vas deferens below the ampulla to form the ejaculatory duct. In the adult gland the main duct forms a series of tortuous coils which are enclosed in a fibrous connective tissue stroma.

Seminal vesicles of adult men show considerable variation in size, shape and internal structure between individuals (PICKER, 1913; NILSSON and BENGMARK, 1962). From various studies (VÖLCKER, 1912; CHWALLA and ZANDANELL, 1958; NILSSON and BENGMARK, 1962) the following dimensions have been determined: average length of about 4.5 cm (range 1.7–5.9 cm), average width of about 1.5 cm (range 0.6–2.2 cm) and an average depth of about 1 cm. Paired gland weight was greatest in young adult males (8–10 g). As with the prostate, seminal vesicle weight declines with increasing age such that in men more than 80 years old the paired gland weight had usually declined to less than 6 g. This age-related decrease in gland weight is probably a result of changing hormonal status in older men.

Various extremes in shape and structure of the seminal vesicles have been described (PALLIN, 1901; PICKER, 1913; NILSSON and BENGMARK, 1962); however, the usually external form is a sacculate, pyramidal gland which lies along the postero-inferior surface of the bladder in the fossa vesiculae seminalis with

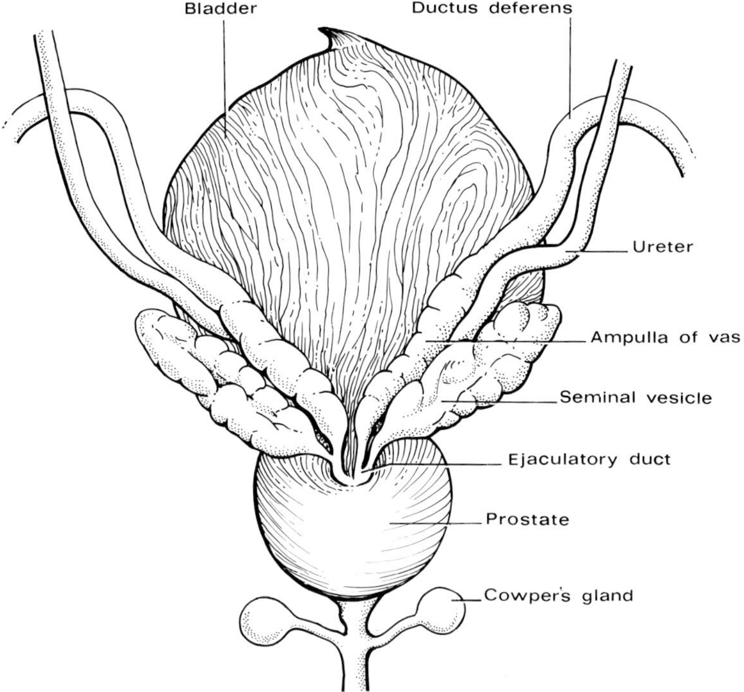

Fig. 51. Diagram of the posterior aspect of the bladder showing its relationship to the prostate, ampulla, seminal vesicles, ureters and ductus defererentia

its base directed backwards, upwards and laterally (Fig. 51). The glands diverge superiorly from each other and are enclosed in a fibromuscular capsule, which also covers the ampullae of the ductus deferens and is firmly attached to the base of the prostate. The seminal vesicles have the following relationship to adjacent structures: the anterior surface is in contact with the posterior wall of the bladder and extends from the distal end of the ureter to the base of the prostate; the posterior surface lies against the anterior wall of the rectum and is separated from it by rectovesical fascia (Denonvilliers fascia); the flat medial surface of each vesicle is in contact with the ampulla of the ductus deferens and at its distal end lies adjacent to the ureters close to where they enter the bladder, and the curved lateral margin is associated with veins of the prostatic venous plexus.

b) Vasculature

Arterial. The seminal vesicles are vascularized by an extensive blood supply which is variably derived from branches of the vesiculodeferential, middle rectal, inferior vesical and occasionally the superior rectal arteries (FRÄNKEL, 1901; CLEGG, 1955; HOLLINSHEAD, 1966). The vesiculodeferential and inferior vesical arteries usually provide the principal arterial supply; the deferential artery may send a small branch to the seminal vesicle close to its point of contact with the ductus deferens and the middle rectal artery often sends a branch anterior to the rectovesical fascia providing an additional supply. Arteries to the seminal vesicles form an extensive anastomosis around the base of the gland. From this anastomosis branches pass to supply posterior-superior and inferior regions of the glands and also their anterior provinces (FRÄNKEL, 1901).

Venous. Venous blood from all regions of the seminal vesicles drains to the vesical plexus (HOLLINSHEAD, 1966), along with venous return from the bladder, and then to the vesicoprostatic plexus which lies within the fascial sheath of the prostate (Sect. B.VII.2.b). Here it is pooled with venous blood returning from the prostate and penis, and drains to the internal iliac veins as described in Sect. B.VII.2.b.

Lymphatics. Lymph from the seminal vesicles drains with efferent vessels from the prostate and bladder to the internal and external iliac nodes (HOLLINS-HEAD, 1966; GRAY, 1973).

c) Innervation

Nerves supplying the seminal vesicles have similar origins to those of the prostate (Sect. B.VII.2.c). Efferent sympathetic fibres to the smooth muscle of the seminal vesicle originate in the lower thoracic and upper lumbar segments of the spinal cord and descend via the pelvic plexus to the prostatic plexus, where bundles of fibres are carried in small branches from the prostatic nerves to the seminal vesicles. Afferent fibres from the seminal vesicles presumably join other pelvic afferents and parasympathetic fibres in the pelvic plexus, and pass with the pelvic splanchnic nerves to sacral spinal segments S2, S3 and S4. Observations on seminal vesicle innervation have been made by FRÄNKEL (1901), HOVELACQUE (1931), SCHLYVITSCH and KOSINTZEW (1939), and HOLLINS-HEAD (1966).

3. Cytological Features

Human seminal vesicles are tubulosaccular glands which consist of a series of irregular, interconnecting sacculations formed by folds of stromal connective tissue branching into the lumen of the main duct (BLOOM and FAWCETT, 1975; AUMÜLLER, 1979). Primary folds, lined by epithelium, form secondary and terti-ary branches which extend deep into the lumen of the main duct. These branches unite at various levels to form a network of interconnecting ridges and crests which in turn create the irregular sacculations and diverticulae that extend peripherally from the central lumen. From the floor of each peripheral diverticu-lum, groups of small tubular or tubulo-alveolar glands penetrate into the perive-sicular stroma and smooth muscle coat. The depth and morphology of this glandular layer varies with its location in the gland. Close to the distal blind end of the seminal vesicle these glandular invaginations form a thin layer of wide, flattened alveoli but with increasing proximity to its neck and excretory duct the glandular layer becomes thicker and the glands form dense aggregations of long, narrow tubules which penetrate deeply into the periductal smooth muscle layer (WATZKA, 1943; BARGMANN, 1977; AUMÜLLER, 1973, 1979). Depth

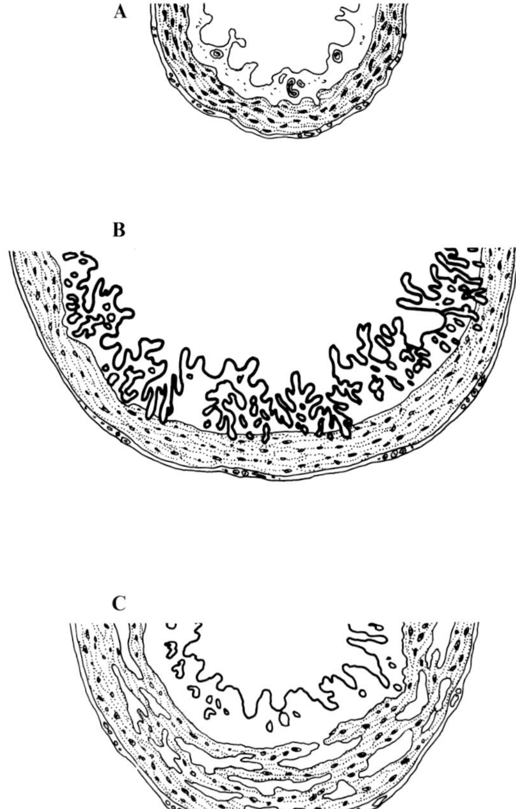

Fig. 52 A–C. Age-related changes in the structure of the seminal vesicle. Transverse sections through the wall of the seminal vesicle of **A** neonate, **B** young adult – about 25 years and **C** an old adult – about 75 years, showing the changing relationships between periglandular stromal connective tissue (*unshaded*) and smooth musculature (*stippled*), and the secretory activity of the glandular epithelium (*upper solid line*) with increasing age. (Redrawn from AUMÜLLER, 1979)

of the mucosa is also influenced by levels of circulating androgens, and age-related changes in the secretory epithelium appear to be a direct response to changes in the balance of circulating steroid hormones, in particular androgens.

The peripheral glandular region forms the primary region of secretory activity in the human seminal vesicles, although histological and cytochemical observations indicate that the epithelium lining the surfaces of the perilumenal diverticulae may also have a secretory capacity (AUMÜLLER, 1979).

Age-related changes in the structure of the seminal vesicles have been observed in older men (Fig. 52). Gland size is usually reduced (see Sect. B.VII.2.a), and there is an obvious decrease in the thickness of the glandular layer and an increase in stromal connective tissue, changes probably resulting from declining testoserone production with age. Reduced stromal folding also commonly occurs causing a loss in area of the perilumenal diverticulae and sacculations.

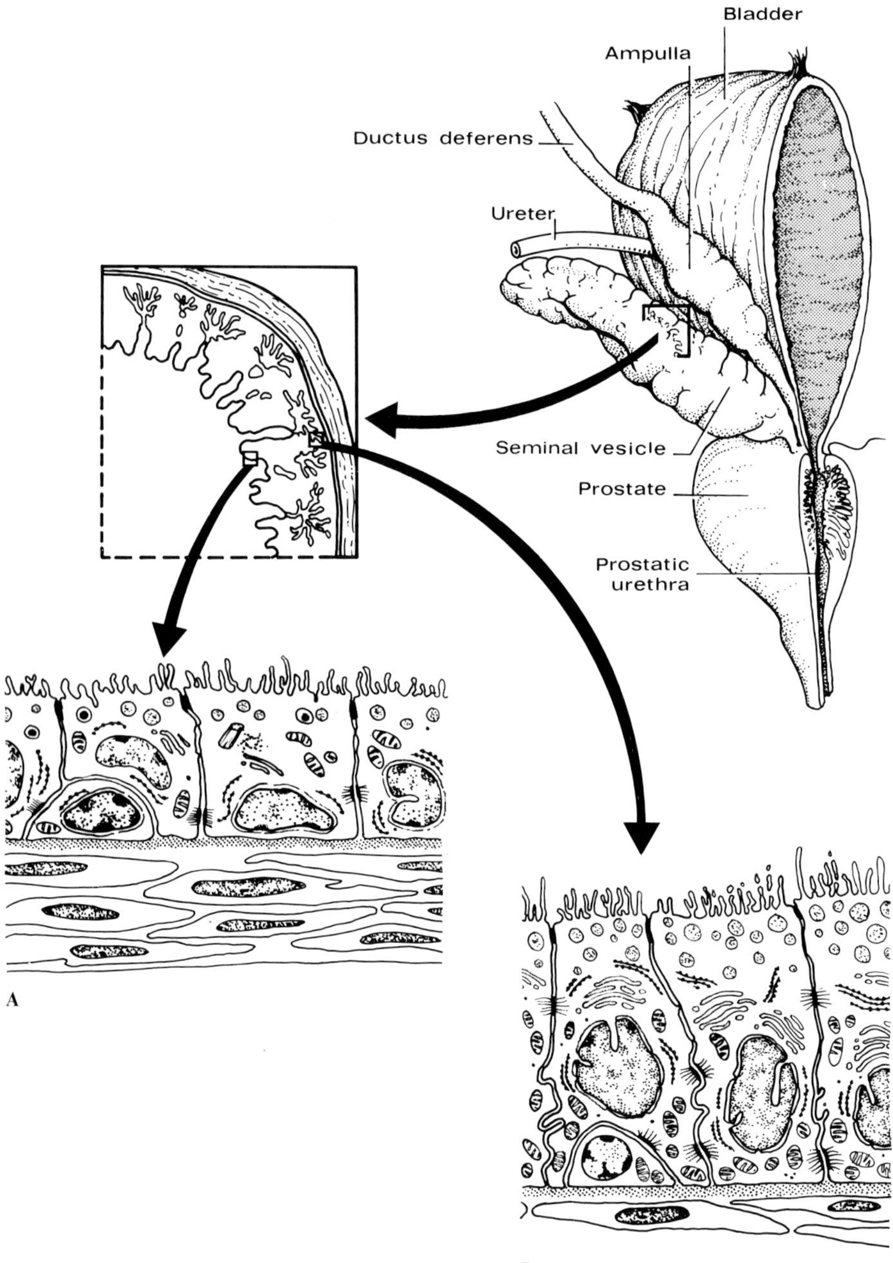

Fig. 53 A, B. Diagram showing the internal structure and cytological features of the seminal vesicles. Principal duct cells lining the ridges and creasts of the main duct **A**. Principal secretory cells lining the glandular regions of the seminal vesicle **B**

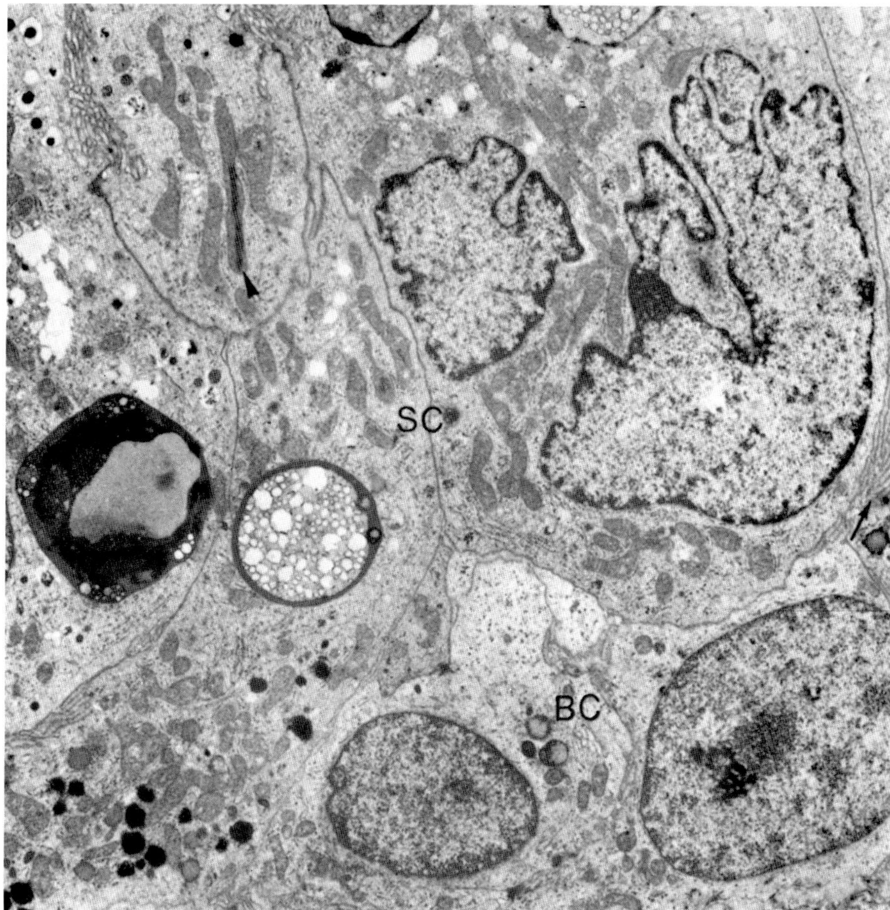

Fig. 54. Low-magnification electron micrograph of an oblique section through the secretory epithelium of human seminal vesicle. The smooth round nuclei of the basal cell (*BC*) contrast with the irregular, indented nuclei of the principal secretory cells (*SC*), and there is a noticable difference in the density of intracellular organelles between the two cell types. Membrane invaginations (*arrow*), intramitochondrial inclusions (*arrowhead*) and heteromorphic dense bodies are common features of the principal secretory cells. (Courtesy of G. Aumüller.) ×4500

a) Epithelium

Two basic types of epithelia line the inner surfaces of the seminal vesicles. A pseudostratified cuboidal or low columnar epithelium covers the folds and cavities of the central duct and its diverticulae, and a simple columnar secretory epithelium, containing a few small basal cells interspersed between tall columnar principal cells, lines the tubular and tubulo-alveolar glands in the peripheral zone (Figs. 53, 54). Principal and basal cells are the only confirmed cell types present in these two epithelia (Riva, 1967; Aumüller, 1979), although Stieve (1930) described a third, as yet unconfirmed, cell type which has no attachment to the basement membrane. The latter, however, are possibly basal cells, similar to those observed by RIVA (1967), which are positioned above, rather than on, the basal lamina and attached to it by only a few fine cytoplasmic processes.

Principal Cells. Principal cells are common to both epithelial types. Although probably derived from similar precursor cells they show distinct ultrastructural features which differ to such an extent that AUMÜLLER (1979) distinguishes principal cells of the seminal vesicles into *principal secretory cells* associated with the epithelium of the peripheral tubular glands and *duct cells,* which line the folds, crests and ridges of the diverticulae and sacculations.

Principal secretory cells are tall, columnar cells 15–25 µm high and 6–10 µm wide, which appear hexagonal in cross-section and form a simple columnar epithelium containing only a few basal cells (Fig. 54). These principal cells are prominent in the tubular glands adjacent to the neck of the seminal vesicle and are similar in structure to the principal cells which line the secretory epithelium of the ampulla (AUMÜLLER and BRUHL, 1977).

Histological and ultrastructural features of these cells (WATZKA, 1943; BRANDES, 1966; AUMÜLLER, 1979) confirm their capacity potential as active secretory cells. As in secretory cells of the epididymis (see Sect. B.IV.3) and other glandular tissues, the secretory principal cells of the seminal vesicles show a distinct compartmentalization of specialized regions of function. Apical, supranuclear, perinuclear and basal regions have been described (AUMÜLLER, 1979).

Each principal secretory cell contains an ovoid nucleus, oriented in the direction of the long axis of the cell. One to three nucleoli are present in each nucleus and the chromatin is condensed peripherally into electron-dense clumps (Fig. 54). The apical compartment of each cell contains a foamy cytoplasm with 'basophilic secretory granules' (FRAZÃO, 1949) and between this and the perinuclear zone lies an extensive Golgi region. FRAZÃO (1949) recognized a secretory cycle in the principal secretory cells, which has since been confirmed in ultrastructural studies by AUMÜLLER (ibid). Many histological specimens of human seminal vesicle are taken from donors suffering from urogenital disease and care should be taken in extrapolating from these observations, since it is possible that they may not represent the normal morphology of the human seminal vesicle epithelium.

RIVA (1967) and AUMÜLLER (1973, 1979) have published the only detailed studies on the ultrastructure of human seminal vesicle, but there is general agreement between them in their observations. The basal surface of each principal cell lies on a thick basal lamina and the basal plasma membrane is attached by a few sparsely distributed hemidesmosomes (Fig. 55). The basal and perinuclear compartments contain aggregations of rough endoplasmic reticulum closely associated with mitochondria, and occasional lysosomes, lipofuscin granules and lipid droplets. The lateral plasma membrane associated with the basal compartment of each cell is characterized by a complex pattern of interdigitations with adjacent cells. Towards the apex of each cell the lateral membrane becomes smooth and is joined to adjacent cell membranes by an extensive apical tight junction, and together with a small subapical macula adherens forms

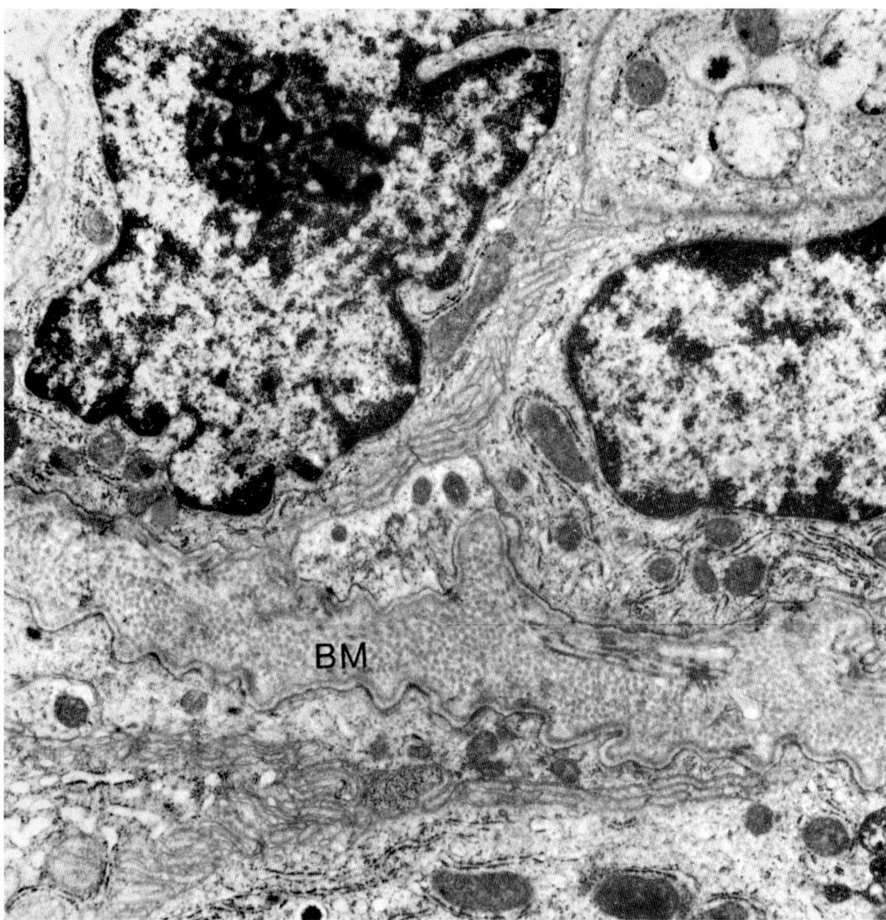

Fig. 55. Basal compartment of principal secretory cells in the epithelium of human seminal vesicle and their relationship to the basement membrane (*BM*). Note the complex interdigitations of the basal lateral cell membranes of adjacent principal cells and the dense aggregations of collagen fibres, shown in cross-section, in the basement membrane. (Courtesy of G. AUMÜLLER.) ×15000

a seal which creates a luminal and intra-epithelial compartment within the gland.

The supranuclear compartment contains extensive arrays of rough endoplasmic reticulum situated beneath a prominent series of flat cisernae and dense aggregations of vesicles containing secretory material, which together form the Golgi system (Fig. 56). The extent of the Golgi apparatus varies considerably between principal cells, a characteristic used by AUMÜLLER (1979) to distinguish normal, juvenile and exhausted principal cells in relation to the cell cycle. The apical region of each principal secretory cell often bulges into the lumen and the associated cytoplasm contains dense aggregations of round electron-dense,

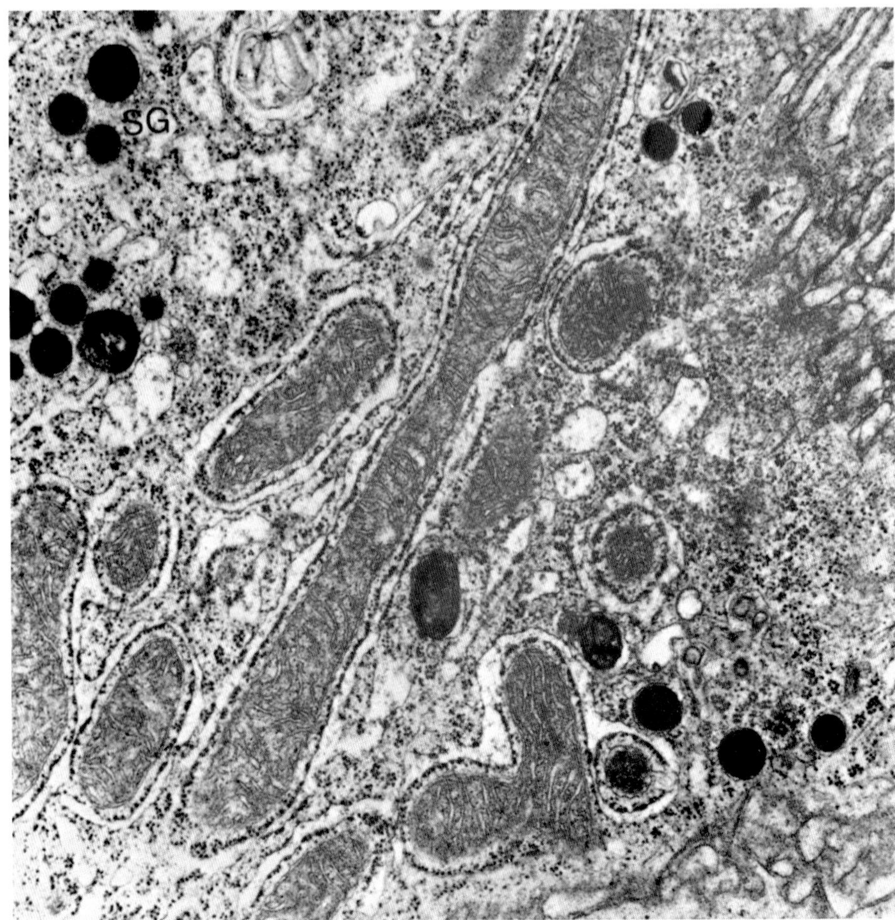

Fig. 56. Supranuclear compartment of a principal cell showing extensive mitochondrion-associated arrays of rough endoplasmic reticulum. Dense membrane-bound secretory granules (*SG*) can be seen adjacent to profiles of Golgi cisternae. (Courtesy of G. AUMÜLLER.)
× 24000

membrane-bound vesicles derived from the Golgi system (RIVA, 1967; AU-MÜLLER, 1979). These secretory vesicles are 0.15–0.28 μm in diameter and sometimes appear to coalesce beneath the apical plasma membrane (Fig. 57).

Secretion from these vesicles occurs by exocytosis. The vesicular membrane fuses with the apical plasma membrane and the secretory products are extruded directly into the lumen. Accumulations of dense amorphous material, which resemble the aggregated contents of intracellular secretory granules, are usually present in the luminal contents of the glands. The apical surface of principal secretory cells is covered with long, slender microvilli about 1 μm in length which extend into the lumen of the gland (Fig. 57). Smooth and coated vesicles, secretory vacuoles and apical aggregates of microfilaments are associated with

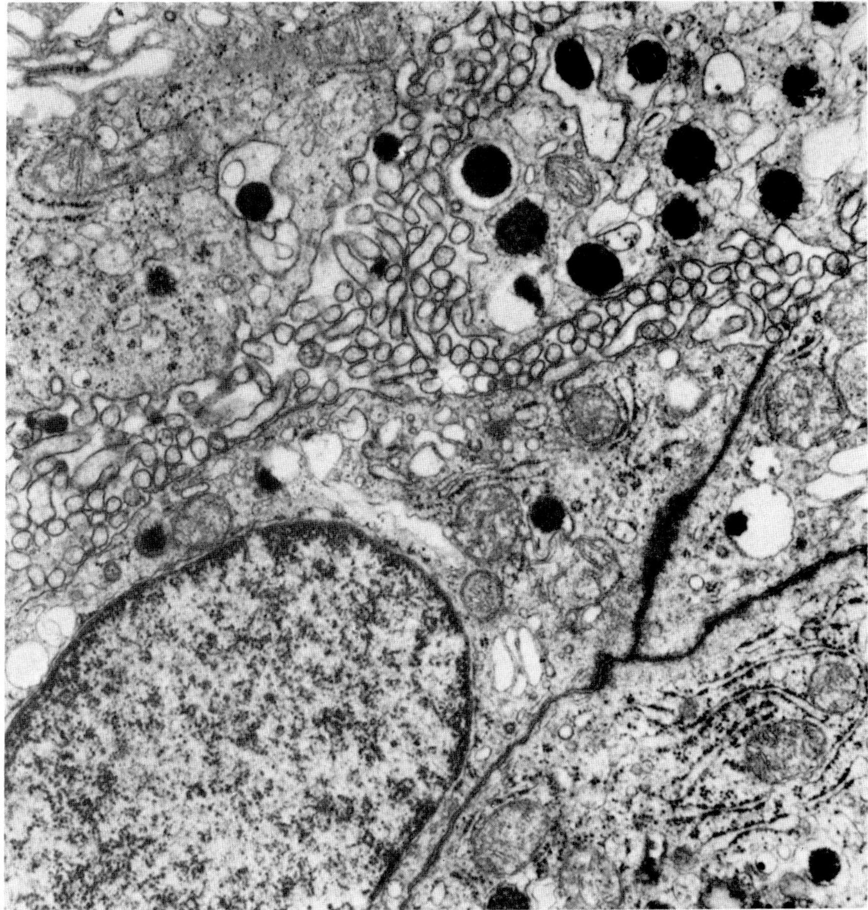

Fig. 57. Oblique section through the apical region of several principal cells showing the lumen and apical microvilli, clusters of ribosomes and profiles of granular endoplasmic reticulum, and apical aggregations of membrane-bound secretory granules. Several extruded granules can be seen within the lumen. (Courtesy of G. AUMÜLLER.) ×23 000

the microvilli. Other cellular inclusions such as lysosomes, membrane-bound granules with polymorphic contents, multivesicular bodies and lipid droplets are not common in principal secretory cells but lipofuscin granules are frequently observed (Fig. 58).

Principal duct cells are restricted to the epithelium associated with the internal surface folds of the gland and in particular around the central duct and its diverticulae (RIVA, 1967; AUMÜLLER, 1979). As with the principal secretory cells, duct cells extend from the basal lamina to the lumen. These cells are cuboidal or low columnar in shape, 8–12 μm high, and, like the secretory cells, display a compartmentalization of cellular organelles (Fig. 59). The main cell component is a large, ovoid, lobulated nucleus containing a small nucleolus.

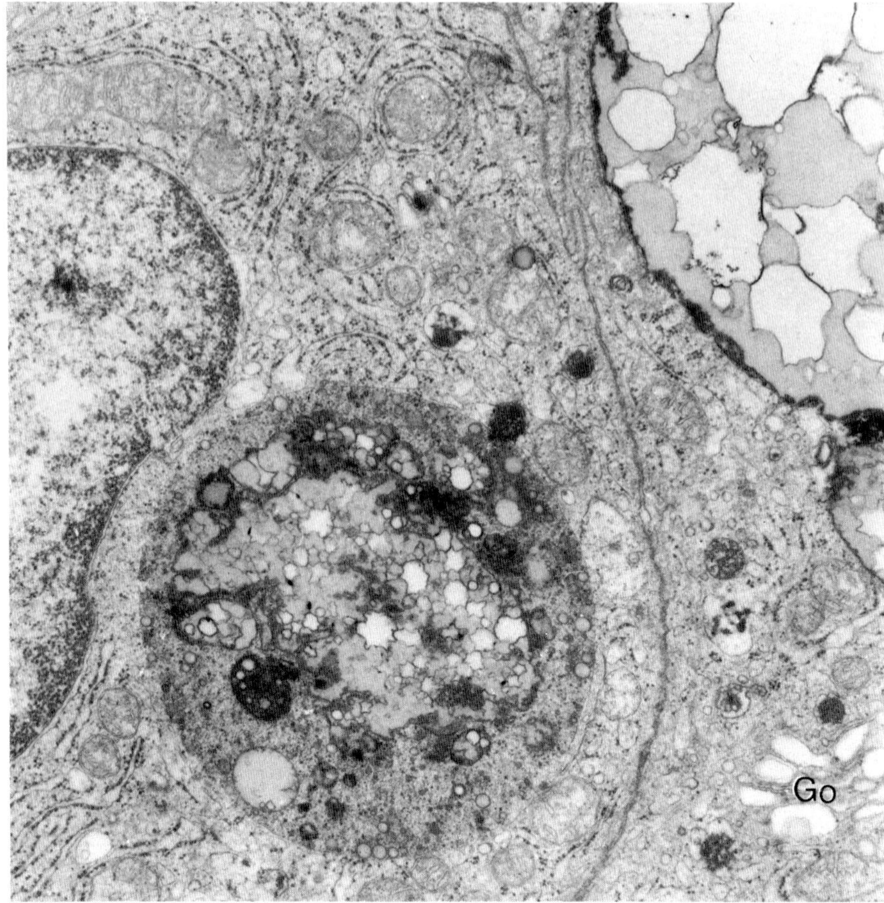

Fig. 58. High-magnification electron micrograph of the Golgi region (*Go*) of a principal secretory cell showing a large lipofuscin inclusion adjacent to the nucleus. (Courtesy of G. AUMÜLLER.) ×22000

In general, the ultrastructure of the duct cell resembles that of the secretory cell, but the intracellular organelles are less numerous and the cells appear to show little evidence of secretory activity. Mitochondria and rough endoplasmic reticulum are sparsely distributed in the perinuclear cytoplasm and multivesicular bodies, lysosomes, and lipofuscin granules are rare. The supranuclear region contains a narrow zone of rough endoplasmic reticulum positioned beneath a few cisternae and smooth vesicles which comprise the substance of the Golgi system. The apical region above the Golgi apparatus contains sparse aggregations of secretory vesicles and vacuoles with electron-dense matrices, a few mitochondria and multivesicular bodies. In contrast to the principal secretory cells, the apical surface of the duct cells contains only a few short microvilli and occasional interdigitations are found along the lateral plasma membrane (see Figs. 53, 59).

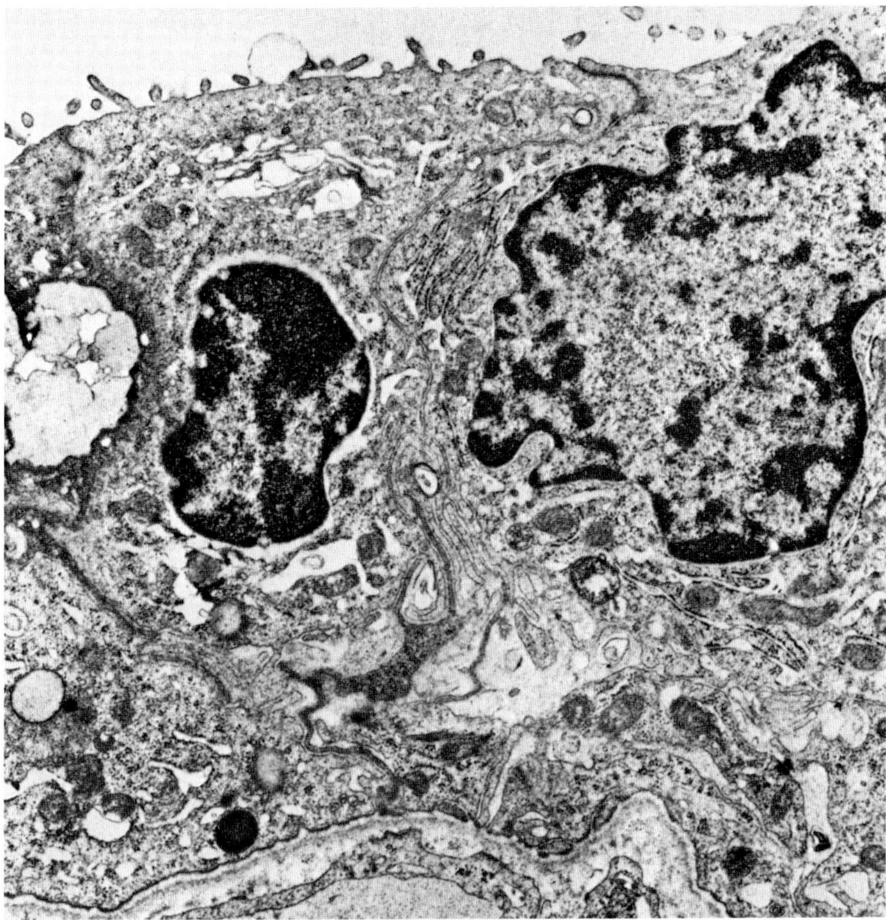

Fig. 59. Electron micrograph showing the structure of principal duct cells lining the internal surface folds of the central duct and its diverticulae. The duct cells are cuboidal and devoid of secretory granules. (Courtesy of G. AUMÜLLER, 1979) × 14400

Basal Cells. These cells are found in both epithelial types of the seminal vesicles but appear in larger numbers in the pseudostratified epithelium lining the ridges and crests of the diverticulae (RIVA, 1967; AUMÜLLER, 1979). They have similar structural features to basal cells found in epithelia of the other male accessory glands. Most basal cells lie against the basal lamina and are sparsely distributed amongst the principal cells of the epithelium (Fig. 54). They vary in shape from pyramidal cells, 7–8 µm in diameter, containing rounded nuclei, to flattened cells 3–5 µm thick containing lenticulate nuclei. The nuclei of basal cells contain little or no heterochromatin and nucleoli are rare. These cells are typically devoid of secretory material, mitochondria are few and elements of rough endoplasmic reticulum and Golgi complex are sparse and inconspicuous. The function of these cells is unknown but, as suggested for the epididymis, they may represent a stem cell population for renewal of epithelial cells.

b) Lamina Propria

The lamina propria consists of an inner narrow basal lamina surrounded by a layer of connective tissue which is interposed between the secretory epithelium and the inner smooth muscle layer of the seminal vesicles. This submucosal, or perhaps more correctly, subepithelial (AUMÜLLER, 1979), connective tissue forms a continuous layer around each seminal vesicle containing small bundles of smooth muscle cells which intermingle with connective tissue cells and irregular layers of collagen and elastin fibres. This layer extends into the folds and ridges adjacent to the central lumen to form the supporting framework for these structures. Connective tissue associated with the folds and ridges is devoid of smooth muscle cells; fibroblasts, plasma cells, mast cells and macrophages are the only cellular components in this layer. These cells lie interspersed between dense aggregations of collagen and elastin fibres. The basal lamina forms a continuous, dense amorphous layer about 500 Å thick (Fig. 55), which lies subjacent to epithelium and closely follows its basal contours (RIVA, 1967). Dense aggregations of argyrophilic elastin fibres form a distinct layer beneath the basal lamina.

Elastin fibres begin to form in the stromal connective tissue of the human seminal vesicles at puberty (VITALI-MAZZA, 1956) and in the adult glands regional differences occur in the distribution of these fibres. Elastin fibres are sparse or absent from the connective tissue ridges around the orifice of each gland, although they occur in the stromal tissue enclosing the tubular glands in this region. In contrast, elastin fibres are more abundant in the stromal connective tissue plate around the central region of the gland, where they are arranged in dense meshworks, and in the subepithelial connective tissue of the cul-de-sac (AUMÜLLER, 1979).

Distinct age-related changes have been described in the structure and organization of the subepithelial connective tissue in the seminal vesicles of man (VITALI-MAZZA, 1956; WITTSTOCK and KIRSCHNER, 1970). In general, connective tissue is sparse in younger men but abundant in older men (KUROSAWA, 1930). Proliferation of connective tissue elements begins at about 30 years (WITTSTOCK and KIRSCHNER, 1970). Between 30 and 40 years, connective tissue invades the adjacent smooth muscle layer and gradually replaces the smooth muscle cells. This process of replacement continues until about 60 years and then between 60 and 80 years of age, it is followed by hyaline degeneration of the connective tissue elements (VITALI-MAZZA, 1956). Concomitant changes occur in gland structure with age (Fig. 52). The dense network of folds and crests which characterize the activity-secreting gland are gradually replaced by thin-walled cysts and diverticulae in older men. These changes are predominantly caused by degeneration and fragmentation of the connective tissue elements, which form the supporting framework for periductal folds and crests. The causes of cyst development in seminal vesicles of older men have not been satisfactorily explained. Although challenged by WITTSOCK and KIRSCHNER, (1970), OBERN-

DORFER (1901) has suggested that cysts and diverticulae develop because of complete or partial obstruction of the channels connecting deep tubular glands to the central duct. OBERNDORFER (1901) further suggested that the obstructions arise from reduction in smooth muscle tissue around the gland and from its replacement by connective tissue which occurs predominantly during senile involution of the seminal vesicles.

c) Muscularis

Enclosing the epithelium and lamina propria is a thick sheath of smooth muscle which is itself enveloped by the outer adventitial layer of the wall of the seminal vesicle. Smooth muscle around the seminal vesicles has traditionally been described as comprising two distinct layers: outer longitudinal and inner circular layers (FRÄNKEL, 1901; AKUTSU, 1903). Recent detailed observations (VITALI-MAZZA, 1956; DÜLLMAN, 1967), particularly those derived from polarized light studies of thick sections (AUMÜLLER, 1973; AUMÜLLER and BRUHL, 1977), have provided a new concept of the structural organization of seminal vesicle smooth muscle. The complexity of AUMÜLLER's (1973) descriptions stands in marked contrast to the more simplistic two-layer descriptions of earlier workers. Smooth muscle layers vary in number from 2 to 10 per transverse section of the muscularis and these layers differ in thickness from 20 to 100 μm. Perhaps the most striking feature of AUMÜLLER's (1973) observations is the realization of an extreme irregularity in the organization and interrelationship of the bundles of smooth muscle fibres. Instead of being arranged in a distinct longitudinal or circular array, they occur in circular, spiralling or longitudinal bundles which change in orientation and thickness as they weave through the muscularis to produce an irregular pattern of flat, interlacing ribbons. Around the tubular glands, fine secondary and tertiary ramifications extend from the adjacent smooth muscle bundles to enclose these structures in a basket-like meshwork of muscle fibres.

In structure and function, human seminal vesicle smooth muscle cells resemble those found in other accessory glands of the male reproductive system. The cells exhibit the usual spindle shape morphology, approximately 150–300 μm long and 5–7 μm in diameter, and in contraction become irregular in shape and twisted helically. The nucleus resembles a rounded cylinder and contains several nucleoli. A dense meshwork of elastin and reticular fibres, produced by the smooth muscle cells (Ross, 1971), surrounds each cell and forms attachments to the external lamina of the plasma membrane causing indentations at these attachment sites. Contractile filaments form the major component of the sarcoplasm with mitochondria and rough endoplasmic reticulum interspersed between myofilament bundles. The myofilaments insert into dense plaques associated with the inner surface of the sarcolemma and vesicle invaginations (caveoli) are common in the plasma membrane between adjacent dense plaques. Golgi apparatus, mitochondria and rough endoplasmic reticulum are usually found concentrated in the cone of juxtanuclear sarcoplasm, which extends from each pole of the nucleus.

An unusual form of intercellular contact occurs in smooth muscle cells of the seminal vesicles, and also the prostate (see Sect. B.VII). Knob-like protrusions from each cell extend into similarly-shaped indentations in adjacent cells to form an intimate "ball and socket" connection. The external elastin and reticular fibre lamina is absent from the surface of each cell at this site of contact and the two cell membranes become very closely apposed, separated only by an intercellular space of about 200 Å. These intercellular connections may function to provide synchronization and coordination of smooth muscle activity during ejaculation.

As in the prostate (see Sect. B.VII.3.c) smooth muscle cells of the seminal vesicles are characterized by a propensity to undergo distinct regressive changes with age. These regressive changes are first obvious with the light microscope as aggregations of intercellular pigment granules. VITALI-MAZZA (1956) has shown an age-dependent relationship with these degenerative processes by demonstrating an absence of pigment granules in smooth muscle cells of prepubertal and early pubertal males but an increasing incidence of granules with advancing age after puberty. The first structural signs of degeneration seem to be the appearance and gradual accumulation of glycogen particles. This is followed by dense aggregation of glycogen, dilation of rough endoplasmic cisternae, dissociation of ribosomes from the reticular membrane and a gradual disappearance of cytoplasmic organelles. In more advanced stages of degeneration, most of the cytoplasmic components are replaced by lipid droplets, lysosomes, membrane whorls and coarse aggregations of glycogen which form large, homogeneous condensations of lipopigment in the disintegrating smooth muscle cells.

The causes of dedifferentiation of smooth muscle cells in the ageing seminal vesicle remain to be elucidated. BURNSTOCK (1970) and FLICKINGER (1972) have shown that normal differentiation of these smooth muscle fibres is androgen-dependent and that a decrease in circulating levels of androgen results in dedifferentiation and a transient redifferentiation of these cells into connective tissue elements, which then acquire large accumulations of lysosomes and begin to degenerate (AUMÜLLER, 1973). The androgen dependence of differentiation in these cells suggests that either reduced peripheral levels of androgen or a loss of androgen sensitivity by these cells in older men may be a contributing factor to cell degeneration.

The peripheral layer of adventitia forming the outer fibrous sheath of the seminal vesicles comprises elastin and collagen fibre bundles, fibroblasts and adipocytes interspersed by occasional groups of smooth muscle cells. The latter are derived from the outer layer of the muscularis and form an intimate association with the larger adventitial blood vessels. The adventitial layer contains the ganglia of the deferential prostatic plexus and transmits the vascular and lymphatic networks which supply and drain the various layers of the wall of the seminal vesicles.

VII. Prostate

1. Development

The embryonic development of the prostate has been described in detail by various investigators (LOWSLEY, 1912; MCNEAL, 1972; GLENISTER, 1962;

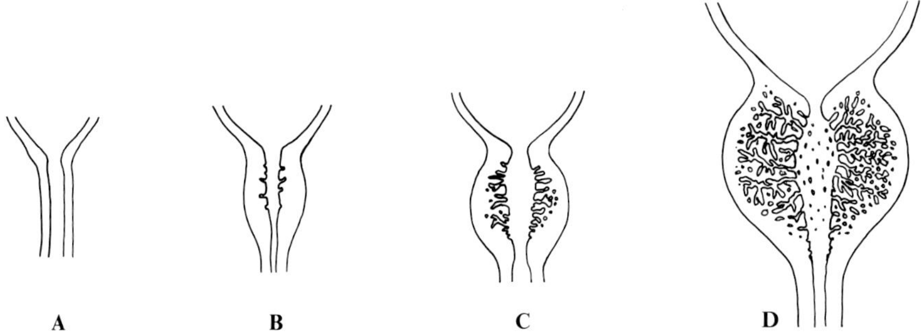

Fig. 60 A–D. Morphological changes in the prostate during development at **A** 8 weeks old, **B** approximately 12 weeks old, **C** 12 months old and **D** about 20 years old. During development invagination of the urethral lining forms the gland primordia. These primordia proliferate and enlarge and become secretory in the adult

AUMÜLLER, 1979). Close to the point of entry of the mesonephric and paramesonephric ducts into the urogenital sinus, the sinus epithelium invaginates to form a series of bud-like gland primordia which enlarge and proliferate around the urogenital sinus to enclose the definitive prostatic urethra (Fig. 60). The onset of this development occurs at about the 3rd month (10–12 weeks) of fetal life when the embryo is 50–55 mm Crown Rump Length (AUMÜLLER, 1979).

Initially a few gland anlagen develop lateral to and below the entrance of the mesonephric and paramesonephric ducts, and subsequently prostatic buds appear in superiolateral and ventral positions. The position, number and pattern of growth of these glandular primordia, which enlarge and extend into the surrounding mesenchyme, show considerable variation. In most individuals by about 16 weeks of fetal life the ventral group of glands rapidly cease development and regress either to form vestigial remnants or to become completely obliterated.

Subsequently the number of gland primordia increases at each of the remaining sites (JOHNSON, 1920) and branching and lumen formation occurs. Proliferation of glandular tissue changes the appearance of the developing prostate from a few tubules interspersed between a large amount of fibromuscular stromal tissue, evident in the early stages of prostate development, to a thinner shell of stroma and stromal septae enclosing and subdividing the proliferating masses of glandular prostatic tissue at term (Fig. 60).

Although the prostate is not functional until puberty, secretory activity has been observed in the developing prostate as early as 26 weeks of gestation (ZONDEK and ZONDEK, 1971, 1975). The factors which influence the onset of this secretory activity or the proliferation of fetal prostatic tissue are as yet unknown.

During prenatal development, changes have been observed in the structure of the prostatic epithelium. Postnatal growth and development of the prostate is usually subdivided into five distinct periods (STIEVE, 1930; ANDREWS, 1951; AUMÜLLER, 1979). The perinatal phase, which extends from the last month of gestation until about the end of the first postnatal month, is regarded as a period of growth and differentiation of the prostate and in particular the prostatic epithelium. MOORE (1936) reported that about 10% of developing acini were lined by two or three layers of cuboidal or columnar cells whereas the remainder were lined by a squamous epithelium which showed regressive changes during the first postnatal month, when the superficial layers of cells are sloughed and replaced by a stratified columnar epithelium. Growth and differentiation of the prostate during this period is believed to be influenced by fetal androgens, which are known to increase in concentration during the third trimester of gestation (REYES et al., 1974; FOREST and CATHIARD, 1975) and which persist until the 3rd month postpartum. Reduced levels of androgens in the neonate coincide with the second period in postnatal development, the involution phase, during which regressive changes are observed in the squamous epithelium (MOORE, 1936) which is sloughed and replaced by a stratified columnar epithelium. Little growth or differentiation occurs in the prostate during subsequent prepubertal years – the infantile resting period – when circulating levels of androgens are low.

However, in about the 10th year prostatic growth recommences and the prostate starts to acquire its definitive shape (AUMÜLLER, 1979).

The pubertal differentiation and maturation phases are perhaps the most important, in a functional sense, for the prostate. During this period from puberty, at about 12 years old, until full sexual development has occurred at about 20 years of age, the prostate completes its differentiation and development, acquiring its definitive shape and fully functional glandular epithelium (STIEVE, 1930; MOORE, 1936). Pubertal differentiation reflects growth and development of glandular and stromal components of the prostate under the influence of increasing circulating levels of androgen.

Discussion of prostatic development would not be complete without reference to the controversy that exists concerning the origin and differentiation of the various regions of the prostate. It has been generally accepted since the comprehensive study of LOWSLEY (1912) that glandular tissue in the prostate is derived from five embryonically distinct regions and that the mature prostate contains five corresponding lobes of glandular tissue: two lateral lobes and median, posterior and anterior (ventral) lobes (NETTER, 1954). However, in the definitive state, apart from the posterior lobe, which is isolated by stromal tissue, the prostate is not a lobate organ and it is not possible, either visually or functionally, to clearly distinguish median, lateral or anterior lobes. These terms in the adult prostate, though widely used, merely imply general regions and not necessarily the embryonic origins of glandular tissue in the prostate.

More recently the trend has been to disregard the various designations of lobate regions within the glandular tissue of the prostate (MCNEAL, 1972, 1978; BLACKLOCK and BOUSKILL, 1977). Instead a more acceptable approach to morphological subregions of the prostate has been proposed (MCNEAL, 1972, 1978) which distinguishes two morphologically distinct zones – a central and peripheral zone – in the prostate using histological criteria (see Sect. C.VII.3). The central zone, representing about one-third of the prostate, consists of a cone of tissue which extends from the neck of the bladder to the colliculus seminalis and incorporates the median and posterior lobes of LOWSLEY (1912). The peripheral zone contains the remaining glandular tissue of the prostate including the lateral lobes and part of the posterior lobe of Lowsley. The peripheral zone encloses most of the central zone tissue and extends distally to enclose the lower region of the prostatic urethra below the colliculus seminalis. Ducts from the central zone drain via the proximal portion of the prostatic urethra into the prostatic sinuses which lie lateral to the base of the colliculus seminalis. Ducts draining the glandular tissue of the peripheral zone empty into the regions of the prostatic sinuses lying adjacent to the columnar portion of the colliculus seminalis.

2. General Anatomy

a) Anatomical Relationships

The prostate is the largest accessory sex organ of the male and, in keeping with its size, contributes more than 60% of the fluid volume of the ejaculate. In the normal male the prostate weighs about 20 g and measures approximately 4 cm in length, 3–5 cm in width across the base and 2 cm in depth (GRAY, 1973; AUMÜLLER, 1979), but gland size is variable and dependent on the age and hormonal status of the individual. The adult prostate is cone-shaped and comprises an outer fibromuscular capsule and inner glandular and stromal tissues which enclose the initial (prostatic) part of the urethra, from which the prostate develops (see Sect. B.VII.1). The base of the prostate abuts against the inferior surface of the bladder and the inverted apex extends distally to contact the fascial sheath covering the superior surface of the urogenital diaphragm in close relation to the sphincter urethrae, the deep transverse perineal muscles and levator prostatae. The prostate is traversed obliquely by the ejaculatory ducts and encloses the utriculus masculinus (utriculus prostaticus) – the distal remnant of the paramesonephric ducts – and the colliculus seminalis.

The prostate is positioned low in the true pelvis immediately above the urogenital diaphragm and about 2 cm behind the inferior border of the pubic symphysis. The anterior and lateral surfaces of the prostate are attached to the symphysis pubis and pubic arches by puboprostatic ligaments which form the inferior wall of the retropubic space (space of Retzius) (NETTER, 1954; HOLLINSHEAD, 1966; GRAY, 1973). Posteriorly, the prostate is related to the seminal vesicles and the distal ends of the ductus deferens (Fig. 51) and to the anterior wall of the rectal ampulla, from which it is separated only by the rectal fascia and thin layers of connective tissue comprising the rectovesical septum or Denonvillier's fascia (HOLLINSHEAD, 1966). The close relationship between the prostate and the rectum is of considerable clinical importance since per rectal digital palpation of the prostate is used routinely to examine the gland for dystrophy or dysfunction. The inferolateral surfaces of the prostate are closely associated with the anterior fibres of levatores ani – the levatores prostatae – which are separated from the prostate by venous plexuses lying within the lateral portion of a fibrous sheath enclosing the gland. This fibrous sheath is only vascularized laterally and anteriorly, where it is in apposition to and continuous with the puboprostatic ligaments. Inferiorly the sheath merges with fascia covering the deep surface of the sphincter urethrae, deep transverse perineal muscles and the perineal body. Posteriorly, the sheath is avascular and arises from the fusion of two layers of peritoneum to form the rectovesical fascia which extends up over the posterior surface of the seminal vesicles and fuses with the peritoneal floor of the rectovesical pouch (GRAY, 1973).

b) Vasculature

Arterial. It is generally agreed that the principal arterial supply to the prostate is derived from the inferior vesical artery, a branch of the anterior trunk of the internal iliac artery (FLOCKS, 1925; CLEGG, 1955; BANCHIETTI et al., 1956; AUMÜLLER, 1971; DUCLOS et al., 1972). Usually a single pair of independent branches, the prostatic arteries, originate from the inferior vesical arteries and divide close to the prostate to give further branches which penetrate the gland. However, a number of major and minor variations in arterial supply to the prostate have been described. CLEGG (1955) found that in 32% of individuals the prostatic arteries were derived from the superior vesical artery and BANCHIETTI et al. (1956) described three major variations in the origin of the blood supply to the prostate, which, in addition to the usual inferior vesical origin, also included arterial branches either solely derived from the obturator artery or partly from the inferior vesical artery via its obturator branches. Minor branches from the middle rectal and internal pudendal arteries sometimes supply the inferior region of the prostate (NETTER, 1954; GRAY, 1973) with occasional additional branches from the vesiculodeferential, middle rectal and umbilical arteries (HOLLINSHEAD, 1966).

These variations in arterial supply to the prostate can, to some extent, be explained by variations in the origins of the main arterial branches of the internal iliac artery (GRAY, 1973). The inferior vesical artery frequently arises in common with the middle rectal artery, which has been observed to anastomose with inferior and superior rectal branches and to interconnect with branches of the inferior vesical artery. Obturator artery supply to the prostate is usually derived from its intrapelvic vesicle branch, which may replace the inferior vesical artery and its associated prostatic branches.

Within the prostate, branches of the prostatic arteries and associated minor arterial vessels are arranged in a regular pattern of distribution of capsular and periurethral vessels (FLOCKS, 1925; AUMÜLLER, 1971). The capsular vessels make contact with posterolateral surfaces of the prostate and form an extensive arterial network in the capsule which supply the outer portion of the prostate, corresponding generally to the peripheral zone of glandular tissue (MCNEAL, 1972). Capsular vessels penetrate to the urethral tissues only in the region of the colliculus seminalis. Urethral vessels penetrate the prostate close to the bladder neck at the vesicoprostatic junction and pass distally in close association with the urethra.

These peri-urethral vessels provide blood supply to the central zone of the prostate, neck of the bladder and periurethral tissue, forming an inner vascular plexus around the prostatic urethra. Minor branches, when present, from the middle rectal and internal pudendal arteries enter the inferior segment of the prostate and augment the arterial supply of the urethral vessels to the distal region of the prostate. Anastomoses may occur between these branches and the urethral plexus of the prostatic arteries.

Flocks (1925) considers that capsular and urethral arterial circulations are essentially isolated systems and that the amount of anastomosis between these two groups of vessels is not sufficient for one system to provide the other with an alternative blood supply to the adjacent area in a situation of obstruction to either vascular province. This rationale has been used clinically as a means to control prostatic hyperplasia, which is usually confined to the periurethral (central) zone of the prostatic tissue, by ligating the urethral branches of the prostatic arteries. However, the effect of this treatment on the structure of the prostate and prostatic urethra, and its efficacy in controlling benign prostatic enlargement, is poorly documented.

Venous. Venous blood from deep and superficial regions of the prostate drains to the plexus of Santorini (Santorinus, 1724; Aumüller, 1979), which is formed by the association of numerous intra- and extracapsular veins. From the prostatic plexus, venous blood flows to the adjacent vesicoprostatic (pudendal) plexus, which lies within the fascial sheath along the ventrolateral surface of the prostate adjacent to the inferior border of pubic arch and pubic symphysis. The vesicoprostatic plexus also receives a major contribution from the deep dorsal vein of the penis (Netter, 1954; Hollinshead, 1966; Last, 1978). This plexus communicates superiorly with the vesical plexus, which also receives some venous drainage from the prostate and the internal pudendal vein, and is usually drained laterally by several vesical veins which commonly unite to form a single trunk before joining the internal iliac vein.

Lymphatics. An extensive network of lymphatic channels and vessels are associated with the prostate and prostatic urethra (Bruhns, 1904; Parker, 1936; Netter, 1954; Ivanov, 1970). The distribution and drainage pattern of prostatic lymphatic vessels appear to follow closely the pattern of distribution of the blood supply to the prostate and may, therefore, vary greatly between individuals. Lymph channels and minor lymphatic vessels unite to form a few larger vessels which drain laterally to the external iliac lymph nodes and to the internal iliac and sacral nodes. Efferent vessels from the superior and posterolateral surfaces of the prostate are numerous and drain via larger efferent trunks to the three groups of external iliac nodes. The few efferent vessels which drain the lateral and anterior surfaces of the gland merge with lymphatic vessels from the membranous urethra and form trunks which drain to the internal iliac and sacral nodes. An alternative drainage route to the internal iliac nodes is via lymph vessels which accompany the vesical branch of the obturator artery and, less commonly, prostatic lymph drains to the superior rectal nodes or to nodes of the gluteal region. Interconnecting channels may also occur between prostatic lymphatics and those of the rectum, bladder, vas deferens and seminal vesicles (Hollinshead, 1966). Minor vessels have also been observed to cross the lateral surface of the rectum and drain to presacral and lateral sacral nodes, which lie adjacent to the middle sacral and lateral sacral arteries in the concavity of the sacrum (Netter, 1954).

c) Innervation

Motor activity of prostatic smooth muscle is controlled by sympathetic innervation from spinal segments T11, T12, L1 and L2. Sympathetic fibres descend from these spinal segments through the pre-aortic plexus and abdominal chains to aggregate in the superior hypogastric plexus (Mitchell, 1935; Schlyvitsch and Kosintzew, 1939). Fibres to the vas deferens branch from this plexus but remaining fibres continue via the inferior hypogastric plexuses to the pelvic plexus, where they join afferent and parasympathetic fibres of sacral origin. Efferent and afferent fibres to the prostate and related parts of the reproductive tract descend to the prostatic plexus and associate into relatively large nerves which enter the base and sides of the gland. Smaller branches from these nerves supply the seminal vesicles, ejaculatory ducts, urethra and bulbo-urethral glands. Prior to and during ejaculation, sympathetic fibres stimulate constriction of the sphincter vesicae at the bladder neck (Kimura et al., 1975), preventing retrograde ejaculation, and are responsible for contraction of prostatic smooth muscle forcing prostatic fluids into the prostatic urethra (Marberger, 1974). Parasympathetic innervation has not been conclusively demonstrated in the prostate except by virtue of the parasympathetic control of the penile vasculature during sexual arousal which transforms the prostatic urethra into a "pressure chamber at ejaculation" (Marberger, 1974).

Most, perhaps all, afferent fibres from the prostate accompany the pelvic parasympathetics from the pelvic plexus and enter the sacral nerves S_2, S_3 and S_4 via the pelvic splanchnic nerves (nervi erigentes) (Hollinshead, 1966). The observations of Cady and Deakins (1933) that chronic prostatic infections may give rise to referred pain in cutaneous sacral segments over the gluteal region and upper posterior region of the thigh confirms the pathways taken by pain afferents from the prostate. The prostate contains a variety of sensory nerve endings including end bulbs and genital corpuscles located in the interstitial connective tissue and free nerve endings in the glandular epithelium. These are supported by an extensive network of non-myelinated fibres associated with small sympathetic ganglia (Bloom and Fawcett, 1975).

3. Cytological Features

The human prostate consists of a series of 30–50 small compound tubulo-alveolar or tubulosaccular glands which are irregular in size and set in dense swathes of stromal connective tissue. These swathes radiate from the region of the colliculus seminalis towards the periphery of the gland where they blend with the dense connective tissue capsule investing the prostate (Stieve, 1930; Bloom and Fawcett, 1975; Bargmann, 1977; Aumüller, 1979). Secretions from the prostatic glands are carried to the prostatic urethra by 15–30 collecting ducts which open into the prostatic sinuses along each side of the colliculus seminalis.

The prostatic urethra is subdivided into two segments (McNeal, 1972). The proximal segment extends from the sphincter vesicae, around the neck of the bladder, to the base of the colliculus seminalis, which penetrates through the posterior wall of the urethra. It contains the urethral glands, which arise in this region, and is enclosed by a thick cylinder of muscle. The distal segment, described as the prostatic portion, contains the openings for the prostatic ducts, the utriculus prostaticus (or utriculus masculinus) and incorporates the colliculus

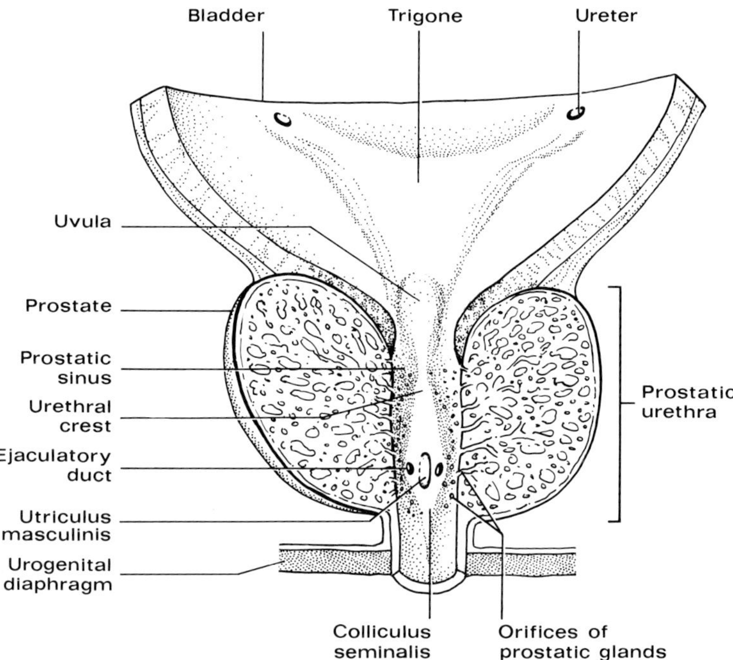

Fig. 61. Coronal section through the bladder and prostate to show the relationship of these two structures and the morphological features of the posterior walls of the bladder and the prostatic urethra

seminalis and the urethral crest, which extend distally into the membranous urethra, as contributing components to the structure of its dorsal wall.

The utriculus prostaticus varies in morphology between individuals from a small cyst-like organ to a glandular structure resembling, in morphology, the prostatic or urethral glands (STIEVE, 1930). Set deep within the substance of the prostate, the utriculus is lined by prostatic epithelium arranged in folds which enclose glandular invaginations (BLOOM and FAWCETT, 1975). It opens into the prostatic urethra via a round or cleft-like orifice, up to 2 mm long, situated in the centre of the colliculus seminalis (AUMÜLLER, 1979). Although often regarded simply as a vestigial remnant of the paramesonephric duct, recent observations suggest that it may be a functional accessory gland in the male (BLOOM and FAWCETT, 1975).

On each side of the utricular orifice is a small opening, less than 1 mm in diameter, which marks the outlet of each ejaculatory duct (Fig. 61), through which the testicular, epididymal and vesicular products are forced at ejaculation. As indicated previously (see Sect. B.VI), the ejaculatory ducts form the short common collecting ducts for the proximal components of the genital tract which extend from the point of confluence of the duct of the seminal vesicle and the ampulla of the ductus deferens (Fig. 51). Throughout most of its length each ejaculatory duct is lined by simple or pseudodstratified columnar epithelium with the mucosa thrown into fine longitudinal folds which extend deep into the lumen surrounded only by a connective tissue sheath. At the distal end of each duct, close to its opening into the urethra, the epithelium often becomes "transitional" in structure. Glandular invaginations which occur along the dorsomedial wall of each duct may function as accessory seminal vesicles (BLOOM and FAWCETT, 1975). The ejaculatory ducts are easily recognized from the surrounding prostatic tissue by a lower epithelial height and a more uniform arrangement of the associated connective tissue sheath (AUMÜLLER, 1979).

a) Epithelium

Like the seminal vesicle epithelium, the epithelium lining the prostate (Fig. 62) varies in appearance depending on its position within the prostatic glands, its secretory activity and the size of the acinus which it lines (RÖHLICH, 1938; AUMÜLLER, 1979). Each prostatic gland comprises a complex glandular component which opens into the prostatic urethra via a relatively straight main collecting duct. The secretory portion of each prostatic gland is usually highly irregular in appearance. Large sacculations or diverticulae, which may appear cystic, join the main collecting duct by shorter secondary intralobular ducts. These diverticulae are interconnected by narrow segments of branching tubules which often form the blind terminal segments of the glands (BLOOM and FAWCETT, 1975; AUMÜLLER, 1979). The epithelium is associated with fine branching folds and papillae which extend from the walls of the tubules, diverticulae and cystic cavities, and protrude deep into the lumina of these structures. Thin cores of connective tissue provide a structural support for these folds. In transverse and oblique section these folds appear as isolated clumps of glandular tissue floating, apparently unattached, within the lumen.

The prostatic epithelium is usually pseudostratified or simple columnar (STIEVE, 1930; FERNER and ZAKI, 1969; BLOOM and FAWCETT, 1975; AUMÜLLER et al., 1976) but variations have been observed which depend on plane of section, height of the epithelium and location within the prostate. RÖHLICH (1938) has reported the presence of zones of stratified epithelium in the prostate and low cuboidal and even squamous epithelial cells lining the large alveolar cavities.

A variety of cell types has been described in the glands of the prostate and within the transitional zones along the terminal prostatic ducts (Fig. 62), which form the main collecting duct of each prostatic gland. In the glandular region of the prostate the epithelium contains mostly principal secretory cells and basal cells interspersed with a few enterochromaffin cells (FEYRTER, 1951; AUMÜLLER et al., 1976). The cytology of the glandular epithelium is variable both between and within individuals, due mainly to changes related to age and hormonal status of the individual and also to the secretory activity of individual cells (STIEVE, 1930; RÖHLICH, 1938; NARBAITZ, 1974).

The uniform cytology of the glandular epithelium of the prostate is in contrast to the epithelial structure of the terminal prostatic connecting ducts, especially in the transitional zone between the secretory portion of the glands and the prostatic urethra. AUMÜLLER et al. (1976) distinguished four different zones along these terminal ducts. The most distal zone, designated zone 1, is situated around the orifice of each duct. Its epithelium, a stratified columnar epithelium interspersed with a few basally situated enterochromaffin and stellate small granu-

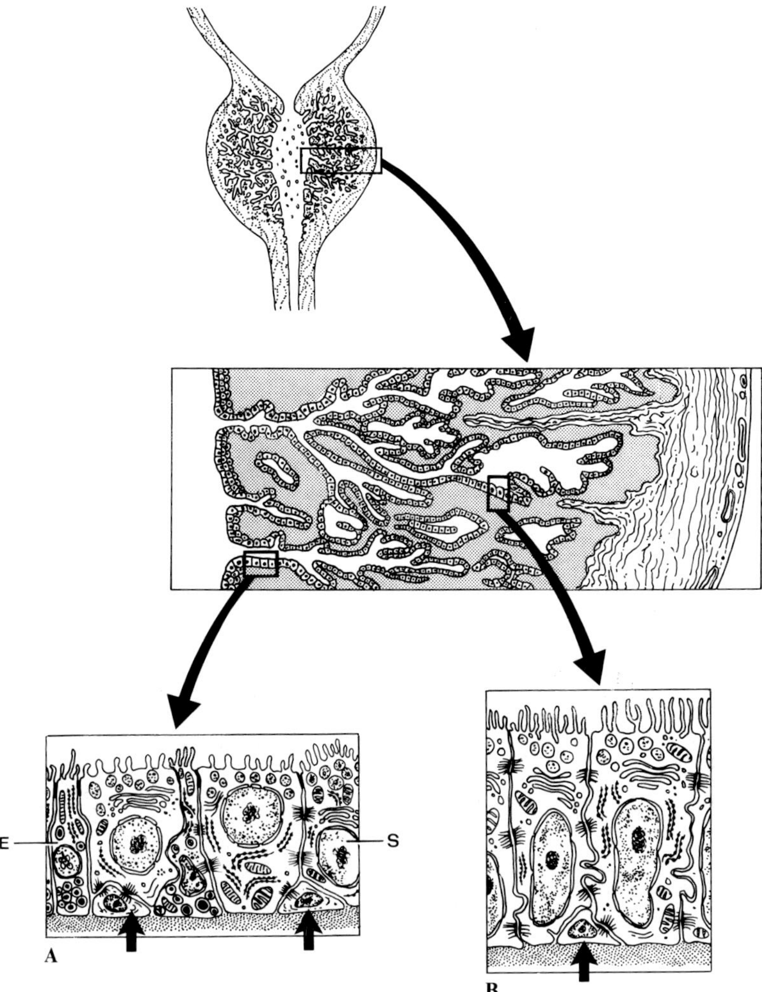

Fig. 62 A, B. Diagram showing the internal structure and cytological features of the prostate. **A** Cuboidal epithelium lining the preterminal segment of the prostatic ducts contains sialomucin (*S*), enterochromaffin (*E*) and basal cells (*arrows*); **B** columnar secretory epithelium lining the prostatic glands containing principal secretory cells and basal cells (*arrow*)

lated cells, merges into the adjacent urethral epithelium, which it resembles. The adjacent proximal zone forms a junction between urethral and prostatic secretory epithelium and is intermediate in structure between these two epithelial types. Zone 3, which coincides with the wider proximal portion of the prostatic ducts, contains a few shallow diverticulae lined by an epithelium consisting of large number of enterochromaffin cells interspersed by isolated sialomucin secretory cells (Fig. 63). Finally, the most proximal zone is lined by an epithelium which is intermediate in structure between zone 3 and the normal secretory epithelium of the prostate. Zone 4 epithelium contains principal secretory cells

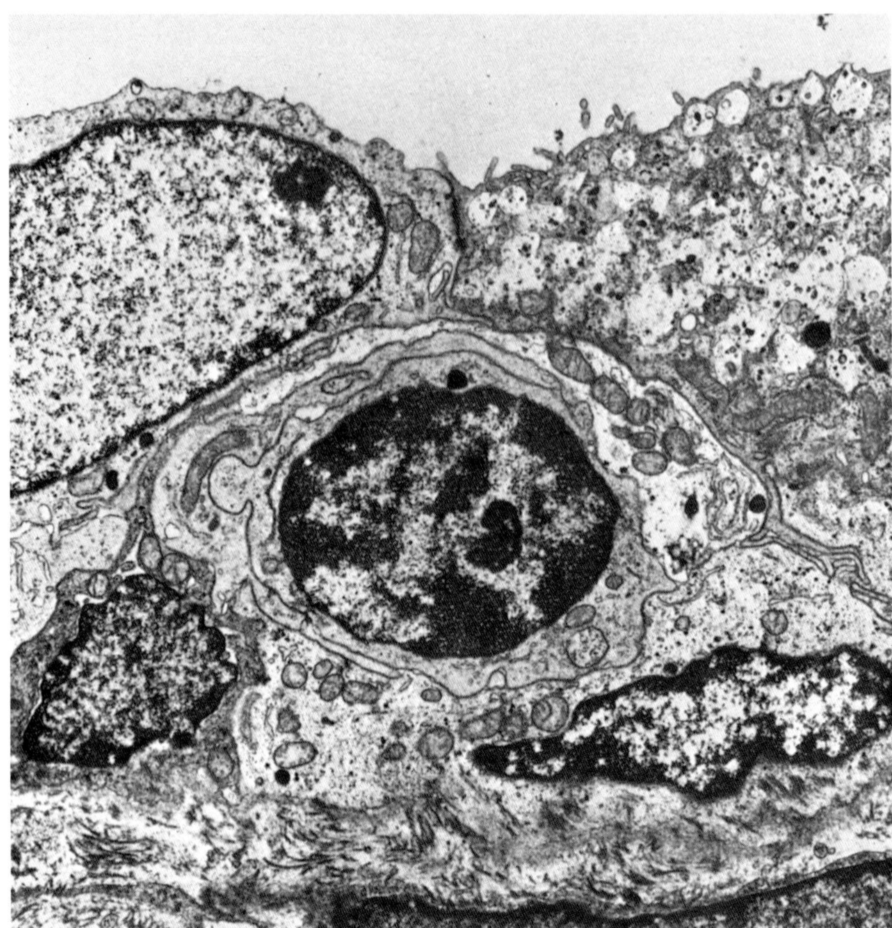

Fig. 63. Cuboial principal cells in the secretory epithelium of a human prostatic acinus. (Courtesy of G. AUMÜLLER.) ×7500

and basal cells. Enterochromaffin cells are numerous distally but occur less frequently in the proximal part of this zone.

The secretory epithelium of the prostate is dependent on androgen for its continued function. Experimental treatments, such as castration, which reduce the levels of circulating androgen cause regression of the secretory epithelial cells and a concomitant reduction in size and associated loss of function of the prostate.

Principal Secretory Cells. As indicated previously, the secretory epithelium lining the acini varies in height due to a variety of age, location and hormonally related factors. Previous studies have suggested the existence of different types of principal secretory cells, based on morphological criteria, which occur together within the same acinus (FISHER and SIERACKI, 1970; KASTENDIECK, 1977). These observations indicated a secretory cell cycle with the various cell types representing stages in the secretory cycle, including renewing stem cell populations of basal cells, immature non-secreting cells, mature secretory glandular cells, non-secretory glandular cells and degenerating glandular cells. Based on further observations, AUMÜLLER et al. (1976) described cells along the prostatic gland ducts which resembled very closely KASTENDIECK's (1977) non-secretory gland cells. These cells are similar to the principal duct cells of the seminal vesicles and were named ductal cells by AUMÜLLER et al. (1976). Four intracellular regions are recognized in the gland cells of the human prostate (KASTIENDIECK, 1977; AUMÜLLER, 1979): a basal region, perinuclear and supranuclear regions and an apical zone (Fig. 64).

The secretory epithelium lining the acini of human prostatic glands contains cells which range in appearance from low cuboidal (Fig. 63) to tall columnar (Fig. 64). Each principal secretory cell has a basally situated, ovoid, heterochromatin-rich nucleus, 5–7 µm in diameter, and a variety of cytoplasmic organelles stratified within the intracellular regions of the cells (Fig. 64).

Principal secretory cells are 10–20 µm high and 7–10 µm wide. These cells are responsible for the synthesis and secretion of a colourless, slightly acidic secretion (MANN, 1964) containing large concentrations of several proteolytic enzymes, including a highly active fibrolysin, β-glucuronidase and a diastase, citric acid (480–2680 mg/100 ml), acid phosphatase (3500–4500 units/ml) and unusually high concentrations of zinc. This active secretory function is reflected in the structural components of these cells.

Basal Cells. Basal cells in the glandular epithelium of the prostate, like those present in the epithelia of other parts of the reproductive tract (see Figs. 41, 54), are situated along the basal lamina squeezed in between principal secretory cells (Fig. 64). Prostatic basal cells are flattened, cuboidal or pyramidal in shape and measure about 5 µm in height and 10 µm wide. Occasionally, as in the seminal vesicle epithelium, cells are observed which resemble vasal cells both in size and nuclear morphology but which have little or no contact with the basal lamina. The identity of these cells has not yet been confirmed (MAO and ANGRIST, 1966) but they may be degenerating principal secretory cells rather than displaced basal cells.

Basal cells are usually attached to the basal lamina by extensive systems of hemidesmosomes and often form an intimate association with adjacent principal cells by means of extensive infoldings and interdigitations of their lateral plasma membranes.

These cells are characterized by a prominent indented ovoid nucleus, with its long axis along the basal lamina, conspicuous nucleoli and a sparse, electron-dense cytoplasmic matrix containing few organelles (Fig. 64). As in other epithelia, basal cells show little evidence of synthetic or secretory activity and the low incidence of mitotic activity in the mature epithelium (SINOWATZ et al., 1977) appears to contradict the suggestion that basal cells function as a stem cell population which produce replacements for degenerating principal cells.

Large numbers of free ribosomes and polyribosomes occur scattered throughout the basal cell cytoplasm and their presence has been interpreted by MAO

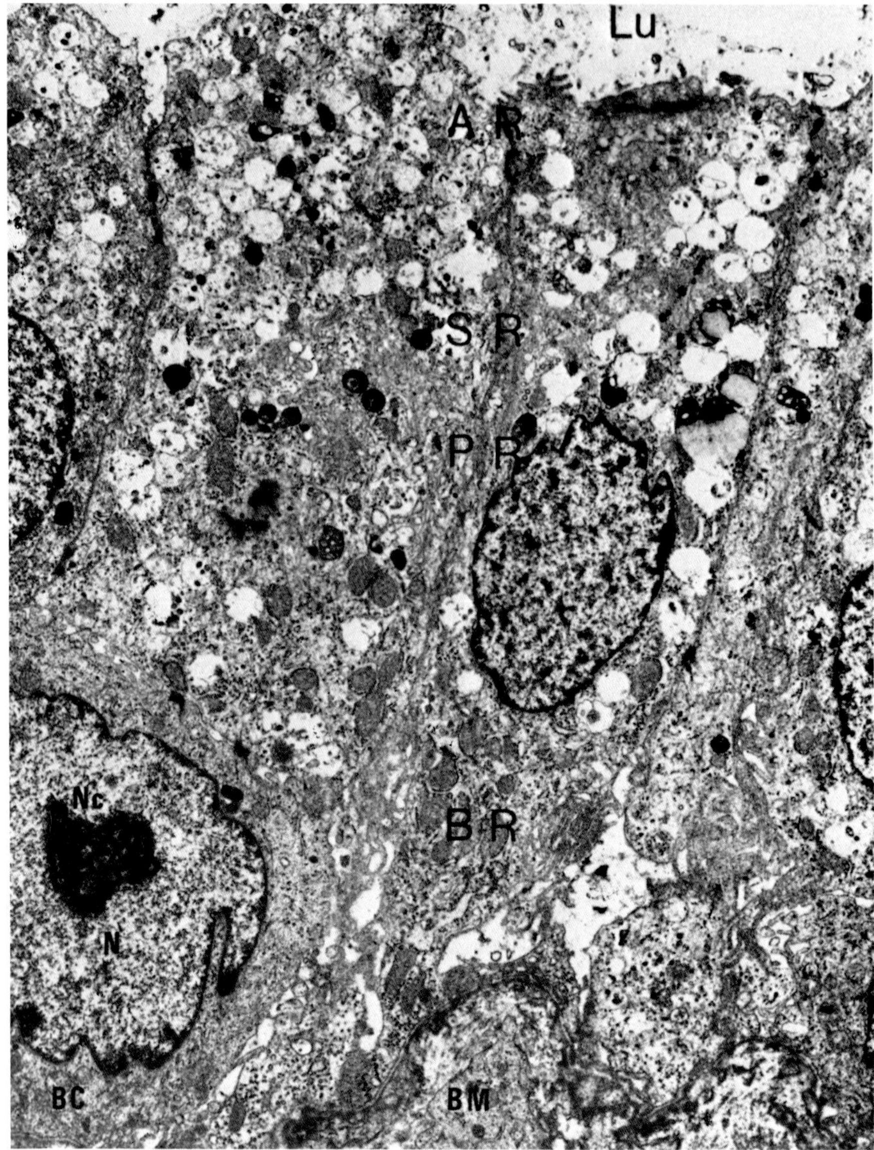

Fig. 64. Low-magnification electron micrograph showing columnar principal cells, basement membrane (*BM*) and a basal cell (*BC*), containing a large nucleus (*N*) and prominent nucleolus (*Nc*), in the secretory epithelium of the human prostate. Four intracellular compartments between the basement membrane and the lumen (*Lu*) are shown: *BR*, basal region; *PR*, perinuclear region; *SR*, supranuclear region; and *AR*, apical region. (Courtesy of G. AUMÜLLER.) ×5500

and ANGRIST (1966) as an indication that basal cells are undifferentiated or growing cells. Endoplasmic reticulum is represented by a few membrane profiles and the Golgi apparatus usually appears as a very poorly developed system of cisternae and vesicles. Mitochondria are widely dispersed through the cytoplasmic matrix, where they may often occur in small clusters. Microfilaments, about 50 Å in diameter, occur in small, dense aggregates scattered through the cytoplasm, and microtubules are present, often associated in distinct aggregates. Lysosomes, multivesicular bodies, glycogen and lipid droplets comprise the remaining organelles and these are sparsely distributed through the cytoplasm.

Principal Duct Cells. These replace the principal secretory cells in the pseudostratified epithelium lining the prostatic collecting ducts (Fig. 62) in the region of the colliculus (AUMÜLLER, 1979). Duct cells are columnar in shape and contain large, oval, usually centrally situated nuclei, dense networks of filaments and microtubules, a well-developed supranuclear Golgi system associated with aggregates of vesicles, large numbers of mitochondria, free ribosomes and glycogen particles and dense profiles of rough endoplasmic reticulum. Adjacent duct cells are intimately associated along their lateral surfaces by complex interdigitations and infolds of the lateral plasma membrane and by numerous desmosomes and a narrow apical junctional complex.

Enterochromaffin Cells. These cells have been identified and described at both light and electron microscope levels (FEYRTER, 1951; DIXON et al., 1973; KAZZAZZ, 1974; HÅKANSON et al., 1974; AUMÜLLER et al., 1976) and have been shown to occur in high densities in the prostatic urethra and in the epithelium which lines the distal portion of the prostatic ducts. Prostatic enterochromaffin cells are usually elongated with an irregular outline caused by branching processes which extend from the apical surface of the cell towards the lumen (Fig. 62). These cells contain basally situated oval nuclei, scattered aggregates of mitochondria and other organelles such as rough endoplasmic reticulum, ribosomes and microfilaments. A well-developed Golgi system and profiles of smooth endoplasmic reticulum are located in the supranuclear region of each cell and the apical plasma membrane sends long microvilli-like projections towards luminal surface of the epithelium. The most characteristic feature of these cells, which identifies them as enterochromaffin like, is the presence of large numbers of electron-dense membrane-bound granules with dark cores (Fig. 65) which vary in size from 1000–1700 Å (AUMÜLLER, 1979). As in other neuro-endocrine cells, these granules are thought to be condensed aggregations of endocrine secretory material.

A second endocrine-like cell, the stellate small granule cell has been identified in the human prostatic urethral epithelium associated with the openings of the prostatic ducts into the urethra (CASANOVA et al., 1974; AUMÜLLER et al., 1976). These slender, stellate cells lie along the basal lamina and send out long dendritic processes between adjacent epithelial cells. These cells contain lysosomes and a well-developed Golgi system associated with round, membrane-bound electron-dense granules (Fig. 66) which are distinctly smaller than those

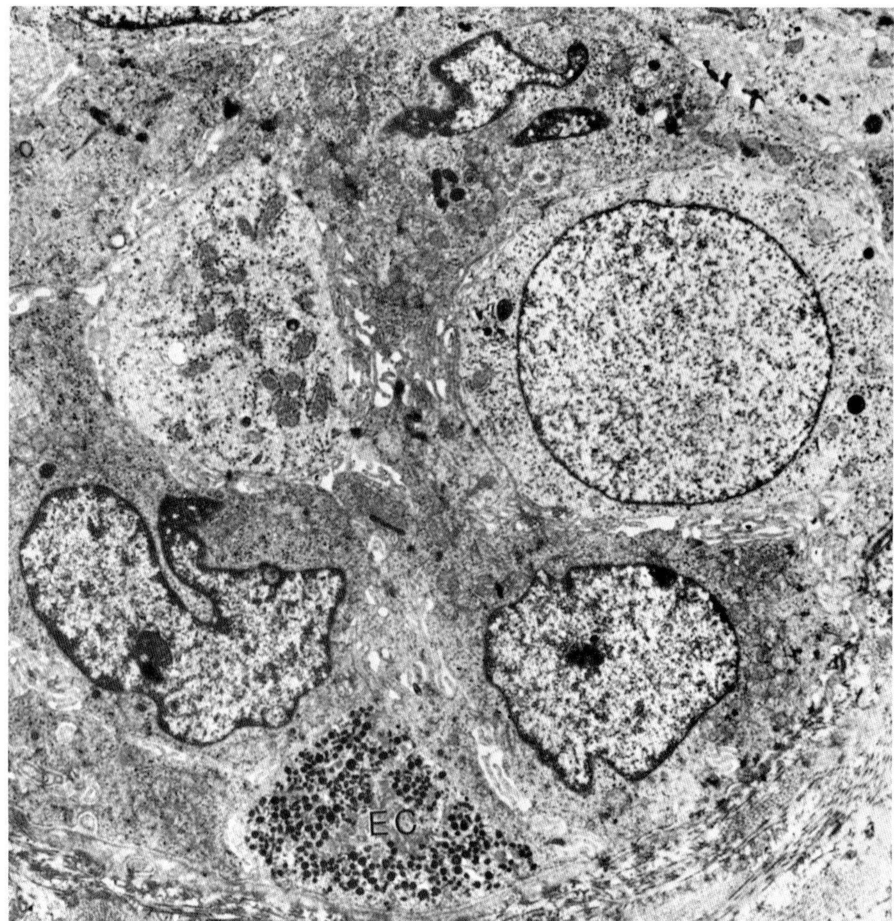

Fig. 65. Tangential section through the base of a prostatic acinus showing an enterochromaffin cell (*EC*), containing large aggregates of darkly staining cytoplasmic secretory granules, lying against the basement membrane. (Courtesy of G. AUMÜLLER.) ×4500

present in the enterochromaffin cells, measuring between about 150 and 800 Å in diameter (CASANOVA et al., 1974; AUMÜLLER et al., 1976).

Composition of the granules and the functional significance of these cells remains to be established. It has been suggested that the enterochromaffin-like cells may control the afferent arm of a reflex responsible for activating urethral smooth muscle (RAMSDALE, 1974) and that the stellate small granule cells produce urogastrone, a component of male urine which inhibits gastric secretion (AUMÜLLER, 1979).

Sialomucin Cells. As with the neuro-endocrine cells of the prostatic duct epithelium, the function of the sialomucin secretory cells has not been defined. They occur in the central collicular region where, with enterochromaffin cells, they form a major component of the prostatic duct epithelium in zone 3 (Fig. 62).

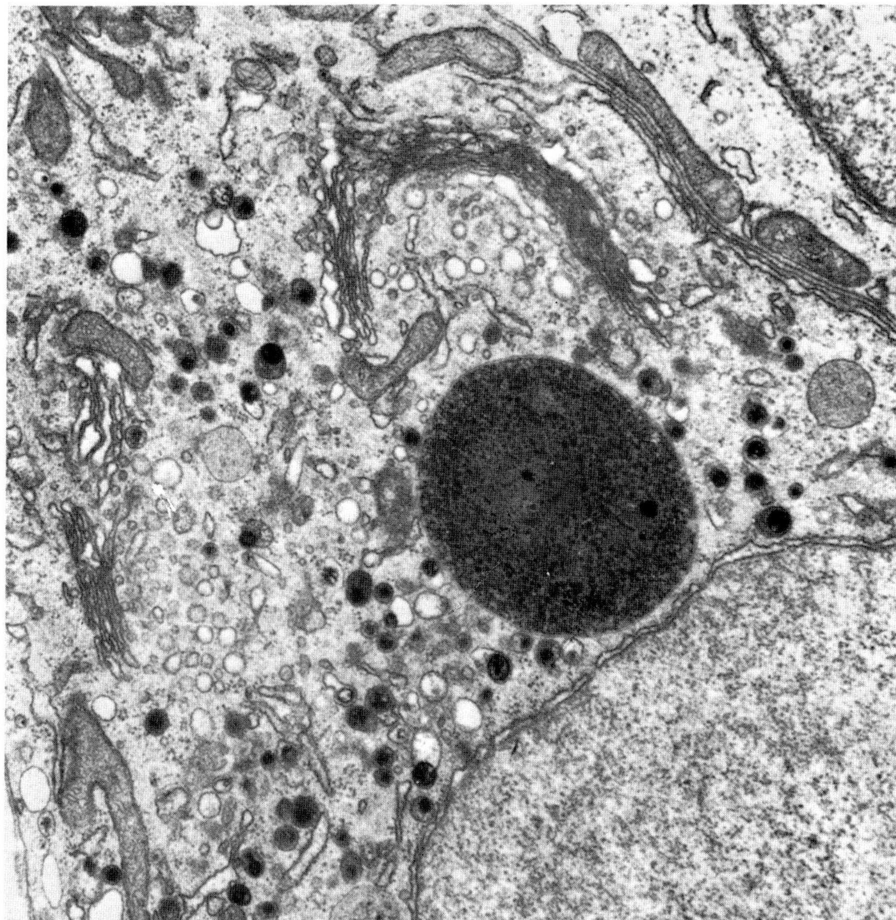

Fig. 66. High magnification electron micrograph of a stellate, small granule-containing endocrine cell showing profiles of Golgi cisternae, mitochondria, various forms of lysosomes and secretory granules. (Courtesy of G. AUMÜLLER.) ×32750

They are cuboidal or low columnar in shape, about 15 µm high and contain an ovoid basal nucleus with marginal or eccentric nucleolus. These cells contain large quantities of glycogen and rough endoplasmic reticulum in their basal compartments, numerous mitochondria, and 600–850 Å membrane-bound secretory vesicles which are closely associated with profiles of rough endoplasmic reticulum in the supranuclear region (AUMÜLLER, 1979). The contents of the secretory vesicles show characteristic variations in homogeneity and electron density.

b) Lamina Propria

The lamina propria of the prostate typically consists of two parts: a smooth inner basal lamina 700–1000 Å thick and a peripheral layer of connective tissue elements. The peripheral layer varies in structure from a thin capsule, formed by a delicate network of reticular fibres (MARBET, 1948), around each prostatic acinus to a thick layer of collagen and elastin fibre bundles loosely arranged into an irregular meshwork around each terminal prostatic duct. Flat, irregularly shaped fibroblasts and smooth muscle cells are common elements within this layer, which gradually blends at its periphery with the swathes of intra- and interlobular smooth muscle and connective tissue. These form the interacinar septae, and the stromal sheaths which encapsulate and separate the prostatic lobules.

c) Muscularis

The stroma of the prostate is formed by three layers: the lamina propria, a connective tissue layer described in the previous section; an outer capsular layer of connective tissue; and an intermediate layer of muscular tissue – the muscularis – which forms the bulk of the stromal tissue (BLOOM and FAWCETT, 1975). At its apex, the prostate is closely associated with condensations of skeletal muscle which are components of the sphincter urethrae and the sling-like levatores prostatae, and are innervated by the pudendal nerve.

The arrangement of smooth muscle in the prostate has led to a zonal classification of the muscularis into periductal, interlobular, intralobular and perivascular components (MOORE, 1936). AUMÜLLER (1971) has, however, shown that this compartmentalization is to some extent contrived because of the continuity that exists between these smooth muscle compartments.

Prostatic smooth muscle has a distinct pattern of distribution. Deep to the connective tissue capsule of the gland is a dense subcapsular sheath of smooth muscle fibres with a predominantly circular orientation. Bundles of smooth muscle fibres arranged into radially oriented trabeculae extend from the subcapsular sheath as an irregular network between the lobules of the prostate towards the periurethral smooth muscle which encloses the colliculus seminalis and is continuous with the internal layer of the detrusor muscle of the bladder.

From these radial trabeculae, thinner branches of stromal tissue enter the substance of each lobule to form the intralobular septa, which provide a supporting framework for the intralobular glands. These intralobular septa are similar in arrangement to the interlobular trabeculae but contain fewer smooth muscle elements and comparatively more connective tissue components. The prostatic ducts are ensheathed by large bundles of longitudinally and circularly arranged smooth muscle fibres interspersed with bundles of collagen and elastin fibres in an amorphous extracellular matrix (AUMÜLLER, 1979).

Inside the lobules each acinus is enclosed in a thin capsule of smooth muscle fibre bundles separated by aggregates of stromal connective tissue. These bundles form sweeping arcs of smooth muscle fibres around each acinus, an arrangement that AUMÜLLER (1979) has suggested would ensure that equal pressure is conveyed to all parts of the acinus on contraction at ejaculation. A thin veil of elastin fibres separates the smooth muscle fibres from the periacinar collagen fibre bundles (STIEVE, 1930).

The smooth muscle cells which form the muscularis of the prostate are similar in structure to those already described for the seminal vesicles (see Sect. B.VI.3.c), and to smooth muscle cells in general (NAGASAWA and MITO, 1967). Each cell is 60–100 µm long and 46 µm wide (AUMÜLLER, 1979) and contains a lightly crenated nucleus, 8–12 µm in length. The size and shape of the nucleus appears to vary with the state of contraction of the cell. The nucleus of each cell is centrally placed and contains a small inconspicuous nucleolus and some peripheral aggregations of heterochromatin. Most of the cytoplasmic organelles are concentrated in a fibre-free zone of cytoplasm at either end of the nucleus. Age-dependent degeneration of prostatic smooth muscle cells is often associated with gradual accumulations of lipid droplets and glycogen granules in this zone (AUMÜLLER, 1979). Most of the cell cytoplasm is occupied by longitudinally arranged bundles of 60 Å diameter filaments which form the contractile apparatus of each cell. These filament bundles usually extend the length of each cell but at various places along the cell membrane decussated bundles can be observed attached to dense submembranous plaques of condensed fibrous proteins. The areas of plasma membrane between these plaques are characterized by numerous vesicular invaginations. Around each cell is a thin (500 Å) lamina sheath derived from material which resembles matrix of the basal lamina. Outside this layer, collagen and elastin fibres form an irregular meshwork which encloses each cell. These fibres often appear to be directly attached to the outer surface of the muscle cell plasma membrane.

The ratio of various connective tissue elements in the stroma of the prostate shows some regional differences (AUMÜLLER, 1971). Elastin fibres are fewer in peripheral regions of the gland but are numerous in the collicular region, where they are concentrated in dense networks of fibres parallel to the surface of colliculus. Collagen fibres form a stable framework throughout the gland, following the lines of smooth muscle fibres, but they appear more numerous in peripheral regions of the gland.

The ratio of stromal tissue elements in the prostate is also age dependent (KRATTER, 1950; AUMÜLLER, 1979). As in the seminal vesicle (see Sect. B.VI.3.c), increasing age results in degenerative changes in the prostatic stroma which leads to a decrease in the numbers of smooth muscle cells and a reduction in elastin fibre content of the stroma accompanied by increased densities of fibroblasts, macrophages, inflammatory cells and collagen fibres. Degenerative changes which are frequently observed in smooth muscle cells and fibroblasts include the accumulation of pigment granules, lipid droplets and glycogen granules, proliferation of rough endoplasmic reticulum, dilation of the Golgi cisterna, degeneration of cytoplasmic organelles and the appearance of dense and myelin bodies within the cells.

VIII. Bulbo-urethral and Urethral Glands

1. Derivation and Development

The bulbo-urethral (COWPER's) and urethral (LITTRÉ's) glands are derivatives, like the prostate, of the urogenital sinus. These glands are not as extensively developed as the prostate but they appear to follow a similar sequence in their embryogenesis although, in contrast to the prostate, information on their development is sparse.

The bulbo-urethral glands originate as paired endodermal outpouchings of the membranous urethra. These outpouchings evaginate into the surrounding mesoderm, which later condenses to form the smooth and striated muscle associated with the glands and the adjacent musculature of the urogenital diaphragm and sphincter urethrae. Few details are available on the subsequent development of the bulbo-urethral glands. Assuming that the sequence of development is similar to that of the closely related prostate, it could be expected that the bulbo-urethral glands undergo a period of active cell proliferation and differentiation in the perinatal period, during which the glands enlarge and the tubulo-alveolar primordia from the urethral outpouches proliferate and form numerous branches, followed by a period of quiescence or slow growth and then a pubertal growth phase, induced by increasing androgen levels at puberty. During this phase the glands enlarge and commence their normal adult secretory activity. As with other accessory glands of male reproduction, androgens are required to maintain normal structure and function of the bulbo-urethral gands.

The urethral glands are derived from a series of evaginations of the urethral epithelium, which are usually restricted to the roof of the penile urethra. There appear to be no published accounts of the embryogenesis or the perinatal and postnatal development of these glands, nor is there evidence to indicate if the urethral glands in man are dependent on circulating androgens for their development or continued function in the adult.

2. General Anatomy

In the adult male, the bulbo-urethral glands are two small, rounded glandular structures, 0.4–1 cm in diameter (Hollinshead, 1966), which lie within the musculature of the urogenital diaphragm at either side of the urethra, in close relation to the sphincter urethrae and the deep transverse perineus muscle and beneath or adjacent to the base of the bulb of the penis. Each gland is connected to the urethra by an excretory duct about 3 or 4 cm long (Sikorski, 1977), which usually penetrates the superficial fascia of the urogenital diaphragm (perineal membrane), passes into the substance of the bulb of the penis and enters the floor of the bulbous urethra just lateral to midline. Variations to this pattern exist; in a few individuals the ducts have been observed to enter the membranous rather than the bulbous urethra.

As stated in Sect. B.VIII.1, the urethral glands develop as outpouchings of the roof of the penile urethra. However, perhaps because of the constraints imposed by the peri-urethral connective tissue fascia, the urethral glands are not as extensively developed in the adult as the other glandular derivatives of the urethral epithelium. Each definitive urethral gland can be subdivided into two distinct parts: an outer system of branched tubular glands, from which the thin, watery mucous of the urethral glands is secreted, and an inner collecting chamber or recess, the *lacuna of Morgagni,* which connects peripherally to the tubular glands and opens centrally into the urethra.

Blood supply to the bulbo-urethral glands is from branches of the deep artery to the penis and that to the urethral glands is via small penetrating branches from the dorsal artery of the penis (HOLLINSHEAD, 1966; LASINSKI and SIKORSKI, 1975). Both these main arteries are terminal branches of the internal pudendal artery.

Venous drainage of the urethral glands is via the deep dorsal vein of the penis to the prostatic venous plexus. Venous drainage from this plexus to the internal iliac vein has been described previously (see Sect. B.VII.2.b). Most of the venous blood from the bulbo-urethral glands is drained by the internal pudendal veins although a minor volume drains to the deep dorsal vein of the penis, which communicates with the internal pudendal vein close to the prostatic plexus. The internal pudendal veins begin as venae comitantes of the internal pudendal artery that unite to form a single vessel, which then drains into the internal iliac vein.

Lymph drainage from the bulbo-urethral glands accompanies that from the membranous urethra in lymphatic vessels associated with the internal pudendal artery. These vessels drain mostly to internal iliac lymph nodes although a few may pass to external iliac nodes. Lymph from the urethral glands mostly drains in lymphatic vessels of the penile urethra to the deep inguinal lymph nodes and less commonly to the external iliac nodes.

3. Cytological Features

Few cytological studies have been made of the bulbo-urethral and urethral glands and no ultrastructural details are available. Consequently, information from brief accounts given in various texts have been combined to provide the data for this section.

The bulbo-urethral glands consist of large glandular lobules separated by trabeculae of stromal connective tissue and enclosed in a thick capsule (HOLLINSHEAD, 1966; BLOOM and FAWCETT, 1975). The lobules of glandular tissue measure 1–3 mm in diameter and each is drained by an interlobular duct, which in turn drains into the main secretory duct.

Externally the glands are enclosed in a thick layer of skeletal muscle derived from the deep perineal and bulbocavernosus muscles.

The glandular tissue consists of compound tubulo-alveolar glands. The tubules and interconnecting ducts have irregular diameters and the terminal secreting portions are tubular or alveolar in shape, or occasionally cyst-like dilatations. The glands are lined by a simple epithelium, which varies in height from columnar in the tubular portions to cuboidal or sometimes squamous in distended alveoli and the cystic dilatations. Principal secretory cells resemble mucous-secreting gland cells with basally situated nuclei and numerous cytoplasmic granules and secretory droplets. The connective tissue stroma which separates the lobules of glandular tissue consists of fibro-elastic tissue containing a few muscle fibres. Smooth and skeletal muscle fibres are numerous in the major interlobular septae.

The smaller intralobular ducts are lined by a simple cuboidal secretory epithelium. These ducts unite and drain into the main secretory duct, which is lined by a pseudostratified epithelium in its proximal region but gradually changes distally into a stratified columnar epithelium, similar to the lining of the urethra (BLOOM and FAWCETT, 1975; COPENHAVER et al., 1978). Isolated patches of secretory cells occur along the main duct, especially in its proximal region.

Blood vessels which supply the glandular tissue are carried in the capsular connective tissue. These send secondary branches along the septae, which terminate as capillary beds around the glandular tissue of the lobules.

The bulbo-urethral glands secrete a mucoid exudate rich in sialic acids which appears to function as a lubricant for the urethral epithelium at ejaculation.

The two structural components of the urethral glands, the lacunae of Morgagni and their associated glands of Littré, have different epithelial linings. The branched tubular glands of Littré extend deep into the stroma and are lined by a simple columnar epithelium of mucous-secreting cells.

The deep irregular outpocketings which comprise the lacunae of Morgagni are lined by a stratified columnar epithelium, similar to the urethral epithelium, which is occasionally interspersed by small isolated islands of mucous cells like those of the tubular glands. The secretion of the urethral glands is similar to that of the bulbo-urethral glands and it probably functions to lubricate the penile urethra.

Acknowledgments. Many people contributed to the preparation of this chapter. In particular we wish to thank Professors G. AUMÜLLER, E. BUSTOS-OBREGON, ANITA P. HOFFER, A.F. HOLSTEIN and E.C. ROOSEN-RUNGE for providing illustrations and for their kind permission to use them. We also thank SUE SIMPSON for preparing line illustrations; TERRY MARTIN for assistance with photography; ROBYN PEAKE and ELIZABETH WALSH for tissue preparations and ultramicrotomy; JEAN CODDINGTON, NOLA JONES and CHRISTINE WITTON for typing the manuscript; and MEREDITH and MARGARET TAYLOR for assistance with referencing and proof-reading.

References

Afzelius BA (1976) A human syndrome caused by immotile cilia. Science 193:317–319

Akutsu S (1903) Beiträge zur Histologie der Samenblasen nebst Bemerkungen über Lipochrome. Virchows Arch 168:467–485

Alford FP, Baker HWG, Burger HG, de Kretser DM, Hudson B, Johns M, Masterton JP, Patel YC, Rennie CG (1973) Temporal patterns of integrated plasma hormone levels during sleep and wakefulness. 2. follicle stimulating hormone, luteinizing hormone, testosterone and oestradiol. J Clin Endocrinol Metab 37:848–854

Amoss M, Burgus R, Blackwell R, Vale W, Fellows R, Guillemin R (1971) Purification, amino acid composition and N-terminus of the hypothalamic LRF of ovine origin. Biochem Biophys Res Commun 44:205–210

Andrews GS (1951) The histology of the human foetal and prepubertal prostates. J Anat (Lond) 85:44–54

Aoki A, Fawcett DW (1978) Is there a local feedback from the seminiferous tubules affecting activity of the Leydig cells? Biol Reprod 19:144–158

Aumüller G (1971) Zur Gefäß- und Muskelarchitektur der menschlichen Prostata. Z Anat Entwicklungsgesch 135:88–100

Aumüller G (1973) Zur funktionellen Morphologie der Bläschendrüse. Habilitationsschrift, Heidelberg

Aumüller G (1976) Fine structure of monkey (Macaca mulatta) male accessory sex glands, juvenile and adult. Z Mikrosk Anat Forsch 90:545–556

Aumüller G (1979) Prostate gland and seminal vesicles. In: Bargmann W (ed) Handbuch der mikroskopischen Anatomie des Menschen, vol VII/6. Springer, Berlin Heidelberg New York

Aumüller G, Bruhl B (1977) Über den Bau der Ampulla ductus deferentis des Menschen. Verh Anat Ges 71:561–564

Aumüller G, Metz W, Grube D (1976) Elektronen- und Fluoreszenz-mikroskopische Untersuchungen an der menschlichen Prostata. Verh Anat Ges 70:895–903

Baker HWG, Burger HG, de Kretser DM, Hudson B, O'Connor S, Wang C, Mirovics A, Court J, Dunlop M, Rennie GC (1976) Changes in the pituitary-testicular system with age. Clin Endocrinol (Oxf) 5:349–372

Banchietti FR, Gambetta G, Marzolla S (1956) La vascularizzatione arteriosa della prostata. Ricerche anatomo-radiologiche Urologia 23:1–10

Bargmann W (1977) Histologie und mikroskopische Anatomie des Menschen. 7. Aufl Thieme, Stuttgart

Battaglia G (1956) Prime osservazioni sui movimenti dell'epididimo del ratto in culture organotipiche rotanti. Bol Soc Ital Biol Sper 32:265–267

Baumgarten HG, Falck B, Holstein AF, Owman C, Owman T (1968) Adrenergic innervation of the human testis, epididymis, ductus deferens and protate: a fluorescence microscopic and fluorimetric study. Z Zellforsch Mikrosk Anat 90:81–95

Baumgarten HG, Holstein AF, Rosengren E (1971) Arrangement, ultrastructure and adrenergic innervation of smooth musculature of the ductuli efferentes, ductus epididymidis and ductus deferens of man. Z Zellforsch 120:37–79

Bedford JM (1963) Morphological changes in rabbit spermatozoa during passage through the epididymis. J Reprod Fertil 5:169–177

Bedford JM (1965) Changes in fine structure of the rabbit sperm head during passage through the epididymis. J Anat 99:891–906

Bedford JM (1966) Development of the fertilizing ability of spermatozoa in the epididymis of the rabbit. Exp Zool 163:319–326

Bedford JM (1975) Maturation, transport and fate of spermatozoa in the epididymis.

In: Hamilton DW, Greep RO (eds) Handbook of physiology, sect 7, vol 5, pp 303–317. Williams & Wilkins, Baltimore

Beford JM (1977) Evolution of the scrotum. The epididymis as the prime mover? In: Calaby JH, Tyndale-Biscoe CH (eds) Reproduction and evolution. Australian Academy of Science, Canberra, pp 171–182

Bedford JM (1978) Anatomical evidence for the epididymis as the prime mover in the evolution of the scrotum. Am J Anat 152:483–508

Bedford JM, Calvin H, Cooper GW (1973) The maturation of spermatozoa in the human epididymis. J Reprod Fertil [Suppl] 18:199–213

Bennett G, Leblond CP, Haddad A (1974) Migration of glycoprotein from the Golgi apparatus to the surface of various cell types as shown by autoradiography after labelled fucose injection into rats. J Cell Biol 60:258–284

Benoit J (1926) Recherches anatomiques, cytologiques et histophysiologiques sur les voies excrétice du testicle, chez les mammifères. Arch Anat Histol Embryol (Strasb) 5:173–412

Bergh A, Helander HF, Wahlquist L (1978) Studies on factors governing testicular descent in the rat – particularly the role of gubernaculum testis. Int J Androl 1:342–356

Berthold R (1849) Transplantation der Hoden. Arch Anat Physiol Wiss Chem Med 16:42–46

Blacklock NJ, Bouskill K (1977) The zonal anatomy of the prostate in man and in the rhesus monkey (Macaca mulatta). Urol Res 5:163–167

Blandau RJ, Rumery RE (1964) The relationship of swimming movements of epididymal spermatozoa to their fertilizing capacity. Fertil Steril 15:571–579

Blaquier JA (1971) Selective uptake and metabolism of androgens by rat epididyms. The presence of a cytoplasmic receptor. Biochem Biophys Res Commun 45:1076–1082

Blaquier JA (1975) The influence of androgens on protein synthesis by cultured rat epididymal tubules Acta Endocrinol (Kbh) 79:403–414

Bloom W, Fawcett DW (1975) A textbook of histology, 10th ed. Saunders, Philadelphia

Bouin P, Ancel P (1903) Recherches sur les cellules interstitielles du testicule des mammiferes. Arch Zool (Stockh)1:437–523

Brady RO (1951) Biosynthesis of radioactive testosterone in vitro. J Biol Chem 193:145–148

Braithwaite JL (1952) The arterial supply of the male urinary bladder. Br J Urol 24:64–69

Brandes D (1966) The fine structure and histochemistry of prostatic glands in relation to sex hormones. Int Rev Cytol 20:207–276

Brandes D (1974) Fine structure and cytochemistry of male sex accessory organs. In: Brandes D (ed) Male accessory sex organs – structure and function in mammals. Academic Press, New York, pp 18–114

Brandt H, Acott TS, Johnson DJ, Hoskins DD (1978) Evidence for an epididymal origin of Bovine sperm forward motility protein. Biol Reprod 19:830–835

Bremner WJ, Paulsen CA (1974) Two pools of luteinizing hormone in the human pituitary: Evidence from constant administration of luteinizing hormone-releasing hormone. J Clin Endocrinol Metab 39:811–815

Brooks DE, Hamilton DW, Malleck AH (1974) Carnitine and glycerylphosphorylcholine in the reproductive tract of the male rat. J Reprod Fertil 36:141–160

Brueschke EE, Bruns M, Maness JH, Wingfield JR, Mayerhofer K, Zaneveld LJD (1974) Development of a reversible vas deferens occlusive devise. I. Anatomical size of the human and dog vas deferens. Fertil Steril 25:659–672

Bruhns C (1904) Untersuchungen über die Lymphgefäße und Lymphdrüsen der Prostata des Menschen. Arch Anat Physiol 1904:330–349

Burgos MH (1964) Uptake of colloidal particles by cells of the caput epididymis. Anat Rec 148:517–525

Burke WR, Aten RF, Eisenfeld AJ, Lytton B (1977) Androgen binding in human testis. J Urol 118:52–57

Burnstock G (1970) Structure of smooth muscle and its innervation. In: Bulbring E, Brading AF, Jones AW, Tomita T (eds) Smooth muscle. Arnold, London, pp 1–66

Bustos-Obregon E, Holstein AF (1976) The rete testis in man: ultrastructural aspects. Cell Tiss Res 175:1–15

Cady LD, Deakins R (1933) Studies of skin manifestations of visceral disease: I. The viscero-sensory aspect of prostato-vesiculitis. J Urol 30:123–137

Calvin HI, Bedford JM (1971) Formation of disulphide bonds in the nucleus and accessory structures of mammalian spermatozoa during maturation in the epididymis. J Reprod Fertil [Suppl] 13:65–75

Cameo MS, Blaquier JA (1976) Androgen controlled specific proteins in rat epididymis. J Endocrinol 69:47–55

Carmel PW, Araki S, Ferrin M (1976) Pituitary stalk portal blood collection in rhesus monkeys: Evidence for pulsatile release of gonadotrophin-releasing hormone (GnRH). Endocrinology 99:243–248

Casanova S, Corrado F, Vignoli G (1974) Endocrine-like cells in the epithelium of the human male urethra. J Submicr Cytol 6:435–438

Catt KJ, Dufau ML, Neaves WB, Walsh PC, Wilson JD (1975) LH-hCG receptors and testosterone content during differentiation of the testis in the rabbit embryo. Endocrinology 97:1157–1163

Chang MC, Hunter RHF (1975) Capacitation of mammalian sperm: biological and experimental aspects. In: Hamilton DW, Greep RO (eds) Handbook of physiology, sect 7, vol 5, pp 339–351. Williams & Wilkins, Baltimore

Christensen AK (1975) Leydig cells. In: Hamilton DW, Greep RO (eds) Handbook of physiology, sect 7, vol 5, pp 57–94. Williams & Wilkins, Baltimore

Christensen AK, Mason NR (1965) Comparative ability of seminiferous tubules and interstitial tissue of rat testes to synthesize androgen from progesterone-4-^{14}C in vitro. Endocrinology 76:646–656

Chwalla R, Zandanell E (1958) Untersuchungen über die Samenblasengröße bei Prostatikern, über die diffuse Prostatahyperplasie und die Samenblasenhyperplasie. Urol Int 1:199–242

Clegg EJ (1955) The arterial supply of the human prostate and seminal vesicles. J Anat (Lond) 89:209–219

Clermont Y (1963) The cycle of the seminiferous epithelium in man. Am J Anat 112:35–51

Clermont Y (1972) Kinetics of spermatogenesis in mammals. Seminiferous epithelium cycle and spermatogonial renewal. Physiol Rev 52:198–236

Comhaire F, Kunnen M (1975) Selective retrograde venography of the internal spermatic vein: A conclusive approach to the diagnosis of varicocele. Andrologia 8:11–24

Cooper TG, Hamilton DW (1977) Phagocytosis of spermatozoa in the terminal region and gland of the vas deferens of the rat. Am J Anat 150:247–268

Copenhaver WM, Kelly DE, Wood RL (1978) Bailey's Textbook of Histology, 17th ed. Williams & Wilkins, Baltimore

Crabo B (1965) Studies on the composition of epididymal content in bulls and boars. Acta Vet Scand 6 [Suppl]5:1–94

Danzo RJ, Orgebin-Crist MC, Toft DO (1973) Characterization of a cytoplasmic receptor for 5α-dihydrotestosterone in the caput epididymis of intact rabbit. Endocrinology 92:310–317

David K, Dingermanse E, Freud J, Laquer E (1935) Über krystallinisches männliches Hormon aus Hoden (Testosteron), wirksamer als aus Harn oder aus Cholesterin bereitetes Androsteron. Z Physiol Chem 233:281–282

Dawson RWC, Rowlands JW (1959) Glycerylphosphorylcholine in the male reproductive organs of rats and guinea pigs. O J Exp Physiol 44:26–34 de Kretser DM (1967a) The fine structure of the testicular interstitial cells in men of normal androgenic status. Z Zellforsch 80:594–609

de Kretser DM (1967b) Changes in the fine structure of the human testicular interstitial cells after treatment with human gonadotrophins. Z Zellforsch 83:344–358

de Kretser DM (1969) Ultrastructural features of human spermiogenesis. Z Zellforsch 98:477–505

de Kretser DM (1974) The management of the infertile male. Clin Obstet Gynaecol 1:409–427

de Kretser DM, Burger HG (1972) Ultrastructural studies of human Sertoli cells in normal men and males with hypogonadotrophic hypogonadism before and after gonadotrophic treatment. In: Saxena BB, Beling CG, Gandy HM (eds) Gonadotrophins. Wiley, New York, pp 640–656

de Kretser DM, Catt KJ, Paulsen CA (1971) Studies on the in vitro testicular binding of iodinated luteinizing hormone in rats. Endocrinology 88:332–337

de Kretser DM, Burger HG, Hudson B (1974) The relationship between germinal cells and serum FSH levels in males with infertility. J Clin Endocrinol Metab 38:787–793

de Kretser DM, Burger HG, Hudson B, Keogh EJ (1975) The HCG stimulation test in men with testicular disorders. Clin Endocrinol (Oxf) 4:591–596

de Kretser DM, Kerr JB, Paulsen CA (1975) The peritubular tissue in the normal and pathological human testis. An ultrastructural study. Biol Reprod 12:317–324

de Kretser DM, Bremner WJ, Burger HG, Eddie L, Hudson B, Keogh EJ, Lee VWK (1977) Control of FSH secretion. Excerpta Med Int Congr Ser No 402, 1:398–403

Dixon JS, Gosling JA, Ramsdale DR (1973) Urethral chromaffin cells. Z Zellforsch 138:397–406

Dorfman RI, Menon KMJ, Forchielli E (1968) Biosynthesis of testosterone in testis. Res Steroids 3:15–31

Dorrington JH, Armstrong DT (1975) Follicle stimulating hormone stimulates estradiol-17 β synthesis in culture Sertoli cells. Proc Natl Acad Sci USA 72:2677–2681

Dorrington JH, Roller NF, Fritz IB (1975) Effects of follicle stimulating hormone on cultures of Sertoli cell preparations. Mol Cell Endocrinol 3:57–70

Duclos JM, Chanzy M, Alexandre JH (1972) Contribution à l'étude de la vascularisation prostatique. Arch Anat Pathol 20:355–358

Dufau ML, Hsueh AJ, Cigorraga S, Baukal AJ, Catt KJ (1978) Inhibition of Leydig cell function through hormonal regulatory mechanisms. In J Androl [Suppl] 2:193–239

Düllman J (1967) Konstruktionsanalytische Untersuchungen am Ureter und der Glandula vesiculosa des Rhesusaffen. Acta Anat (Basel) 68:344–360

Dym M (1973) The fine structure of the Monkey (Macaca) Sertoli cell and its role in maintaining the blood-testis barrier. Anat Rec 175:639–656

Dym M (1974) The fine structure of monkey Sertoli cells in the transitional zone at the junction of the seminiferous tubules with the tubuli recti. Am J Anat 140:1–26

Dym M (1976) The mammalian rete testis – a morphological examination. Anat Rec 186:493–524

Dym M, Fawcett DW (1970) The blood-testis barrier in the rat and the physiological compartmentation of the seminiferous epithelium. Biol Reprod 3:308–326

Dym M, Fawcett DW (1971) Further observations on the numbers of spermatogonia, spermatocytes and spermatids connected by bridges in the mammalian testis. Biol Reprod 4:195–215

Dym M, Romrell LJ (1975) Intraepithelial lymphocytes in the male reproductive tract of rats and rhesus monkeys. J Reprod Fertil 42:1–7

Dyson AL, Orgebin-Crist MC (1973) Effect of hypophysectomy, castration and androgen replacement upon the fertilizing ability of rat epididymal spermatozoa. Endocrinology 93:391–402

Ebner V von (1902) Männliche Geschlechtsorgane. In: Koelliker A (Hrsg) Handbuch der Gewebelehre des Menschen, 6. Aufl. Bd. III. S 402–505. Engelmann, Leipzig

Edwardson JA, Gilbert D (1975) Sensitivity of selfpotentiating effect of luteinizing hormone-releasing hormone to cycloheximide. Nature 255:71

Eliasson R, Mossberg B, Camner P, Afzelius BA (1977) The immotile-cilia syndrome. N Engl J Med 297:1–6

Fawcett DW (1975) Ultrastructure and function of the Sertoli cell. In: Greep RO, Hamilton DW (eds) Handbook of physiology, sect 7, vol 5. pp 21–55. Baltimore, Williams & Wilkins

Fawcett DW, Burgos MH (1960) Studies on the fine structure of the mammalian testis. II. The human interstitial tissue. Am J Anat 107:245–269

Fawcett DW, Hollenberg RD (1963) Changes in the acrosome of the guinea pig spermatozoa during passage through the epididymis. Z Zellforsch 60:276–292

Fawcett DW, Neaves WB, Flores MN (1973) Comparative observations on intertubular lymphatics and the organization of the interstitial tissue of the mammalian testis. Biol Reprod 9:500–532

Ferner H, Zaki CH (1969) Mikroskopische Anatomie des Hodens und der ableitenden Samenwege. In: Alken CE, Dix VW, Goodwin WE, Wildbolz E (eds) Handbuch der Urologie Bd. 1, S 410–475. Springer, Berlin Heidelberg New York

Feyrter F (1951) Über das urogenitale Helle-Zellen-System des Menschen. Z Mikrosk Anat Forsch 57:324–344

Ficher M, Steinberger E (1968) Conversion of progesterone to androsterone by testicular tissue at different stages of maturation. Steroids 12:491–506

Fisher ER, Sieracki JC (1970) Ultrastructure of human normal and neoplastic prostate. Pathology Annu (Lond) 5:1–26

Flickinger CJ (1967) The postnatal development of the Sertoli cells of the mouse. Z Zellforsch 78:92–113

Flickinger CJ (1972) The fine structure of the interstitial tissue of the rat prostate. Am J Anat 134:107–126

Flickinger CJ (1973) Regional variations in endoplasmic reticulum in the vas deferens of normal and vasectomized rats. Anat Rec 176:205–224

Flocks RH (1925) The arterial distribution within the prostate gland. Its role in transurethral prostatic resection. J Urol 37:524–548

Forest MG, Cathiard AM (1975) Pattern of plasma testosterone and Δ^4 androstenedione in normal newborns: evidence for testicular activity at birth. J Clin Endocrinol Metab 41:977–980

Fournier S (1966) Distribution of sialic acid in the genital system of adult normal and castrated Wistar rats. Compt Rend Soc Biol 160:1087–1090

Frankel AI, Eik-Nes KB (1970) Metabolism of steroids in the rabbit epididymis. Endocrinology 87:646–652

Fränkel M (1901) Die Samenblasen des Menschen mit besonderer Berücksichtigung ihrer Topographie, Gefäßversorgung und ihres feineren Baues. Hirschwald, Berlin

Frazão JV (1949) Aspects histophysiologiques de la vésicule séminale humaine. Arch Port Sci Biol 10:95–98

Free MJ, Jaffe RA, Jain SK, Gomes WR (1973) Testosterone concentrating mechanism in the reproductive organs of the male rat. Nature New Biol 244:24–26

French FS, Ritzen EM (1973) A high-affinity androgen-binding protein (ABP) in rat testis: evidence for secretion into efferent duct fluid and absorption by epididymis. Endocrinology 93:88–95

Frenkel G, Peterson RN, Davis JE, Freund M (1974) Glycerylphosphorylcholine and carnitine in normal human semen and in post-vasectomy semen: differences in concentrations. Fertil Steril 25:84–96

Friend DS, Farquar MG (1967) Functions of coated vesicles during protein absorption in the rat vas deferens. J Cell Biol 35:357–376

Gaddum P, Glover TD (1965) Some reactions of rabbit spermatozoa to ligation of the epididymis. J Reprod Fertil 9:119–130

Gledhill BL, Gledhill MP, Rigler R, Ringertz NR (1966) Changes in deoxyribonucleoprotein during spermatogenesis in the bull. Exp Cell Res 41:652–665

Glenister RW (1962) The development of the utricle and of the so-called middle or median lobe of the human prostate. J Anat (Lond) 96:443–455

Glover TD (1969) Some aspects of function in the epididymis. Int J Fertil 14:216–221

Glover TD, Nicander L (1971) Some aspects of structure and function in the mammalian epididymis. J Reprod Fertil 13:39–70

Gray H (1973) Gray's Anatomy, 35th ed Warwick R, Williams P (eds). Longman. Edinburgh

Griswold MD, Solari A, Tung PS, Fritz IB (1977) Stimulation by follicle stimulating hormone of DNA synthesis and of mitosis in cultured Sertoli cells prepared from testes of immature rats. Mol Cell Endocrinol 7:151–165

Gunsalus GL, Musto NA, Bardin CW (1978) Immunoassay of androgen binding protein in blood: A new approach for study of the seminiferous tubule. Science 200:66

Hagenas L, Ritzen EM (1976) Impaired Sertoli cell function in experimental cryptorchidism. Mol Cell Endocrinol 4:25–34

Håkanson R, Larsson LL, Sjöberg NO, Sundler F (1974) Amine-producing endocrine-like cells in the epithelium of urethra and prostate of the guinea pig. A chemical, fluorescence histochemical, and electron microscopic study. Histochemistry 38:259–270

Hall PF, Irby DC, de Kretser DM (1969) Conversion of cholesterol to androgens by rat testis: comparison of interstitial cells and seminiferous tubules. Endocrinology 84:488–496

Hamilton DW (1971) Steroid function in the mammalian epididymis. J Reprod Fertil [Suppl] 13:89–97

Hamilton DW (1972) The mammalian epididymis. In: Balin H, Glasser S (eds) Reproductive biology. Excerpta Medica. Amsterdam, pp 268–337

Hamilton DW (1975) Structure and function of the epithelium lining the ductuli efferentes, ductus epididymidis, and ductus deferens in the rat. In: Hamilton DW, Greep RO (eds) Handbook of physiology, sect 7, vol 5, pp 259–301. Williams & Wilkins, Baltimore

Hamilton DW, Cooper TG (1978) Gross and histological variations along the length of the rat vas deferens. Anat Rec 190:795–810

Hamilton DW, Fawcett DW (1970) In vitro synthesis of cholesterol and testosterone from acetate by rat epididymis and vas deferens. Proc Soc Exp Biol Med 133:693–695

Hamilton DW, Jones AL, Fawcett DW (1969) Cholesterol biosynthesis in the mouse epididymis and ductus deferens: a biochemical and morphological study. Biol Reprod 1:167–184

Hansson V, Ritzen EM, French FS, Nayfeh S (1975a) Androgen transport and receptor mechanisms in testis and epididymis. In: Hamilton DW, Greep RO (eds) Handbook of physiology, sect 7, vol 5, pp 173–201. Williams & Wilkins, Baltimore

Hansson V, Ritzen EM, French FS, Weddington SC, Nayfeh SC (1975b) Testicular androgen binding protein (ABP): Comparison of ABP in rabbit testis and epididymis with a similar androgen binding protein (TeBG) in rabbit serum. Mol Cell Endocrinol 3:1–20

Harrison RG, Barclay AE (1948) The distribution of the testicular artery (internal spermatic artery) to the human testis. Br J Urol 20:57–66

Heidenhain M, Werner F (1924) Über die Epithelzellen des Corpus epididymidis beim Menschen. Z Anat Entwickl-Gesch 72:556–608

Heller CG, Clermont Y (1964) Kinetics of the germinal epithelium in man. Recent Prog Horm Res 20:545–575

Hemeida NA, Sack WO, McEntee K (1978) Ductuli efferentes in the epididymis of the boar, goat, ram bull and stallion. Am J Vet Res 39:1892–1900

Hoffer AP (1976) The ultrastructure of the ductus deferens in man. Biol Reprod 14:425–443

Hoffer AP, Greenberg J (1978) The structure of the epididymis, efferent ductules and ductus deferens of the guinea pig: A light microscope study. Anat Rec 190:659–678

Hoffer AP, Hamilton DW, Fawcett DW (1973) The ultrastructure of the principal cells and intraepithelial leucocytes in the initial segment of the rat epididymis. Anat Rec 175:169–202

Hollinshead WH (1966) Anatomy for surgeons, vol 2: The thorax, abdomen and pelvis. Harper & Row, New York

Holstein AF (1969) Morphologische Studien am Nebenhoden des Menschen. In: Bargmann W. Doerr W (eds) Zwanglose Abhandlungen aus dem Gebiet der normalen und pathologischen Anatomie. Thieme, Stuttgart

Holstein AF (1976a) Ultrastructural observations on the differentiation of spermatids in man. Andrologia 8:157–165

Holstein AF (1976b) Structure of the human epididymis. In: Hafez ESE (ed) Human semen and fertility regulation in men. Mosby, Saint Louis, pp 23–30

Horstmann E (1962) Die Elektronenmikroskopie des menschlichen Nebenhodenepithels. Z Zellforsch Mikrosk Anat 57:692–699

Hoskins DD, Casillas ER (1975) Function of cyclic nucleotides in mammalian spermatozoa. In: Hamilton DW, Greep RO (eds) Handbook of physiology, sect 7, vol 5, pp 453–460. Williams & Wilkins, Baltimore

Hovelacque A (1931/32) Les vesicules seminales et leur loge. Arch Mal Reins 6:28–51

Howards SS, Johnson A, Jessee S (1975) Micropuncture and microanalytical studies of the rat testis and epididymis. Fertil Steril 26:13–19

Hsu AF, Nankin HR, Troen P (1977) Androgen binding protein in human testis: Effect of age. In: Troen P, Nankin HR (eds) The testes in normal and infertile men. Raven, New York, pp 421–427

Inano H, Machino A, Tamaoki Bl (1969) *In vitro* metabolism of adult rats. Endocrinology 84:997–1003

Ivanov AV (1970) Blood and lymph vessels of the human prostate gland in health and disease. In: Holstein AF, Horstmann E (eds) Morphological aspects of andrology. vol 1, pp 151–152

Jirasek JE (1967) Morphogenesis of the genital system in the human. In: Blandau RJ, Bergsma D, Paul NW (eds) Morphogenesis and malformation of the genital system. Alan R. Liss, New York, pp 13–40

Johnson AL, Howards SS (1977) Hyperosmolality in intraluminal fluids from hamster testis and epididymis: A micropuncture study. Science 195:492–493

Johnson FP (1920) The later development of the urethra in the male. J Urol 4:447–503

Jost A, Vigier B, Prepin J, Perchelet JP (1973) Studies on sex differentiation in mammals. Recent Prog Horm Res 29:1–35

Jost A, Magre S, Cressent M (1974) Sertoli cells and early testicular differentiation. In: Mancini RE, Martini L (eds) Male fertility and sterility. Academic Press, New York, pp 1–11

Josso N, Picard J, Tran D (1977) The antimullerian hormone. Recent Prog Horm Res 33:117–163

Kastendieck H (1977) Ultrastrukturpathologie der menschlichen Prostatadrüse: Cyto- und

Histomorphogenese von Atrophie, Hyperplasie, Metaplasie, Dysplasie und Carcinom. Veröffentl. aus der Pathologie, H 106. Fischer, Stuttgart.

Kazzazz BA (1974) Argentaffin and argyrophil cells in the prostate. J Pathol 112:189–193

Kelch RP, Jenner MR, Weinstein R, Kaplan SL, Grumbach MM (1972a) Estradiol and testosterone secretion by human, simian and canine testes, in males with hypogonadism and in male pseudohermaphrodites with the feminizing testes syndrome. J Clin Invest 51:824–839

Kelch RP, Grunbach MM. Kaplan SL (1972b) Studies on the mechanism of puberty in man. In: Saxena BB, Beling CG, Gandy HM (eds) Gonadotropins. Wiley, New York, pp 524–534

Kerr JB, de Kretser DM (1975) Cyclic variations in Sertoli cell lipid content throughout the spermatogenic cycle in the rat. J Reprod Fertil 43:1–8

Kerr JB, Rich KA, de Kretser DM (1979) Alterations of the fine structure and androgen secretion of the interstitial cells in the experimentally cryptorchid rat testis. Biol Reprod 20:409–422

Kimura Y, Miyata K, Adachi K, Kisaki N (1975) Peripheral nerves controlling the closure of internal urethral orifice during ejaculation. Urol Int 30:218–227

Kohengkul S, Tanphaichtir V, Muangmun V, Tangphaichtir N (1977) Levels of L-carnitine and L-O-acetylcarnitine in normal and infertile human semen: a lower level of L-O-acetylcarnitine in infertile semen. Fertil Steril 28:1333–1339

Kratter V (1950) Modificazioni strutturali dello stroma della prostata umare nelle varie eta. Arch Ital Anat Istol Pat 23:3–25

Kurosawa T (1930) Beitrag zur Pathologie der Samenblase. Virchows Arch 274:594–605

Lacy D (1960) Light and electron microscopy and its use in the study of factors influencing spermatogenesis in the rat. J Microscop Soc 79:209–225

Ladman AJ (1967) The fine structure of the ductuli efferentes of the opossum. Anat Rec 157:559–576

Ladman AJ, Young WC (1958) An electron microscopic study of the ductuli efferentes and rete testis of the guinea pig. J Biophys Biochem Cytol 4:219–226

Langerhans P (1875) Über die accessorischen Drüsen der Geschlechtsorgane. Virchows Arch [Pathol Anat] 61:208–228

Lasinski W, Sikorski A (1975) La vascularisation arterielle des glandes bulbo-urétrales humaines. Bull Assoc Anat 175:167–171

Last RJ (1978) Anatomy: Regional and applied, 6th ed. Churchill Livingstone, Edinburgh

Levine N, Marsh DJ (1971) Micropuncture studies of the electrochemical aspects of fluid and electrolyte transport in individual seminiferous tubules, the epididymis and the vas deferens in rats. J Physiol (Lond) 213:557–570

Lipsett MB, Wilson H, Kirschner MA, Korenman SG, Fishman LM, Sarfaty GA, Bardin CW (1966) Studies on Leydig cell physiology and pathology: Secretion and metabolism of testosterone. Recent Prog Horm Res 22:245–281

Lording DW, de Kretser DM (1972) Comparative ultrastructural and histochemical studies of the interstitial cells of the rat testis during fetal and postnatal development. J Reprod Fertil 29:261–270

Lowsley OS (1912) The development of the human prostate gland with reference to the development of other structures at the neck of the urinary bladder. Am J Anat 13:299–349

Macleod J, Pazianos A, Ray B (1966) The restoration of human spermatogenesis and of the reproductive tract with urinary gonadotropins following hypophysectomy. Fertil Steril 17:7–23

Maddock WO, Nelson WO (1952) The effects of chorionic gonadotrophin in adult men: Increased estrogen, 17-ketosteroid excretion, gynecomastia, Leydig cell stimulation and seminiferous tubule damage. J Clin Endocrinol Metab 12:985–1007

Mancini RE, Vilar O, Donini P, Perez-Lloret A (1971) Effect of human urinary FSH and LH on the recovery of spermatogenesis in hypophysectomized patients. J Clin Endocrinol Metab 33:888–895

Maneely RB (1959) Epididymal structure and function: a historical and critical review. Acta Zool (Stockh) 40:1–21

Mann T (1964) The biochemistry of semen and of the male reproductive tract. Methuen, London

Mao P, Angrist A (1966) The fine structure of the basal cell of the human prostate. Lab Invest 15:1768–1782

Marberger H (1974) The mechanisms of ejaculation. In: Coutinho EM, Fuchs F (eds) Physiology and genetics of reproduction. Plenum Press, London, part 3, pp 99–110

Marbet T (1948) Über die Gitterfasern in der menschlichen Prostata. Acta Anat (Basel) 5:380–391

Marquis NR, Fritz IB (1965) Effects of testosterone on the distribution of carnitine, acetyl-carnitine and carnitine acetyltransferase in tissues of the reproductive system of the male rat. J Biol Chem 240:2197–2200

Martan J, Risley PL, Hruban Z (1964) Holocrine cells of the human epididymis. Fertil Steril 15:180–187

McNeal JE (1972) The prostate and prostatic urethra: A morphologic synthesis. J Urol 107:1008–1016

Mc Neal JE (1978) Origin and evolution of benign prostatic enlargement. Invest Urol 15:340–345

Means AR, Huckins C (1974) Coupled events in the early biochemical actions of FSH on the Sertoli cell of the testis. In: Dufau ML, Means AR (eds) Hormone binding and target cell activation in the testis. Plenum, New York, pp 145–165

Means AR, Fakunding JL, Huckins C, Tindall DJ, Vitale R (1976) Follicle stimulating hormone, the Sertoli cell and spermatogenesis. Recent Prog Horm Res 32:477–525

Mitchell GAG (1935) The innervation of the kidney, ureter testicle and epididymis. J Anat (Lond) 70:10–32

Mitchell GAG (1938) The innervation of the ovary, uterine tube, testis and epididymis. J Anat (Lond) 72:508–517

Montorzi NM, Burgos MH (1967) Uptake of colloidal particles by cells of the ductuli efferentes of the hamster. Z Zellforsch 83:58–69

Moore KL (1973) The developing human: clinically oriented embryology. Saunders, Philadelphia

Moore RA (1936) The evolution and involution of the prostate gland. Am J Pathol 12:599–624

Morita I (1966) Some observations on the fine structure of the human ductuli efferentes. Arch Histol Jpn 26:341–356

Muggli R, Baumgartner HR (1972) Pattern of membrane invagination at the surface of smooth muscle cells of rabbit arteries. Experientia 28:1212

Nagasawa J, Mito S (1967) Electron microscope observations on the innervation of the smooth muscle. Tokohu J Exp Med 91:277–293

Nagy F, Edmonds RH (1975) Cellular proliferation and renewal in the various zones of the hamster epididymis after colchicine administration. Fertil Steril 26:460–468

Narbaitz R (1974) Embryology, anatomy and histology of the male sex accessory glands. In: Brandes D (ed) Male accessory sex organs – structure and function in mammals. Academic Press, New York, pp 3–17

Netter FH (1954) The CIBA collection of medical illustrations, vol 2: Reproductive system. Oppenheimer E (ed) CIBA Pharmaceutical Products Inc., Summit, New Jersey, pp 1–286

Nicander L (1957a) On the regional histology and cytochemistry of the ductus epididymids in the rabbit. Acta Morphol Neerl Scand 1:99–118

Nicander L (1957b) Studies on the regional histology and cytochemistry of the ductus epididymids in stallions, rams and bulls. Acta Morphol Neerl Scand 1:337–362

Nicander L (1965) An electron microscopical study of absorbing cells in the posterior caput epididymis of rabbits. Z Zellforsch 66:829–847

Nickerson M (1970) Drugs inhibiting adrenergic nerves and structures innervated by them. In: Goodman LS, Gilman A (eds) The pharmacological basis of therapeutics. London, MacMillan, pp 549–584

Nilsson S, Bengmark S (1962) The human seminal vesicle. A morphogenetic and gross anatomic study with special regard to changes due to age and to prostatic adenoma. Acta Chir Scand [Suppl] 296:1–96

Norberg K-A, Risley PL, Ungerstedt U (1967) Adrenergic innervation of the male reproductive ducts in some mammals. I. The distribution of adrenergic nerves. Z Zellforsch 76:278–286

Oberndorfer S (1901) Beiträge zur Anatomie und Pathologie der Samenblasen. Zeiglers Beitr. Pathologie 31:325–346

Odell WD, Swerdloff RS, Jacobs HS, Hescox MA (1973) FSH induction of sensitivity to LH: one cause of sexual maturation in the male rat. Endocrinology 92:160–165

Ohno S (1977) Control of meiotic process. In: Troen P, Nankin HR (eds) The testis in normal and infertile men. Raven Press, New York, pp 1–8

Orcini L, Perrelet A (1973) Membrane-associated particles: increase at sites of pinocytosis demonstrated by freeze-etching. Science 181:868–869

Orgebin-Crist MC (1967) Maturation of spermatozoa in the rabbit epididymis: fertilizing ability and embryonic mortality in does inseminated with epididymal spermatozoa. Ann Biol Anim Biochim Biophys 7:373–389

Orgebin-Crist MC (1969) Studies on the function the epididymis. Biol Reprod [Suppl] 1:155–175

Orth J, Christensen AK (1978) Autoradiographic localization of specifically bound ^{125}I-labelled follicle stimulating hormone on spermatogonia of the rat testis. Endocrinology 103:1944–1951

Paloma A (1949) Radical cure of varicocele by a new technique: preliminary report. J Urol 61:604–607

Pallin G (1901) Beiträge zur Anatomie und Embryologie der Prostata und der Samenblasen. Arch Anat Physiol Anat Abt 1901:134–176

Parker A (1936) The lymph vessels from the posterior urethra, their regional lymph nodes and relationships to the main posterior abdominal lymph channels. J Urol 36:538–556

Parvinen M, Hansson V, Ritzen EM (1980) Functional cycle of rat sertoli cells: Differential binding and action of FSH at various stages of the spermatogenic cycle. In: Steinberger A (ed) Proceedings of 6th Testis Workshop, Raven, New York, pp 425–432

Paufler SK, Foote RH (1968) Morphology, motility and fertility of spermatozoa recovered from different areas of ligated rabbit epididymides. J Reprod Fertil 17:125–137

Paulsen CA (1966) The effect of human menopausal gonadotrophin on spermatogenesis in hypogonadotrophic hypogonadism. Excerpta Med Int Congr Ser 112:398–407

Paulsen CA (1974) The Testis. In: Williams RH (ed) Textbook of endocrinology, 5th ed, pp 323–367. Saunders, Philadelphia

Paulsen CA, Gordon DL, Carpenter RW, Gandy HM, Drucker WD (1968) Klinefelter's syndrome and its variants: a hormonal and chromosomal study. Recent Prog Horm Res 24:321–363

Pearson OJ, Tubbs PK (1967) Carnitine and derivatives in rat tissue. Biochem J 105:593–963

Pederson H, Rebbe H (1975) Absence of arms in the axoneme of immotile human spermatozoa. Biol Reprod 12:541–544

Pelleniemi LJ, Niemi M (1969) Fine structure of the human foetal testis. Z Zellforsch 99:507–522

Pelliniemi LJ, Dym M, Durand M, Gunsalus GL, Musto NA, Bardin CW, Fawcett DW (1979) Localization of immunoreactive androgen binding protein in caput epididymis of the rat. Proc Am Soc Androl 4:28

Picker R (1913) Über den Bau der menschlichen Samenblasen. Anat Anz 44:377–381

Pickering AJMC, Fink G (1976) Priming effect of luteinizing hormone releasing hormone: In vitro and in vivo evidence consistent with its dependence upon protein and RNA synthesis. J Endocrinol 69:373–379

Podesta EJ, Rivarola MA (1974) Concentration of androgens in whole testis, seminiferous tubules and interstitial tissue of rats at different stages of development. Endocrinology 95:455–461

Popovic NA, McLeod DG, Borski AA (1973) Ultrastructure of the human vas deferens. Invest Urol 10:266–277

Ramos AS, Dym M (1977) Ultrastructure of the ductuli efferentes in monkeys. Biol Reprod 17:339–349

Ramsdale DR (1974) Further observations on urethral chromaffin cells. An electron microscope study. Cell Tiss Res 148:499–504

Reid BL, Cleland KW (1957) The structure and function of the epididymis I. The histology of the rat epididymis. Aust J Zool 5:223–246

Reyes FI, Boroditsky RS, Winter JSD, Faiman C (1974) Studies on human sexual development. II. Fetal and maternal serum gonadotropin and sex steroid concentrations. J Clin Endocrinol Metab 38:612–617

Rich KA, de Kretser (1977) Effect of differing degrees of destruction of the rat seminiferous epithelium on levels of serum FSH and androgen binding protein. Endocrinology 101:959–968

Rich KA, Kerr JB, de Kretser DM (1979) Evidence for Leydig cell dysfunction in rats with seminiferous tubule damage. Mol Cell Endocrinol 13:123–135

Risley PL (1958) The contractile behaviour *in vivo* of the ductus epididymidis and vasa efferentia of the rat. Anat Rec 130:471

Riva A (1967) Fine structure of human seminal vesicle epithelium. J Anat (Lond) 102:71–86

Rivarola MA, Podesta EJ, Chemes HE (1972) In vitro testosterone ^{14}C metabolism by rat seminiferous tubules at different stages of development: formation of 5α-androstandiol at meiosis. Endocrinology 91:537–542

Röhlich K (1938) Über die Prostatasekretion. Z Mikrosk Anat Forsch 43:451–465

Roosen-Runge EC (1961) The rete testis in the albino rat: its structure, development and morphological significance. Acta Anat (Basel) 45:1–29

Roosen-Runge EC, Holstein AF (1978) The human rete testis. Cell Tiss Res 189:409–433

Ross MH, Long IR (1966) Contractile cells in human seminiferous tubules. Science 153:1271–1273

Ross R (1971) The smooth muscle cell. II. Growth of smooth muscle in culture and formation of elastic fibers. J Cell Biol 50:172–186

Rowley MJ, Teshima F, Heller CG (1970) Duration of transit of spermatozoa through the human male ductular system. Fertil Steril 21:390–396

Santen RJ (1975) Is aromatization of testosterone to estradiol required for inhibition of luteinizing hormone secretion in man. J Clin Invest 56:1555–1563

Santen RJ, Bardin CW (1973) Episodic LH secretion in man: Pulse analysis, clinical interpretation, physiologic mechanism. J Clin Invest 52:2617–2628

Santorinus JD (1724) Observations anatomicae. Cap. X. pp 181–182. Venetiis apud. Jo Baptistam Recurti

Savard K, Dorfman RI, Poutasse E (1952) Biogenesis of androgens in the human testis. J Clin Endocrinol Metab 12:935

Schally AV, Arimura A, Baba Y, Nair RHG, Matsuo H, Redding TW, Debeljuk L, White WF (1971) Isolation and properties of the FSH and LH-releasing hormone. Biochem Biophys Res Commun 44:1566–1571

Schlyvitsch B, Kosintzew A (1939) Über die Morphologie der Rami viscerales plexus pudendi (Nervi pelvici) beim Menschen. Z Anat Entwickl-Gesch 109:421–441

Scott TW, Wales RG, Wallace JC, White IG (1963) Composition of ram epididymal and testicular fluid and the biosynthesis of glycerylphosphorylcholine by the rabbit epididymis. J Reprod Fertil 6:49–59

Setchell BP, Waites GMH (1975) The blood-testis barrier. In: Hamilton DW, Greep RO (eds) Handbook of physiology, sect 7, vol 5, pp 143–172. William & Wilkins. Baltimore

Sikorski A (1977a) Efferent ducts of the bulbo-urethral glands in man. Folia Morphol (Warsz) 36:69–76

Sikorski A (1977b) Macroscopic structure of the bulbo-urethral glands of man. Arkh Anat Gistol Embriol 72:27–31

Sinowatz F, Chandler JA, Pierrepoint CG (1977) Ultrastructural studies on the effect of testosterone, 5α-dihydrotestosterone and 5α-androstane-3α, 17α-diol on the canine prostate cultured *in vitro*. J Ultrastruct Res 60:1–11

Slaunwhite WR, Samuels LT (1956) Progesterone as a precursor of testicular androgens. J Biol Chem 220:341–352

Sniffen RC (1950) The testis (i) The normal testis. Arch Pathol 50:259–284

Solari AJ, Tres LL (1970) Ultrastructure and biochemistry of the nucleus during male meiotic prophase. In: Rosemberg E, Paulsen CA (eds) The human testis. Plenum. New York, pp 127–138

Steinberger A, Steinberger E (1976) Secretion of an FSH inhibiting factor by cultured Sertoli cells. Endocrinology 99:918–921

Steinberger E (1971) Hormonal control of mammalian spermatogenesis. Physiol Rev 51:122

Stieve H (1930) Männliche Genitalorgane In: Möllendorf WV (Hrsg) Handbuch der Mikroskopischen Anatomie des Menschen, vol VII, part 2, pp 1–399, Springer, Berlin

Suzuki F, Nagano T (1978) Regional differentiation of cell junctions in the excurrent duct epithelium of the rat testis as revealed by freeze-fracture. Anat Rec 191:503–520

Tindall DJ, Miller DA, Means AR (1977) Characterization of androgen receptor in Sertoli cell-enriched testis. Endocrinology 101:13–23

Tillinger KG (1957) Testicular-morphology. Acta Endocrinol (Kbh) [Suppl] 30:1–192

Turner TT (1979) On the epididymis and its function. Invest Urol 16:311–321

Valladares LE, Payne AH (1979) Induction of testicular aromatisation by luteinizing hormone in mature rats. Endocrinology 105:431–436

Vitali-Mazza (1956) Le modeficazioni strutturali delle vescichette seminali nelle varie eta. Riv Anat Pathol 11:739–761

Völcker F (1912) Chirurgie der Samenblase. In: Bruhns PV (Hrsg) Neue deutsche Chirurgie, Enke, Stuttgart

Waites GMH, Moule GR (1961) Relation of vascular heat exchange to temperature regulation in the testis of the ram. J Reprod Fertil 2:213–224

Watzka M (1943) Zur Kenntnis der menschlichen Samenblase. Z Mikrosk Anat Forsch 54:396–418

Wettstein R, Sotelo JR (1967) Electron microscope serial reconstruction of the spermatocyte I nuclei at pachytene. J Microsc 6:557–576

Witschi E (1951) Gonad development and function. Recent Prog Horm Res 6:1–23
Wittstock G, Kirchner J (1970) Zur Biomorphose der Samenblase unter besonderer Berücksichtigung der chronischen Spermatocystitis. Virchows Arch [Pathol Anat] 351:12–20
Wollesen F, Swerdloff RS, Odell WD (1976) LH and FSH responses to luteinizing hormone releasing hormone in normal, adult human males. Metabolism 25:845–863

Young WC (1931) A study of the function of the epididymis. III. Functional changes undergone by spermatozoa during their passage through the epididymis and vas deferens in the guinea pig. J Exptl Biol 8:151–162

Zondek LH, Zondek Th (1971) The foetal and neonatal prostate in congenital malformation of the urinary tract. Virchows Arch [Pathol Anat] 354:197–208
Zondek LH, Zondek TH (1975) The fetal and neonatal prostate. In: Goland M (ed) Normal and abnormal growth of the prostate. Thomas, Springfield, pp 5–28

Quantitative Morphology of the Prostate and Epididymis

G. Bartsch and H. P. Rohr

With 32 Figures

A. Introduction

In general, morphologic evaluation of tissue and cells of the male accessory sex organs, especially of human biopsy specimens, is based on a qualitative description obtained at the light- and/or electron-microscopic level. This descriptive morphology is of primary and undisputed importance, e.g., for diagnosis in pathology. A considerable amount of biochemical data is now available; the morphological information about the ultrastructural changes of the male accessory sex organs has been restricted to descriptive findings.

However, to establish structure-function relationships, these morphological methods should be complemented by quantitative techniques that would yield objective and reproducible values for any morphological structure allowing statistically defined comparisons. This can be achieved by stereological methods.

Stereology, a term coined by the International Society of Stereology in 1961, is based on geometric probability and allows quantitation of three-dimensional structures by extrapolation from measurements of their two-dimensional cross sections. Morphometry is the application of stereological axioms (Elias et al., 1971; Rohr et al., 1976; Weibel et al., 1966; Weibel, 1969), which allows quantitation of the volume (V), the surface (S), and number (N) of tissue and cell components by light and/or electron microscopy (Fig. 1).

We would like to stress, however, that stereology will only be a valuable complement to the qualitative and therefore subjective description of cell structure and its alterations. Stereology will never replace this qualitative type of information.

B. Theoretical Basis of Stereology

I. Symbols and Definitions

For basic stereological symbols we refer to Fig. 2. Stereological analyses include the evaluation of the volume, the surface, and the number of tissue and cell components as nuclei, mitochondria, microbodies, rough endoplasmic reticulum, smooth endoplasmic reticulum, or the Golgi apparatus. The values for a given component i are expressed as densities that relate its volume, surface,

Volume ↘
Surface → of ⟨ Tissue and / cell components
Number ↗

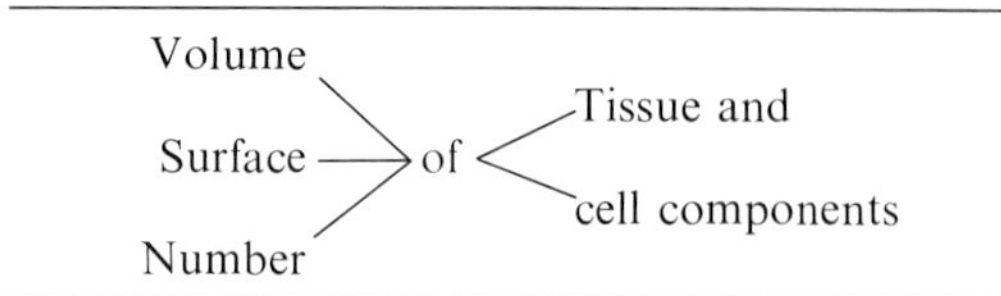

Fig. 1. Quantitative morphology: stereology

V_{Vi} = volume density of component i

Symbols used for its calculation:
P_i = test points lying over component i
P_T = total number of test points
P_{Pi} = relative amount of test points lying over component i

S_{Vi} = surface density of component i

Symbols used for its calculation:
I_i = intersection points between test line system and membrane traces of component i
L_T = total length of test line system
I_L = intersection points between the *unit* test length and the membrane traces of component i (= intersection density)

N_{Vi} = numerical density of component i

Symbols used for its calculation:
N_i = number of profiles of component i per test area (A_T)
A_T = total test area
N_{Ai} = number of profiles of component i per *unit* test area (= area density)

Fig. 2. Basic stereological symbols

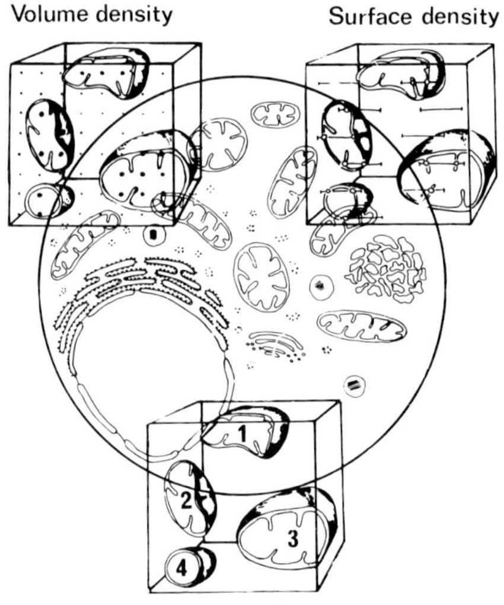

Fig. 3. Measurements of the three main parameters. Volume density (V_V):fraction of test points (P_P) lying over profiles of a given particle equals volume density (V_V)($P_P = V_V$). Surface density (S_V): from the intersection density (I_L) of membrane traces with test lines the surface density (S_V) is calculated. Numerical density (N_V): number of profiles (1–4) in the test area (A_T) is converted into N_V by a formula including correction factors for shape and inhomogeneous distribution

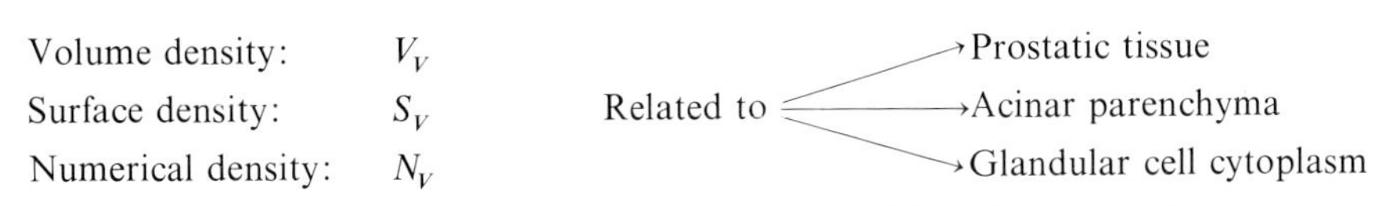

Volume density: V_V
Surface density: S_V Related to   →Prostatic tissue
Numerical density: N_V →Acinar parenchyma
                                                  →Glandular cell cytoplasm

Fig. 4. Parameters that can be determined (prostatic gland)

or number to the unit volume of a given reference space (BOLENDER, 1974) (Fig. 3). Accordingly, a component i may be analyzed in terms of it:

Volume density (V_{Vi}) = the volume of the component i within the unit volume of a given reference space

Surface density (S_{Vi}) = the surface of the component i within the unit volume of a given reference space

Numerical density (N_{Vi}) = number of the component i within the unit volume of a given reference space

By application of appropriate calculations these densities can be related to different reference spaces, as is shown for the prostatic gland in Fig. 4. Usually, the following reference spaces are used: unit volume of organ tissue, unit volume of organ-specific cells, unit volume of cytoplasm, or absolute volume of organ-specific cells.

II. Basic Stereological Equations

1. Volume Density

How can the volume density be determined? The French geologist DELESSE (1847) stated:

Let us consider a rock of such a type that surface areas of the sections made through a particle mineral by a series of parallel planes are equivalent to those made by one specified sectional plane through the rock. This occurs more or less when the rock can be said to be homogeneous. It is easy to see that the volumes of the component minerals are related to each other as the proportions of the corresponding surface areas on a single section.

In other words, DELESSE proved that volume fraction (= volume density, V_{Vi}) of a component i is equal to the areal fraction (= areal density, A_{Ai}) occupied by the profiles in plane through the object under study:

$$V_{Vi} = A_{Ai}$$

GLAGOLEFF (1933) and CHALKLEY (1943) extended DELESSE's principle by establishing the basis for the so-called point-counting procedure by superimposing over the sample section a point network (lattice). They found that the fraction of test points (P_{Pi}) is equal to its volume density (V_{Vi}) $(P_P \rhd V_V$ in Fig. 3):

$$V_{Vi} = P_{Pi} = \frac{P_i}{P_T}$$

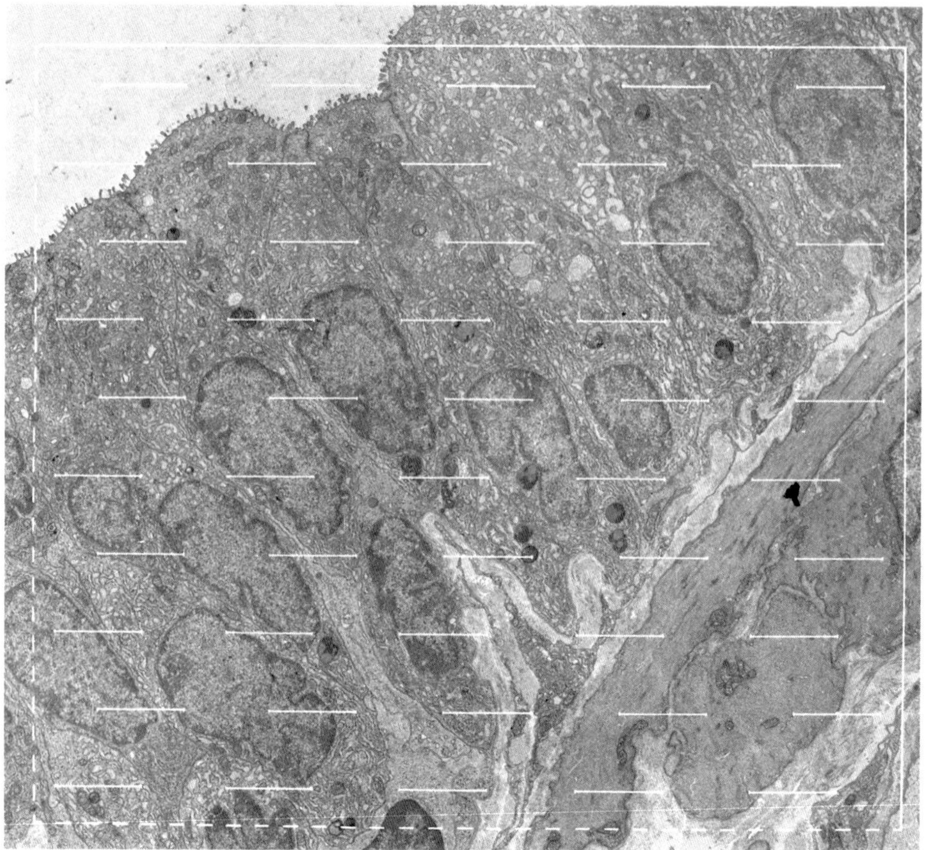

Fig. 5. Detail of glandular cell (ventral prostatic lobe, rat ×1300) with superimposed multipurpose test lattice. The multipurpose test system consists of 50 test lines and 100 test points, which are represented by both ends of the test lines.

whereby P_i = the points over the profiles of a given component i and P_T = the total number of test points per test area.

In practice, the volume density of tissue and cell components, e.g., of prostatic gland, can be determined by superimposing a systematic set of test points over micrographs of cross sections (Fig. 5). Then, the test points lying over the different components, e.g., the nuclei, have to be counted. On the micrograph represented in Fig. 5, the total test point set (P_T) consists of 100 points, 10 points of which lie over the nuclei (P_N). This gives the nuclei a point density (P_{PN}), i.e., volume density (V_{VN}), of 0.1 (see also Fig. 6).

2. Surface Density

Tomkeieff (1945) demonstrated that the surface density (S_{Vi}) can be calculated from the number of intersection points formed by the membrane traces of the structure i with a test line system superimposed on sample sections as

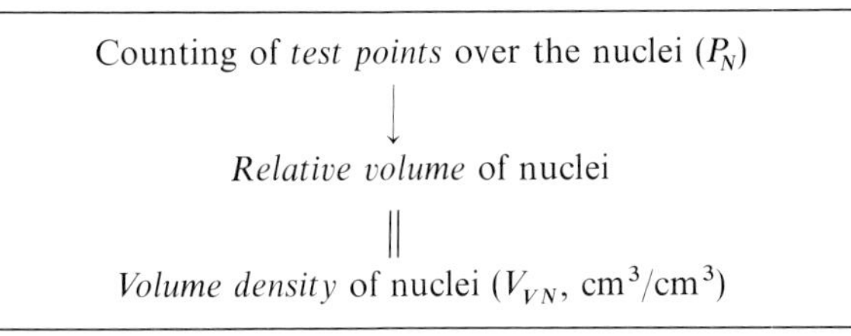

Fig. 6. From "point counting to volume density"

demonstrated in Fig. 5 ($I_L \rhd S_V$ in Fig. 3):

$$S_V = 2 \cdot \frac{I_i}{L_I} = 2 \cdot I_L$$

whereby I_i = the number of intersection points between the test line system and the membrane traces of structure i and L_T = the total length of the test line system per test area.

3. Numerical Density

The numerical density (N_{Vi}) of a structure i can be evaluated according to WEIBEL and GOMEZ (1962) by counting the number of particle profiles (N_i) in the test area (A_T) ($N_A \rhd N_V$ in Fig. 3):

$$N_{Vi} = \frac{K}{\beta} \cdot \frac{N_{Ai}^{3/2}}{V_{Vi}^{1/2}}$$

whereby:

$$N_{Ai} = \frac{K_i}{A_T}$$

and N_{Ai} = the number of profiles of a given component i per unit test area (= areal density), V_{Vi} = the volume density of a given component i (evaluated by point counting), K = the size distribution factor, and β = the shape factor.

For spherical particles, such as nuclei, the shape factor β is usually well definable, whereas for complicated structures, e.g., for distorted mitochondria, the reliability of calculations is reduced. Therefore, the values for the numerical densities must be regarded as estimates in most cases.

In summary, it should be emphasized (as demonstrated in Fig. 3) that stereological analysis is based on:
Counting of points for evaluation of volume densities (V_V)
Counting of intersection points for evaluation of surface densities (S_V)
Counting of particle profiles for evaluation of numerical densities (N_V)

III. Preconditions for Stereological Analysis

a) The structure to be analyzed must be distributed homogeneously in the reference space. Compared to other organs, the liver is one of the most homogeneous objects for stereology. However, zonal differences within the lobule have been shown in animals for several biochemical and morphological parameters (Loud, 1968; Reith et al., 1976) and have to be taken into consideration for related studies.

b) The study must be done on a representative number of strictly randomized sections or micrographs so that statistical analysis can be performed. As a rule the standard error for a given compartment i should be less than 10% of the mean, otherwise the sampling volume has to be increased (Weibel, 1973).

c) For the determination of volume of surface densities, the cellular compartments can be simple or complicated structures, discrete or continuous, large or small, or variable in size (Weibel, 1974). However, for the determination of the numerical density the shape of the cellular component in question must be geometrically definable.

d) The choice of an appropriate method and procedure for tissue fixation as well as for embedding (shrinkage!) is of primary importance in stereological analysis. Bolender (1974) proposed a standardized fixation procedure and en bloc staining for better identification of cellular structures as well as for the sampling of electron micrographs. Such a procedure allows a better assignment of the different morphological criteria to the cellular components.

IV. Stereological Procedure

1. General Stereological Model

In any attempt to describe cellular structure quantitatively, a stereological model for the organ or the cell in question must be elaborated. Such stereological models can be useful in relating structural changes to cellular function since a close relationship exists between morphology and biochemistry (Stäubli et al., 1969).

Therefore, a short, general analytical approach to such a stereological model will be outlined (see also Bolender, 1974). To establish a stereological model that guarantees the most possible flexibility in respect to the different possible experimental designs, the organ or the cell under analysis must be divided into morphologically clearly defined components or compartments. The term "compartment" is defined as the aggregate of all the elements of a given component (Bolender, 1974). In stereological analysis of a given organ, this is usually divided into two major portions: the extracellular space and the organ-specific cells. The cells obviously can be subdivided into the nuclear and the various cytoplasmic compartments, in which all spaces and membranes can be included. An example of a stereological model is given in Fig. 7.

Such a general design of the stereological model allows to relate the determined values to different reference systems. Usually, the following reference systems are used:

A cubic centimeter of the organ
A cubic centimeter of the organ-specific cell
A cubic centimeter of cellular cytoplasm and the volume of an average "mononuclear" organ-specific cell (Weibel, 1969)

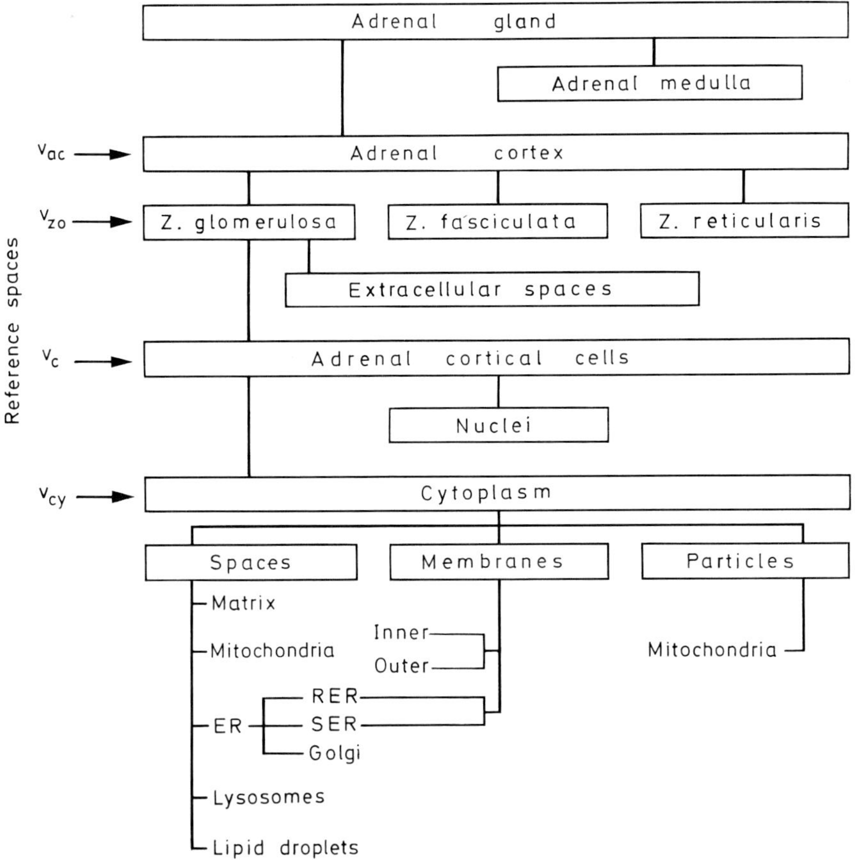

Fig. 7. Stereological model of the adrenal cortex, showing its division into the different tissue and cell compartments. *ER*, endoplasmic reticulum; *RER*, rough endoplasmic reticulum; *SER*, smooth endoplasmic reticulum

Sometimes, the introduction of additional reference systems, such as a cubic centimeter of mitochondria or a cubic centimeter of rough and/or smooth endoplasmic reticulum, may be desirable. Finally, it may be useful to convert stereological volumes to weights. However, in such a case the specific gravity of the analyzed organ must be known. For the determination of the specific gravity of an organ we propose the method of SCHERLE (1970).

To exclude influences by changes in cellular or tissue volume (extracellular space) the reference system "average mononuclear cell" is appropriate in most stereological studies. Absolute as well as relative values (volumes, surfaces, number) of the different cellular components can be evaluated.

2. Morphological Criteria

Strict morphological criteria must be established in analyzing organs or cells by stereological methods. Usually, no problems arise in identifying the extracellular components. In most cases, the extracellular space needs no further subdivision. However, for the organ-specific cellular components several criteria must be introduced. The rough and the smooth endoplasmic reticulum and the transitional zones (depending on the experimental design) must be taken into consideration under certain circumstances. Furthermore, special attention must also be given to the determination of the volume and surface densities of the rough and smooth endoplasmic reticulum. Preferably, only test points over the lumina of the endoplasmic reticulum should be counted. However, sometimes, e.g., when the rough endoplasmic cisternae are flattened, areas of the rough endoplasmic reticulum, including therefore the intercisternal spaces, can be evaluated.

For the counting of the intersections of the test lines with the different membrane traces some well-defined assumptions should be considered. Usually, all the intersections of test lines with perpendicularly cut membrane surfaces are counted for the determination of the corresponding surface densities. Therefore, the calculated values for the surface densities are too low and must be corrected (Reith et al., 1976). For more detailed information on these morphological assumptions we refer the reader to Weibel (1973), Bolender (1974), Reith et al. (1976), and Rohr et al. (1976).

3. Sampling

The sampling must be done according to strict criteria of randomization. For instance, the electron micrographs are made by photographing in regular steps in the same corner of the supporting copper grid. For further sampling techniques we refer the reader to Weibel (1973).

To establish baseline data for a given organ or a cell type by stereological methods, evidence should be given that the organ is homogeneous throughout. Otherwise, regional differences should be taken into consideration. The determination of a representative sample size for the different parameters at each sampling level can be done by the approach proposed by Weibel (1969).

4. Multistage Sampling

The cell compartments cannot be determined at a single stage of magnification since they represent a broad range of sizes and frequencies (e.g., nuclei and microbodies). Therefore, the sampling must often be done at different magnification levels (light and/or electron microscopy) to establish an adequate relationship between the size of the components to be analyzed by stereological methods and the test systems.

5. Test Systems (Point and/or Line Sets)

The test systems (see also Weibel, 1973; Rohr et al., 1976) should be chosen to count cellular components with the best possible economy. The test systems and the primary magnification of the films or film plates should be adapted in such a way that the diameter of the components under consideration more or less equals the distance between the test points. To adjust the magnification to the test systems for evaluating surface densities, see WEIBEL (1969). However, this problem is not definitely solved. Empirically, the magnification should be adjusted so that the membranes under consideration can easily be identified.

6. Stereological Model of the Prostatic Gland

To evaluate the prostatic gland and its components in stereological terms, a morphometric model of the prostate was developed (BARTSCH et al., 1975a; 1977). Figure 7 shows how the ventral lobe of the rat prostate was divided into morphologically defined compartments. Essentially, the model has two major divisions – the interacinar tissue (IT), including connective tissue, blood vessels, nerves, and smooth muscle fibers, and the acinar parenchyma (AP), including the lumina of the acini (AL) and the glandular epithelial cells. The latter were divided into the nuclei and the various cytoplasmic compartments.

Three magnification levels are used in the determination of the different parameters listed as follows:

Level I,   primary magnification 1:90 (light microscopy)
Level II,   primary magnification 1:1300 (electron microscopy)
Level III, primary magnification 1:4100 (electron microscopy)

V. Stereological Calculations

1. Level I

Counted: test points on:

$$P_C{}^1 \quad \text{(fine lattice, } P_T = 1089)$$
$$P_{AL}{}^1 \quad \text{(coarse lattice, } P_T = 121)$$
$$P_{IT}{}^1 \quad \text{(coarse lattice, } P_T = 121)$$

Calculated: $$P_P = \tfrac{1}{9} P_C + P_{AL} + P_{IT}$$
$$P_{AP} = \tfrac{1}{9} P_C + P_{AL}$$

Volume densities of C, AL, or IT in prostate (P) and acinar parenchyma (AP):

$$AL: \ V_{VAL,P} = \frac{P_{AL}}{P_P}$$

$$C: \ V_{VC,P} = \frac{P_C}{9 \cdot P_P}$$

$$V_{VAL,AP} = \frac{P_{AL}}{P_{AP}}$$

$$V_{VC,AP} = \frac{P_C}{9 \cdot P_{AP}}$$

2. Level II

Counted:
$$P_N^{II}$$
$$P_{IT}^{II} \qquad P_T = 100$$
$$P_{AL}^{II}$$

and the number of nuclear profiles (N_N^{II}) within the test are A_T.

Calculated:
$$P_C = P_T - (P_{IT}^{II} + P_{AL}^{II}).$$

Volume density of nuclei (N) in acinar cell (C):

$$V_{VN,C} = \frac{P_N^{II}}{P_C} = \frac{P_N^{II}}{P_T - (P_{IT}^{II} + P_{AL}^{II})}$$

The numerical density of the nuclei ($N_{VN,C}$) was calculated according to Weibel and Gomez (1962).

$$N_{VN,C} = \frac{1}{\beta} \cdot \frac{(N_{AN,C})^{3/2}}{(V_{VN,C})^{1/2}}$$

whereby

$$N_{AN,C} = \frac{N_N^{II}}{A_T} \frac{P_T}{P_C^{II}}$$

3. Level III

Counted:

coarse test points ($P_T = 121$)

$$P_N^{III} + P_{IT}^{III} + P_{AL}^{III}$$
$$P_{RER}^{III}$$

Fine test points ($P_T = 1089$)

$$P_G^{III}$$
$$P_M^{III}$$
$$P_{LY}^{III}$$
$$P_F^{III}$$
$$P_{GS}^{III}$$

I_{RER} = the intersections of both horizontal and vertical 22 coarse lines with rough endoplasmic reticulum. N_M = the number of mitochondrial profiles per test area (A_T).

Calculated:

$$P_{CYT} = P_T - (P_N^{III} + P_{IT}^{III} + P_{AL}^{III})$$
$$P_{CYT} = P_{RER}^{III} + \tfrac{1}{9}(P_G^{III} + P_M^{III} + P_{LY}^{III} + P_F^{III} + P_{GS}^{III})$$

The volume of, e.g., rough endoplasmic reticulum (RER) in cytoplasm (CYT):

$$V_{V\,RER,CYT} = \frac{P_{RER}^{III}}{P_{CYT}}$$

$$\text{or } \quad V_{V\,M,CYT} = \frac{P_M{}^{III}}{9 \cdot P_{CYT}}$$

Surface density of *RER* in cytoplasm (*CYT*):

$$S_{V\,RER,CYT} = \frac{2 \cdot I_{RER}}{L_{T,CYT}} = \frac{I_{RER}}{d \cdot P_{CYT}}$$

The numerical density of mitochondria ($N_{VM,CYT}$) was calculated according to WEIBEL and GOMEZ (1967):

$$N_{VM,CYT} = \frac{1}{\beta} \cdot \frac{(N_{AM,CYT})^{3/2}}{(V_{VM,CYT})^{1/2}}$$

whereby

$$N_{AM,CYT} = \frac{N_M{}^{II}}{A_T} \cdot \frac{P_T}{P_{CYT}{}^{II}}$$

4. Absolute Values

The mean single volume of "average prostatic acinar cell" (V_C) was calculated as follows:

$$V_C = \frac{1}{N_{VN,C}}$$

The volume of mitochondria (*M*) per average cell was then obtained as:

$$V_{M,C} = V_{VM,C} \cdot V_C$$

and the average volume of a single mitochondria (*M*) as:

$$V_M = \frac{V_{VM,CYT}}{N_{M,CYT}}$$

and finally the mean number of mitochondria per acinar cell as:

$$N_{M,C} = \frac{N_{VM,C}}{N_{VN,C}}$$

5. Smooth Muscle Cells (*SM*)

Stage I ($\times 4100$)

$$P_{SM} \quad = P_T - P_{EX} = \sum P_{COMP} + P_N$$
$$\sum P_{COMP} = P_{MF} + P_G + P_M + P_{RER} + P_{VES}$$
$$P_{SMCYT} = P_T - (P_{EX} + P_N)$$

$$P_{COMP,SMCYT} = \frac{P_{COMP}}{P_{SMCYT}}$$

e.g.,

$$P_{G,SMCYT} = \frac{P_G}{P_{SMCYT}} = \frac{P_G}{P_T - (P_{EX} + P_N)}$$

C. Ventral Prostatic Lobe of the Rat

I. Light-Microscopic Analysis

As shown in Fig. 8 the glandular part contributes 75% of the whole ventral prostatic lobe; the acinar lumina represent 52% of the rat ventral prostatic lobe and the glandular cells 23%. The stromal part (=interacinar tissue) amounts to 25% of the whole glandular volume.

II. Ultrastructural Findings

The glandular cells show in the apical pole well-defined secretory granules containing condensed secretory material. The luminal border of the plasma membrane shows minute cytoplasmic projections or microvilli. In the supra-nuclear region, the well-developed Golgi apparatus and numerous cisternae of the rough endoplasmic reticulum can be seen (Fig. 9) in between lysosomes.

III. Stereological Data

As shown in Fig. 10, the rough endoplasmic reticulum makes up 31% of the unit volume of cytoplasm; the Golgi apparatus amounts to 8%. The

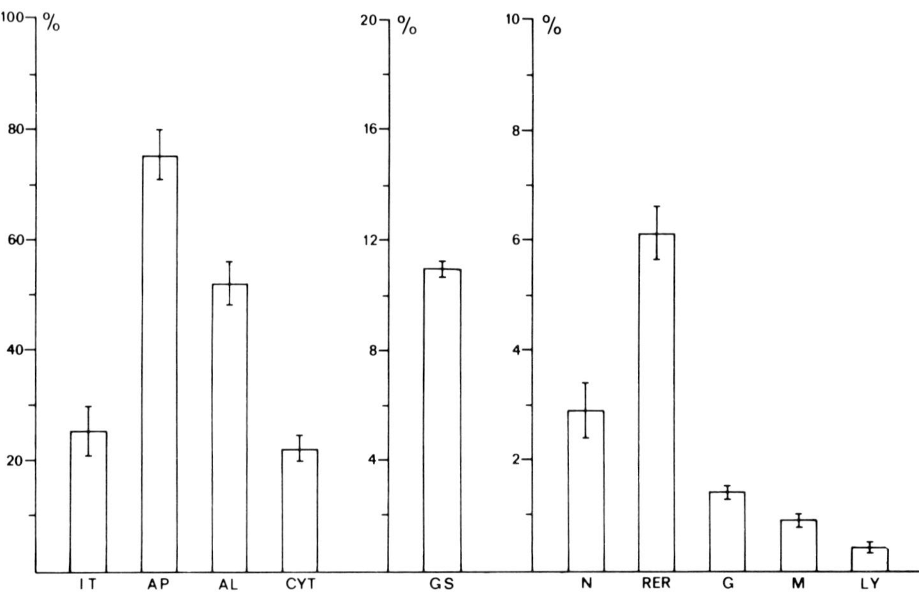

Fig. 8. Tissue compartments and glandular cell compartments of the ventral prostatic lobe are expressed as a percentage of the total prostatic gland volume. SEM is indicated. *IT*, interacinar tissue; *AP*, acinar parenchyma; *AL*, acinar lumina; *CYT*, cytoplasm; *GS*, ground substance; *N*, nucleus; *RER*, rough endoplasmic reticulum; *G*, Golgi apparatus; *M*, mitochondria; *LY*, lysosomes

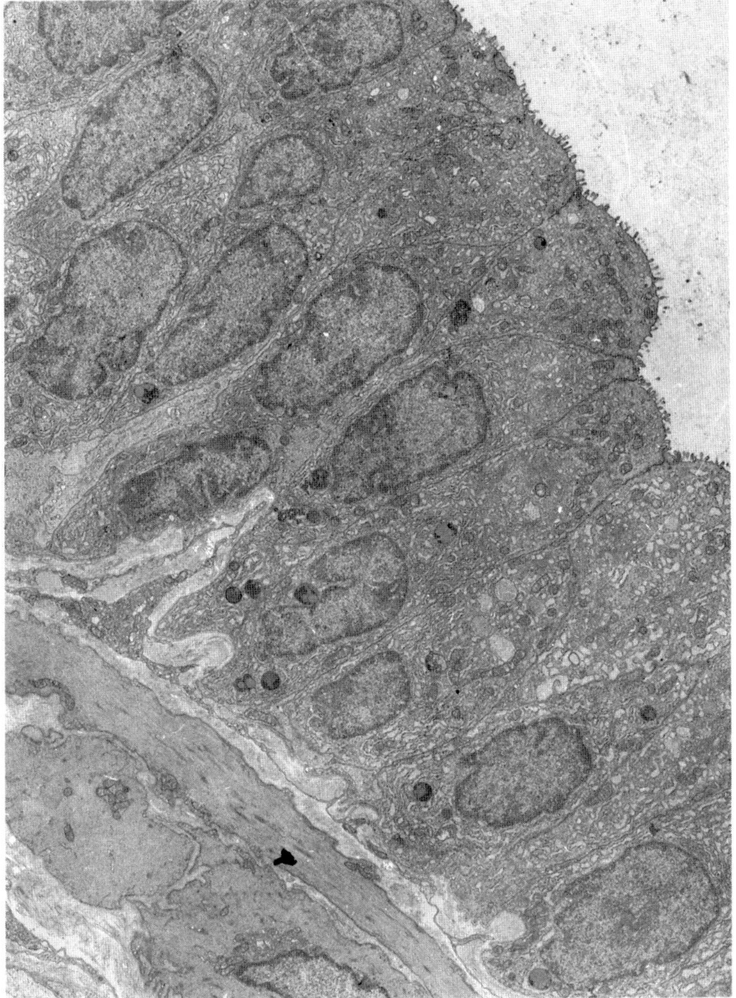

Fig. 9. Low-power electron micrograph of a glandular cell of the rat ventral prostatic lobe

compartement of lysosomes is defined as containing primary lysosomes and secretory granules.

IV. Experimental Applications on the Ventral Prostatic Lobe

Using this approach of the first quantitative data of the prostatic gland, the influence of various steroids on the fine structure of the glandular prostatic cell was studied. Two examples are demonstrated.

The administration of 17-ethyl-19-nortestosterone in a daily dosage of 180 µg/day for 3 months leads to a reduction of the acinar parenchyma, the

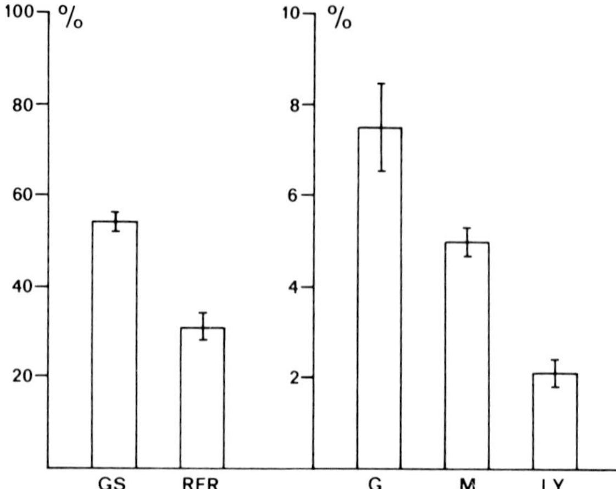

Fig. 10. Volumes of the glandular cell (*VPL*) compartments are expressed as a percentage of the total glandular cell cytoplasm volume. SEM is indicated

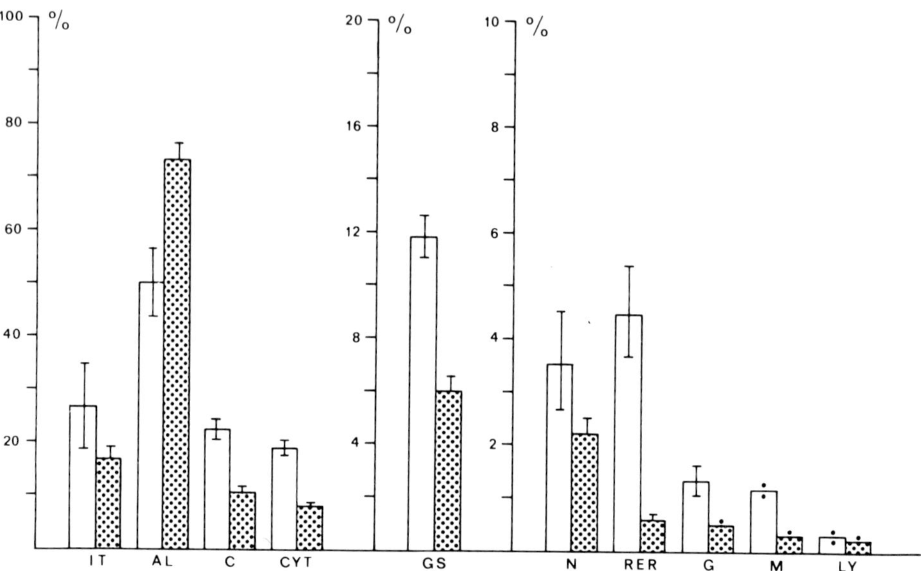

Fig. 11. Tissue components and glandular cell compartments of the ventral prostatic lobe are expressed as a percentage of the total prostatic gland volume. The values of the progestin-treated animals are stippled. SEM is indicated. *IT*, interacinar tissue; *AL*, acinar lumina; *C*, acinar cell; *CYT*, cytoplasm; *GS*, ground substance; *N*, nucleus; *RER*, rough endoplasmic reticulum; *G*, Golgi apparatus; *M*, mitochondria; *LY*, lysosomes

glandular cell, and its various subcellular compartments. The volume density of the interacinar tissue is not changed. Related to the unit volume of prostatic tissue, there is a significant decrease of the acinar parenchyma, the nucleus, and the cytoplasm as well as of the various subcellular organelles of the glandular

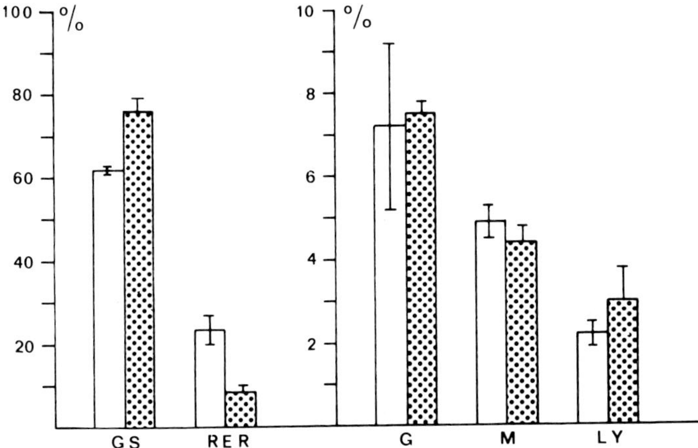

Fig. 12. Volumes of the glandular cell compartments are expressed as a percentage of the total glandular cell cytoplasm volume. The values of the progestin-treated animals are stippled. SEM is indicated. *GS*, ground substance; *RER*, rough endoplasmic reticulum; *G*, Golgi apparatus; *M*, mitochondria; *LY*, lysosomes

cell (Fig. 11). Related to the unit volume of cytoplasm, there is a significant decrease of the rough endoplasmic reticulum, while the volume densities of the Golgi apparatus, the mitochondria, and lysosomes remain constant (Fig. 12).

The administration of tamoxifen for 28 days in a daily dosage of 0.6 mg/kg body weight leads to an activation of the acinar parenchyma, the glandular cell, and the cellular compartments. As shown in Fig. 13 the volume density of the glandular cells related to the unit volume of prostatic tissue ($=100\%$) is increased by 45% compared to that of the controls, whereas the volume density of the acinar lumina becomes significantly smaller in amount. The relative volume of interacinar tissue has not changed.

Related to the unit volume of cytoplasm, the volume density of the rough endoplasmic reticulum is decreased (0.47, controls: 0.58), while that of the Golgi apparatus (0.17), the mitochondria (0.06), and the lysosomes and secretory droplets (0.03) are elevated (controls: Golgi apparatus 0.10, mitochondria 0.05, lysosomes and secretory droplets, 0.02 (Fig. 14).

V. Discussion of the Experimental Applications

The prostatic glandular cells depend on androgen stimulation for the maintenance of their structural and functional integrity. Biochemical studies suggest that RNA synthesis and the following synthesis and secretion of the prostatic fluid is stimulated and controlled not directly by testosterone but by metabolites of testosterone, mainly 5-α-dihydrotestosterone (BRUCHOVSKY and WILSON, 1968). In vitro incubations of rat prostate slices (ANDERSON and LIAO, 1968), ventral prostate homogenates (BRUCHOVSKY and WILSON, 1968), and ventral prostate organ cultures (BAULIEU et al., 1968) confirmed that 5-α-dihydrotestosterone and 5-α-androstanedione are the two main metabolites of testos-

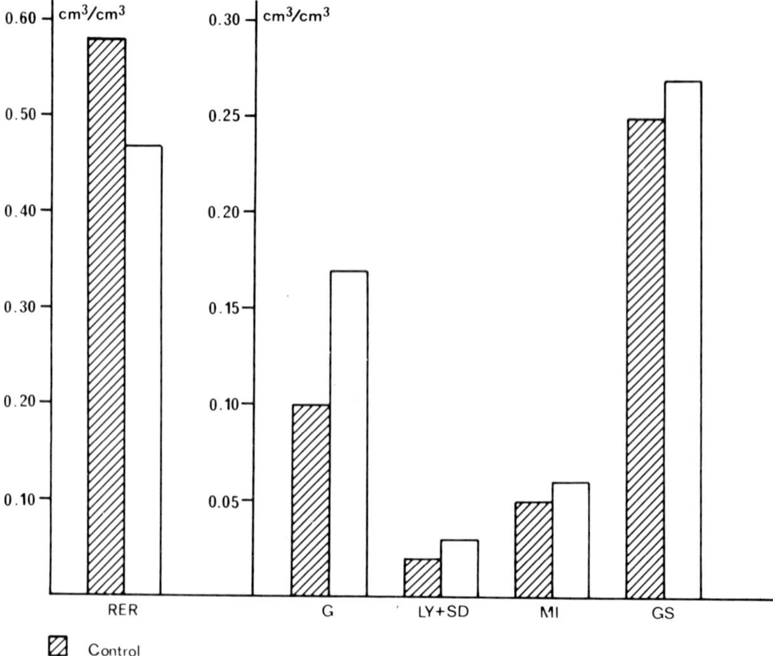

Fig. 13. Effect of tamoxifen on volume densities of cellular components per unit of prostatic cellular cytoplasm. *RER*, rough endoplasmic reticulum; *G*, Golgi apparatus; *LY*, lysosomes; *SD*, sectory droplets; *MI*, mitochondria; *GS*, ground substance

terone. The conversion of testosterone by 5-α-reductase to 5-α-dihydrotestosterone is performed in isolated ventral prostatic nuclei (Bruchovsky and Wilson, 1968). However, other authors have found a high activity of 5-α-reductase in the microsomal fraction (Kowarski et al. 1969; Robel, 1971).

The fine structure of the ventral prostatic gland of the rat after stimulation of the hypothalamic-pituitary gonadal axis by administration of tamoxifen is similar to that after high dosage testosterone treatment in the adult male rat (Gysin-Kellerhals, unpublished). The stereological data suggest a proliferation of the glandular epithelium. This fact is demonstrated by a significant increase of the volume density of the glandular cells and its nuclei as well as by a significant increase of the number of nuclear profiles of the glandular cells. Compared to the adult male rat treated with a high dosage of testosterone (Gysin-Kellerhals, unpublished), in the tamoxifen-treated group the activation of the glandular cell is more extensive.

In the administration of progestins two factors have to be considered. On the one hand, it is well known that the administration of progesterone in a high dose suppresses the gonadotropic hormones, thus reducing the circulating levels of testosterone (Sundsfjord et al., 1971). On the other hand, Baulieu et al. (1968) found that estrogens, progesterone, and cyproterone are possibly competitors of 5-α-dihydrotestosterone binding to cytoplasmic and nuclear receptor proteins. In this way, progestin inhibits testosterone and its active

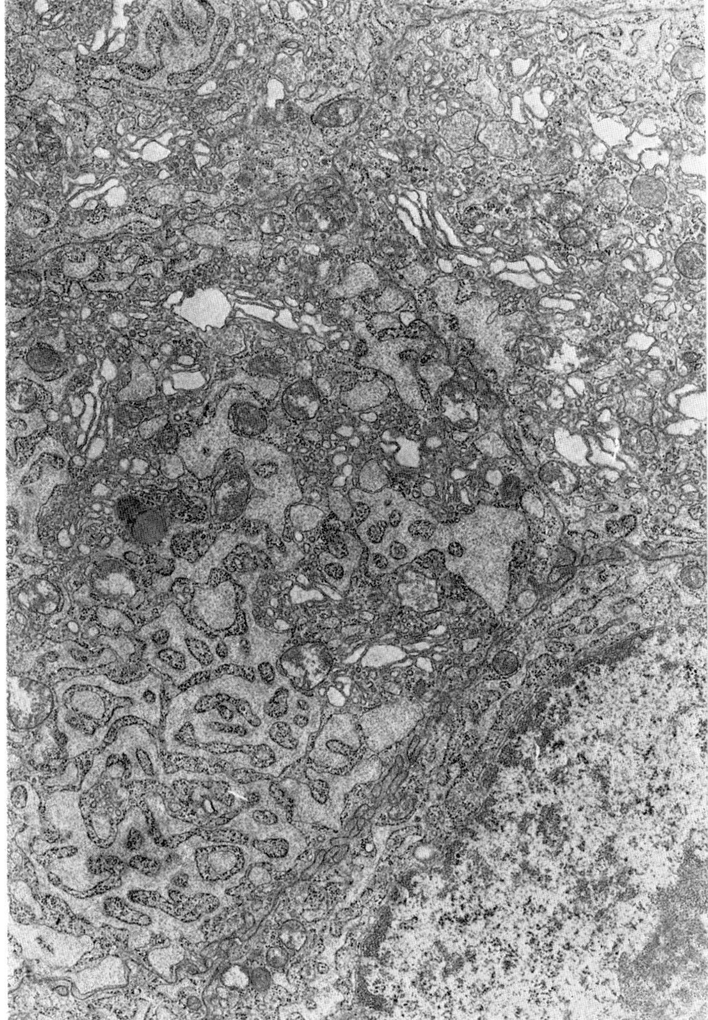

Fig. 14. Electron micrograph. The secretory activity of the prostatic glandular cells is increased. The rough endoplasmic reticulum (*RER*) is well developed; many Golgi areas can be seen. × 4100

metabolites from RNA transcription of nuclear DNA with the following protein and enzyme synthesis on the ribosomes of the rough endoplasmic reticulum.

The fine structure of the ventral prostatic gland of the rat observed in our own study after long-term administration of a low dose of progestin is not similar to that found by HELMINEN and ERICSSON (1972), BRANDES (1966), and BRANDES and GROTH (1962) after castration or administration of a high dose of estrogen.

Whereas castration or estrogen administration is followed by a marked and sustained collapse and depletion of the rough endoplasmic reticulum and by a diminution and a fragmentation of the Golgi apparatus (Helminen and Erics-son, 1972), our morphometric findings after 3 months of progestin adminis-tration support the assumption of persistence of the cell compartments in-volved in enzyme and protein synthesis. Secretion still occurs in the glandular cell. The morphometric data show a diminution of the prostatic gland, its cell, and its organelles. The cytoplasm-nuclear ratio remains unchanged. The per-centage of the cell compartments (related to the unit volume of cytoplasm), except the rough endoplasmic reticulum, remains unchanged. From these mor-phometric data, we may conclude that the fine structural integrity of the nucleus, the cytoplasm, and its compartments is not affected.

D. Dog Prostate (Normal and Spontaneous Hyperplasia)

Prostate glands classified as normal were tubuloalveolar glands that ra-diated from their duct opening into the urethra. The glandular cells varied from cuboidal to columnar with basally located oval nuclei. The alveoli were separated by a dense stroma that contains blood capillaries, nerves, collagen fibers, and smooth muscle cells. Prostates were considered to have glandular hyperplasia when there was an obvious increase in the amount of glandular epithelium and when each of the lobules was larger and had more elaborate branchings. Sometimes, a cystic hyperplasia with atrophic areas of glandular, epithelium could be demonstrated (for details of nomenclature, see de Klerk et al., 1979).

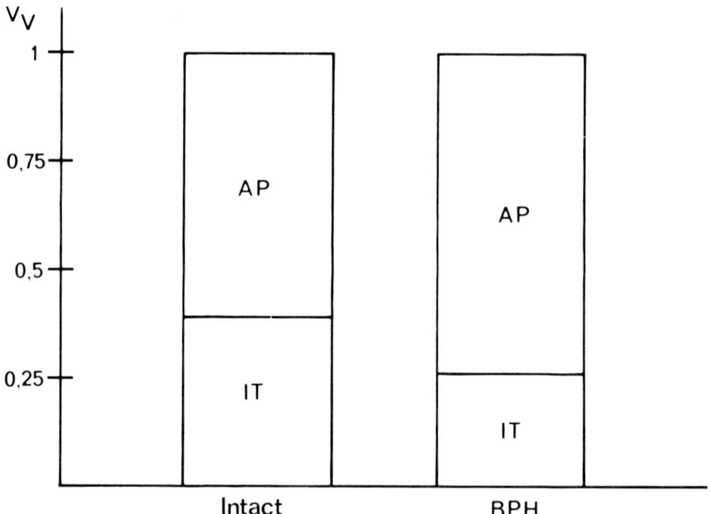

Fig. 15. Volume densities of the glandular and stromal part in the normal dog prostate and spontaneous dog prostatic hyperplasia. *AP*, acinar parenchyma; *IT,* interacinar tissue; *BPH*, benign prostatic hyperplasia

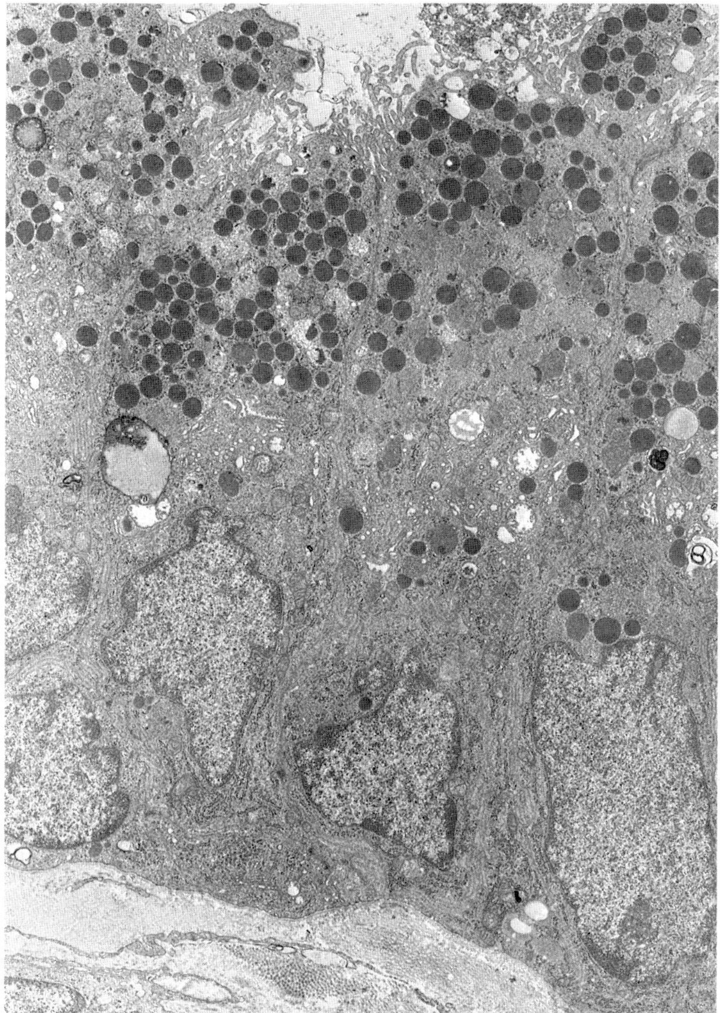

Fig. 16. Electron micrograph of glandular cells of the dog prostate

I. Light-Microscopic Analysis

Whereas the relative amount of the stromal tissue in the normal dog prostate was estimated to comprise 38%, in spontaneous benign prostatic hyperplasia (BPH) a volumetric amount of 25% is indicated; in benign prostatic enlargement of the dog, a statistically significant increase of the glandular part is observed (normal dog: 62%, BPH, 75%); as seen from the absolute results, there is a statistically significant increase of the glandular part whereas the stromal part has not changed in BPH tissue compared to the normal dog. (Fig. 15).

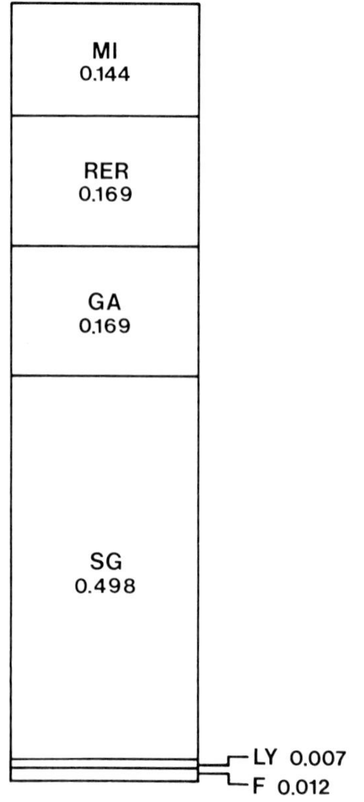

Fig. 17. Volumes of the glandular cell compartments are expressed as a percentage of the total glandular cell cytoplasm volume. *MI*, mitochondria; *RER*, rough endoplasmic reticulum; *GA*, Golgi apparatus; *SG*, secretory granules; *LY*, lysosomes; *F*, fat droplets

II. Electron Microscopy

The glandular epithelial cells are of cuboid or columnar shape. The nuclei occupy the basal portion of the cells, mostly supranuclear, a well-developed rough endoplasmic reticulum as well as the Golgi apparatus can be seen; large quantities of ribosomes are dispersed in the cytoplasm. Numerous electron-dense secretory granules occur in the apical portion of the cell (Fig. 16). The smooth muscle cells are similar to those observed in the normal human prostate.

III. Stereological Analysis

Related to the glandular cell cytoplasm, the rough endoplasmic reticulum as well as the Golgi apparatus represent 7% of the cytoplasm (Fig. 17). The compartment of secretory granules amounts to 20%, whereas the volume density of the mitochondria is 6%. Related to the unit volume of smooth muscle cell cytoplasm, the volumetric amount of the rough endoplasmic reticulum has been estimated to comprise 7% of the whole cytoplasm (mitochondria 2%, vacuoles and vesicles 1%).

E. Human Prostate

One of the most serious restrictions when performing stereological studies on human biopsy specimens is the small amount of tissue available. Therefore, a light-microscopic stereological analysis of needle biopsy material cannot be performed. Nevertheless, the determination of the volumetric tissue composition of a distinct biopsy specimen can be of great importance for the biochemist. Such results can complement in a decisive way biochemical results. Contrary to needle biopsies, light- and electron-microscopic stereological analysis is possible on surgical biopsy specimens. In view of the difficulties (inhomogeneity of material) encountered in stereological analysis of human biopsy specimens in contrast to experimental studies on animals, the following strategies may be considered (Fig. 18) (ROHR et al., 1975):

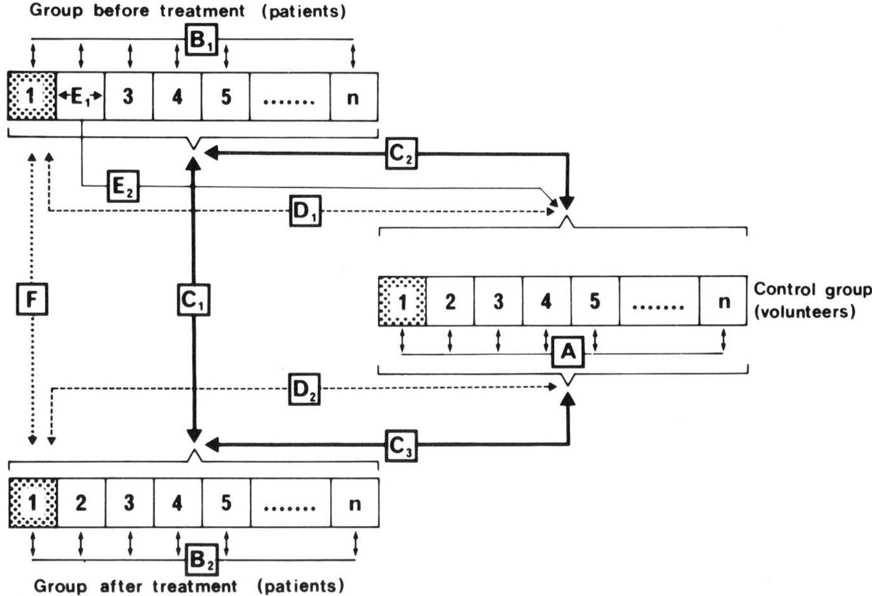

Fig. 18. Schematic representation of possible strategies for comparative stereologic evaluation of human biopsy specimens (see text)

1. Evaluation of a healthy volunteer group as performed in the present study, in which the mean and the physiologic variations are calculated. In addition, each individual of this group may be compared with the mean of the whole group and/or with any single individual of this group (evelution A).
2. Evaluation of a number of individual patients before and after treatment, as in 1 (evaluation B_1 and B_2)

3. Comparison of an entire group of patients before and after treatment with strict consideration of variability (evaluation C_1)
4. Comparison of a normal volunteer group with a group of patients before (evaluation C_2) and after treatment (evaluation C_3)
5. Comparison of every single patient before and after treatment with the mean of the volunteer group (evaluations D_1 and D_2)
6. In focal cell alterations, the specific lesion may be compared to the rest of the parenchyma in a given biopsy (evaluation E_1) and the control group (evaluation E_2)
7. Evaluation of a single patient compared morphometrically before and after treatment (evaluation F)

According to our experience, stereological analysis on human material is – if at all – of restricted diagnostic value. However, stereological analyses can be of primary importance in time-sequence studies to obtain some further information about the pathogenesis of a disease.

In considering special sample strategies, it was previously shown by Hess et al. (1973) and Rohr et al. (1976) that a stereological analysis is also successful with needle biopsies; so far the stereological methods are also practicable for studying the normal human prostatic gland. Currently, there is neither descriptive nor quantitative ultrastructural morphological information on the normal human prostatic gland since biopsies of so-called noncompressed areas of prostatic gland exhibiting BPH or uninvolved areas of carcinomatous gland are not representative of the normal human prostate in the 3rd decade of life.

I. Materials

1. Normal Human Prostate

Using a Vim-Silverman needle, perineal prostate biopsies were performed in five young male volunteers aging 21–29 years who had undergone vasectomy. All five patients had no previous history of disease in the genitourinary tract, especially no history of inflammation of the prostate. The testosterone, 17-β-estradiol, luteinizing hormone (LH), follicle-stimulating hormone (FSH), and prolactin levels in all five patients were within the normal range, indicating no pathologic lesions in the pituitary-gonadal system of these patients.

2. Benign Prostatic Hyperplasia

Portions of specimens obtained by suprapubic prostatectomy from five patients were used. All five patients had a history of long-standing bladder neck obstruction symptoms and received no endocrine therapy for BPH. The weight of the enucleated adenoma ranged from 70 to 95 g.

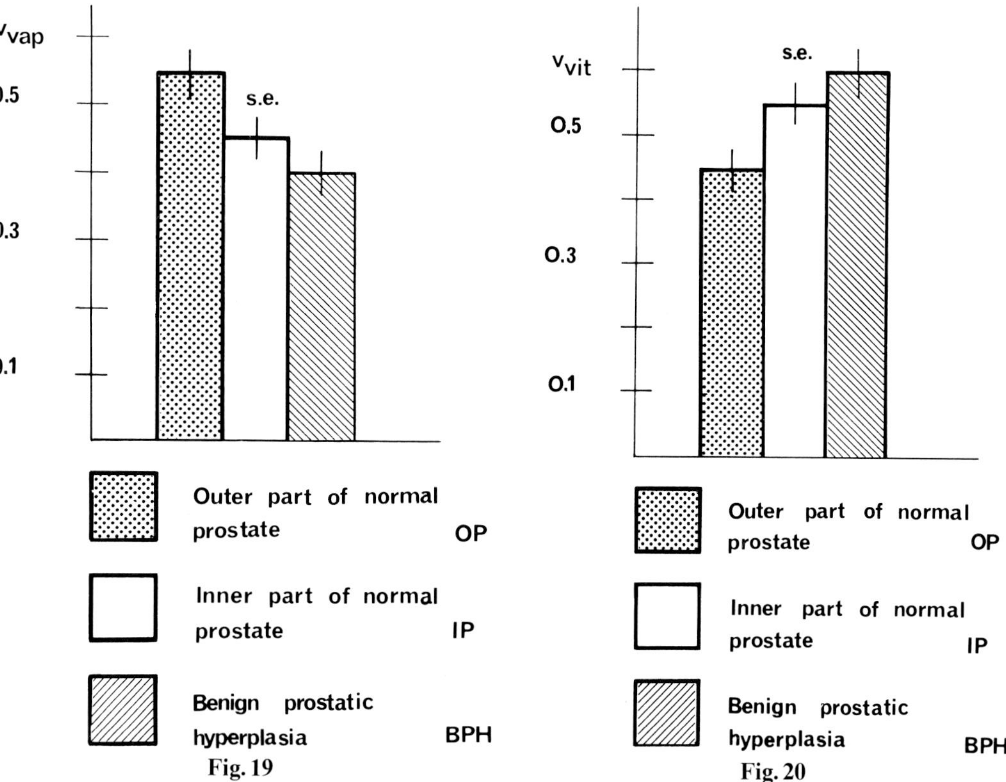

Fig. 19. Volume densities of the glandular part in the normal human prostate (inner and outer part) and BPH

Fig. 20. Volume densities of the stromal (= fibromuscular part) in the normal human prostate (inner and outer part) and BPH

II. Results

1. Light-Microscopic Analysis

As shown in Fig. 20, the glandular portion of the inner part of the normal prostate contributes 45% of the tissue of the inner part, whereas in the outer part it represents 55%.

The volumetric amount of the stromal tissue is higher in the inner part of the normal human prostate (inner part: 55%, outer part: 45%). Compared to the normal human prostate in benign prostatic hyperplasia, a statistically significant increase of the stromal tissue and a statistically significant decrease of the glandular part compared to the normal human prostate is indicated (Figs. 19 and 20).

2. Ultrastructural Findings

In the normal human prostate the glandular cells are mostly of long, columnar shape. In the apical region numerous electron-dense secretory drop-

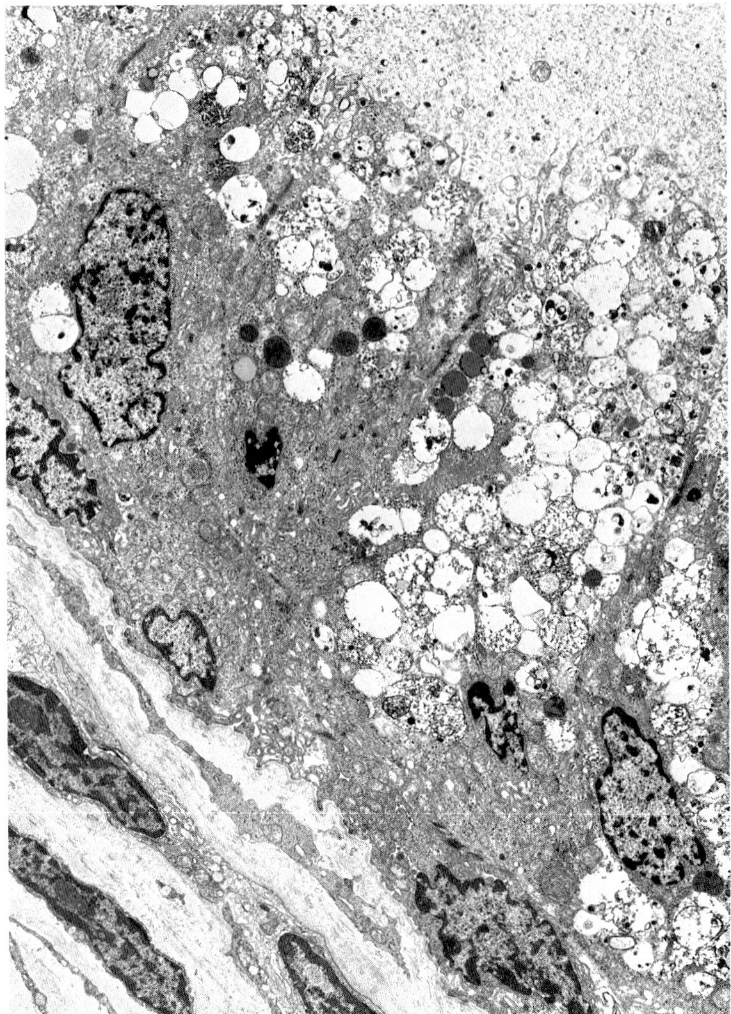

Fig. 21. Glandular cells of the normal human prostate; note the large amount of secretory droplets and lysosomes

lets and lysosomes can be observed. A moderate number of mitochondria are interspersed between rough endoplasmic reticulum and the Golgi apparatus (Fig. 21). In benign prostatic hyperplasia the glandular cells are reduced in height, the amount of secretory droplets is diminished, whereas the rough endoplasmic reticulum, Golgi apparatus, and mitochondria do not differ significantly from the normal human prostate (Fig. 22).

The smooth muscle cells in the normal human prostate are spindle-shaped. Most of the organelles are located near the nucleus or in small clusters in the cell periphery. The largest portion of the cytoplasm is occupied by myofilaments. The rough endoplasmic reticulum consists of a few profiles of mem-

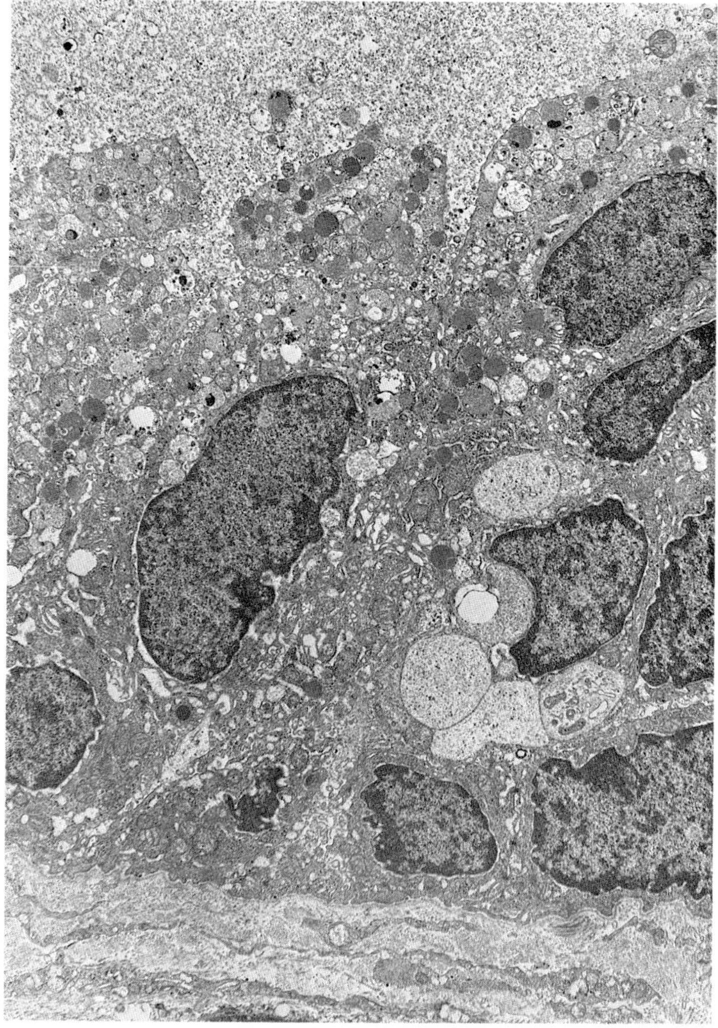

Fig. 22. Glandular cells in BPH; the cells are smaller in height, and the amount of secretory droplets seems to be reduced

branes, a great part is often seen devoid of ribosomes, sometimes a small Golgi apparatus, and mitochondria can be observed (Fig. 23). Contrary to these findings, in benign prostatic hyperplasia the perinuclear zone is markedly increased. The abundant rough endoplasmic reticulum shows enlarged cisternae, studded with ribosomes. The Golgi apparatus is also enlarged and contains more vesical than cisternal elements (Fig. 24).

3. Ultrastructural-Microscopic Analysis

Data for the various glandular and smooth muscle cell compartments are given in Figs. 25 and 26. Related to the unit volume of glandular cell cyto-

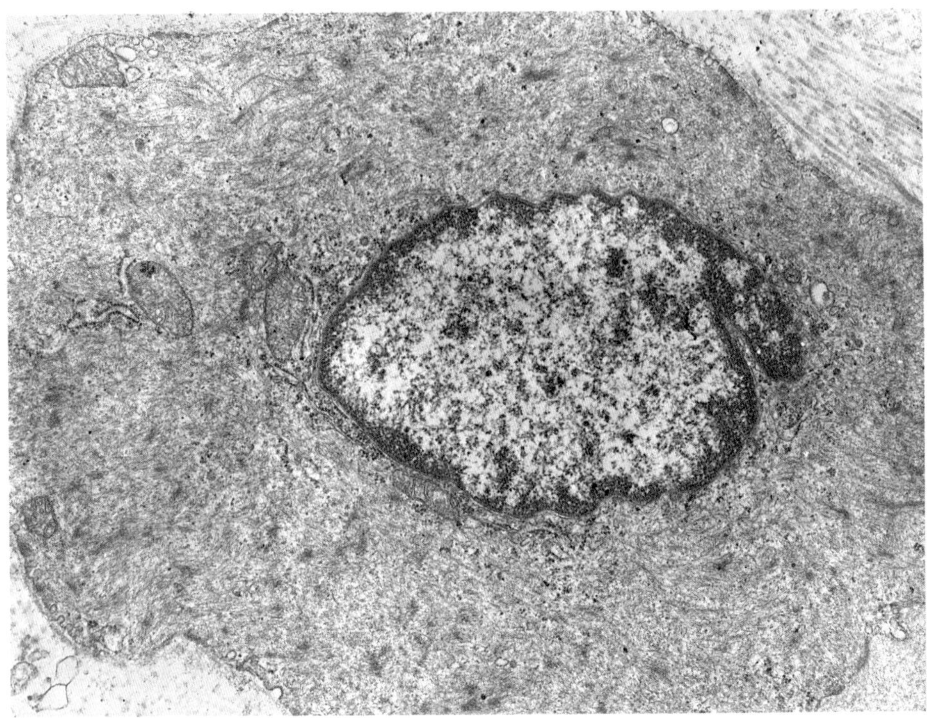

Fig. 23. Smooth muscle cell in the normal human prostate

plasm in the normal human prostate, the volume fraction of secretory droplets and lysosomes was estimated to comprise 35% of the whole cytoplasm (rough endoplasmic reticulum 13%, Golgi apparatus 4%, mitochondria 5%) (Fig. 25). Regarding the smooth muscle cell, in benign prostatic hyperplasia compared to the normal human prostate, there is a statistically significant increase in the volume fraction of the rough endoplasmic reticulum, mitochondria, and Golgi apparatus (normal 5%, BPH 13%) (Fig. 26).

In comparing the light-microscopic analysis of the rat ventral prostatic lobe to that of the dog prostate, the volumetric amount of the glandular cells in the dog prostate is two times greater than in the rat (ventral prostatic lobe). In the normal human prostate the volumetric amount of the glandular part was calculated to be 55% of the outer part or 45% of the inner part of the prostate. Regarding the stromal tissue, there is no difference betwen the dog and the normal human prostate but a striking difference compared to the rat ventral prostatic lobe, where stromal development seems to be sparse (25%). The quantitative measurements of spontaneous dog and human prostatic hyperplasia show that the dog hyperplasia is primarily a glandular disease, whereas human BPH reflects more stromal activation.

As shown by the electron-microscopic measurements in the normal human and dog prostate, there is similarly a great volumetric amount of secretory

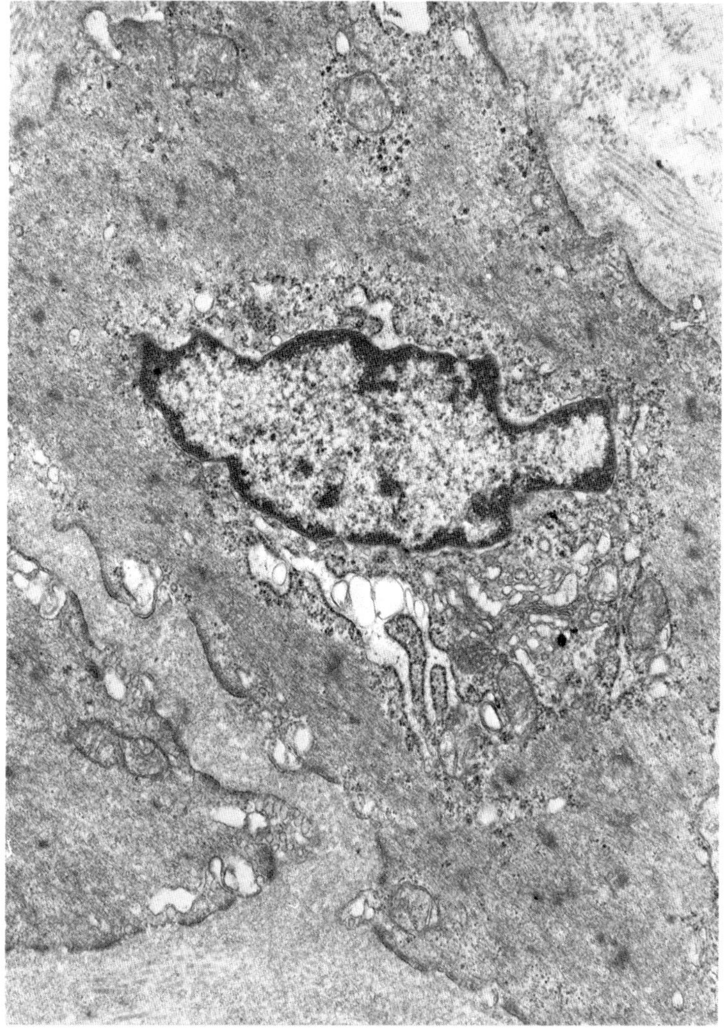

Fig. 24. Smooth muscle cell in BPH; an enlargement of the rough endoplasmic reticulum, Golgi apparatus, and mitochondria can be seen

granules. In comparing the data of the rough endoplasmic reticulum, in the rat there is a higher amount than in the normal human and dog prostate. Conversely, the amount of secretory granules is higher in the dog and human prostate than in the rat (ventral prostatic lobe).

Although dog and human prostatic hyperplasia show similarities (natural history, early castration prevents its occurrence, both show in tissue high 5-α-dihydrotestosterone concentrations), these stereological data demonstrate that they are quite different as seen from their tissue distribution. Once more it should be stressed that the dog BPH resembles a glandular hyperplasia, where-

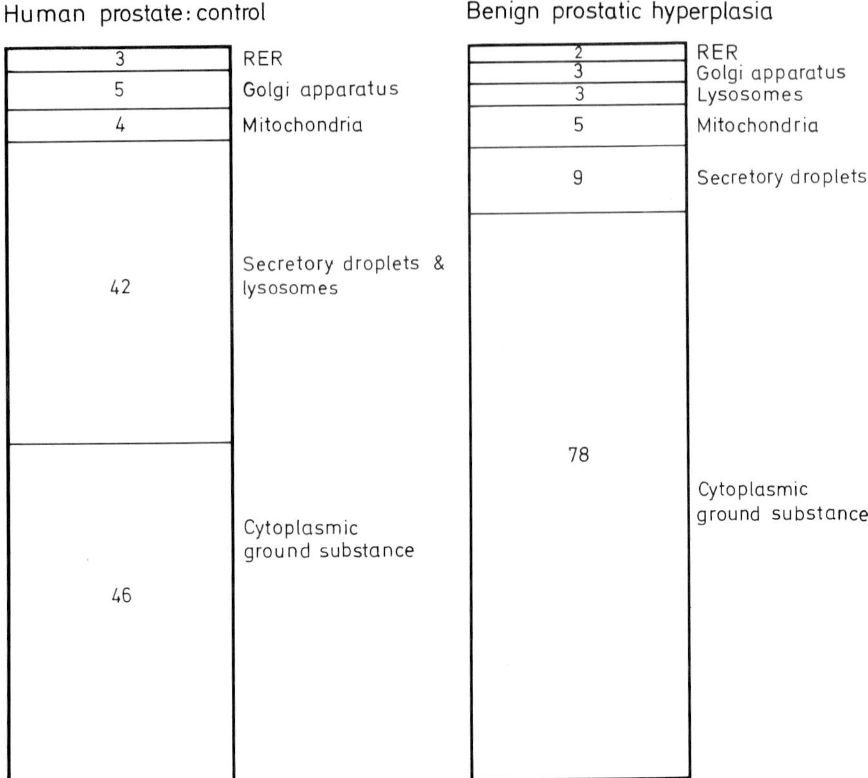

Fig. 25. Volumes of the glandular cell compartments are expressed as a percentage of the total glandular cell cytoplasm. The values of BPH are indicated. SEM is indicated.

as human BPH is primarily due to stromal overgrowth. In extending the concept of achieving an animal model of human BPH, special interest should be given to the fact that experimentally induced dog BPH in castrated animals has been shown by Walsh and Wilson (1976) and more recently by de Klerk et al. (1979).

E. Epididymis

In recent years the epididymis has been a subject of interest to physiologists and biochemists, particularly with respect to the various aspects of the epididymal function (Bedford, 1972; Brooks et al., 1974; Cavazos, 1958; Dawson and Rowlands, 1959; Djøseland et al., 1974; Gaddum and Glover, 1965; Jones, 1974; McGadey et al., 1966; Rajalakshimi and Prasad, 1969; Riar et al., 1973; Waites and Setchell, 1969). Subsequent to the initial ultrastructural studies, numerous descriptive reports on ultrastructural changes of the epididymis in various animal species have been published (Faehrmann

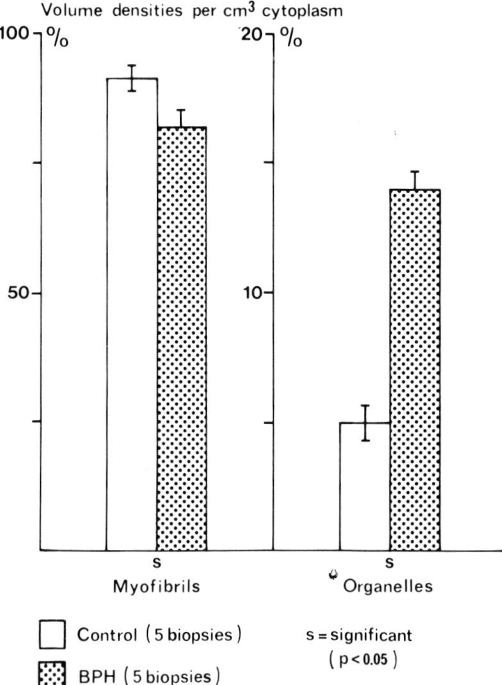

Fig. 26. Volumes of the smooth muscle cell compartments are expressed as a percentage of the total smooth muscle cell cytoplasm (volume densities per cm³ cytoplasm). The values of BPH are indicated. *Open columns;* control (five biopsies); *stippled columns,* BPH (five biopsies); *s,* significant ($P < 0.05$). SEM is indicated

and SCHUCHARDT, 1966; GLOVER and NICANDER, 1971; HAMILTON et al., 1969; ORGEBIN-CRIST, 1967). Although a considerable amount of biochemical data is now available, the above-cited morphological information about the ultrastructural changes of the epididymis and the epithelial cells has been restricted to descriptive findings.

I. Stereological Model

To evaluate the epididymis and its components in stereological terms, a stereological model of the rat epididymal head was developed (BARTSCH et al., 1978). Figure 27 shows how the epididymal head of the rat was divided into morphologically defined compartments. Essentially, the model has two major divisions – the interductular tissue (IT), including connective tissue, blood vessels, nerves, and smooth muscle fibers, and the ductus epididymidis (DE), including the lumina of the ductus and the epithelial cells. These were divided into the nuclei and the various cytoplasmic compartments. The basal cells and clear cells were excluded by descriptive morphology from the principal cells and regarded as compartments of the interductular tissue.

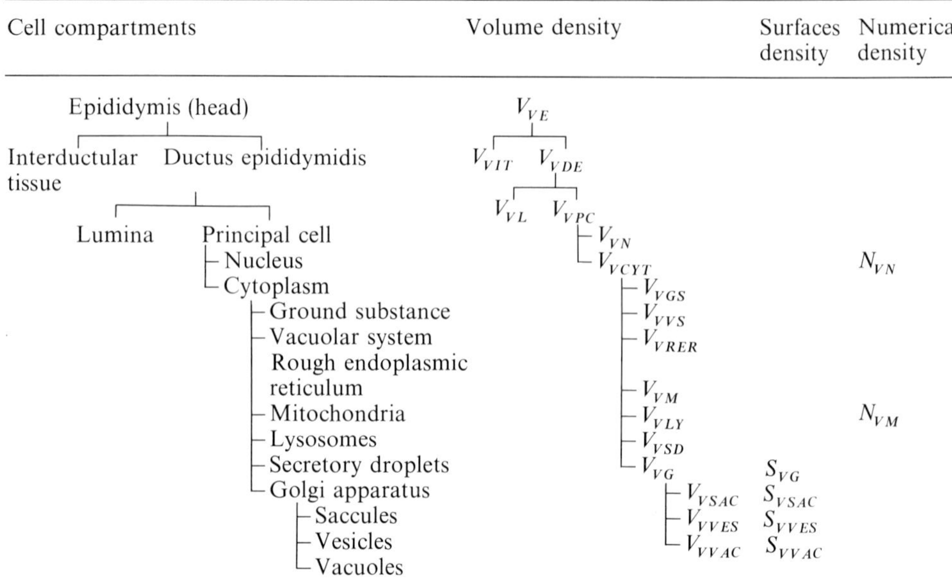

Fig. 27. Stereological model of the epididymis (head)

The stereological analysis was performed at several magnification levels. Three magnification levels are used in the determination of the different parameters as follows:

Level I,   primary magnification 1:200 (light microscopy).
Level II, primary magnification 1:1200 (electron microscopy).
Level III, primary magnification 1:3400 (electron microscopy).

II. Epididymal Head of the Rat

The light-microscopic analysis of the rat epididymal head related to the unit volume of epididymal tissue ($=100\%$) shows that this part of the epididymis consists of 18% principal cells and 26% interductular tissue, whereas the lumina of the epididymal duct makes up a volume density of 54% (Fig. 28). Related to the unit volume of principal cell cytoplasm, there is a great volume density of the rough endoplasmic reticulum (10%), of the smooth endoplasmic reticulum (12%), and of the Golgi apparatus (3%) (Fig. 29).

III. Experimental Applications

The following two experimental applications on the epididymal head demonstrate the effect of the synthetic progestin ethinylnorgestrienone (R 23 23, Roussel, France) and the effect of long-term hypophysectomy.

The administration of the synthetic progestin ethinylnorgestrienone for 3 months in low dosage shows an inactivation of the principal cell and its

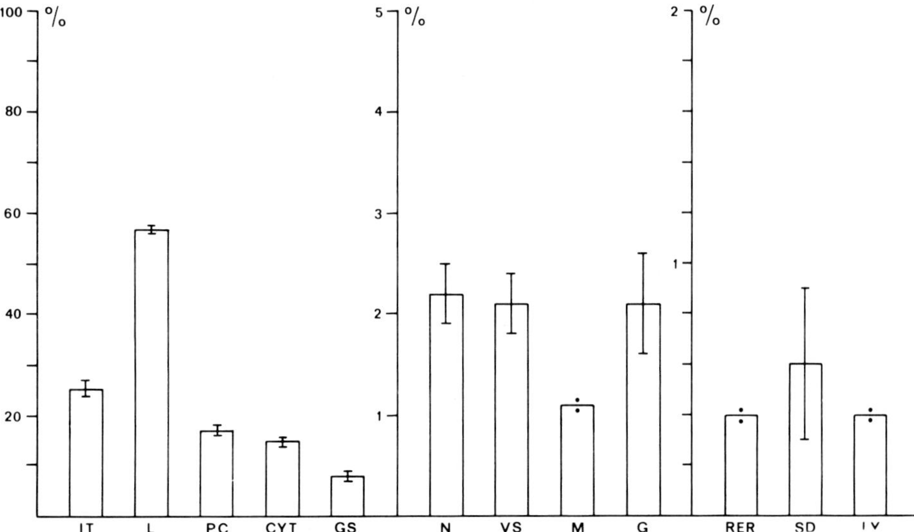

Fig. 28. Tissue components and principal cell compartments of the epididymal head are expressed as a percentage of the total epididymal head volume. SEM is indicated. *IT,* interacinar tissue; *L,* lumina; *PC,* principal cell; *CYT,* cytoplasm; *GS,* ground substance; *N,* nucleus; *VS,* vacuolar system; *M,* mitochondria; *G,* Golgi apparatus; *RER,* rough endoplasmic reticulum; *SD,* secretory droplets; *LY,* lysosomes

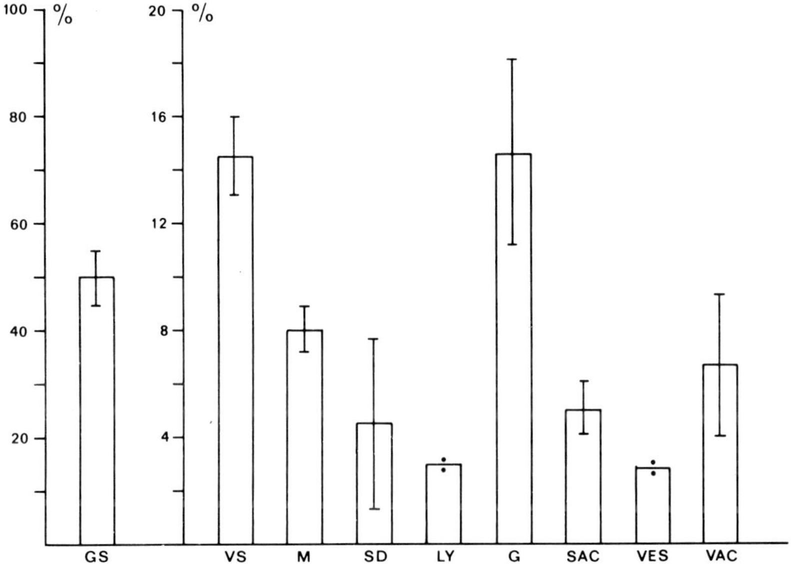

Fig. 29. Volumes of the principal cell compartments are expressed as a percentage of the total principal cell cytoplasm volume. SEM is indicated. *GS,* ground substance; *VS,* vacuolar system; *M,* mitochondria; *SD,* secretory droplets; *LY,* lysosomes; *G,* Golgi apparatus; *SAC,* saccules; *VES,* vesicles; *VAC,* vacuoles

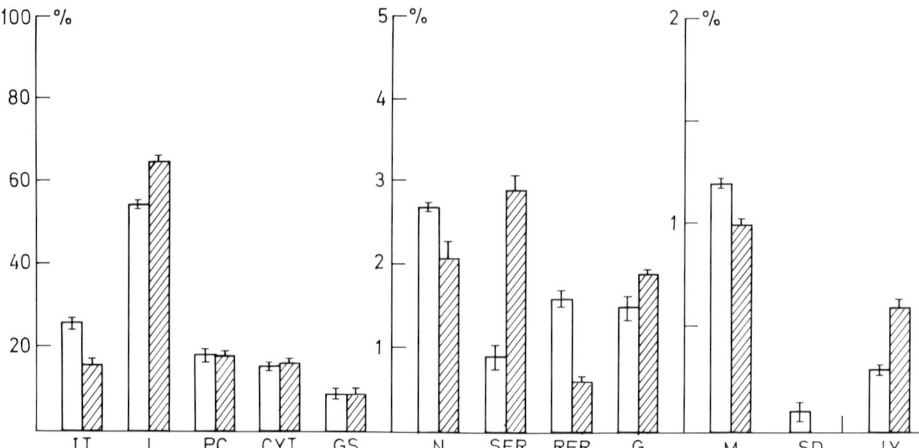

Fig. 30. Tissue components and principal cell compartments of the epididymal head are expressed as a percentage of the total epididymal head volume. SEM is indicated. Stippled columns: R 23 23-treated group. *IT*, interacinar tissue; *L*, lumina; *PC*, principal cell; *CYT*, cytoplasm; *GS*, ground substance; *N*, nucleus; *SER*, smooth endoplasmic reticulum; *RER*, rough endoplasmic reticulum; *G*, Golgi apparatus; *M*, mitochondria; *SD*, secretory droplets; *LY*, lysosomes

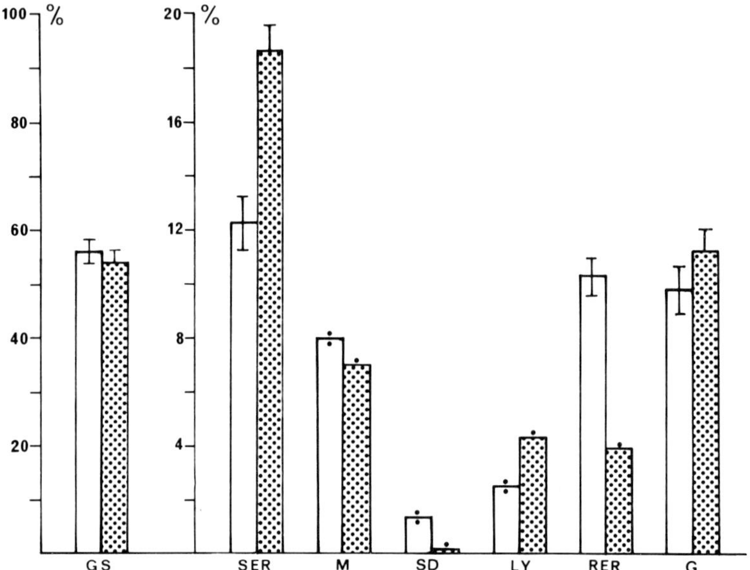

Fig. 31. Volumes of the principal cell compartments are expressed as a percentage of the total principal cell cytoplasm volume. SEM is indicated. Stippled columns: R 23 23-treated group. *GS*, ground substance; *SER*, smooth endoplasmic reticulum; *M*, mitochondria; *SD*, secretory droplets; *LY*, lysosomes; *RER*, rough endoplasmic reticulum; *G*, Golgi apparatus

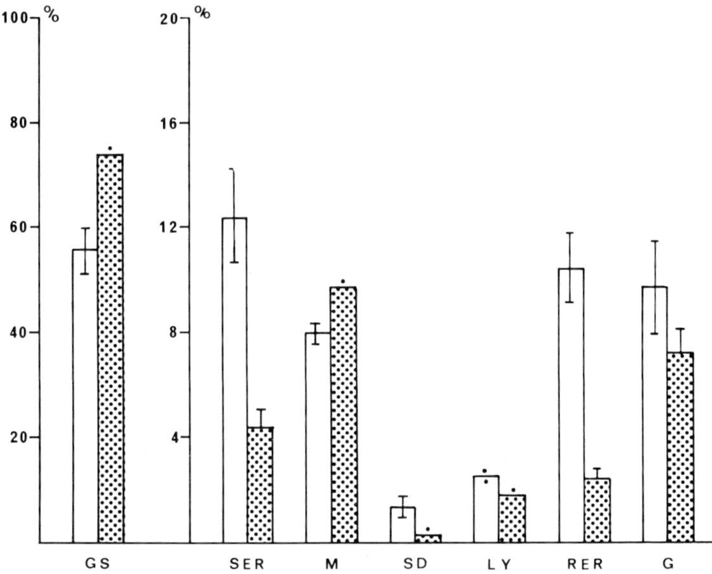

Fig. 32. Volumes of the principal cell compartments are expressed as a percentage of the total principal cell cytoplasm volume. The values of the hypophysectomized animals are stippled. SEM is indicated. *GS*, ground substance; *SER*, smooth endoplasmic reticulum; *M*, mitochondria; *SD*, secretory droplets; *LY*, lysosomes; *RER*, rough endoplasmic reticulum; *G*, Golgi apparatus

various compartments, possibly involved in the various functions of this part of the epididymis. Related to the unit volume of epididymal tissue, there is a significant decrease of the interductular tissue, whereas that for the lumina of the ductus epididymidis is significantly higher. The volume density of the glandular epithelium remains unchanged (Fig. 30). Related to the unit volume of cytoplasm, there is a significant decrease of the rough endoplasmic reticulum and a significant increase of the smooth endoplasmic reticulum, whereas the volume densities for the Golgi apparatus and the mitochondria remain unchanged (Fig. 31). These stereological data suggest an impaired membrane flow process in the principal cells after administration of the synthetic progestin ethinylnorgestrienone. However, a transformation of the rough endoplasmic reticulum membranes with a concomitant loss of attached ribosomes to smooth endoplasmic reticulum membranes cannot be excluded by these data.

Contrary to these findings, the stereological data of the epididymal head following long-term hypophysectomy show an involution of the ductus epididymidis, the epithelium cells, and their organelles. Related to the unit volume of principal cell cytoplasm, the rough and smooth endoplasmic reticulum, secretory droplets, and lysosomes are significantly diminished, whereas the volume density of the Golgi apparatus and of the mitochondria remains constant (Fig. 32).

IV. Discussion of the Experimental Applications

Epididymal function and plasma composition are dependent on testosterone (Gaddum and Glover, 1965; Hamilton and Fawcett, 1970). The epididymal head receives testosterone from two different sources: the circulating testosterone and the tubular testosterone (Glover, 1974). In performing a long-term hypophysectomy a deprivation of all sources of androgens can be achieved. The morphological aspects of the epididymal epithelium after castration have been well documented by light- and electron-microscopic studies (Allen and Slater, 1958; Cavazos, 1958). At the electron-microscopic level, a regression of the various organelles due to castration and a recovery during testosterone replacement therapy has been seen. The stereological data of the epididymal head following hypophysectomy show an involution of the ductus epididymidis, the epithelial cells, and their organelles. From the stereological data, we see a diminution of the rough and smooth endoplasmic reticulum, secretory droplets, and lysosomes, whereas the volume densities of the mitochondria and Golgi apparatus remain unchanged.

G. Conclusion and Outlook

Ten examples have been presented to show how stereology can be used to obtain information from light-microscopic slides and electron micrographs of normal and pathologically altered prostatic and epididymal tissue. How useful is this new morphological method in achieving collaboration between the clinician, the biochemist, and the morphologist for studying the normal and pathologically altered prostate and epididymis?

In attempting to relate morphological and biochemical data, the quantitative morphological data permit determination from intact tissue of the relative and also partially the absolute amounts of tissue and cell compartments of these glands. For example, a microsomal fraction of the rat prostatic tissue containing rough endoplasmic reticulum and the Golgi apparatus would be expected in the normal rat prostatic gland to contain a volume fraction of about 80% rough endoplasmic reticulum and 20% Golgi apparatus. In the application model in which the progestin 17-ethyl-19-nortestosterone is administered, a shift of this relationship could be expected (55% rough endoplasmic reticulum, 45% Golgi apparatus). Under some restrictions, quantitative morphological data can also be obtained from homogenates, thus making it possible to compare the stereological data of the homogenates to the cell fractions (Bolender, 1974). The same calculations can be performed for epididymal tissue.

These quantitative morphological data allow us to elaborate a subcellular reaction pattern of the male accessory sex organs under physiologic and pathologic conditions. They permit us to study the effect of steroids and drugs on the male accessory sex organs, thus providing an objective and reproducible method for evaluating the efficacy of drugs and steroids in influencing the growth of these glands. With special sampling strategies, it was previously shown that a stereological analysis is also successful with biopsy samples (ROHR et al., 1976; HESS et al., 1973). Stereological methods would also be practicable in the study of human prostatic and epididymal tissue.

When comparing the prostatic glandular cells of healthy young men with those of men suffering from benign prostatic hyperplasia (BPH), a definite inactivation of the prostatic glandular cell in human BPH was indicated (BARTSCH et al., 1979b). In contrast, the results of stereological analysis of the smooth muscle cells of the stromal tissue of the prostate of healthy young men and of men with BPH show an activation of the smooth muscle cells in BPH (BARTSCH et al., 1979b). Therefore, an activation of the secretory activity, namely, synthesis of collagen and mucopolysaccharides, can be assumed. A similar reaction pattern of the smooth muscle cell was observed in castrated dogs following high-dosage administration of estrogen during a 3-week period (ROHR et al., 1981). Most probably, the activated smooth muscle cell is one of the most important keys in the morphogenesis of human BPH. However, the factors that activate the smooth muscle cells are still unknown. If we assume that cellular events (prostatic glandular cell: protein and enzyme synthesis and resultant secretion) are related to morphologically defined compartments and known biochemical factors (e.g., testosterone metabolism, C_{19} steroids, acid phosphatase), the usefulness of morphology in this example of a known target cell inside the male hypothalamic pituitary-gonadal system could only be expanded in developing techniques that allow quantification of cellular structure.

By means of stereological methods a differentiation of the two parts of the prostate (glandular and stromal) as well as a differentiation of the various cells (glandular cells, smooth muscle cells) is possible, whereas biochemical methods fail. Therefore, especially in the example of the human prostate with a high volumetric amount of stromal tissue, it must be expected that subcellular fractions derived from homogenized tissue will contain a large amount of organelles and membranes from cells other than the glandular cells. Such considerations may be very important for the biochemist and are possibly responsible for the contradictory biochemical results obtained from human prostatic tissue homogenates, especially in BPH. In extending this concept, there is possibly another source of information for the biochemist working on testosterone metabolism in BPH, including RNA and DNA metabolism of the prostatic cell nuclei. The amount of the volume fraction of the glandular cell nuclei is very low (about 5%) and is greatly contaminated with nuclei of activated smooth muscle cells. In other words, in a fraction of prostatic cell nuclei, one can anticipate that there will be about the same amount of glandular cell nuclei as stromal cell nuclei, such as fibroblasts and smooth muscle cells. Such a fact should be recalled to the biochemist's mind.

Stereological methods can be very helpful in interdisciplinary work. Such methods will become increasingly important. However, some serious hurdles have to be overcome and certain warnings observed in the stereological day-to-day work in order not to discredit this quantitative morphological approach. Finally, it must be stressed again that both stereology and description should complement each other as much as possible.

References

Allen JM, Slater JJ (1958) A chemical and histochemical study of acid phosphatase in the epididymis of normal, castrate and hormone replaced castrate mice. Anat Rec 130: 731–745

Anderson KM, Liao S (1968) Selective retention of dihydrotestosterone by prostate nuclei. Nature 219:277–279

Bartsch G (1977) Stereology, a new quantitative morphological approach to study prostatic function and disease. Eur Urol 3:85–92

Bartsch G, Rohr HP (1977) Ultrastructural stereology: A new approach to the study of prostatic function. Invest Urol 14:301–306

Bartsch G, Fischer E, Rohr HP (1975a) Ultrastructural morphometric analysis of the rat prostate (vetral lobe). Urol Res 3:1

Bartsch G, Hindermann Ch, Rohr HP (1975b) The effect of a synthetic progestine on the fine structure of rat prostate (ultrastructural-morphometric analysis). Exp Urol Pathol 23:188–202

Bartsch G, Oberholzer M, Holliger O, Weber J, Weber A, Rohr HP (1978) Stereology – A new quantitative morphological method to study epidymal function. Andrologia 10:31–42

Bartsch G, Müller HR, Oberholzer M, Rohr HP (1979a) Light microscopic stereological analysis of the normal human prostate and of benign prostate hyperplasia. J Urol 122, 487

Bartsch G, Frick J, Rüegg I, Bucher M, Holliger O, Oberholzer M, Rohr HP (1979b) Electron microscopic stereological analysis of the normal human prostate and of benign prostate hyperplasia. J Urol 122, 481

Baulieu EE, Lasnitzki I, Robel P (1968) Metabolism of testosterone and action of metabolites on prostate glands grown in organ culture. Nature 219:1155

Bedford JM (1972) Sperm transport and fertilization. Biology of reproduction. Excerpta Medica, Amsterdam, pp 338–392

Bolender RP (1974) Stereological analysis of the guinea pig pancreas. J Cell Biol 61:269

Brandes D (1966) The fine structure and histochemistry of prostatic glands in relation to sex hormones. Int Rev Cytol 20:207–276

Brandes D, Groth DP (1961) Fine structure of rat prostatic complex. Exp Cell Res 23:159

Brooks DE, Hamilton DW, Mallek AH (1974) Carnitine and glycerylphosphorylcholine in the reproductive tract of the male rat. J Reprod Fertil 36:141–160

Bruchovsky N, Wilson JD (1968) The conversion of testosterone to 5-α-androstan-17-β-ol-3-one by rat prostate in vivo and in vitro. J Biol Chem 243:2012

Cavazos LF (1958) Effects of testosterone proprionate on histochemical reactions of epithelium of rat ductus epididymis. Anat Rec 132:209–227

Chalkley HW (1943) Method for the quantitative morphologic analysis of tissues. J Nat Cancer Inst 4:47

Dawson RM, Rowlands JW (1959) Glycerylphosphorylcholine in the male reproductive organs of rats and guinea pigs. Q J Exp Physiol 44:26–34

De Klerk DP, Coeffey DS, Ewing LL, McDermott IR, Reiner WG, Robinson CH, Scott WW, Strandberg JD, Talalay P, Walsh PC, Wheaton LG, Zirkin BR (1979) A comparison of spontaneous and experimentally induced canine prostatic hyperplasia. J Clin Invest 64, 842

Delesse MA (1847) Procédé mécanique pour déterminer la composition des roches. CR Acad Sci (Paris) 25:544

Djøseland O, Hannson V, Haugen HN (1974) Androgen metabolism by rat epididymis. 2. Metabolic conversion of 3H-testosterone in vitro. Steroids 23:397–410

Elias H, Hennig A, Schwartz DE (1971) Stereology: Applications to biomedical research. Physiol Rev 51:158

Faehrmann W, Schuchardt E (1966) Licht- und elektronenmikroskopische Untersuchungen am Nebenhodengangepithel der Ratte vor und nach der Geschlechtsreifung. Z Mikrosk Anat Forsch 74:337–362

Gaddum P, Glover TD (1965) Some reactions of rabbit spermatozoa to ligation of the epididymis. J Reprod Fertil 9:119–130

Glagoleff AA (1933) On the geometrical methods of quantitative mineralogic analysis of rocks. Trans Inst Econ Mineral (Moscow) 59

Glover TD (1974) Recent progress in the study of male reproductive physiology: Testis stimulation, sperm formation, transport and maturation (Epididymal); semen analysis, storage and artificial insemination. In: Reproductive physiology. MTP International Review of Science. Vol 8. Butterworths University Park Press

Glover TD, Nicander L (1971) Some aspects of structure and function in the mammilian epididymis. J Reprod Fertil [Suppl] 13:39

Hamilton DW, Jones AL, Fawcett DW (1969) Cholesterol biosynthesis in the mouse epididymis and ductus deferens: A biochemical and morphological study. Biol Reprod 1:167

Hamilton DW, Fawcett DW (1970) In vitro synthesis of cholesterol and testosterone from acetate by rat epididymis and vas deferens. Proc Soc Exp Biol Med 133:693

Helminen HJ, Ericsson JLE (1972) Ultrastructural studies on prostatic involution in the rat. Changes in secretory pathways. J Ultrastruct Res 40:152–166

Hess FA, Weibel ER, Preisig R (1973) Morphometry of dog liver. Normal base line data. Virchows Archiv [Cell Pathol] 12:303–317

Jones R (1974) The effects of artificial cryprorchidism on the composition of epididymal plasma in the rabbit. Fertil Steril 25:432–438

Kowarski A, Shalf J, Migeon CJ (1969) Concentration of testosterone and dihydrotestosterone in subcellular fractions of liver, kidney's prostate and muscle in the male dog. J Biol Chem 244:5269–5273

Loud AV (1968) A quantitative stereological description of the ultrastructure of normal rat liver parenchymal cells. J Cell Biol 37:27

Martan J, Allen JM (1964) Morphological and cytochemical properties of the holocrine cells in the epididymis of the mouse. J Histochem Cytochem 12:628–639

McGadey J, Baillie AH, Ferguson MM (1966) Histochemical utilisation of hydroxyteroids by the hamster epididymis. Histochemie 7:211–217

Orgebin-Crist MC (1967) Maturation of spermatozoa in the rabbit epididymis: Fertilizing ability and embryonic mortality in dogs inseminated with epididymal spermatozoa. Ann Biol Anim Biochem Biophys 7:373–389

Rajalakshmi M, Prasad MRN (1969) Changes in sialic acid in the testis and epididymis of the rat during the onset of puberty. J Endocrinol 44:379–385

Reith A, Barnard T, Rohr HP (1976) Stereology of cellular reaction patterns. Crit Rev Toxicol 4:219

Riar SS, Setty SB, Kar AB (1973) Studies on the physiology and biochemistry of mammilian epididymis: Biochemical composition of epidididymis: A comparative study. Fertil Steril 24:255–363

Robel P (1971) Karolinska Symposium: Research methods in reproductive endocrinology. Steroid hormone metabolism in responsive tissues in vitro. Acta Endocrinol (Kbh) 113:279–281

Rohr HP, Lüthy L, Gudat F, Oberholzer M, Gysin C, Stalder G, Bianchi L (1975) Stereology: A new supplement to the study of human liver biopsy specimens. In: Popper H, Schaffner F (eds) Progress in liver diseases, vol. V. Grune & Stratton, New York

Rohr HP, Oberholzer M, Bartsch G, Keller M (1976) Morphometry in experimental pathology (methods, baseline data and applications). Int Rev Exp Pathol 15:233

Rohr HP, Naef HF, Holliger O, Oberholzer M, Ibach B, Weissbach L, Bartsch G (1981) The effect of estrogen on stromal growth of the dog prostate. In press, U Res

Scherle W (1970) A simple method for volumetry of organs in quantitative stereology. Mikroskopie 26:57

Stäubli W, Hess R, Weibel ER (1969) Correlated morphometric and biochemical studies on the liver. II. Effects of phenobarbital on rat hepatocytes. J Cell Biol 42:92

Sundsfjord JA, Aakvaag A, Norman N (1971) Reduced plasma testosterone and LH in young men during progesterone administration. J Reprod Fertil 26:263–265

Tomkeieff SI (1945) Linear intercepts, areas and volumes. Nature 155:107
Waites GMH, Setchell BP (1969) Physiology of the epididymis. Adv Reprod Physiol 4:27–33
Walsh PC, Wilson JD (1976) The induction of prostatic hypertrophy in the dog with androstendiol. J Clin Invest 57:1093
Weibel ER (1969) Stereological principles for morphometry in electron microscopic cytology. Int Rev Cytol 26:235
Weibel ER (1973) Stereological techniques for electron microscopic morphometry. In: Hayat MA (ed) Principles and techniques of electron microscopy, Vol 3. Van Nostrand Reinhold, New York
Weibel ER (1974) Selection of the best method in stereology. J Microsc 100:261
Weibel ER, Gomez DM (1967) A principle for counting tissue structures on random sections. J Appl Physiol 17:343
Weibel ER, Kistler GS, Scherle WF (1966) Practical stereological methods for morphometric cytology. J Cell Biol 30:23

Etiology of Fertility Disturbances in Man

M. Glezerman

With 2 Figures

A. Introduction

Approximately 10% of all marriages are involuntarily childless; in about a third of the cases the male partner bears the responsibility for the infertility problem. The development of sensitive radio-ligand assays enabling accurate measurement of gonadotropins and steroids in plasma and the availability of GNRH, clomiphene citrate, and purified gonadotropin preparations as well as hormone receptor studies have provided powerful tools for evaluation of hypothalamus, pituitary, and testes and enabled precise localization of the lesion along the endocrine axis in many patients (GLEZERMAN et al. 1978 a).

Embryologic studies, development of cytogenetic techniques and cytogenetic surveys of infertile males, electron microscopy, bacteriology, sexology, and psychology are only some of the disciplines that have provided a deeper insight into the physiology and pathophysiology of male reproduction. Algorithmic schemes have been useful to define and classify some groups of patients according to etiology and localization of reproductive dysfunction. They have also helped to designate appropriate management to those responsive to treatment and to define those for whom restoration of fertility is not achievable by means available to date (LUNENFELD and GLEZERMAN, 1977).

Testicular function may be impaired due to an inherent or acquired defect of steroidogenesis or spermatogenesis or to inadequate stimulation of these functions by pituitary or hypothalamus. The former situation is defined as primary testicular failure and the latter as secondary testicular failure. However, in a large number of patients, infertility is due neither to primary nor to secondary testicular dysfunction but to extratesticular factors affecting reproductive performance. These can be various diseases, environmental influences, infections, immunologic disturbances, sexual dysfunction, psychological problems, etc.

We shall attempt to classify the etiology of male infertility into the basic groups of primary testicular failure, secondary testicular failure, and extratesticular failure. Anatomopathologic situations e.g., varicocele, and malformations of sperm-conveying structures related to fertility have not been included in this classification and will be dealt with elsewhere in this volume.

B. Primary Testicular Failure

I. Genetic Abnormalities

1. Sertoli-Cell-Only Syndrome

In 1947 DE CASTILLO et al. described an entity known as "germinal cell aplasia" or "Sertoli-cell-only syndrome." Individuals with this condition are usually phenotypic males with adequate androgenization. On testicular biopsy the seminiferous tubules are devoid of germ cells and lined by Sertoli cells only. It stands to reason that the ejaculate is azoospermic. Germinal cell aplasia seems to occur rather frequently.In a series of 1294 consecutive cases of male infertility, DUBIN and AMELAR (1971) observed this condition in 2.7% of the patients. Among azoospermic patients, this condition has been shown to account for approximately one-third of cases (CHANDLEY et al. 1976). Hormonal evaluation reveals normal LH levels but highly elevated FSH values due to lack of inhibin (see below). This defines the patients as hypergonadotropic and not responsive to fertility-restoring treatment. The chromosomal pattern may be either normal or abnormal (KJESSLER, 1966; CHANDLEY et al. 1975). It has been postulated that in these individuals migration of primordial germ cells from the yolk sac and hind gut to the gonadal ridges had been impaired by gene action in the early embryonal life. MINTZ (1957) described this condition in certain mutant strains of the mouse, and the extrapolation to the human seems logic. However, there is no direct evidence for congenital absence of germinal cells from the testes. Acquired complete destruction, i.e., a nongenetic etiology, may be present in some patients.

2. Maturation Arrest

Spermatogenesis is a continuous process stimulated by pituitary gonadotropins and testicular androgens. Germ cells undergo six developmental stages from spermatogonia to spermatozoa. These changes comprise three phases: proliferation of spermatogonia, two reduction divisions (meioses), and spermatohistogenesis, i.e., the metamorphosis of spermatid to spermatozoa. The duration of this process in man is 74 ± 5 days (HELLER and CLERMONT, 1964). Maturation of germinal cells is qualitatively and probably quantitatively determined by genes. In some cases, depression or arrest of spermatogenesis at various stages can be brought about by gene mutations, the chromosomal pattern of the individual being either normal or abnormal (SKAKKEBAEK et al. 1973).

During the process of spermatogenesis, a substance is produced that selectively inhibits FSH secretion by the pituitary gland. The existence of this substance has been postulated by MCCULLAGH (1932) and named thereafter "inhibin." JOHNSEN (1970) speculated that the cytoplasmic rest that is lost by the maturing spermatid contains inhibin. The cytoplasmic body is either phagocytosed by the Sertoli cell while inhibin is transported through the cytoplasm of this cell to the peritubular lymph labyrinth, or it is cast off in the epididymis where inhibin gains access to the peripheral circulation. On the basis of cell culture studies, STEINBERGER and STEINBERGER (1976) have postulated that inhibin is an active product of the Sertoli cell. Inhibin has been demonstrated as a peptide-rich fraction of the rete testis fluid of rats (SETCHELL and JACKS, 1974). Probably due to high dilution and low sensitivity of assay methods, inhibin has not yet been demonstrated in the peripheral circulation. It stands to reason that maturation arrest may have either normal or elevated FSH values dependent on the stage prior to which development of sperm cells is arrested. The ejaculates are mostly azoospermic or contain fragments of sloughed immature cells. FRANCHIMONT et al. (1972) showed that azoospermic patients in whom spermatogenesis was arrested prior to the spermatid stage had elevated FSH levels, while maturation arrest beyond the spermatid stage did not affect FSH levels.

Probably not all cases of maturation arrest are due to genetic mutations. One may assume that in some cases inadequate gonadotropic stimulation may be the cause of this condition. However, differential diagnosis may be attempted only retrospectively and following treatment with human gonadotropins (GLEZERMAN and LUNENFELD, Chap. 6).

3. Structural Defects of Spermatozoa

In man, approximately 25%–30% of ejaculated spermatozoa exhibit light microscopically distinguishable morphologic abnormalities. If the percentage of abnormal spermatozoa in a given ejaculate is higher, fewer cells will be able to penetrate the cervical mucus properly (PERRY et al. 1977) and fertility may be impaired. Electron microscopy enables us to study distinct malformations and to define the cell organelles responsible. Structural malformations of spermatozoa causing reduced fertilizing capacity arise most probably through gene mutations affecting the late stages of spermatogenesis. The chromosomal pattern is usually normal although translocations have been observed in patients with severe teratospermia (LUNENFELD et al. unpublished data).

II. Chromosomal Abnormalities

Chromosomal abnormalities may impair somatic development of an individual without affecting his reproductive capacity, may affect testicular function without exerting other severe adverse effects on the individual, or may cause a variety of phenotype defects including somatic abnormalities and testicular failure. The majority of chromosomal aberrations with adverse effects on male fertility affect the sex chromosomes. Abnormal autosomal patterns affecting the phenotype leaving the reproductive capacity intact will in most cases not lead to procreation because of the individual's usual inability to enter into a normal sexual relationship. The incidence of chromosomal aberrations in infertile males has been estimated in numerous clinical surveys and has been reported to range from 2.2% to almost 20% (Table 1).

1. Additional X Chromosomes (Klinefelter's Syndrome)

The most common chromosomal abnormality in infertile males is the 47 XXY type. This additional X chromosome is responsible for a syndrome that was described in 1942 by KLINEFELTER, REIFENSTEIN, und ALBRIGHT and

Table 1. Frequency of chromosomal aberrations in infertile patients.

Authors	Year	No. of patients	Frequency of chromosomal aberrations (%)
Chandley et al.	1972	1599	2.2
Glezerman et al.	1980	333	3.3
Kjessler	1972	1263	6.2
van Zyl et al.	1975	596	11.0
Hendry et al.	1976	204	13.5
de Kretser et al.	1972	56	19.6

Table 2. Clinical features in XXY and XY/XXY Klinefelter's syndrome (Paulsen et al., 1968).

Symptoms	Affected patients (%)	
	XXY	XY/XXY
Small testes	99	73
Azoospermia	93	50
Decreased testosterone	79	33
Scarce facial hair	77	64
Increased gonadotropins	75	33
Gynecomastia	55	33
Microphallus	41	21

is named after the first author. One in every 400 live-born males is affected. Including variations of the classic syndrome the incidence is 7% in infertile patients and 20%–23% in azoospermic males (Koulischer and Schoysman, 1974; Glezerman et al., 1980). Virtually all patients have azoospermia and atrophic testes, and most patients have elevated FSH levels. The classic syndrome also includes gynecomastia and various degrees of impaired androgenization. Some 30 karyotype variations of Klinefelter's syndrome have been described, the most common being the 46 XY/47 XXY mosaic. Nasr et al. (1971) described isolated fertile patients carrying this mosaicism. Paulsen et al. (1968) calculated the distribution in percent of typical symptoms for 47 XXY and 46 XY/47 XXY patients (Table 2). An important finding is a decreased testosterone level concomitant with an elevated gonadotropin level in nearly 80% of the patients. Steinberger (1977) pointed out that patients with Klinefelter's syndrome become hypoandrogenic in a very slow and insiduous fashion and must therefore be followed carefully to initiate androgen substitution therapy when required. Fertility restoration is obviously not possible.

2. Additional Y Chromosomes and Y Chromosome Abnormalities

The usually employed screening technique for chromosomal abnormalities in the male consists mainly of nuclear sexing, i.e., staining of exfoliated buccal mucous cells and demonstration of Barr bodies. The number of Barr bodies is always one less than the number of X chromosomes present in the individual. Normal women and XXY men thus show one Barr body while in normal men no Barr bodies are present. In individuals with additional Y chromosomes, nuclear sexing will be negative, and if no further evaluation is performed, the patient's abnormal chromosomal pattern will remain undiscovered. The reported incidence of 0.2%, similar to the incidence of Klinefelter's syndrome, is probably lower than the true incidence of this abnormality. The phenotypic expression is much more variable than in the 47 XXY condition. Spermatogenesis may be normal; gonadotropin and steroid values show wide variations between individuals. Usually, affected males are tall and pustular acne is frequent, both a probably effect of the additional Y chromosome. The often cited social maladaptation of Klinefelter males is probably more attributable to XYY individuals. Actually, the incidence of affected males in a prison population was reported to have been tenfold higher than in newborn male babies (HOOK, 1973). In some patients fertility is not impaired; in some infertile patients fertility may be restored therapeutically. However, the question of heredity has to be considered and the desirability of procreation discussed.

The significance of Y chromosome abnormalities in infertile males is not clear. Some authors reported on abnormal Y chromosomes in infertile patients (VAN WIJCK, 1962; HENDRY et al., 1976) while others have observed this variety in fertile males (BENDER and GOOCH, 1961).

3. Noonan's Syndrome (Male Turner's Syndrome)

The typical Turner syndrome is characterized by a female phenotype with a 45 XO chromosomal pattern and typical physical features including webbed neck, short stature, congenital heart disease, cubitus valgus, streak ovaries, and elevated gonadotropin levels. In Noonan's disease these physical characteristics (with the exception of streak ovaries) coincide with normal male genotype and male features (FRACCARO et al. 1961). Cryptorchidism is common. Gonadotropins are usually elevated and testosterone levels decreased. However, some cases of descended testes and almost normal testicular function have been described (SUMMIT, 1973).

4. Autosomal Abnormalities and Translocations

Autosomal abnormalities have been associated with impaired fertility in man. In his study of 1263 infertile males, KJESSLER (1972) found 11 balanced autosomal translocations and 3 cases with extra markers. CHANDLEY et al. (1975) compared the incidence of chromosomal aberrations among 1599 infertile males with 1560 normal men (Table 3). They found translocations and extra markers in 0.8% of their patients compared to 0.1% in the normal population. The most common direct cause for infertility in patients with translocations seems to be teratospermia or maturation breakdown. It is interesting to note that in human as well as in other species (CHANDLEY et al. 1972, CACHEIRO et al., 1974) gametogenesis in females is not or only rarely affected by translocations. CHANDLEY et al. (1972) reported a family pedigree of 9/22 translocations in

Table 3. Frequency of occurrence of chromosomal abnormalities among subfertile men (N = 1599) compared with that among a control population of adult men (N = 1560) (Chandley, 1976).

Abnormality	Subfertile group		Control group	
	No.	Frequency/1000	No.	Frequency/1000
47 XXY	16	10.00	1	0.64
47 XYY	3	1.88	3	1.92
47 XY with additional marker	4	2.50	0	0
Chromatin neg.	19	11.88	6	3.85
Autosomal translocation	9	5.63	2	1.28
Total	51	31.89	12	7.69

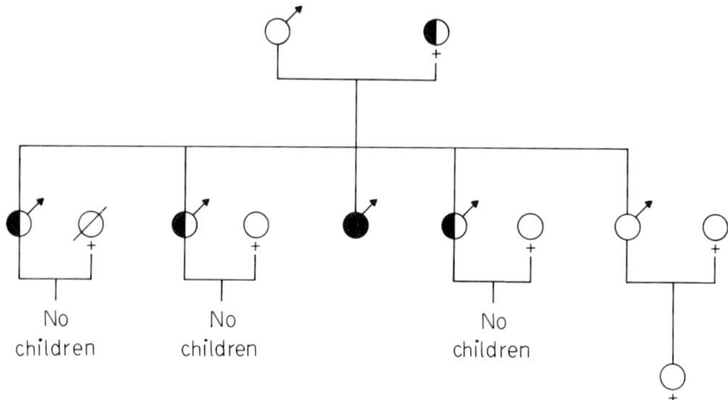

Fig. 1. Family pedigree of 9/22 translocation heterozygote. ♀, untested female; ♂, normal male; ♀, balanced female heterozygote; ♂, balanced male heterozygote; ♂, unbalanced male heterozygote; ♀, deceased female. (Chandley et al. 1972)

which a fully fertile female with balanced heterozygocity had three sons with balanced heterozygocity, all of whom were involuntarily sterile. Another son was an unbalanced heterozygote and one son was normal and fertile (Fig. 1). Another family pedigree of 1/18 translocations (Fig. 2) reported in the same study demonstrated the possible correlation between heterozygote translocation and embryonic/fetal wastage through probable chromosomal imbalance in the spermatozoa or ovum. A male heterozygote transmitted the abnormality to one son and one daughter (the proband). His wife had two additional miscarriages. The affected son impregnated his wife three times but two pregnancies resulted in abortions. His semen was completely normal but meiotic studies of testicular biopsy material revealed chromosomal abnormalities compatible with his abnormal chromosomal condition. The daughter was pregnant four times, and all pregnancies resulted in abortions. In the only abortus examined, the abnormal chromosomal constitution could be verified.

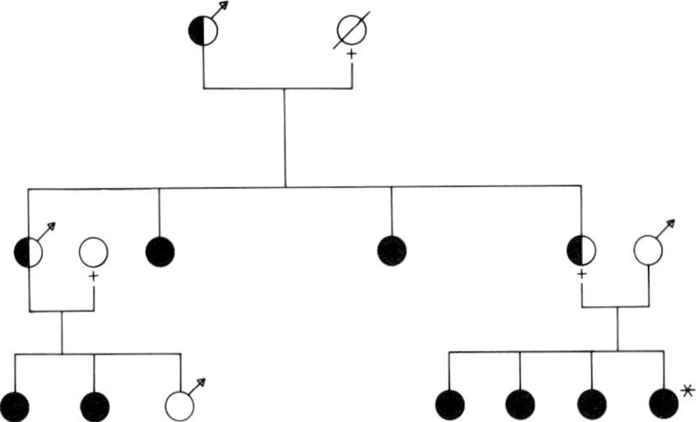

Fig. 2. Family pedigree of 1/18 translocation heterozygote. ♀, normal female; ♂, normal male; ♀, female heterozygote; ♂, male heterozygote; ●, untested abortus; ●*, unbalanced abortus; ♀̶, deceased female. (CHANDLEY et al. 1972)

Reciprocal translocation may thus lead to impaired spermatogenesis or to fetal wastage, the former mechanism being the more common. Considering the manifold expressions of chromosomal abnormalities and the higher than expected incidence in infertile males, the chromosomal evaluation should be included in the search of etiology in infertile males. Employing only nuclear sexing, FERGUSON-SMITH et al. (1957) showed that 1%–3% of men attending infertility clinics had abnormal sex chromosome constitutions.

III. Developmental Abnormalities

1. Congenital Anorchism

Congenital absence of testes is a rather rare condition and less than 100 cases have been reported to date (GLENN and MCPHERSON, 1971). Prepubertally the situation is usually misdiagnosed as cryptochidism. Postpubertally individuals manifest classic features of eunuchoidism including female-type fat-muscle and hair distribution, high-pitched voice, normal but small external genitalia, and empty scrotum. The chromosomal pattern is 46 XY and hormonal evaluation reveals the hypergonadotropic status with elevated LH and FSH levels and very low testosterone levels. The Wolffian duct system is developed and the Müllerian ducts are supressed. Differentiation of Wolffian ducts and suppression of Müllerian ducts commonly occur before the 20th week of intrauterine life and depend on a morphogenic substance secreted by the fetal testes for supression of Müllerian ducts and adequate androgenization for development of Wolffian ducts. The complete regression of Müllerian ducts coinciding with normal development of Wolffian ducts, masculinization of the urogenital sinus, and developmental of a normal, albeit small phallus allows the assumption that testicular material existed during the first half of intrauterine life and degenerated thereafter for unknown reasons.

Diagnosis does not require surgical exploration. By means of the HCG test (LUNENFELD and GLEZERMAN, Chap. 5 and 6 in this volume), the existence of testicular tissue can be documented regardless of its location. HCG is administered intramuscularly every 5 days for 3 weeks (5000 IU), and testosterone levels are measured in plasma. Rising testosterone levels point to ectopic testicular tissue, the localization of which may then be explored surgically. If testosterone levels remain unchanged, congenital anorchism may be safely assumed and further evaluation is not necessary. Fertility-restoring therapy is obviously not possible.

2. Cryptorchidism

The incidence of cryptorchidism in the adult population is about 0.5%. Cryptorchidism is a notorious cause of infertility. Van Zyl et al. (1975) found no cases of undescended testes among patients with a sperm density of greater than 20 million/ml, whereas the incidence among males with a sperm density of less than 20 million/ml was 9%. Woodhead et al. (1973) reported that one of three men who had previously been treated for unilateral cryptorchidism later was infertile. Hecker and Hienz (1967) reported that of 346 patients in whom unilateral cryptorchidism remained uncorrected 226 were infertile (65.3%). Adult males in whom both testes are outside the scrotum after puberty are always infertile. Individuals have azoospermia and highly elevated plasma FSH levels. Since Leyding cell function is usually not affected by ectopic testicular localization, the patients are normally virilized. Treatment for cryptorchidism is indicated for three main reasons:

1. The frequency of tumors in maldescended testes in adults has been estimated to be about 45 times greater than in normally descended gonads (Dubin and Amelar, 1977).
2. Males with empty scrotum are quite probably handicapped in their psychosexual development.
3. Timely and adequate treatment of cryptorchidism is mandatory as a prophylactic measure for later fertility potential.

Since irreversible changes begin to take place in a testicle that remains outside the scrotum beyond the age of 5, treatment has to be initiated earlier. The diagnosis and management of cryptorchidism in childhood is beyond the scope of this presentation and is dealt with elsewhere in this handbook. In adult patients with cryptorchidism, the risk of malignant degeneration in an irreversibly infertile testicle seem to outweigh the retained steroidogenic potential. We feel that ectopic testes in the adult should be removed. In case of bilateral cryptorchidism, the implantation of testes protheses and androgen substitution therapy may be the proper management. In cases of unilateral cryptorchidism, the decision concerning removal will be easier.

3. Intersexuality

Intersexuality if a fascinating topic but cannot be reviewed within the framework of this presentation. Psychological intersexuality such as transsexualism is evaluated psychosocially, cytogenetically and hormonally, and managed surgically and endocrinologically. Fertility is usually not of primary concern for these hapless patients.

Morphologic intersexuality as a phenomenon in a male infertility clinic is rather rarely encountered. A chromosomal etiology is present in the syndrome of "mixed gonadal dysgenesis." The most common karyotype is 45 XO/46 XY. The phenotypic expression is various. Müllerian structures are never completely suppressed, and a uterus, vagina, and at least one fallopian tube are virtually always present. One of the the gonads is a testicle and the other a streak structure (DAVIDOFF and FEDERMAN, 1973). Only a minority of affected individuals are sufficiently virilized to be reared as males. They are azoospermic and hypergonadotropic; on testicular biopsy no germinal cells can be found. No fertility-restoring therapy can be offered to these patients, and the removal of the testis should be considered seriously since one of four patients who are reared as males will develop a testicular tumor (WALSH, 1977).

Another expression of intersexuality associated with abnormalities in sex chromosomes is the so-called sex reversal syndrome. The incidence has been estimated to be 1 in 9000 new born males (DE LA CHAPELLE, 1972). These patients exhibit typical features of Klinefelter's syndrome, including male phenotype, atrophic testes, gynecomastia, and azoospermia. The genotype is 46 XX. WACHTEL et al. (1976) demonstrated an H-Y antigen in these patients, indicating that this syndrome is one more variety of Klinefelter's syndrome. The patients are azoospermic, hypergonadotropic, and irreversibly sterile. Androgen substitution therapy has to be considered in some cases. Genotypic females who present as phenotypic males in an infertility clinic are rather a curiosity. In most of these cases the adrenogenital syndrome will be the underlying etiology. On the other hand, patients with the most common expression of male pseudohermaphroditism, namely, the testicular feminization syndrome, will turn to female infertility clinics since these individuals are invariably reared as females. This entity will be discussed below.

IV. Defective Androgenization

Throughout life, adequate androgenization in the male is of paramount importance. Testosterone levels in the 14–18-week-old fetus are in the adult range and are indispensable for the development of male sex organs and the determination of a hypothalamic secretory pattern compatible with the requirements for gonadotropin secretion in later adult life. Postpubertally secreted testosterone promotes the development of secondary sex characteristics, exerts metabolic and psychic effects, stimulates the function of accessory sexual glands, plays an important role in the hormonal feedback mechanism, and is crucial for the process of spermatogenesis. Inadequate testosterone secretion in intrauterine life will therefore lead to ambiguous genitalia, and in the more severe forms, to male pseudohermaphroditism. Postpubertally, inadequate androgenization will lead to eunuchoidism (as expressed by inadequate development of secondary sex characteristics) and to spermatogenic testicular failure.

1. Inadequate Androgen Synthesis

Inadequate or failed androgen synthesis as a primary failure of Leydig cells to produce testosterone in adequate amounts in spite of sufficient LH stimulation occurs among others under the following conditions:

1. In primary anorchism: congenital anorchism was discussed previously. It is assumed that in congenital anorchism testicular tissue must have been present in early intrauterine life to account for supression of Müllerian structures and development of Wolffian ducts. Primary anorchism would imply that a functional testicular substance was absent a priori. Theoretically, individuals should have developed Müllerian ducts, whereas the Wolffian duct system should be absent. Thus, individuals should present as *gonadless* phenotypic females with a 46 XY karyotype. Search of the literature did not reveal reports of such cases.
2. In some cases of Klinefelter's syndrome: this condition was discussed previously.
3. In cases of enzymatic defects involving enzymes unique to the pathway of androgen synthesis: 17,20 desmolase (Zachman et al., 1972) and 17-β-*OH*-steroid dehydrogenase (Goebelsman et al. 1973): this condition has to be differentiated from the adrenogenital syndrome since enzymes involved in adrenal hormone synthesis are not affected and adrenal hyperplasia does not occur. According to the severity of the enzymatic defect, all stages from complete male hermaphroditism to mild hypospadias can be encountered. Since the morphogenic substance of the testes is secreted normally, the Müllerian duct system is invariably supressed. Walsh (1977) stated that fertility had not been reported to occur in patients with these enzymatic abnormalities. Both enzymatic defects are inherited either as autosomal-recessive or X-linked recessive traits.
4. In certain cases of male menopause: this entity is discussed elsewhere in this volume by Lunenfeld, Eshkol and Glezerman (Chap. 17 in this volume).

2. Inadequate Androgen Utilization (Androgen Insensitivity)

Androgen insensitivity should properly not be included in the framework of primary testicular failures. The substrate for both spermatogenesis, i.e., seminiferous tubules and steroidogenesis, i.e., Leydig cells, are a priori intact. However, testosterone produced by the Leydig cells in proper amounts and of adequate biologic properties does not exert its manifold effects due to an inability of hormone receptors to respond. Thus, in the complete form of androgen insensitivity, the so-called testicular feminization syndrome, individuals develop as phenotypic females. In less severe forms, phenotypic females have partial Wolffian duct development and ambiguous genitalia (Lubs et al. 1959). Since patients suffering from testicular feminization syndrome and from Lubs syndrom are reared as females, these entities will not be discussed here. Patients with milder expressions of androgen insensitivity, however, will be reared as males and may come to male infertility clinics. The symtomatology is directly related to the degree of deficient virilization, and among the broad spectrum of expressions at least three entities may be distinguished:

1. Gilbert-Dreyfus et al. (1957) described familial pseudohermaphroditism expressed by micophallus, severe hypospadias, gynecomastia, and azoospermia. The syndrome bears the name of the first author.
2. Reifenstein's syndrome (Reifenstein, 1947; Wilson et al., 1974; Amrhein et al., 1977; Glezerman et al., 1978a) consists of microtestes, gynecomastia, hypospadias, azoospermia, and various degrees of virilization deficiency.
3. The mildest form of androgen insensitivity is probably Rosewater's syndrome, characterized by gynecomastia and infertility (Rosewater et al., 1965). Androgen insensitivity in all its forms is X-linked recessive or male-limited autosomal inheritable. The patients are azoospermic, have atrophic testes, are hypergonadotropic, and irreversibly sterile.

V. Acquired "Primary" Testicular Failure

Acquired primary testicular failure could be defined as a condition in which testicular function has been changed by exogenous influences to such an extent that hormonal stimulation does not lead to the restoration of its functional capacity. Such a situation can occur following orchitis. Systemic infections may spread by the hematogenic or other routes to the testicles and cause this complication; possible causes are varicella, Bang's disease, malaria, syphilis, spotted fever, leprosy, infectious mononucleosis, filariasis, and others. However, the infection that is of practical importance and is notorious for its role in producing irreversible testicular damage in man is post-mumps orchitis, If mumps occurs before puberty, orchitis is a very rare complication. Postpubertal mumps, however, is relatively often followed by orchitis (according to DERRICK and DAHLBERG, 1976 in 18% of cases). The occurrence of this complication does not seem to be related to the severity of parotitis and may even develop without obvious involvement of the parotid glands. Fortunately, orchitis occurs most commonly unilaterally. In these cases the prognosis for fertility remains relatively good. Following bilateral orchitis with consequent testicular atrophic changes, irreversible testicular damage is the rule. It is only occasional that atrophy does not follow orchitis, and spermatogenesis recovers within 2–3 months (AMELAR and DUBIN, 1977). Atrophic testes are not necessarily diminished in size and may even be enlarged; the consistency is firm. The histologic appearance is characterized by distintegration of testicular structures, diminished tubular diameter, severe hyalinization of tubular walls and germinal epithelium, and complete lack of spermatogenetic elements. Leydig cells are usually not affected. Secondary to destruction of the germinal epithelium and lack of adequate feedback, FSH levels are elevated while LH levels are in the normal range. Patients are irreversible sterile. It has been stated that a similar picture may be the result of an autoimmune disease (GÜNTER, 1972).

C. Secondary Testicular Failure

Secondary testicular failure is a term that implies that normal function potential of the testes is not expressed due to insufficient stimulation by gonadotropins. Failed gonadotropin secretion may be result of pituitary or hypothalamic insufficiency and may involve the secretion of LH, FSH, or both. By definition, patients suffer from hypogonadotropic hypogonadism. Dysfunction of the pituitary-hypothalamic axis can be further differentiated with the aid of clomiphene citrate and GNRH (LUNENFELD and GLEZERMAN, Chap. 7).

I. Hypothalamic Failure

The Laurence-Moon-Biedl syndrome may be an expression of generalized hypothalamic insufficiency. KATZNELSON et al. (1974) examined two cousins demonstrating the classic picture of hypogonadism, obesity, short stature, mental retardation, retinitis pigmentosa, and diabetes mellitus. Leydig cell insufficiency was proved to be secondary by the HCG test (LUNENFELD et al., 1973). Employing the GNRH test, pituitary responsiveness was demonstrated. Normal response to ACTH stimulation but lack of diurnal variation of plasma cortisol in association with feedback disorders as demonstrated by negative short dexamethasone suppression test and metapyrone test indicated additional endocrine disorders secondary to hypothalamic insufficiency. Inheritance of the disease is most probably autosomal recessive.

Isolated hypothalamic failure to secrete GNRH will prevent the synthesis of pituitary gonadotropins and consequently lead to hypogonadotropic hypogonadism. Affected individuals fail to enter puberty and manifest typical features of eunuchoidism. Plasma gonadotropins and testosterone are in the prepubertal range and administration of clomiphene citrate fails to cause elevation of gonadotropin levels, as it would in prepubertal boys (BOYAR et al., 1973). The selective gonadotropin deficiency may occur sporadically or be inherited as an autosomal-dominant trait (SANTEN and PAULSEN, 1973). If anosmia coincides with hypogonadotropic hypogonadism, the entity is referred to as Kallman's syndrome (KALLMAN et al., 1944). Father-to-son transmission has been reported (MERRIAM et al., 1977). A variety of congenital defects may be associated with hypothalamic hypogonadism. The most common defect of the central nervous system apart from anosmia is congenital deafness, the most common somatic defect is cleft lip and/or palate, and the most common associated genital defect is cryptorchidism. Congenital defects seen in association with hypogonadotropic hypothalamic hypogonadism are compiled in Table 4. It has to be remembered that incomplete penetrance is a feature of this disorder. Relatives of the patients may be fertile but exhibit associated somatic defects.

Hypothalamic hypogonadotropic hypogonadism may be one expression of secondary hypothalamic lesions, such as neoplasms, inflammations, injury, and degenerative disorders. The severe general symptomatology of these entities will make the associated infertility a problem of secondary concern and is therefore not discussed here.

II. Pituitary Failure

Panhypopituitarism may be due to pituitary tumors, infection, and infiltrative processes and is a consequence of radiative or surgical ablation. In cases of prepubertal panhypopituitarism, growth retardation and deficiency symptoms of adrenal and thyroid involvement are the major clinical features. Postpubertal panhypopituitarism is expressed initially by reduced libibo, potency, and fatigue. As the extent of the lesion increases, deficiency symptomatology of other endocrine axes follow.

Pituitary failure expressed by selective insufficiency to secrete one or both gonadotropic hormones (FSH and LH) has occasionally appeared in the literature but has not been sufficiently substantiated. One syndrome that may be due to selective LH deficiency is referred to as the "fertile eunuch syndrome" (PASQUALINI and BURR, 1950). It is, however, still a matter of discussion whether pituitary failure is indeed the primary etiology of this syndrome. Patients are characterized by eunuchoid features associated with normally or low to normally

Table 4. Congenital defects seen in association with hypogonadotropic hypogonadism: (WINTER and SHERINS, 1977).[a]

Central nervous system	Somatic	Genital
Cranial nerve defects I, III, IV, V, VI, VIII (*mainly anosmia and deafness*)	*Cleft lip*	*Cryptorchidism*
	Cleft palate	Microphallus
Color blindness	Bifid uvula	Hypospadias
Colobomas	Phocomelia	
Retinitis pigmentosa	Short 4th metacarpal	
Mental retardation	Polydactly	
Seizures	Hypotonia	
Cerebellar ataxia		

[a] The most commonly occurring defects are in italics.

sized testes, presence of active spermatogenesis despite absence or scarcity of Leydig cells, and androgenic response (clinical or chemical or both) to administered HCG. McGULLAGH et al. (1953) and FAIMAN et al. (1968), among others, believe that selective LH deficiency is the underlying cause. MAKLER et al. (1977) have shown in two cases of fertile eunuch syndrome that GNRH administration results in significant secretion of FSH and LH by the pituitary gland, indicating normal functional capacity. Following HCG administration, testosterone levels rose to normal values; estradiol levels, however, remained low. Finally, no rise of FSH and LH could be observed after administration of clomiphene citrate during 3 weeks, indicating hypothalamic nonresponsiveness to chemical stimuli. Based on these results, the authors proposed a hypothesis, which bases the features of the fertile eunuch syndrome primarily on decreased estrogen production. Since estrogens are crucial for the synthesis and maintenance of hormone receptors, the impaired steroidal milieu may be responsible for inadequate functioning of the hypothalamus-pituitary-gonad axis.

Testicular function may be impaired due to excessive secretion of other pituitary hormones interfering with spermatogenesis and/or steroidogenesis and/or utilization. It has been demonstrated that prolactin, if secreted in excess, can cause anovulation and luteal insufficiency in the female. Prolactin supression therapy restores ovulatory cycles in most cases. In men, some authors (KRAUSE, 1978) have demonstrated correlations between prolactin levels and gonadotropin levels, while others (SEGAL et al., 1976; GLEZERMAN, unpublished data) could not confirm these observations. Equally equivocal were correlations between prolactin levels and sperm density (SEGAL et al., 1976; FONZO et al., 1977). Although elevated prolactin levels have been associated with impotency, testosterone levels are usually not influenced (FONZO et al., 1977). Increased prolactin secretion has been shown to occur following the administration of certain compounds (phenothiazines, reserpin, methyldopa, TSH) and may be an early sign of pituitary tumors. Galactorrhea may be associated in some cases but occurs more rarely than in the female. The observation of elevated prolactin levels in a patient requires meticulous screening for pituitary tumors, including tomography of the sella turcica and examination of visual fields. Since prolactin secretion is physiologically controlled by a hypothalamic-inhibiting factor, increased prolactin secretion by the pituitary gland may be an early sign of hypothalamic insufficiency, which should be evaluated.

Promising results with drugs inhibiting prolactin secretion in anovulatory females have prompted investigators to employ prolactin-inhibiting agents, mainly bromergocryptine, to treat male infertility (THORNER and BESSER, 1978). Good results were reported in hyperprolactinemic oligospermic males (SAIDI et al., 1977) and in normoprolactinemic oligospermic males (MONTANARI and VOLPE, 1978). The beneficial effect of prolactin-inhibiting agents in hyperprolactinemic impotency is impressive (FONZO et al., 1977).

D. Extratesticular Disturbances of Male Fertility

I. Infections

Infections of the genital tract have been shown to be associated with impaired fertility in man. Acute orchitis may lead to permanent damage of the germinal epithelium. Epididymitis, seminal vesiculitis, and prostatitis may be followed by strictures and scars in sperm-conveying structures, leading in most severe cases to azoospermia. Finally, infections of secondary sex glands may impair the secretory pattern of these glands and thus cause changes in the proper composition of seminal fluid. Seminal morphology, motility, and longevity may consequently be affected (LINDHOLMER, 1974; DEL PORTO and DERRICK, 1975). A high percentage of coiled spermatozoal tails (more than 20%) has been associated by ELIASSON (1977a) with prostatic infection. Genital tract infection may be completely asymptomatic and is sometimes detected only by meticulous clinical examination combined with biochemical and cytologic studies. Rectal palpation is an integral part of the physical examination of the patient. Details are described elsewhere in this volume. Laboratory evaluation includes exfoliative cytology of urinary sediments and of expressed prostatic secretions and bacteriologic cultures. Nevertheless, the diagnosis of inflammatory processes in the secondary sex glands is difficult due to the paucity of symptoms. In many patients with chronic prostatitis, no pathologic changes can be detected by rectal palpation. The presence of leukocytes in seminal fluid or in expressed prostatic secretions does not necessarily prove infection if numbered below 20 leukocytes per high-power field. Following sexual intercourse, the leukocyte count in expressed prostatic secretion may even surpass this limit without pathologic significance. Still, sufficient evidence is available to associate urogenital infection with leukocyte counts. MORTON (1968) considered more than 5×10^6 leukocytes/ml seminal fluid as definite evidence for urogenital infection. Usually, exfoliative cytology is employed in combination with palpatory findings to assess prostatic and seminal vesicle infections. The upper limit of leukocytes per high-power field in expressed prostatic secretions is considered to be 10 by MEARES (1973) and 20 by ELIASSON (1977b) and DERRICK and DAHLBERG (1976).

The differentiation between leukocytes and immature sperm cells, especially Sa and Sb spermatids, may be difficult. COUTURE et al. (1976) proposed a staining technique that enables better differentiation due to specifically staining of acrosome caps and accentuating cytoplasmic granules in polymorphonuclear leukocytes. The incidence of positive bacteriologic cultures of semen from nonsymptomatic infertile males was reported to be as high as 50% (GROSSEBAUER and KADEN, 1970). However, not all of the bacterial organisms, especially grampositive isolates, are considered to be pathogens (MEARS, 1973).

1. Gonorrhea

In recent years gonorrheic infections have increased in many parts of the world due to undertreatment, inadequate self-treatment, and occurrence of resistant strains. *Neisseria* infections may be complicated by invasion of periurethral glands with consequent healing and stricture formation. In untreated cases, the incidence of urethral strictures has been reported to be as high as 14% (DERRICK and DAHLBERG, 1976). The stricture may cause recurrent uterine tract infections including prostatitis, seminal vesiculitis, and epididymitis by providing facilities for bacterial colonization. Another complication of gonorrhea is ductal obstruction. Among 1294 cases of male infertility evaluated by AMELAR and DUBIN (1973), 4.4% had ductal obstructions, the majority of which followed gonorrheic infections.

2. Tuberculosis

Genital tuberculosis primarily affects prostate and seminal vesicles. In some 60% of cases, the epididymis is involved (DERRICK and DAHLBERG, 1976). Obstruction of sperm-conveying structures is the rule. Fortunately, tuberculotic infection of the genital tract is a rarity today thanks to currently available modes of therapy.

3. Smallpox

PHADKE et al. (1973) reported that some 80% of patients suffering from smallpox eventually develop obstructive epididymitis. In Europe and North America, this disease has been virtually eliminated. In some Asian countries, notably India, obstructive azoospermia as a sequela of smallpox is still a rather often encountered etiology of infertility.

4. Viral Infections

Post-mumps orchitis has been previously discussed. Other viral infections, such as mononucleosis, hepatitis, may cause depression of spermatogenesis. However, normal semen is usually obtained following a recovery period of 3–12 months. It has been speculated that not the viral infection per se but accompanying hyperpyrexia is responsible for suppressed sperm output in man. In studies of volunteers this concept was substantiated almost half a century ago (MACLEOD and HOTCHKISS, 1941).

5. T Mycoplasma Infections

T mycoplasma are commonly found in the urogenital tract of both females and males. There is still much controversy as to the role of these microorganisms in human infertility. Nongonococcal urethritis has been associated in 40%–60% of cases with T mycoplasma (Ambrose and Taylor, 1952; Shepard, 1956). Habitual abortions have been associated with colonization of T mycoplasma in 30%–40% of cases by Gnarpe and Friberg (1972) and Horn et al. (1974). T mycoplasma have been shown to occur more frequently in semen and cervical secretions of couples with unexplained infertility than in normal couples (Gnarpe and Friberg, 1972). DeLouvois et al. (1974), however, could not confirm these findings. Furthermore, Patton and Taymor (1975) could find no correlation between results of postcoital tests and mycoplasma colonization.

The observation by Mardh and Westrom (1976) that pregnant women harbored mycoplasma in their cervical secretions more often than nonpregnant women does not seem to contradict the possible role of mycoplasma in infertility since colonization may have occurred following conception.

Fowlkes et al. (1975) provided electron-microscopic evidence for the association of T mycoplasma with human spermatozoa. They demonstrated that mycoplasma adhere to the midpiece of spermatozoa in large numbers and form fibrin-like structures between tail and midpiece. Consequently, the tails of the spermatozoa become coiled. This may result in decreased motility, longevity, and reduced penetrability through cervical mucus. Spermatozoa that succeed in penetrating the cervical mucus column will transport mycoplasma into the uterine cavity. This might explain the relatively high incidence of habitual abortions associated with mycoplasma infections. Finally, a direct effect of mycoplasma upon the normal metabolism of spermatozoa is possible. Tetracyclines, especially doxycycline, have been shown to be very effective in the eradication of mycoplasma infections.

6. Trichomonas vaginalis

Derrick and Dahlberg (1976) observed seminal contamination with *Trichomonas* in as many as 89% of 190 infertile males as compared to 30% in a fertile control group. *Trichomonas* has been shown to cause spermatozoal agglutination and may thus interfere with motility and reduce the actual number of sperm cells that are available to penetrate the cervical mucus on their way to the oviduct. Walther (1973) reported decreased spermatozoal motility associated with *Trichomonas* infection of the semen. Metronidazole is a very efficient compound for the treatment of *Trichomonas* infections in both females and males.

7. Candida albicans

Candida albicans is encountered occasionally in semen of infertile patients. Sperm agglutination and clumping is observed if colonies are numerous. The effect upon spermatozoa is comparable to that of *Trichomonas* infection. Nystatin (Mycostatin) is the drug of choice to combat this infection.

8. Reiter's Syndrome

Bacterial urethritis associated with bilateral conjunctivitis and polyarthritis has been referred to as Reiter's syndrome. The causative organism is not know.

Chlamydia and mycoplasma have been named but not proved. Reduced spermatozoal motility is sometimes observed.

II. Stress

Stress and emotional tension may have deleterious effects on fertility (URRY, 1977). This fact has been known in animals for a long time. HUGGINS et al. (1939) reported that often during the first weeks of a dog's cage life transient testicular atrophy occurred. MESCHAKS (1955) observed reduced fertility in bulls that has been transported a long distance by truck. Following surgery in animals and humans, testosterone levels have been observed to be decreased in spite of unchanged LH levels (NAKASHIMA et al., 1975). Androgen secretion is reduced in men under combat training (ROSE et al., 1969) and in racing cyclists during a race (ISRAEL, 1969).

Thermal stress is known for its detrimental effect upon spermatogenesis. Cryptorchidism exposes the testes to an internal body temperature that is more than 2° C higher than the normal intrascrotal temperature. Irreversible damage of germinal epithelium is the rule in the postpubertal age group. Febrile infections may cause transient spermatogenetic suppression. Tight underwear or frequent hot baths may interfere with scrotal ventilation and thus increase the intrascrotal temperature, leading to thermal testicular stress. A similar effect is exerted by large varicoceles that lead to stasis of venous blood at the internal body temperature within the scrotum (GLEZERMAN et al., 1976b).

In thermal stress the effect is probably exerted directly upon the gonads and caused by the changed thermal environment. In emotional stress a more complicated mechanism must underlie the changes observed in testicular function. The detrimental effect of stress upon the gonads could be exerted through testosterone inhibition, suppression of spermatogenesis, or alteration of the testicular blood supply. Biogenic amines have been shown to be intimately involved in these processes. The reader is referred to the excellent review by URRY (1977).

III. Radiation

Rapidly dividing cells, such as germinal cells, are more susceptible to irradiation-induced damage than cells in the resting phase. Relatively low doses of radioactivity will damage spermatogonia, while larger dosis applied directly to spermatozoa will cause little or no effect upon motility, viability, or metabolism. (Possible chromosomal mutations, however, may interfere with fertilizing capacity. Data available to date are insufficient to allow conclusions to be drawn concerning this aspect.) Leydig cells and Sertoli cells are relatively insensitive to ionizing radiation. The radiation effect is dose related in both the intensity and duration of the radiation. Following irradiation, gradual depopulation of the seminiferous tubules may ensue, reflecting the loss of progeny of damaged spermatogonia. The loss of spermatogonia after irradiation seems to be due to direct destruction rather than to inhibition of mitosis or premature maturation (OAKBERG, 1959). However, even considerable damage to the testes following irradiation may be reversible as demonstrated by MacLeod and Hotchkiss (1964).

IV. Drugs

Alkylating agents, such as busulfan and triethylenemelamine, have an effect upon germinal cells similar to radiation. *Cyclophosphamide* may depress spermatogenesis completely, and the choice of this drug in nonmalignant diseases, such as chronic glomerulonephritis and rheumatoid arthritis, should be considered carefully. *Antimetabolites*, such as methotrexate, have been shown to produce chromosomal abnormalities in germinal cells. The uncritical use of these drugs in patients with psoriasis, for instance, should be weighed carefully against the deleterious effects on reproduction.

Similar side-effects are attributed to *colchicine*, a drug used in the therapy of gout and Mediterranean fever. Diphenylhydantoin (*Dilantin*), an antiepileptic drug, has been shown to selectively supress FSH secretion by the pituitary gland with consequent inhibition of spermatogenesis (STEWART-BENTLEY et al., 1976). *Antihypertensive drugs*, such as reserpine, may interfere with the normal ejaculative mechanism.

Testosterone application may lead to spermatogenic suppression due to inhibition of hypothalamic secretion of GNRH. *Diethylstilbestrol (DES)*, ingested by pregnant women, may produce anatomic changes in the genitals of male offspring, and defective spermatogenesis has been observed (GILL et al., 1976).

Marihuana has been associated with chromosomal abnormalities in cultured lymphocytes and lung tissue of smokers (NAHAS, 1975) and with temporary sterility. *Alcohol*, used excessively, may cause liver damage that in turn may impair the liver's ability to metabolize estrogen. Elevated estrogens may then interfere with the feedback mechanism, and reduced gonadotropin secretion by the pituitary gland may ensue with consequent inadequate stimulation of spermatogenesis. Excessive *tobacco* smoking may lead to increased levels of rhodanide in seminal fluid. This substance has been shown to suppress spermatozoal motility (HEHN, 1975).

V. Ejaculatory Problems

Psychosexual problems will be discussed more extensively in Chap. 16. Only ejaculatory problems will be mentioned here:

1. Anorgasmy

Patients suffering from anorgasmy are able to perform normal sexual intercourse, but ejaculation does not occur. In the presence of normal testicular function the patient will be infertile. Sexological therapy is usually rather effective to initiate or restore the ejaculatory pattern. In some cases the use of electrovibrators may be tried to obtain semen for artificial insemination in the female partner (VOGT, 1974; GLEZERMAN and LUNENFELD, 1976).

2. Retrograde Ejaculation

In patients with retrograde ejaculation, semen is ejected backward into the urinary bladder instead of being ejaculated through the meatus externus urethrae. This abnormality can be due to congenital malformations of the bladder neck, may be a sequela of prostatic or bladder neck surgery, may be caused by sympathetic blocking agents, or may be a complication of diabetes.

Diagnosis of retrograde ejaculation is made by the demonstration of spermatozoa in the urine following coitus or masturbation. Attempts to obtain semen can be made either by use of sympathomimetic agents (STEWART and BERGANT, 1974) or by regaining semen from a postcoital urinary specimen with subsequent washing to be used for artificial insemination in the female partner (HOTCHKISS et al., 1955; GLEZERMAN et al., 1976a). KEISERMAN et al. (1974) observed another type of retrograde ejaculation in which the ejaculate is partly propelled antegrade and partly regurgitated into the bladder. All stages of sperm deficiency may thus appear in the seminal analysis, ranging from oligospermia to azoospermia.

References

Ambrose SS Jr, Taylor WW (1952) A study of the etiology, epidemiology and therapy of non-gonoccocal urethritis. Am J Syph Gonorr Ven Dis 37:501

Amelar RD, Dubin L (1973) Male infertility: Current diagnosis and treatment. Urology 1:1

Amelar RD, Dubin L (1977) Other factors affecting male infertility. In: Amelar RD, Dubin L, Walsh PC (eds) Male infertility. Saunders, Philadelphia London Toronto, p 69

Amrhein JA, Klingensmith GJ, Walsh PC, McKusick VA, Migeon CJ (1977) Partial androgen insensitivity. The Reifenstein syndrome revisited. N Engl J Med 297:350

Bender MA, Gooch PC (1961) An unusually long human Y chromosome. Lancet 2:463

Boyar RM, Finkelstein, JW, Witkin M, Kapen S, Weitzmann E, Hellman L (1973) Studies of endocrine function in isolated gonadotropin deficiency. J Clin Endocrinol Metab 36:64

Cacheiro N, Russell LB, Swartout MS (1974) Translocations, the predominant cause of total sterility in sons of mice treated with mutagens. Genetics 76:73

del Castillo EB, Trabucco A, de la Balze FA (1947) Syndrome produced by absence of the germinal epithelium without impairment of the Sertoli or Leydig cells. J Clin Endocrinol Metab 7:493

Chandley AC (1976) Cytogenetics of infertile men. In: Hafez ESE (ed) Human semen and fertility regulation in man. Mosby, St. Louis, p 419

Chandley AC, Christie S, Fletcher J, Frackiewicz A, Jacobs PA (1972) Translocation heterozygosity and associated subfertility in man. Cytogenet Cell Genet 11:516

Chandley AC, Edmond PE, Christie S, Gowans L, Fletcher J, Frackiewicz A, Newton M (1975) Cytogenetics and infertility in man. Results of a five year survey of men attending a subfertility clinic. Part I. Karyotype and seminal analysis. Ann Hum Genet 39:231

Chandley AC, Edmond P, Maclean N, Fletcher J, Watson ES (1976) Cytogenetics and infertility in man. Results of a five year survey of men attending an infertility clinic. II. Testicular histology and meiosis. Ann Hum Genet 40:165

Chapelle A de la (1972) Analytic review: Nature and origin of males with XX sex chromosomes. Am J Hum Genet 24:71

Couture ML, Ulstein M, Paulsen CA (1976) Improved method for differentiating immature germ cells from white blood cells in human semen. Andrologia 8:61

Davidoff F, Federman DD (1973) Mixed gonadal gysgenesis. Pediatrics 52:725

Derrick FC Jr, Dahlberg B (1976) Male genital tract infections and sperm viability. In: Hafez ESE (ed) Human semen and fertility regulation in man. Mosby, St Louis, p 389

Dubin L, Amelar RD (1971) Etiologic factors in 1294 consecutive cases of male infertility. Fertil Steril 22:469

Dubin L, Amelar RD (1977) Surgery for male infertility. In: Amelar, RD, Dubin L, Walsh, PC (eds) Male infertility. Saunders, Philadelphia London Toronto, p 215

Eliasson R (1977a) Semen analysis and laboratory workup. In: Cockett ATK, Urry RL (eds) Male infertility. Grune & Stratton, New York San Francisco London, p 169

Eliasson R (1977b) Seminal plasma, accessory genital glands and infertility. In: Cockett ATK, Urry RL (eds) Male infertility. Grune & Stratton, New York San Francisco London, p 189

Faiman CH, Hoffmann DL, Ryan RJ, Albert A (1968) The "Fertile Eunuch" syndrome: Demonstration of isolated luteinizing hormone deficiency by RIA technique. Mayo Clin Proc 43:661

Ferguson-Smith MA, Lennox B, Mack WS, Stewart JSS (1957) Klinefelter's syndrome: Frequency and testicular morphology in relation to nuclear sex. Lancet 2:167

Fonzo D, Sivieri R, Gallone G, Andriolo S, Angeli A, Ceresa F (1977) Effect of a prolactin inhibitor on libido, sexual potency and sex hormones in men with mild hyperprolactinemia, oligospermia and/or impotence. Acta Endocrinol [Suppl 212] (Kbh) 85:142

Fowlkes DM, Dooher GB, O'Leary WM (1975) Evidence by scanning electronmicroscopy for an association between spermatozoa and T-mycoplasmas in men of infertile marriage. Fertil Steril 26:1203

Fraccaro M, Ikkos D, Londsten J, Luft R, Tillinges KG (1961) Testicular germinal dysgenesis (male Turner's syndrome). Acta Endocrinol (Kbh) 36:98

Franchimont P, Millet D, Vendrely E, Letawe J, Legros JJ, Netter A (1972) Relationship between spermatogenesis and serum gonadotrophin levels in azoospermia and oligospermia. J Clin Endocrinol Metab 34:1003

Gilbert-Dreyfus S, Sebaoun CIA, Belaisch J (1957) Etude d'un cas familial d'androgynoidisme avec hypospadias grave, gynecomastie et hyperoestrogenie. Ann Endocrinol (Paris) 18:93

Gill WB, Schumacher GFB, Bibbo M (1976) Structural and functional abnormalities in sex organs of male offspring of mothers treated with diethylstilbestrol (DES). J Reprod Med 16:147

Glenn JF, McPherson HT (1971) Anorchism: Definition of a clinical entity. J Urol 105:265

Glezerman M, Lunenfeld B (1976) Zur Therapie der männlichen Anorgasmie. Ein Fallbericht. Akutel Dermatol 2:167

Glezerman M, Lunenfeld B, Potashnik G, Oelsner G, Beer R (1976a) Retrograde ejaculation: Pathophysiologic aspects and report of two successfully treated cases. Fertil Steril 27:796

Glezerman M, Rakowszcyk M, Lunenfeld B, Beer R, Goldman B (1976b) Varicocele in oligospermic patients: Pathophysiology and results after ligation and division of the internal spermatic vein. J Urol 115:562

Glezerman M, Lewin S, Bernstein D (1978a) Reifenstein's syndrome – a target cell failure. Andrologia 10:353

Glezerman M, Lunenfeld B, Insler V (1978b) Male infertility. In: Lunenfeld B, Insler V: Diagnosis and treatment of functional infertility. Grosse, Berlin, p 114

Glezerman M, Brook I, Potashnik G, Ben-Aderet N, Insler V (1980) Fertility pattern and reported pregnancies in 333 patients referred to male infertility clinics. In: Proceedings of V° ESCO, Venice B. Salvadori, K. Semm, E. Vadora (Eds) Edizioni Internazionali, Rome p. 495

Gnarpe H, Friberg J (1972) Mycoplasma and human reproductive failure. 1. The occurrence of different mycoplasmas in couples with reproductive failure. Am J Obstet Gynecol 114:727

Goebelsman U, Horton R, Mestman JH, Arce JJ, Nagata Y, Nakamura RM, Thorneycroft IH, Mishell DR Jr (1973) Male pseudohermaphroditism due to testicular 17 β hydroxysteroid dehydrogenase deficiency. J Clin Endocrinol Metab 36:867

Grossgebauer K, Kaden R (1970) Bakteriologische Untersuchungen an menschlichen Ejakulaten. Arch Hyg Bakteriol 154:158

Günther E (1972) Die immunologische bedingte Orchitis. Andrologia 4:157

Hecker WC, Hienz HA (1967) Cryptorchism and fertility. J Pediatr Surg 2:513

Hehn S (1975) Einfluß von Rhodanid auf die Motilität menschlicher Spermatozoen nach verschiedenen Einwirkungszeiten und in verschiedener Konzentration. Andrologia 7:255

Heller CG, Clermont Y (1964) Kinetics of the germinal epithelium in man. Recent Prog Horm Res 20:545

Hendry WF, Polani PE, Pugh RCB, Sommerville IF, Wallace DM (1976) 200 infertile males: correlation of chromosome, histological, endocrine and clinical studies. Br J Urol 47:889

Hook EB (1973) Behavioral implication of the human XYY genotype. Science 179:139

Horn HW Jr, Kundsin RB, Kosasa TS (1974) The role of mycoplasma infection in human reproductive failure. Fertil Steril 25:380

Hotchkiss RS, Pinto AB, Kleegmann S (1955) Artificial insemination with semen recovered from the bladder. Fertil Steril 6:37

Huggins C, Masina MH, Eichelberger L, Wharton JD (1939) Qualitative studies of prostatic secretion. J Exp Med 7:543

Israel S (1969) C-17 ketosteroid excretion in extreme endurance effort. Endocrinologie 54:277

Johnsen SG (1970) The human testes. Plenum Press, New York

Kallman FJ, Schoenfeld WA, Barrera SE (1944) The genetic aspects of primary eunuchoidism. Am J Ment Defic 68:203

Katznelson D, Glezerman M, Saal B, Theodor R, Rotem Y (1974) An attempt to localize the primary lesion in Laurence-Moon-Biedl syndrome. Isr J Med Sci 10:796

Keiserman WM, Dubin L, Amelar RD (1974) A new type of retrograde ejaculation: report of three cases. Fertil Steril 25:1071

Kjessler B (1966) Karyotype, meiosis and spermatogenesis in a sample of men attending an infertility clinic. Monogr Hum Genet 2:1–93

Kjessler B (1972) Facteurs génétiques dans la subfertilité mâle humaine. In: Fécondite et stérilité du mâle. Masson, Paris

Klinefelter HF Jr, Reifenstein EC Jr, Albright F (1942) Syndrome characterized by gynecomastia, aspermatogenesis without A-Leydigism and increased excretion of follicle stimulating hormone. J Clin Endocrinol Metab 2:615

Koulischer L, Schoysman R (1974) Chromosomes and human infertility. I. Mitotic and meiotic chromosome studies in 202 consecutive male patients. Clin Gen 5:116

Krause W (1978) Prolaktinspiegel im Serum bei Patienten mit Störungen der Spermatogenese. Hautarzt 29:77

Kretser DM de, Burger HG, Fortune D, Hudson B, Long AR, Paulsen CA, Taft HP (1972) Hormonal, histological and chromosome studies. J Clin Endocrinol Metab 35:392

Lindholmer C (1974) The importance of seminal plasma for human sperm motility. Biol Reprod 10:533

Louvois J de, Harrison RF, Blades M, Hurley R, Stanley VC (1974) Frequency of mycoplasma in fertile and infertile couples. Lancet 1:1074

Lubs HA Jr, Vilar O, Bergenstal DM (1959) Familial male pseudohermaphroditism with labial testes and partial feminisation: Endocrine studies and genetic aspects. J Clin Endocrinol Metab 19:1110

Lunenfeld B, Glezerman M (1977) Versuch eines algorithmischen Ansatzes zur Diagnose männlicher Fertilitätsstörungen. Akta Dermatol 3:119

Lunenfeld B, Kohen F, Eshkol A, Beer R, Zuckerman Z, Birnboim N, Glezerman M (1973) Evaluation of male infertility by dynamic tests. In: James VHT, Serio M (eds) The endocrine function of the human testis, vol I. Academic Press, New York, p 561

MacLeod J, Hotchkiss RS (1941) The effect of hyperexia upon spermatozoa counts in men. Endocrinology 28:780

MacLeod J, Hotchkiss RS, Sitterson BW (1964) Recovery of male fertility after sterilization by nuclear radiation. JAMA 187:637

Makler A, Glezerman M, Lunenfeld B (1977) The fertile eunuch syndrome – an isolated Leydig cell failure? Andrologia 9:163

Mardh PA, Westrom L (1970) T-Mycoplasmas in the genitourinary tract of the female. Acta Pathol Microbiol Scand [A] 78:367

McCullagh DR (1932) Dual endocrine activity of testes. Science 76:19

McCullagh EP, Beck JC, Schaffenburg CA (1953) Syndrome of eunuchoidism with spermatogenesis, normal urinary FSH and low ICSH ("fertile eunuchs"). J Clin Endocrinol Metab 13:489

Meares EM (1973) Bacterial prostatitis versus "prostatosis". A clinical and bacteriological study. JAMA 224:1372

Merriam GR, Beitins IZ, Bode HH (1977) Father-to-son transmission of hypogonadism with anosmia. Am J Dis Child 131:1216

Meschaks P (1955) The effect of transport on spermatogenesis and excretion of neural steroids in the urine of bulls. Ciba Found Symp Mammalian Germ Cells, p 37

Mintz B (1957) Embryological development of primordial germ cells in the mouse: influence of a new mutation. W J Embryol Exp Morphol 5:396

Montanari GD, Volpe A (1978) Bromocryptine treatment for oligospermia and asthenospermia with normal prolactin. Lancet 1 (No 8056):160

Morton RS (1968) White cell counts in human semen. Their use in the diagnosis of prostatitis with references to uveitis. Br J Ven Dis 44:72

Nahas CG (1975) When friends or patients ask about marihuana. JAMA 233:79

Nakashima A, Koshiyama K, Uozumi T, Monden Y, Hamanaka Y, Kurachi K, Aono T, Mizutani S, Matsumoto K (1975) Effects of general anesthesia and severity of surgical stress on serum LH and testosterone in males. Acta Endocrinol (Kbh) 78:258

Nasr H, Chen JC, Pearson OH, Wieland RG (1971) Chromatin-negative Klinefelter's syndrome with normal testes and serum gonadotropins and testosterone. Fertil Steril 22:761

Oakberg EF (1959) Initial depletion and subsequent recovery of spermatogonia of the mouse after 20 r of gamma rays and 100, 300 and 600 r of X-rays. Radiat Res 11:700

Pasqualini RQ, Burr GE (1950) Sindrome hypoandrogenico con gametogenesis conservada. Classification de la insufficienca testicular. Rev Asoc Med Argent 64:6

Patton WC, Taymor ML (1975) An investigation of the relationship between cervical mycoplasma infection, the post coital test and infertility. Fertil Steril 26:211

Paulsen CA, Gordon DL, Carpenter RW, Gandy HM, Drucker WD (1968) Klinefelter's syndrome and its variants: A hormonal and chromosomal study. Recent Prog Horm Res 24:321

Perry G, Glezerman M, Insler V (1977) Selective filtration of abnormal spermatozoa by the cervical mucus *in vitro*. In: Insler, V, Bettendorf G (eds) The uterine cervix in reproduction. Thieme, Stuttgart, p 118

Phadke AM, Samant NR, Dewal SD (1973) Smallpox as an etiologic factor in male infertility. Fertil Steril 24:802

Porto G del, Derrick FC Jr (1975) Effect of bacteria on sperm motility. Urology 5:638

Reifenstein EC (1947) Hereditary familial hypogonadism. Am Fed Clin Res 3:86

Rose RM, Bourne PG, Poe RO, Mougey EH, Collins DR, Mason JW (1969) Androgen response to stress. II Excretion of testosterone, epitestosterone, androsterone and etiocholanolone during basic combat training and under threat of attack. Psychsom Med 31:418

Rosewater S, Gwinup G, Hamwi GJ (1965) Familial gynecomastia. Ann Intern Med 63:377

Saidi K, Wenn RV, Sharif F (1977) Bromocriptine for male infertility. Lancet 8005:250

Santen RJ, Paulsen CA (1973) Hypogonadotropic eunuchoidism. I. Clinical study of the mode of inheritance. J Clin Endocrinol Metab 36:47

Segal S, Polishuk WZ, Ben-David M (1976) Hyperprolactinemic male infertility. Fertil Steril 27:1425

Setchell BP, Jacks F (1974) Inhibin-like activity in rat testis fluid. J Endocrinol 62:675

Shepar MC (1956) T-form colonies of pleuropneumonia-like organisms. J Bacteriol 71:362

Skakkebaek N, Hultén M, Philip J (1973) Quantification of human seminiferous epithelium. IV. Histological studies in 17 men with numerical and structural autosomal aberrations. Acta Pathol Microbiol Scand [A] 81:112

Steinberger E (1977) Discussion to D.T. Mininberg: Genetic aspects of male infertility. In: Cockett ATK, Urry RL (eds) Male infertility. Grune & Stratton, New York San Francisco London, p 59

Steinberger A, Steinberger E (1976) Secretion of an FSH-inhibiting factor by cultured Sertoli cells. Endocrinology 99:918

Stewart BH, Bergant JA (1974) Correction of retrograde ejaculation by sympaticomimetic medication. Preliminary report. Fertil Steril 25:1073

Stewart-Bentley M, Vergi A, Chang S, Hiatt R, Horton R (1976) Effects of Dilantin of FSH and spermatogenesis. Clin Res 24:101

Summit RL (1973) Noonan syndrome. In: Bergsma D (ed) Birth defects atlas and compendium. National Foundation – March of Dimes. Williams & Wilkins, Baltimore

Thorner MO, Besser GM (1978) Bromocryptine treatment of hyperprolactinemic hypogonadism. Acta Endocrinol (Suppl 216) (Kbh) 88:131

Urry RL (1977) Stress and infertility. In: Cockett ATK, Urry RL (eds) Male infertility. Grune & Stratton, New York San Francisco London, p 145

Vogt HJ (1974) Primäre männliche Anorgasmie. In: Fortschritte der Fertilitätsforschung, Bd II. Grosse, Berlin p 186

Wachtel SS, Koo GC, Breg WR, Thaler HT, Dillard GM, Rosenthal IM, Dosik H, Gerald PS, Saenger P, New M, Lieber E, Miller OJ (1976) Serologic detection of a Y-linked gene in XX males and XX true hermaphrodites. N Engl J Med 295:750

Walsh PC (1977) Endocrine and chromosomal factors associated with infertility. In: Amelar RD, Dubin L, Walsh PC (eds) Male infertility. Saunders, Philadelphia London Toronto, p 33

Walther H (1973) Trichomonas infection, clinical picture; therapy and significance to fertility and sterility. Z Hautkr 48:553

Wijk JAM van, Tijdnik GAJ, Stolte LAM (1962) Anomalies in the Y chromosome. Lancet 1:218

Wilson JD, Harrod MJ, Goldstein JL, Hemsell D, MacDonald PC (1974) Familial incomplete male pseudohermaphroditism; Type I: Evidence for androgen resistance and variable clinical manifestations in a family with the Reifenstein's syndrome. N Engl J Med 290:1097

Winters SJ, Sherins RJ (1977) Endocrine causes of male infertility. In: Cockett ATK, Urry RL (eds) Male infertility. Grune & Stratton, New York San Francisco London, p 79

Woodhead DM, Pohl DR, Johnson DE (1973) Fertility of patients with solitary testes. J Urol 109:66

Zachman M, Vollmin JA, Hamilton W, Prader A (1972) Steroid 17,20 desmolase deficiency: A new cause of male psudohermaphroditism. Clin Endocrinol (Oxf) 1:369

Zyl JA van, Menkveld R, Kotze TJ van, Retief AE, Nierkerk WA van (1975) Oligozoospermia: A seven-year survey of the incidence, chromosomal aberrations, treatment and pregnancy rate. Int J Fertil 20:129

Male Fertility Disorders –
History and Clinical Examination

K. Bandhauer

With 1 Figure

A. History

The first interview with the patient frequently has a decisive influence on the success of his future management. In andrologic care, numerous details of the patient's most intimate life are significant for diagnosis and treatment: a quite exceptional relationship between the physician and his patient is therefore required. It is not infrequently the wife who first drives her husband to seek confirmation of his fertility. Not wishing to be shown up as "inadequate", he may adopt an attitude of denial to his possible inability to procreate and may therefore flatly reject the diagnosis of disordered spermatogenesis. On occasion, it may suffice to point out that impaired fertility is a common condition in the male. Relieving him thus of the conviction that he is alone in his plight often helps to secure the patient's cooperation for further investigation and treatment. At this juncture, it is also worth making an inquiry about the condition of his wife. Documenting her state of investigation will offer, early in the diagnostic process, an opportunity to establish the all-important contact with her gynecologist.

Quite apart from facilitating initial personal introduction, careful history taking may also provide important clues as to the possible causation of impaired fertility. A considerable number of questionnaires and history forms have been developed (Schirren, 1971; Ludvik, 1973; Bandhauer and Koevesdi, 1970), all with the object of making the most carefully directed and accurate inquiries possible from the patient.

Comparison of these forms shows that they are broadly congruent in content and differ only on formal points.

The information to be gleaned from the patient may be divided into four principal sections:
1. Past history of illnesses, injuries, and operations
2. Sexual and marital history (including puberty)
3. Drug history, addiction, nicotine and alcohol consumption, exposure to physical and chemical agents impairing spermatogenesis
4. Urinary symptoms

I. Past History

The history of past illness should be as complete as possible and should include trivial long-standing infections and childhood illnesses. Alterations of spermatogenesis may be brought about by apparently harmless illnesses, such as measles and simple pneumonia, as well by serious infections, such as typhoid, syphilis, and gonorrhoea (see Chap. 3). The deleterious influence of raised temperature and protracted febrile illness on spermatogenesis is well-known. The age factor needs to be taken into consideration in the history of these illnesses since the testicular changes occurring in various infectious diseases of infants and children tend to be reversible, just as prepubertal mumps orchitis is frequently benign and runs a reversible course. After puberty, however, febrile or toxic damage to the spermatogenic system seems to occur more frequently (MacLeod, 1951; Barton and Wiesner, 1952; Schulz and Niermann, 1973; Marberger and Marberger, 1963).

II. Sexual History

The significance of the sexual history reaches far beyond mere determination of the frequency of intercourse. It is not adequate for the partners simply to have determined the time of ovulation in the realization that this is a particularly favorable period for conception. Other factors are of equal importance, such as the extent to which the partners understand each other's sexual needs, their ability to achieve orgasm simultaneously, and the particular technique of intercourse they employ. Coitus in the shadow of a psychological obligation to fertilize is not just characterized by a variable disturbance of libido and potency but actually carries an impaired conception rate, as many physicians with an andrologic interest have observed. Complaints of premature ejaculation are not uncommon among couples with a particularly intense desire to have children, and such couples require corresponding counseling.

III. Drug History

Attention has already been drawn in Chap. 3 to the disturbance of spermatogenesis by various groups of pharmacologic, physical, and chemical agents. In addition, physical and psychological problems influencing the patient's fertility may be gained access to by the frequency with which he takes tranquillizers, hypnotics, stimulants, phenacetin and salicylic acid derivatives, and various other drugs. Excess consumption of alcohol and nicotine should equally be noted and integrated into the eventual therapeutic design.

IV. Urinary Symptoms

No history can makes its proper contribution to the evaluation of impaired male fertility unless it detects urinary symptoms of an inflammatory or obstructive nature. Patients with a urethral stricture are more likely to notice their poor urinary stream than the retarded efflux of their semen with its concomitant poor deposition. Equally, inflammatory symptoms of micturition may be noted more rapidly, and registered as an unpleasant sensation by many patients, than may be only slightly painful ejaculation, such as occurs in genital tuberculosis or in chronic recurrent vesiculoprostatitis.

The significance of recognizing these symptoms lies chiefly in highlighting areas of interest in the examination and further investigation of the urinary tract and in alerting the physician to the possibility of morphological and functional causes of sterility to be found beyond the limits of the genital tract.

In this context, useful information may also be gained by inquiring after the sequence of events at ejaculation as well as the form and color of the ejaculate. Often it is only after the most searching questioning that such symptoms as painful ejaculation, frank blood in the ejaculate or its brownish discoloration (hematospermia), or the total absence of ejaculation are brought to light.

B. Clinical Examination

Examination of the husband in a childless marriage requires both a general clinical examination and attention to possible alterations of the genital tract. The general physique of the patient, his hair distribution, possible obesity or abnormal fat distribution, gynecomastia, dysmorphic stature, and the presence of edema or ascites will need to be noted. Such changes may often enable an early clinical diagnosis, which may then be confirmed by an appropriately restricted series of investigations.

I. Genital Tract

Clinical examination of the external genitalia, prostate, and seminal vesicles should be precise and should take account of the various possible etiologies of male fertility disturbances. Phimosis, hypospadic deformity of the urethra, and Peyronie's disease may not be so pronounced as to result in an absolute barrier to intercourse. They may nevertheless interfere with conception by preventing the proper deposition of semen in the upper vagina.

Quite apart from such technical factors, congenital abnormalities of the penis are accompanied by an increased incidence of abnormal seminal analysis. In an extensive study, SCHIRREN and MOLNAR (1969) were thus able to demonstrate impaired fertility in patients with hypospadias or phimosis, finding a pathologically altered spermiogram in 60% of their group. The relationship between these anatomic and seminal abnormalities has not yet been elucidated.

Palpation of the testicle should assess its size and consistency as well as the presence or absence of infiltration, hydrocele, tumor, etc. HEINKE and DÖPFNER (1960) and LABHART (1971) have developed an instrument (orchidometer) for determining testicular size (Fig. 1). An alternative instrument permitting exact measurements of length and volume has been described by HYNIE (1969).

Assessment of the epididymis may present difficulties. Residual post-inflammatory changes and scarring may be difficult to differentiate from the epididymis distended by obstruction of the vas deferens. Nevertheless, in proven cases of azoospermia, palpation of the epididymis by an experienced urologist may provide clues as to the site of the lesion. The "empty" epididymis may be caused by a primary testicular abnormality or by obstruction of the rete testis,

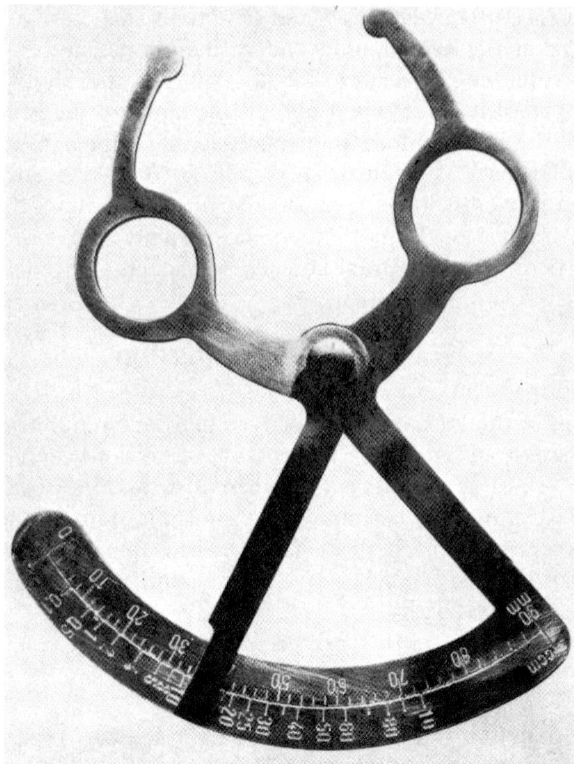

Fig. 1. Orchidometer for determining testicular size

whereas a "full" epididymis suggests an obstruction in the tail of the epididymis
or in the vas deferens.

Assessment of the scrotal contents should on principal always be carried
out with the patient first supine and then erect, chiefly to demonstrate varicocele.

Rectal examination represents an important part of clinical examination
in adrologic practice. Diagnostic parameters that may influence further management include shape, size, and consistency of the prostate and seminal vesicles,
infiltration of the pelvic organs in inflammatory conditions, localized tenderness
on examination, tumors, and last but not least assessment of tone in the anal
sphincter where a neurogenic inadequacy of ejaculation is suspected. Wherever
possible, definite morphological change of the prostate or seminal vesicles should
be related to abnormalities of the semen (fructose, citric acid, motility, etc.)
to put the findings in their broad diagnostic context. An impalpable or extremely
small prostate suggests an endocrine adnormality of hypogonadal type, as do
"absent" seminal vesicles.

II. General Examination

The patient's general clinical appearance not infrequently suggests endocrine
abnormalities whose possible causal role in disordered male fertility may require

consideration. As endocrine disturbances chiefly express themselves in a manifest disproportion of trunk and limb length, clinical assessment of the patient's physical proportions plays a particular role. Comparison of span (distance from forefinger tip to forefinger tip of the outstretched arms) to body height provides a rough guide. Before the 10th year of life, span is normally less than height, whereas it subsequently exceeds it. In the condition of precocious puberty, early fusion of the epiphyses brings about a span that is markedly less than height. Delayed puberty on the other hand produces a span markedly in excess of body height as is also the case in eunuchs and patients with Klinefelter's syndrome and other testicular disorders.

Determination of bone age, and to a lesser extent of dental development, provides further clues as to abnormalities of endocrine development. However, the chief role of these investigations is in relation to childhood and adolescence, and they do not play an important part in assessing disorders of fertility in the adult man.

1. Typical Alterations of Physical Habit with Related Disorders of Spermatogenesis

a) Early (Prepubertal) Castration

Male sex characteristics are absent, the penis is infantile, and the scrotum small and not at all pouchlike. Prostate and seminal vesicles are impalpable. Skin is remarkably fine, wrinkled, and pale. Pubic and axillary hair is absent or only sparsely developed; a beard is equally absent. There is an increased amount of subcutaneous fat, especially in the region of the lower abdomen, hips, and pubic fat pad. The build is tall and eunuchoid (standing giant – sitting dwarf). Genu valgum and a high-pitched voice are prominent features.
Absent sexual function

b) Late (Postpubertal) Castration

Prostate and seminal vesicles are atrophic and barely palpable. Pubic and axillary hair is deficient, as is the beard. There is a marked tendency to adiposity of the lower abdomen, hips, and pubic fat pad.
Absent or reduced sexual function

c) Congenital Hypogonadism: Werner's Syndrome

Mainly apparent with advancing age, this is characterized by premature baldness, generalized atrophy of the musculature, sensory disturbances, and ulceration of the skin. The voice is notably high-pitched and croaking.
Azoospermia or high-grade oligozoospermia

d) Rothmund's Syndrome

This syndrome consists of poikilodermia, alopecia, and cataract formation.
Azoospermia or high-grade oligozoospermia

e) Lawrence-Moon-Biedel Syndrome

This comprises notable obesity, debility, and poly- or syndactyly.
Azoospermia or high-grade oligozoospermia

f) Prader-Labhart-Willi Syndrome

The patients are of short stature, are adipose, and show considerable imbecility. The beard is very poorly developed.
Absent spermatogenesis

g) Klinefelter's Syndrome

In this syndrome all transitional grades from normal male habit to severe eunuchism may be observed. Gigantism, disproportionate leg length, and an excess of ground-to-pubis measurement over pubis-to-crown length or half span are characteristic. There is frequently well-defined gynecomastia, and the beard is poorly developed. The testes are at most bean-sized and are of coarse texture.

These patients are sex-chromatin positive. Chromosome counts most frequently reveal an XXY or XXXY constitution, but other mosaics are possible.
Azoospermia
(To date a single case with high-grade oligozoospermia has been described by Warburg, 1963).

h) "Pseudo-" Klinefelter's Syndrome

This is a condition of hypogonadism with small testes, eunuchism, and dysproportion of stature, as well as gynecomastia. Sex chromatin is absent and there are no mosaics on chromosome count.
Azoospermia

References

Bandhauer K, Koevesdi S (1970) Der Fertilitätsstatus des Mannes. Urol A 9:4, 192
Barton M, Wiesner BP (1952) Significance of testicular exfoliation in male infertility. Br Med J 4791:958
Bowen P, Lee CSN, Migeon CJ, Kaplan NM, Whalley TJ, McKusick VA, Reifenstein EC Jr (1965) Hereditary male pseudohermaphroditism with hypogonadism, hypospadias and gynecomastia. Ann Intern Med 62:252
Heinke E, Doepfner R (1960) Fertilitätsstörungen beim Mann. Somatischer Teil. In: Jadasohns Handbuch der Haut- und Geschlechtskrankheiten. Ergänzungswerk. Bd VI/3. Springer, Berlin Göttingen Heidelberg
Hynie J (1969) Erfahrungen bei der Diagnostik und Therapie andrologischer Störungen. Andrologie 1:155
Klinefelter HF, Reifenstein EC, Albright F (1942) Syndrome characterized by gynecomastia, spermatogenesis without A-leydigism and increased excretion of follicle stimulating hormone. J Clin Endocr 2:615
Labhart A (1971) Klinik der inneren Sekretion, 2. Aufl. Springer, Berlin Heidelberg New York
Lipsett MB, Davis TE, Wilson H, Canfield CJ (1965) Testosterone production in chromatine-positive Klinefelter's syndrome. J Clin Endocr 25:1027
Ludvik W (1973) Erkrankungen der Genitalsphäre des Mannes. In: Alken CE, Staehler W (Hrsg) Klinische Urologie. Thieme, Stuttgart, S 488

MacLeod J (1951) Effect of chickenpox and of pneumonia on semen quality. Fertil Steril 2:6, 253

Marberger E, Marberger H (1963) Veränderungen des Ejakulates bei entzündlichen Veränderungen der männlichen Adnexe. Wien Med Wochenschr 113:153

Prader A, Labhart A, Willi H (1956) Ein Syndrom von Adipositas, Kleinwuchs, Kryptorchismus und Oligophrenie nach myatonieartigem Zustand im Neugeborenenalter. Schweiz Med Wochenschr 86:1250

Reifenstein EC Jr (1947) Hereditary familial hypogonadism (Abstract). Proc Am Med Clin Res 3:86

Schirren C (1971) Praktische Andrologie. Brüder Hartmann, Berlin

Schirren C (1972) Exakte Messung der Hodengröße. Andrologie 4:261

Schirren C, Molnar J (1969) Der Genitalbefund bei andrologischen Patienten. I. Entwicklungsstörungen von Penis und Urethra. Andrologie 1:101

Schulz H, Niermann H (1973) Fertilität und Infektionskrankheiten. Andrologie 5:133

Vischer D, Labhart A, Prader A, Ginsberg J (1971) Das Prader-Labhart-Willi-Syndrom. Syndrom von Myatonie, Oligophrenie, Adipositas, Hypogenitalismus, Hypogonadismus, Diabetes mellitus. In: Pfeiffer EF (Hrsg) Handbuch des Diabetes mellitus, Bd II. Lehmann, München

Warburg E (1963) A fertile patient with Klinefelter's syndrome. Acta Endocrinol (Kbh) 43:12

Zuppinger K, Engel E, Forbes AP, Mantooth L, Claffey J (1967) Klinefelter's syndrome, a clinical and cytogenetic study in 24 cases. Acta Endocrinol [Suppl] (Kbh) 113 ad vol 54

ing the vagina per se. For these patients, even condom intercourse will present a form of unacceptable masturbation and a violation of the biblical injunction against "spilling of the seed needlessly" (Genesis 38:7–10). In these cases, we suggest intercourse using a perforated "Milex pouch." Since a very tiny hole will allow for a physical connection between penis and vagina but will hardly diminish the seminal volume, this simple technical procedure will relieve the conflict of conscience and is generally acceptable to both patient and religious authorities.

If a private area is available on the premises of the clinic or at the office, semen collection is best performed there since semen is then available for immediate evaluation. However, it may be less embarassing for the patient to produce semen at his own home. This is acceptable if the semen can be delivered to the laboratory in less than 45 min (see below). If the patient's home is too far away and masturbation on the premises is not acceptable, we usually suggest renting a hotel room in the vicinity.

The specimen bottle should be supplied by the laboratory. If the specimen container is provided by the patient, the result may be an exotic collection of drug, food, and cosmetic bottles, and the usefulness of the specimen obtained may be subject to doubt. It should be emphasized that only containers be used that were pretested by chemical and biologic studies as to their effects on seminal parameters. Inchiosa (1965) demonstrated that toxic substances may leak through plastic and rubber material used in disposable syringes, and Jaeger and Rubin (1970) showed that plastic bags used for blood storage may be similarly hazardous. Although glass bottles are probably better suited for semen collection, disposable plastic material is certainly cheaper. Some toxicity studies should be undertaken prior to their introduction into laboratory use.

C. Sexual Abstinence Before Collection of the Ejaculate

The period of continence preceding collection of the semen specimen has a remarkable influence on spermatozoal concentration and less effect on motility and morphology (Freund, 1962, 1963). For the sake of standardization, most laboratories specify a period of continence (usually 3–5 days). However, Freund and Peterson (1976) have defended the position of not specifying a set period of abstinence. They have pointedly stressed that a fixed period of continence preceding the collection of the specimen means that the specimen is no longer a random sample of the patient's spermatozoal output at his usual frequency of ejaculation. Thus, the semen sample delivered may not be representative of the patient's semen.

Sperm output observed in longitudinal studies is far from uniform and may vary considerably even in fertile volunteers. Thus, examination of a single semen specimen is of very limited usefulness if the quantitative gametogenic function of the testes is to be assessed. Since both standardization and proper reflection of physiologic conditions are important in the evaluation of the infertile male, it is justified to perform two to four semen analyses prior to diagnosis and treatment. We prefer to examine two semen samples delivered following set periods of continence (4 days) end two samples delivered after intervals similar to regular intervals of intercourse. The two samples following preset abstinence periods are delivered at an interval of at least 6 weeks while the two samples following "physiologic intervals" are delivered during these 6 weeks. Thus, semen output is observed longitudinally within a period approaching three-quarters of a spermatogenic cycle.

The patient should be carefully instructed to protect his specimen from undercooling and overheating. Evaluation of the sample delivered is made following adjustment to 37° C, but mostly at room temperature. We make a point of having the sample received personally by a technician to guarantee the availability of the patient to supply important information regarding the sample. Relevant information is best gained by direct questioning rather than by often incompletely filled out questionnaires. The following information should be obtained from the patient upon receiving the specimen:

1. Mode of production (i.e., masturbation, condom).
2. Length of abstinence before ejaculation.
3. Age of the specimen (i.e., time lapse between collection and delivery).
4. Mode of transport with special regard to possible temperature changes.
5. Whether the ejaculate has been collected completely into the container.

D. Examination of the Ejaculate

Usually the color of the ejaculate is whitish-gray to yellowish and tends more to yellowish the longer the abstinence period is. Although color determination is by no means a test for sexual abstinence, it may nevertheless provide some clue concerning the abstinence interval. Discoloration of the semen may point to genital tract infections if the specimen appears white or yellow (leukocytes) or to bleeding from some point along the tract if the semen is reddish (erythrocytes). Finally, certain drugs such as antibiotics may lead to discoloration.

I. Coagulation and Liquefaction

Immediately after ejaculation, the liquid seminal fluid coagulates and subsequently liquefies within 5–30 min. The physiologic function of this process remains unclear (LUNENFELD and GLEZERMAN, 1981). The coagulation process differs basically from blood coagulation as far as coagulation factors are concerned. The coagulative enzyme in man originates in the seminal vesicle while the liquefying enzyme, seminine, is produced by the prostate gland.

The progress of coagulation or liquefaction may be disturbed. Azoospermia concomitant with complete lack of coagulation would indicate agenesis of the seminal vesicle or occlusion of ejaculatory ducts. If the seminal coagulum fails to liquefy, probably due to poor prostate lytic activity, the persistent coagulum may trap spermatozoa and restrict motility. Thus, observation of coagulation and liquefaction is of considerable importance.

Following liquefaction, the seminal fluid achieves a viscous state. Hyperviscosity may also impair sperm transport. Usually, viscosity is ascertained approximately by observing the ability of the fluid to adapt to the form of the slowly rotated semen container (Zaneveld and Polakovski, 1977) or by pouring it into another jar and observing its ability to fractionate (Amelar et al. 1977). A more accurate method consists of measuring the time necessary for the seminal fluid to form a drop if released from a pipette (Eliasson, 1973). While experienced personnel may gain sufficient information concerning viscosity with the former technique, it may be necessary in some cases to collect more exact information by using the latter technique.

II. Volume

The volume of the seminal fluid averages 2–5 ml. Prolonged sexual abstinence may result in a larger seminal volume. The prostate and epididymal contribution to the seminal fluid usually does not exceed 1 ml. Thus, semen volume is mainly a function of the activity of the seminal vesicles. Inflammatory processes, mainly of this gland and to a lesser extent of the prostate, may lead to hypervolemia with resultant dilution of the cell content. Reduced seminal volume may result from androgen deficiency, may be the consequence of proximal occlusion of the ejaculatory ducts, or may simply reflect incomplete ejaculation or loss of parts of the specimen.

pH determination is easily performed using indicator paper. A pH exceeding 8.0 may suggest acute diseases of the seminal vesicles or may be due to delayed measurement. (Seminal plasma releases CO_2 continuously and consequently pH values increase.) If the pH is below 7, it may be a sign of occlusion of the ejaculatory ducts or of contamination of the semen specimen by urine.

III. Biochemical Analysis

Specific secretory products of the secondary sexual glands may be identified in the seminal plasma. Since these glands are androgen dependent, testosterone levels should be examined whenever abnormal results are obtained. Estimation of zinc, inositol, citric acid, and acid phosphatase may lead to conclusions concerning proper functioning of the prostate gland. Fructose and prostaglandins are specific products of the seminal vesicles, and carnitine and glycerophosphorylcholine (GPC) are rather specific excretions of the epididymis. Thus, examination of these substances may help to identify malfunction of either of these organs.

E. Microscopic Examination

Sperm quality is evaluated immediately after liquefaction of the sample.

I. Motility

Motility is generally evaluated by direct microscopic observation of the semen and is expressed in percentages. The type of movement (progressive or nonprogressive) is assessed, and duration of motility is evaluated by repeated observation within a period of at least 3 h. A motility loss of 10%–20% within 3 h is considered within the normal range. The subjectivity of the evaluation of motility has troubled investigators for many years. Sophisticated methods for objectivization have been proposed: BOTELLA LLUSIA (1956) used graduated glass vessels and measured the time required by sperm cells to travel one end of the vessel to the other. JANICK and MACLEOD (1970) measured the course of sperm cells per unit time on microfilm, and CASTENHOLZ (1974) used the photokymographic approach. JECHT and RUSSO (1973) used a closed-circuit method comprising video tape, digital data display, and a computer. However, all methods aimed at improving objectivity require either considerable amounts of man-hours or remain restricted to highly specialized and well-equipped laboratories.

Recently, MAKLER (1978) developed a new method for objective determination of sperm motility. A special counting chamber of 10-μm depth was designed that provides standard conditions under which samples can be examined. Due to the special design of the chamber, horizontal movement of cells and surface friction is eliminated while all cells are seen on one focal plane. Motility is measured by a multiple-exposure photographic technique using a still camera and a stroboscope. Information gained from films includes:

1. Percentage of motile and nonmotile cells.
2. Individual speed of sperms and mean velocity.
3. Grading of motility.
4. Easy calculation of sperm density expressed in millions per milliliter.

This method seems to be highly accurate with a remarkably good cost/efficiency index. Figure 1 demonstrates a typical semen specimen after 7 consecutive exposures during 1 s. Nonmotile sperm appear much brighter than the motile sperm, which appear as 7-linked chains; their shape indicates direction and distance traveled by each sperm during 1 s. From the direction and length of the chains, the distance traveled by each individual sperm and its progressive speed may be easily calculated.

II. Count

Sperm cell counts are usually performed in a Neubauer of Thoma-Zeiss counting chamber after immobilizing the sperm cells by dilution with distilled water or by immersion of the test tube in hot water. Cells counted in the chamber are multiplied by a factor that is dependent on the dilution and the volume of the chamber. If photokymographic methods one day replace motility evaluation, then separate counting of cells will become superfluous since their concentration may be calculated simultaneously with motility observation.

III. Morphology

Evaluation of sperm morphology is of paramount importance and is best done on a stained specimen. Preparation of a stain using the hematoxylin technique is easy and requires less than 10 min. The Papanicolaou stain is more

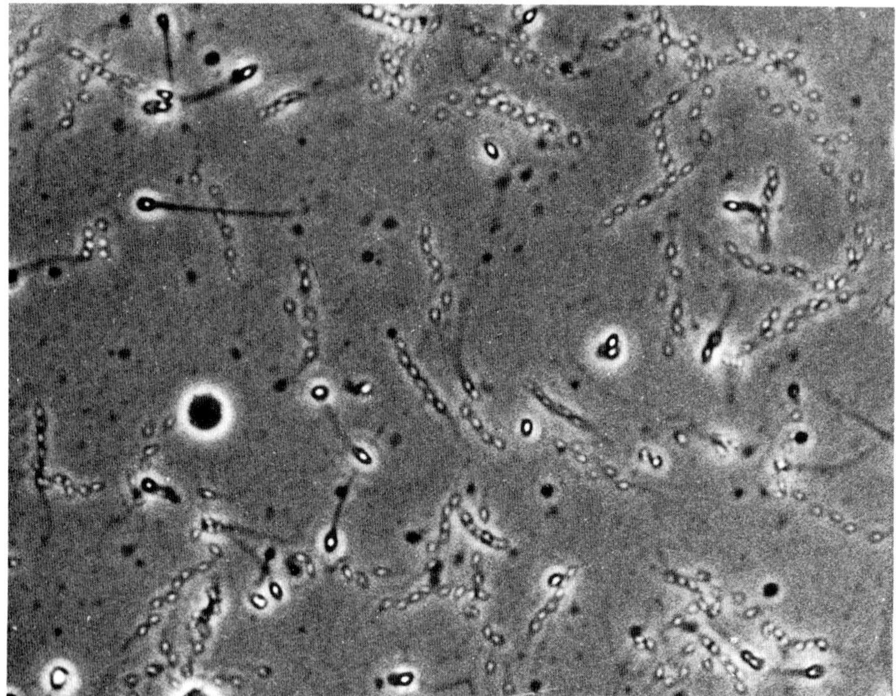

Fig. 1. Evaluation of sperm motility by multiple-exposure photography (phase-contrast microphotograph)

cumbersome, requiring about 30 min and 23 staining steps. However, we find results obtained by this method more accurate and more reliable. The staining procedure is as follows:

1. Prepare semen smear and air-dry.
2. Fix for 5 min in a mixture of 95% alcohol and ether (1:1)
3. Decrease alcohol concentration (80%, 70%, 50%; 10 s each).
4. Hematoxylin (3 min in 80%, 70%, 50%).
5. Rinse in running water for at least 10 min.
6. 0.5% HCl (2 s).
7. Increase alcohol concentrations (50%, 70%, 80%; 10 s each).
8. Orange G (2 min).
9. 95% alcohol (2 s).
10. Polychrome solution (2 min).
11. Wash off excess in three containers of 95% alcohol (5 s each).
12. Absolute alcohol (2 min).
13. Mixture of absolute alcohol and xylene (1:1) (2 min).
14. Xylene (20 min).
15. Dry.

Makler et al. (1980) recently reported on a semiautoanalysis method that permits a fairly good impression of sperm morphology from unstained wet preparations. Figures 2 and 3 are examples obtained by this method.

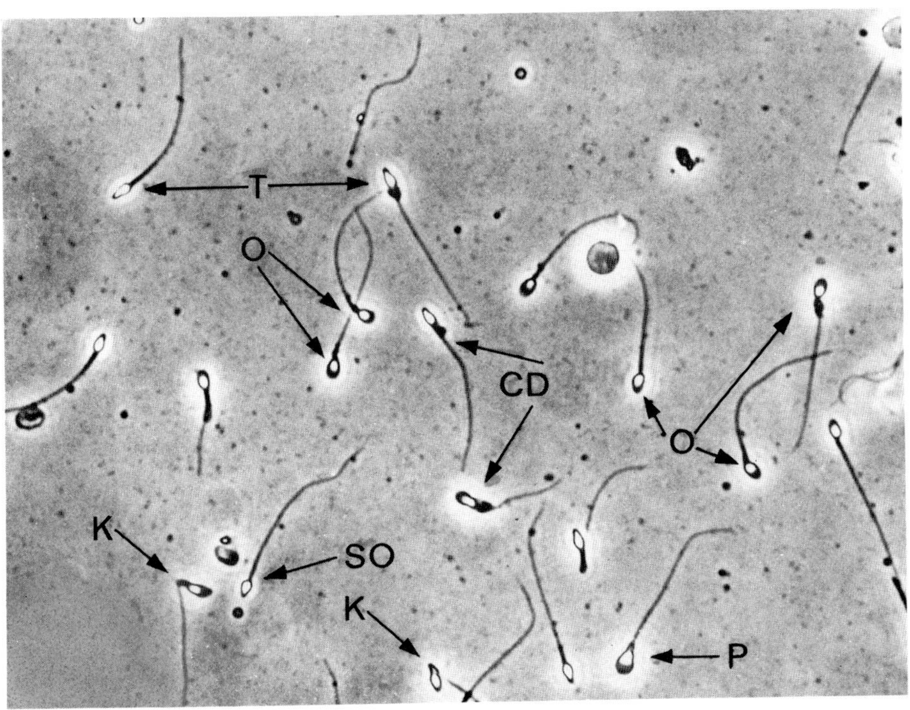

Fig. 2. A phase-contrast microphotograph of normal and abnormal spermatozoa from a wet preparation of immobilized sperm cells. The specimen is unstained. (For technique, see MAKLER et al., 1979.) *O*, oval forms; *SO*, small oval; *T*, tapering; *CD*, cytoplasmic droplets; *P*, piriform; *K*, kinked tails

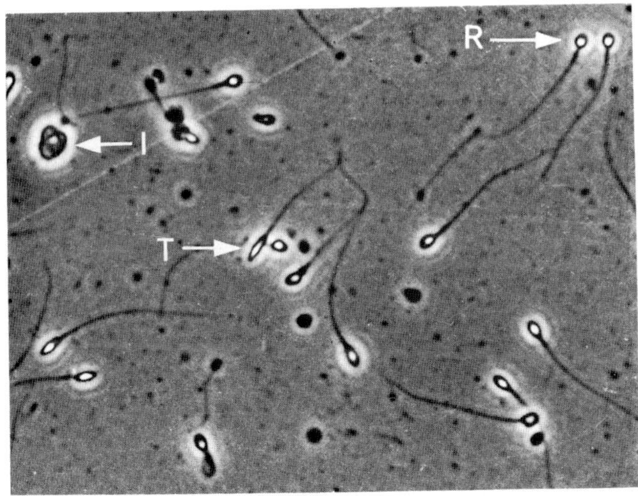

Fig. 3. Microphotograph (see Fig. 2). *T*, tapering; *I*, immature cells; *R*, round forms

For a semen sample to be morphologically normal, it should contain more than 60% normally shaped sperm. These cells have a regular, oval-shaped head, intact midpiece, and uncoiled tail of at least 45 μm. The head width is usually 2–3 μm and head length 3–5 μm. Oval forms may exceed these measurements (large oval) or may be smaller (small oval). It is not clear whether these are physiologic or pathologic variations.

The abnormal forms most often encountered are: amorphous, tapering, piriform, round, and duplicate spermatozoa. Furthermore, immature cells, spermatozoa with cytoplasmic droplets, and tail defects may be observed in a semen specimen. The category of amorphous cells includes a variety of bizarre structural defects of the spermatozoal head. Further subdivisions are of no practical value. Tapering forms exhibit a greatly diminished head width in relation to the head length, which usually exceeds 7 μm. Piriform spermatozoa are characterized by their typical teardrop shape. Round spermatozoa have heads with the same length and width. Duplicate forms are characterized by multiple heads. The category of immature forms includes spermatocytes and spermatids at different stages of development. Spermatogonia are very rarely found in a semen specimen. Spermatozoa with cytoplasmic droplets should actually also be included in the group of immature forms. The category of tail defects includes multiple tails, broken, coiled, and kinked tails.

Oval forms and most of the abnormal forms described above can be seen in Figs. 2 and 3. Electron-microscopic studies may further clarify the mechanism responsible for malformations by providing information on where the cellular organelles originated and the possible developmental stage at which they occur.

Some 60 different morphologic aberrations of mature spermatozoa have been described (MACLEOD, 1964; FREUND, 1966). However, of practical importance are primarily the total proportion of abnormal spermatozoa and some distinct morphologic abnormalities such as tapering forms that are indicative of varicocele (GLEZERMAN et al., 1976), round forms that may suggest failure of acrosome formation (SCHIRREN et al., 1971), and kinked forms that may result from defective spermatogenesis (BARTOOV et al., 1980) or may hint at urogenital infections (O'LEARY and FRICK, 1975; GROSSGEBAUER et al., 1977).

IV. Supravital Staining

The method of supravital staining is mainly used to differentiate between living nonmotile cells and dead cells (necrospermia). Eosin in an aqueous solution cannot penetrate living cell membranes, and stained cells can thus be identified as dead. The method is rather simple. A drop of semen is mixed with a drop of 0.5%–1% eosin solution and thoroughly mixed. After the slide is dried over a flame, it is examined with the oil immersion objective. Normally, less than 10% of spermatozoa are eosin positive.

F. Normal Values

Normal ranges for motility and morphology do not differ for various laboratories. More than 70% motile sperm cells per ejaculate and more than 70% normally configured cells are regarded to be within normal limits (FREUND,

Table 1. Suggested normal values for the concentration of spermatozoa in human semen

Author	Year	Suggested normal value
MACOMBER and SANDERS	1929	60×10^6
WILLIAMS	1964	40×10^6
MACLEOD	1965	20×10^6
VAN ZYL	1972	10×10^6
SCHIRREN	1972	40×10^6
SCHILL	1975	40×10^6
LUDVIK	1976	40×10^6
FREUND and PETERSON	1976	20×10^6
ELIASSON	1977	20×10^6
AMELAR et al.	1977	40×10^6
ZANEVELD and POLAKOVSKI	1977	50×10^6

Table 2. Normal values of semen analysis

Volume	2–5 ml
pH	7.0–7.8
Color	Gray-white-yellow
Liquefaction	Within 40 min
Sperm count	More than 30×10^6/ml
Sperm motility	More than 70% within 1 h; more than 60% after 3 h
Sperm morphology	More than 70% oval cells; less than 6% tapering forms; less than 0.5% immature forms; less than 8% amorphous forms; less than 4% tail defects
Eosin-positive cells	Less than 10% stained cells
Fructose	More than 1 200 µg/ml
Acid phosphatase	More than 100–300 µg/ml
Citric acid	More than 300 mg%
Inositol	More than 1 000 µg/ml
Zinc	More than 500 µg/ml
Glycerophosphorylcholine	More than 5 400 mg%

1962, 1963; JAEGER and RUBIN, 1970; ELIASSON, 1973; FREUND and PETERSON 1976; ZANEVELD and POLAKOVSKI, 1977; LUNENFELD and GLEZERMAN, 1981). However, normal values for sperm concentration are given in rather wide ranges by different authors (Table 1). Nevertheless, in evaluating semen one has to set criteria, at least for the purpose of inter- and intraindividual comparison prior to and following treatment. Taking into account laboratory variations, we consider the values listed in Table 2 normal.

G. Outlook

As sophisticated and valuable as semen analysis may be, one still has to consider it a static test that gives biochemical results and describes spermatozoal behavior in its own medium, the seminal fluid. Semen analysis per se may be indicative of fertilizing capacity but is by no means conclusive (with the exception of azoospermia). Postcoital tests to determine sperm-mucus interaction or even better to determine sperm penetration (INSLER et al., 1977) may add vital information concerning fertility prognosis. Finally, one may speculate that in the not too distant future, in vitro fertilization studies will complete our knowledge of the fertilizing ability of a given semen specimen.

Acknowledgment. The author gratefully acknowledges Dr. A. Makler for the preparation of microphotographs and Prof. V. Insler for his very valuable advice.

References

Amelar RD, Dubin L, Walsh PC (1977) Male infertility. Saunders, Philadelphia London Toronto (1977)

Bartoov B, Eltes F, Lunenfeld B, Weisselberg R (1980) Morphological characteristics of abnormal human spermatozoa using transmission electron microscopy. Arch of Androl. 5:305

Botella Llusia J (1956) Measurement of lineal progression of human spermatozoa as an index of male fertility. Int J Fertil 1:113

Castenholz A (1974) Photokymographische Registriermethode zur Darstellung und Analyse der Spermatozoenbewegung. Andrologia 6:155

Eliasson R (1973) Parameters of male fertility. In: Hafez ESE, Evans TN (eds) Human reproduction. Conception and contraception. Harper & Row, New York, p 39

Eliasson R (1977) Semen analysis and laboratory work up. In: Cockett ATK, Urry RL (eds) Male infertility. Grune & Stratton, New York San Francisco London, p 169

Freund M (1962) Interrelationship among the characteristics of human semen and factors affecting semen-specimen quality. J Reprod Fertil 4:143

Freund M (1963) Effects of frequency of emission on semen output and an estimate of daily sperm production in man. J Reprod Fertil 6:269

Freund M (1966) Standards for the rating of human sperm morphology. A cooperative study. Int J Fertil [Suppl] 11:1

Freund M, Peterson RN (1976) Semen evaluation and fertility. In: Hafez ESE (ed) Human semen and fertility regulation in man. Mosby, St Louis, p 344

Glezerman M, Rakowszcyk M, Lunenfeld B, Beer R, Goldman B (1976) Varicocele in oligospermic patients: Pathophysiology and results after ligation and division of the internal spermatic vein. J Urol 115:562

Grossgebauer K, Hennig A, Hartmann D (1977) Mykoplasmenbedingte Spermatozoen-kopfschäden bei infertilen Männern. Hautarzt 28:299

Heller CG, Clermont Y (1964) Kinetics of the germinal epithelium in man. Recent Prog Horm Res 20:545

Inchiosa MA Jr (1965) Water soluble extractives of disposable syringes. Nature and significance. J Pharm Sci 54:1379

Insler V, Bernstein, D, Glezerman M (1977) Diagnosis and classification of the cervical factor of infertility. In: Insler V, Bettendorf G (eds) The uterine cervix in reproduction. Thieme, Stuttgart, p 265

Jaeger RJ, Rubin RJ (1970) Plasicizers from plastic devices: Extraction, metabolism and accumulation by biological systems. Science 170:460

Janick J, MacLeod J (1970) The measurement of human spermatozoan motility. Fertil Steril 21:140

Jecht EW, Russo JJ (1973) A system for the quantitative analysis of human sperm motility. Andrologia 5:215

Ludvik W (1976) Andrologie. Thieme, Stuttgart

Lunenfeld B, Glezerman M (1981) Diagnose und Therapie männlicher Fertilitätsstörungen. Grosse, Berlin

MacLeod J (1964) Human serology cytology as a sensitive indicator of the germinal epithelium. Int J Fertil 9:281

MacLeod J (1965) The semen examination. Clin Obstet Gynecol 8:15

Macomber D, Sanders MR (1929) The spermatozoa count. N Engl J Med 200:981

Makler A (1978) A new multiple exposure photography method for sperm motility determination. Fertil Steril 30:192

Makler A, Tatcher M, Mohiliver J (1980) Sperm semi-autoanalyses by combination of the MEP and computer techniques. Int J Fertil 25:62

O'Leary WM, Frick J (1975) The correlation of human male infertility with the presence of mycoplasma T-strains. Andrologia 7:309

Schill WB (1975) Moderne Aspekte der andrologischen Therapie. Therapiewoche 25:2762

Schirren CG (1972) Praktische Andrologie. Hartmann, Berlin

Schirren CG, Holstein A, Schirren C (1971) Über die Morphogenese rundköpfiger Spermatozoen des Menschen. Andrologia 3:117

Williams WW (1964) Sterility. The diagnostic survey of the infertile couple. Springfield, Mass (published privately)

Zaneveld LJD, Polakovski KL (1977) Collection and physical examination of the ejaculate. In: Hafez ESE (ed) Techniques of human andrology. Elsevier North-Holland, Amsterdam New York Oxford, p 147

Zyl JA van (1972) A review of the male factor in 231 infertile couples. S Afr J Obstet Gynecol 10:17

Testicular Biopsy

M. Glezerman

With 7 Figures

A. Introduction

Few diagnostic procedures have gained at different times so much popularity and so much condemnation and eventual rehabilitation as the biopsy of the testis. Since the first report of this procedure by Charny (1940), the spectrum of indications has grown steadily. As late as 1969 (Georgescu et al.), rather bizarre indications for testicular biopsy were proposed, reaching from impotency and a variety of endocrine disturbances to obesity and nervous disorders. Eventually, testicular biopsy received its proper position as a diagnostic and prognostic tool in the fertility survey of male infertility. However, analysis of a large amount of material (Garduno and Mehan, 1970; Girgis et al., 1969; Schwarzstein et al., 1975; Scott et al., 1976) permits the conclusion that hormonal and cytogenetic studies may today replace testicular biopsy in a majority of cases. In all hypergonadotropic conditions, such as Sertoli-cell-only syndrome, post-mumps orchitis, Klinefelter's syndrome, etc., testicular biopsy may only confirm an untreatable situation and will thus be of academic interest only. We feel that indication for testicular biopsy should be limited to differential diagnosis between testicular failure and obstruction of sperm-conveying structures in normogonadotropic males. In selected cases and for specific aims, testicular biopsy will provide tissue for electronmicroscopy and for chemical and morphofunctional studies.

Whenever a decision is made to perform testicular biopsy, one should be conscious about possible adverse effects: Rowley et al. (1969) have shown significant decrease in sperm counts in 39 of 100 volunteers following testicular biopsy. These persisted for periods up to 18 weeks. Antisperm antibody formation has been observed by some investigators to occur following testicular biopsy (Hjort et al., 1974), while others did not confirm this finding, rendering this aspect controversial (Noren and Friberg, 1978). However, full knowledge of technique and interpretation of testicular biopsy is of utmost importance for those interested in male fertility.

B. Technique

Usually open bilateral biopsy is preferred, since morphologic differences between the two testes may exist. Needle biopsy is only mentioned to be condemned. Results obtained by this method seem not to be representative and testicular damage may occur unnoticed. Vasography may be performed concomitantly, although some investigators (Amelar et al., 1977) feel that this procedure should be performed only if immediate reconstructive surgery is feasible if indicated.

Testicular biopsy must be performed under strict aseptic conditions with either local or preferably general anesthesia. Following adequate preparation of the scrotal area, the testicle is held firmly by the left hand of the surgeon with the skin stretched tautly over its anterior surface. Special care has to be taken to ascertain that the epididymis is in its proper posterior position to avoid erroneous incision into this structure. The skin is incised longitudinally for a length of 2 cm, and the incision is deepened until the tunica vaginalis appears. When this layer is opened, a few drops of clear fluid will usually emerge. The edges of the tunica vaginalis are picked up with hemostats. Some authors advocate the enlargement of the scrotal incision and opening of the tunica vaginalis to such an extent that the whole testis and epididymis can be examined under vision. We agree with this approach, since inspection of the scrotal content may add valuable information regarding the functional state of the testis. Those who restrict the procedure to testicular biopsy and dispense with complete testicular inspection achieve a fairly good exposure of the testicle by placing a small retractor beneath the tunica vaginalis. The tunica albuginea is then incised transversely at the midportion of the anterior surface. The transverse incision is preferable to the longitudinal one, since this technique will avoid cutting through small superficial transverse branches of the spermatic artery. Very gentle pressure on the testis will now cause protrusion of testicular tissue that may be cut off using either scalpel or sharp scissors. Immediately upon obtaining the grain of tissue, it is placed in a labeled jar with freshly mixed fixation solution. The use of formalin for this purpose is strongly condemned, since this agent will cause shrinkage of tubules, distortion of germ cells, and sloughing of germinal epithelium. Differentiation between maturation stages and evaluation of testicular ultrastructure will thus become impossible. We use Bouin's solution for fixation of testicular material, but solutions such Zenker's, Stieve's, and Cornoy's may also be used. The tunica albuginea is then sutured with 5-0 chromic catgut using an atraumatic needle. The tunica vaginalis is closed with 3-0 chromic catgut, and the skin is approximated with 3-0 plain catgut sutures. The patient may be discharged the following day if general anesthesia has been used or the same day if local anesthesia has been applied.

C. Histologic Evaluation of the Testicular Biopsy

Following proper fixation of the specimen, paraffin sections of 3–6 μm thickness are mounted on slides and stained with one of the following four stains (Howley and Heller, 1966): iron hematoxylin and eosin Y; Masson's tricrome; periodic acid-Schiff (PAS); or Harris' hematoxylin and eosin Y.

Evaluation should begin with an overall assessment of the testicular structures. The tubuli seminiferi of the mature testes exhibit an open lumen if cross-sectioned and contain relatively few spermatozoa. The tubules possess a fine but distinct basal membrane surrounded by connective tissue, the tunica propria. The interstitial tissue between the tubules contains blood vessels, fine lymph vessels, and clumps of Leydig cells. The interstitial tissue with its cell content and structures represents about 20% of the total volume of the mature testis.

Within the seminiferous tubules, all stages of spermatogenesis and mature Sertoli cells will usually be encountered. It is this rich variety of cells that is typical of the mature testis. Tubular size is measured as the internal diameter using an ocular micrometer. At least ten cross-sectioned tubules are measured, and the mean is given in micrometers (the average in the mature testis being 150–250 µm). Meticulous description of the tubular wall must be included in any protocol of testicular biopsy evaluation. An excessive proliferation of the tunica propria, the so-called peritubular fibrosis, may hamper transport of hormones and nutrients across the tubular wall and thus be of paramount importance for prognosis. Hyalinization of the tubular wall, i.e., apparent accumulation of amorphous material, is according to electron-microscopic studies a quantitative augmentation of this process. The material observed is not a new deposited substance but simply represents reduplication and enlargement of existing fibers (BUSTOS-OBREGON and HOLSTEIN, 1973; DEKRETSER et al., 1975; DE-KRETSER and HOLSTEIN, 1976). The Leydig cell population is judged qualitatively and quantitatively, taking into consideration number and size of cells. It should be recalled that Leydig cells usually do not appear in increased numbers following stimulation but proliferate and exhibit hypertrophy rather than hyperplasy (HALLER and LEACH, 1971).

For evaluation of the spermatogenic function, we have found the method described by JOHNSEN (1970) very useful. This method is based on the reasoning

Table 1. A scoring system for the evaluation of the spermatogenetic function of the human testis (JOHNSEN, 1970)

Score 10	Germinal epithelium regularly organized with an open tubular lumen; complete spermatogenesis with many mature spermatozoa seen
Score 9	Many spermatozoa present but germinal epithelium partially disorganized with marked sloughing of immature cells into the lumen or obliteration of lumen
Score 8	Less than five spermatozoa seen in tubule
Score 7	No spermatozoa but many spermatids present
Score 6	No spermatozoa and less than five spermatids present
Score 5	No spermatozoa, no spermatids, but many spermatocytes
Score 4	No spermatozoa, no spermatids, and less than five spermatocytes present
Score 3	Spermatogonia are the only germ cells present
Score 2	No germ cells present; the only cell type observed in the tubule are Sertoli cells
Score 1	No cells in tubular section

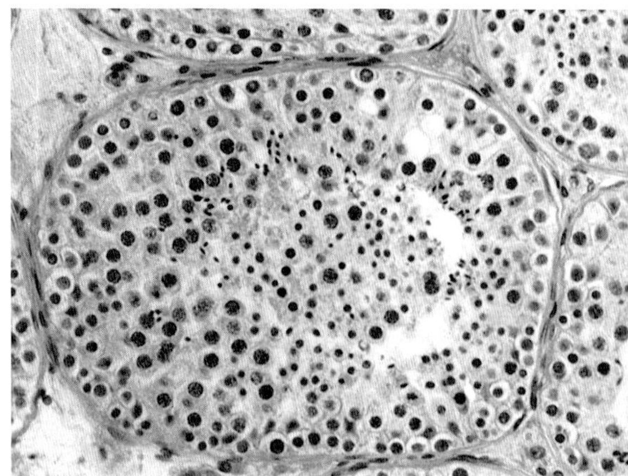

Fig. 1. Normal appearance of testicular biopsy. Note complete spermatogenesis, fine tubular wall, and Leydig cells between tubules

that in progressive degeneration the tubule loses its cell content in a fixed order from the most developed stage to the least developed one (Johnsen, 1967). Accordingly, tubular condition can be described by recording the most mature cell type present in cross sections of as many tubules as possible (Table 1). A mean score can be calculated by multiplication of each score by the number of tubuli present at this specific stage and subsequent division by the total number of tubuli recorded, at least 100. Although this mean score (MS) may be convenient for some correlations, the complete protocol of all score types must be given as the result of evaluation of spermatogenetic function. The complete result of the testicular biopsy will thus include spermatogenetic protocol, description of the tubular wall and interstitial tissue, mean tubular diameter, and overall description of testicular uniformity. Recently, a scoring system was presented that combines most of the above parameters into a single numeric score and also seems to be useful (Makler and Abramovici, 1978).

In normal, mature testis, the spermatogenetic score is at stage 10 in at least 60% of all tubules (Fig. 1). In primary infantilism and eunuchoidism tubular diameter will be greatly diminished, Leydig cell population will be sparse or absent, and tubules will possess a fine tubular wall and will be at a mean stage of 3 (Fig. 2). In Klinefelter's syndrome, tubular diameter is usually diminished, the Leydig cell population may be normal, diminished, or hypertrophic, and the spermatogenetic mean score will be 2 or less (Fig. 3). The tubular membrane may be totally hyalinized or severely fibrotic. A similar picture will usually appear following mumps orchitis (Fig. 4). Spermatogenetic maturation arrest is characterized by normal tubular diameters, normal Leydig cell population and sometimes an unremarkable tubular wall. The spermatogenetic score is always below 7, expressing the maturation arrest at certain spermatogenetic stages (Fig. 5).

A rather obscure condition is the so-called hypospermatogenesis. Here one will find intact qualitative but reduced quantitative spermatogenesis, with normal tubular diameters and Leydig cell population. The tubular wall may be thickened. For some unknown reasons, many of these patients are azoospermic.

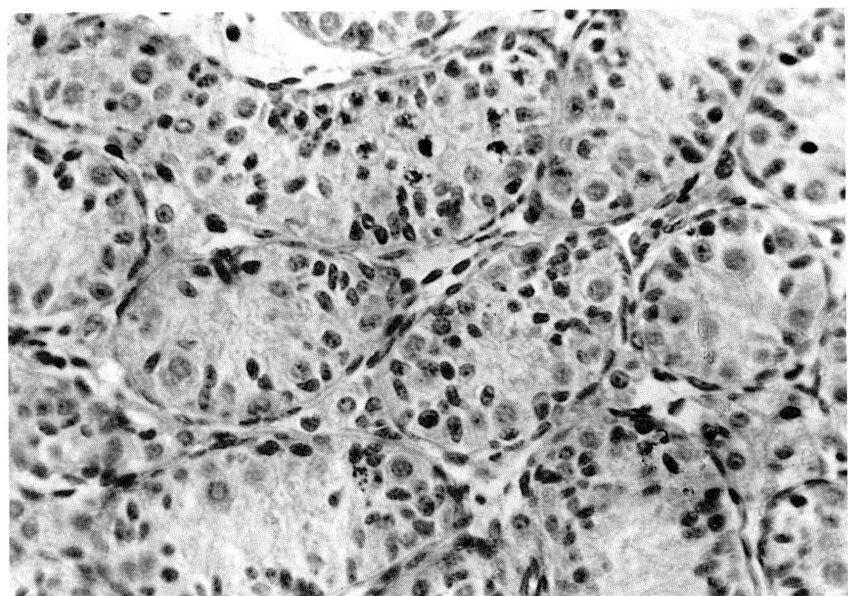

Fig. 2. Infantile testis. Note diminished tubular diameter. Tubules lack lumen and contain Sertoli cells and spermatogonia. Very few primary spermatocytes can be seen. Leydig cell population is sparce

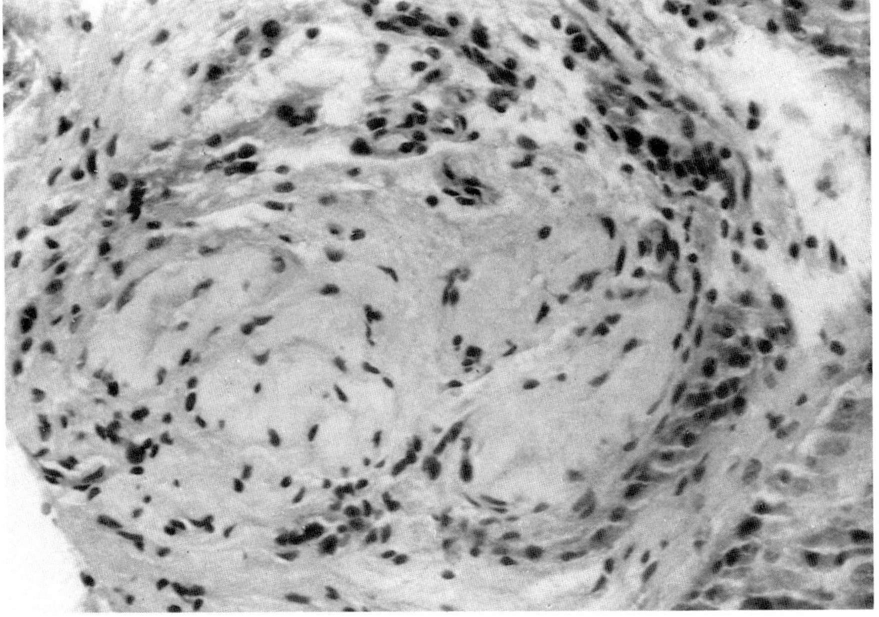

Fig. 3. Klinefelter's syndrome. Tubules are completely hyalinized, and no regular tubular structure can be observed. Leydig cells are abundant and appear in clusters

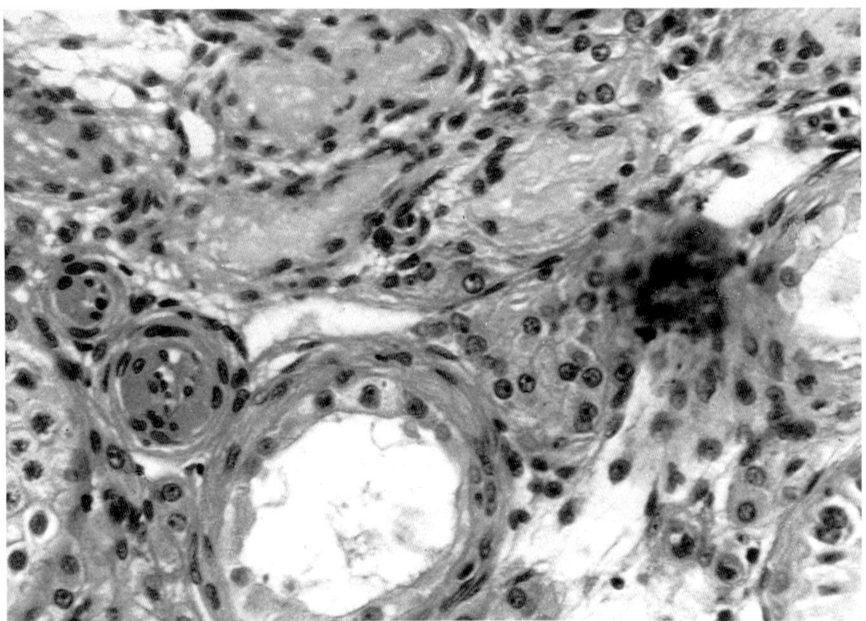

Fig. 4. Post-mumps orchitis. Testicular ultrastructure is severely destroyed. Tubules are either empty or completely hyalinized. Leydig cells appear normal

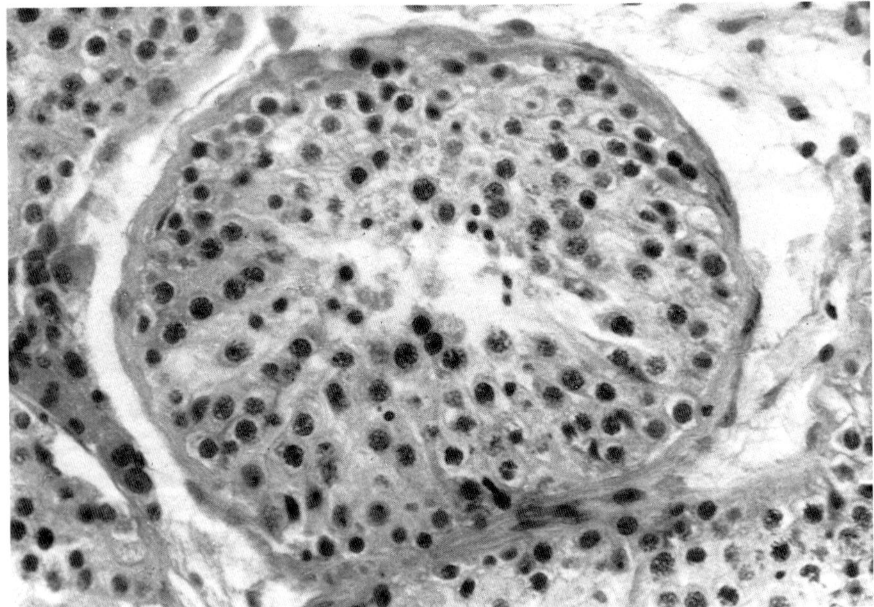

Fig. 5. Spermatogenic arrest. Tubular diameter is normal, and the tubular wall slightly fibrotic. Spermatogenesis does not proceed beyond the spermatid stage

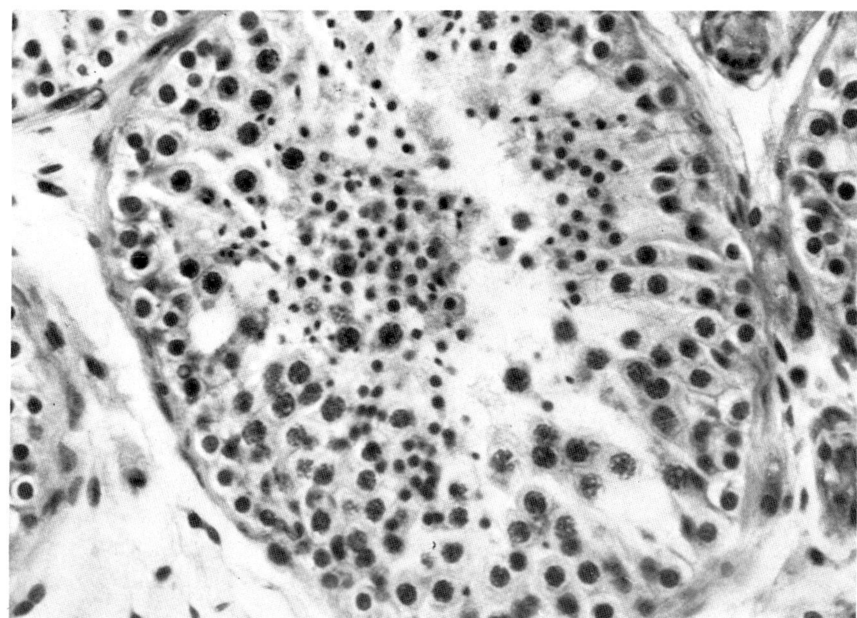

Fig. 6. Sloughing of germinal epithelium. Tubular walls are normal. Complete spermatogenesis can be observed but in disorderly fashion. Young germinal cells are sloughed into the tubular lumen. Leydig cells appear normal

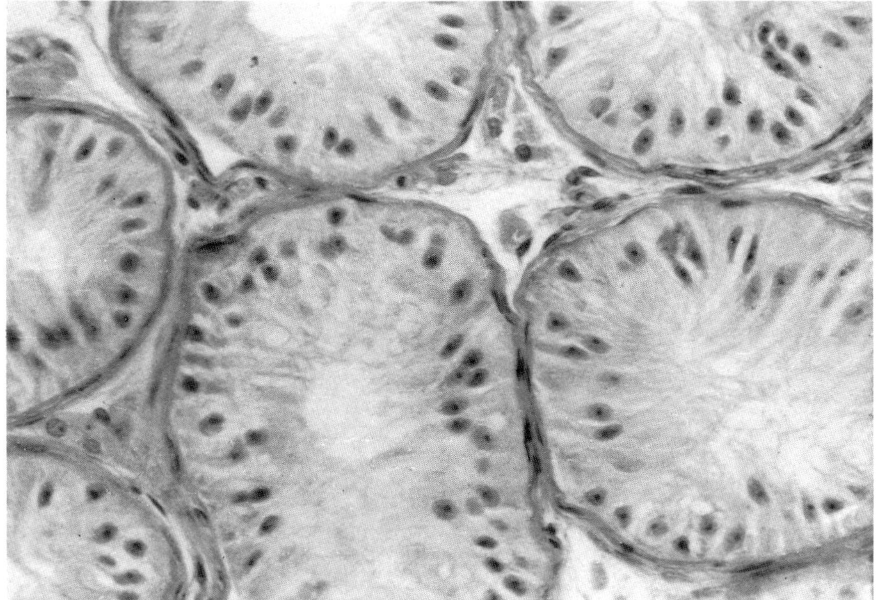

Fig. 7. Sertoli-cell-only syndrome. Tubular diameter is slightly diminished, tubular wall moderately fibrotic, no germ cells can be observed within the tubules. The cells seen are Sertoli cells, which appear normal. Leydig cells are normal

Another interesting condition is the so-called disorganized testis. Tubular walls are sometimes thickened, the tubular diameter is usually normal, and the Leydig cells are of normal appearance. Within the tubules, all stages of spermatogenesis can usually be observed, but immature cells are sloughed into the tubular lumen (Fig. 6). Due to this premature separation of spermatogenic cells, the germinal epithelium may be depleted of distinct populations and appear arrested in its development prior to the stage represented by the sloughed cells. These may sometimes obstruct the tubular lumen, at least partially. Patients usually exhibit oligospermia, and immature cells in the ejaculate are often misinterpreted as leukocytes. It has been pointed out that sloughing of immature germinal cells may be an expression of stress or injury exerted upon the testes.

A not so rare condition encountered on testicular biopsy is the so-called Sertoli-cell-only syndrome (Fig. 7). Tubules are usually of normal size, the tubular wall is normal or slightly fibrotic, and within the tubules only Sertoli cells are observed. Germinal cells are completely absent. Leydig cells appear usually normal. The MS for such tubules is 2.

If focal damage is observed in the biopsy specimen (e.g., focal tubular atrophy, etc.), this condition must be described in addition to the general evaluation protocol as if a separate specimen is being evaluated. Quantitative relations between the two protocols must be stated.

Acknowledgements. Thanks are due to Dr. Amnon Makler for preparation of microphotographs.

References

Amelar R, Dubin L, Walsh PC (1977) Male infertility. Saunders, Philadelphia London Toronto

Bustos-Obregon E, Holstein AF (1973) On structural patterns of the lamina propria of human seminiferous tubules. Z Zellforsch Mikrosk Anat 141:413

Charny CW (1940) Testicular biopsy, its value in male sterility. JAMA 115:1429

Garduno A, Mehan DJ (1970) Testicular biopsy findings in patients with impaired fertility. J Urol 104:871

Georgescu MM, Stoenescu D, Klepsch I, Tache A (1969) Some clinical and hormonal effects of testicular biopsy. Fertil Steril 20:612

Girgis SM, Etriby A, Ibrahim AA, Kahil SA (1969) Testicular biopsy in azoospermia. A review of the last ten years' experience of over 800 cases. Fertil Steril 20:467

Heller CG, Leach DR (1971) Quantification of Leydig cells and measurement of Leydig cell size following administration of human chorionic Gonadotropin to normal men. J Reprod Fertil 25:185

Hjort T, Husted S, Linnet-Jepsen P (1974) The effect of testis biopsy on autosensitisation against spermatozoal antigens. Clin Exp Immunol 18:201

Johnsen SG (1967) The mechanism involved in testicular degeneration in man. Acta Endocrinol [Suppl] (Kbh) 124:17

Johnsen SG (1970) Testicular biopsy score count – a method for registration of spermatogenesis in human testes: Normal values and results in 335 hypogonadal males. Hormones 1:1

Kretser DM de, Kerr JB, Paulsen CA (1975) The peritubular tissue in the normal and pathological human testis. An ultrastructural study. Biol Reprod 12:317

Kretser DM de, Holstein AF (1976) Testicular biopsy and abnormal germ cells. In: Hafez ESE, (ed) Human semen and fertility regulation in men. Mosby, St Louis, p 332

Makler A, Abramowici H (1978) The correlation between sperm count and testicular biopsy using a new scoring system. Int J Fertil 23:300
Norén S, Friberg J (1978) Does testicular biopsy produce sperm agglutinating antibodies? Int J Androl [Suppl] 1:159
Rowley MJ, Heller CG (1966) The testicular biopsy: Surgical procedure, fixation and staining technics. Fertil Steril 17:177
Rowley MJ, O'Keefe KB, Heller CG (1969) Decreases in sperm concentration due to testicular biopsy procedures in men. J Urol 101:347
Schwarzstein L, Premoli F, Aparacio NJ (1975) Testicular biopsy as a selective criterion in hormonal treatment of male infertility. Int J Fertil 20:245
Scott R, Rourke A, Yates A, Sinclair J, Chowdhury S, Shaba J (1976) The results of 100 small tissue biopsies of testes in male infertile patients. Postgrad Med J 52:693

Radiologic Investigation
of Male Fertility Disorders

K. Bandhauer

With 6 Figures

Radiologic investigations play a relatively minor role in the management of disorders of male fertility and should not be regarded as routine. Despite this fact, there may be individual cases in which radiologic examination of the urogenital tract becomes a sine qua non of exact diagnosis.

The following are the principal indications for including radiology in the diagnosis of male fertility disorders:

Demonstration of patency of the spermatic tract
Imaging of pathologic change in the glandular structures of the reproductive system, mainly the seminal vesicles and prostate
Assessment of urethral abnormalities in relation to ejaculatory disorders
Phlebography of varicoceles

A. Demonstration of Patency
in the Spermatic Tract

I. Indications

Vasovesiculography – radiologic examination of the vas deferens and seminal vesicles – allows the patency of the spermatic tract to be established where there is azoospermia in the presence of histologically proven adequate spermatogenesis (obstructive azoospermia). It also allows congenital, inflammatory, or neoplastic lesions of the seminal vesicles to be assessed.

The indications for vasovesiculography need to be kept under stringent review as puncture of the vas deferens carries a definite risk of scarring and therefore of stenosis of the distal spermatic pathway.

II. Technique

Transurethral injection of contrast medium into the ejaculatory ducts (Klotz and Luys, 1962) is now of historical interest only and is hardly ever practiced.

Direct puncture of the scrotal portion of the vas deferens (Belfield, 1913) with centripetal injection of contrast medium into the spermatic tract is the method of choice (Fig. 1).

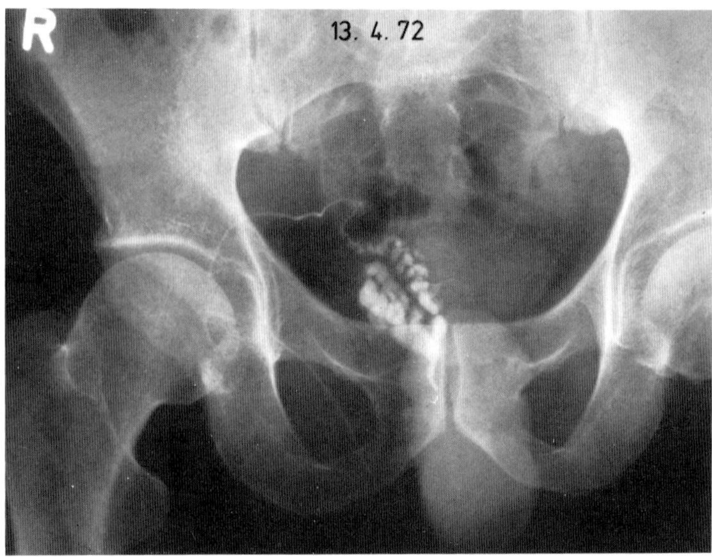

Fig. 1. Normal vasovesiculogram

The vascular supply to the vas deferens should be kept carefully in mind during dissection, which should be gentle and limited so as to avoid the danger of postischemic cicatrization.

Water-soluble contrast media of low concentration (30%) should be employed as more concentrated preparations may be both too viscous for the narrow lumen of the vas deferens and may also cause local irritation. Before the injection of contrast medium, the intracanalicular position of the needle or plastic cannula should be checked by perfusion with saline.

Should contrast spill over into the posterior urethra and thence reach the bladder, the seminal vesicles may be obscured. Therefore, no more than 2 or 3 ml should be injected.

Although epididymography (i.e., central injection of contrast medium) is possible in conjunction with vasography, it is no longer widely employed in the investigation of male fertility disorders: the risk of inflammatory change and scarring in the fine duct of the epididymis is very considerable.

III. Complications

Puncture of the vas deferens invariably leads to fibrosis affecting the muscular coat, the extent of which is, however, variable. As a result, the lumen of the vas deferens becomes narrowed, and if the fibrosis is extensive, there may be impairment of contractility with concomitant spermatic retention.

There is no general agreement as to the position to be occupied by vasography in a planned series of male fertility investigations. Some authors (Winer, 1975 and others) prefer, in cases of azoospermia, to test the patency of the spermatic tract at the time of testicular biopsy, whereas others (Bandhauer, 1977; Klos-

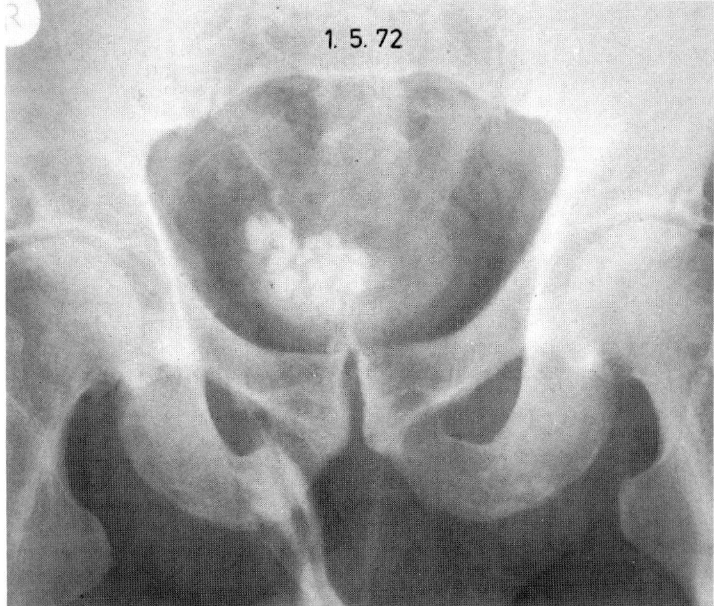

Fig. 2. Moderate dilatation of the right seminal vesicle and ejaculatory duct in a case
of chronic recurrent prostatitis (fructose deficiency – impaired motility)

TERHALFEN, 1977) reserve contrast radiology of the vas deferens for the time
of eventual vasovasostomy or vasoepididymostomy, i.e., after histologic proof
of spermatogenesis. Although in the simultaneous technique time may be saved,
this is frequently at the expense of rather more extensive scarring, which may
represent an obstacle to subsequent operative attempts at recanalization. In
addition, "quick-look" histologic techniques (i.e., frozen section) do not provide
absolute information on spermatogenesis. For this reason, investigation and
treatment of obstructive azoospermia should not be undertaken in a single
operating session (ALTDORFER and HEDINGER, 1977).

B. Imaging of Glandular Structures

In certain selected cases, radiologic imaging of the glandular structures in
the reproductive tract, especially of the seminal vesicles and the prostate, may
be of great significance for the management of disordered male fertility. In
the presence of an abnormal ejaculate (e.g., inadequate motility due to fructose
deficiency), lengthy expensive and fruitless hormone therapy may be avoided,
and the therapeutic strategy decisively redirected, if radiology demonstrates
severe inflammatory or congenital changes in the seminal vesicles or gross cavitation in the prostate (e.g., in genitourinary tuberculosis) (Figs. 2–4). The seminal
vesicles are visualized during vasovesiculography and the prostate during urethrography.

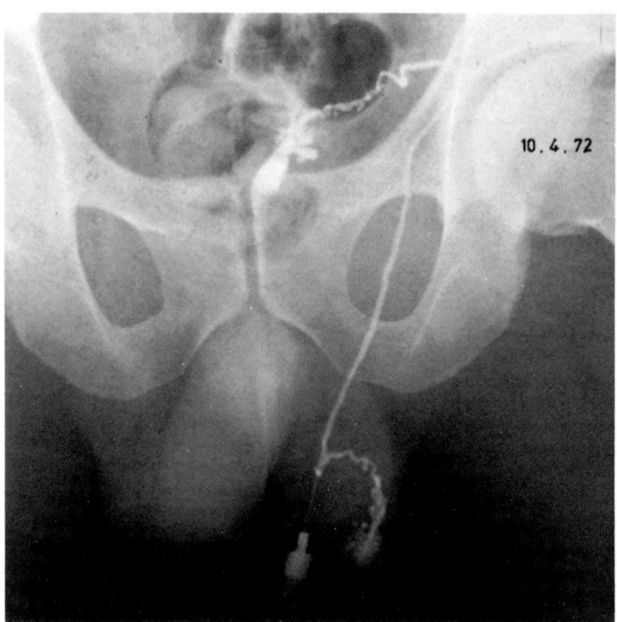

Fig. 3. Marked hypoplasia of the left seminal vesicle and considerable abnormality of the ejaculatory duct in a 30-year-old patient (azoospermia – high-grade fructose deficiency)

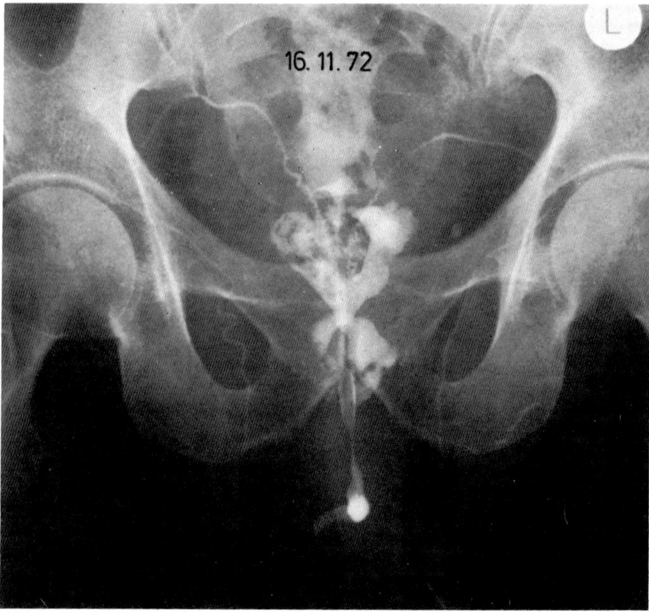

Fig. 4. Marked bilateral change in the seminal vesicles, cavitation in the prostate, and stricture formation in the posterior urethra of a 31-year-old patient after 3 years of medical treatment for a genitourinary tuberculosis (oligozoospermia with marked fructose deficiency and disturbance of ejaculation)

C. Assessment of Urethral Abnormalities

Sub- or infertility in the male may be due to "weakness" of ejaculation, as the semen may reflux out of the vagina instead of being deposited high in the vault. Frequently, abnormalities of the urethra, such as stricture and diverticulum, not only prevent a proper emission but may also lead to progressive inflammatory change in proximal segments of the seminal tract, such as prostate and seminal vesicles. Changes in the urethra must therefore be included among the possible causes of infertility and need to be excluded by urethrography. The latter will also help to exclude abnormalities of the prostate, such as calculi and atrophic conditions (Fig. 5). The indications for this investigation arise from the history, which will suggest obstructive symptoms of micturition and ejaculation.

D. Phlebography of Varicoceles

The diagnosis of varicocele is principally a clinical one and does not require phlebography. If on the other hand retroperitoneal ligation of the internal spermatic vein is to be a therapeutic success, complete obliteration of the vein and its radicles is required. Considering that the venous return from the pampiniform plexus is via several radicles of the internal spermatic vein and since confluence of these radicles may occur at varying levels, radiologic demonstra-

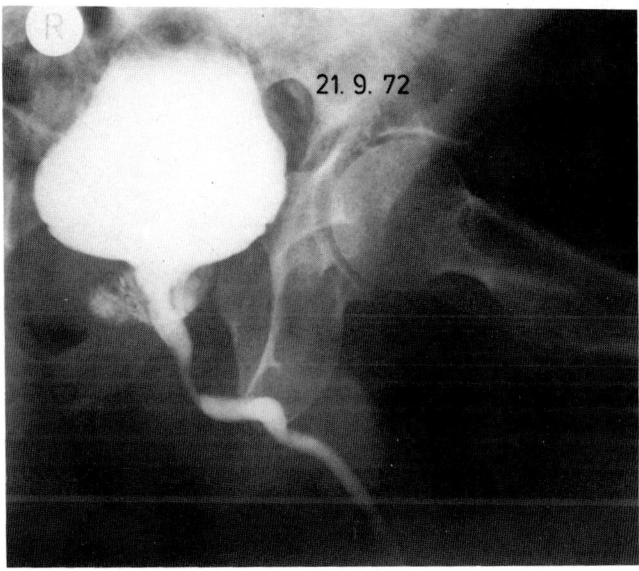

Fig. 5. Extensive reflux into prostatic glands, which have undergone inflammatory change. This 34-year-old patient, whose marriage is childless, has a stricture (probably congenital) of the posterior urethra with subsequent proximal inflammatory change. (moderate oligozoospermia with marked hypomotility and fructose deficiency)

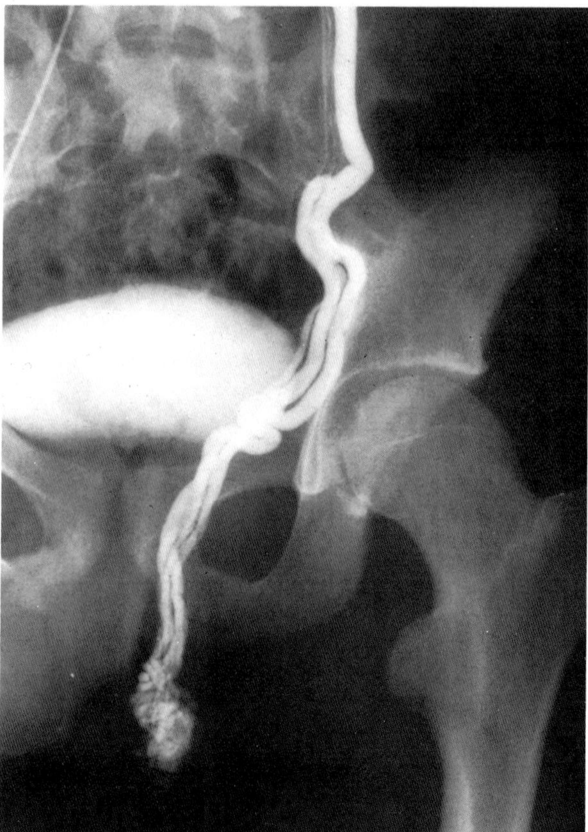

Fig. 6. Large left varicocele in a 27-year-old patient: the left spermatic vein is filled with contrast following pampiniform plexus puncture (pronounced oligozoospermia with hypomotility – childless marriage)

tion of these veins constitutes an important adjunct to radical treatment and therapeutic success. According to Völter et al. (1975), the internal spermatic vein has a double orifice in 30% and a triple one in 3% of the male population. In 70% the left-sided vessel divides into two or three branches in its upper third, and in 30% this division occurs in the middle third. It is for these reasons that internal spermatic phlebography preceding ligation makes an important contribution to the prevention of subsequent recurrence.

The internal spermatic vein may be demonstrated either by caval venography or by the injection of contrast into the pampiniform plexus (Fig. 6). Caval venography and catheterization of the left renal vein may be carried out preoperatively (Combaire and Kunnen, 1976), but this may not show all branches of the vessel. Paminiform plexus puncture is generally carried out immediately preoperatively or as a peroperative procedure and should demonstrate the retroperitoneal efferent plexus of veins in its entirety (Knöner et al., 1974).

References

Altdorfer J, Hedinger Chr (1977) Diagnostische Probleme der Hodenbiopsie. Verhandl Ber d Dtsch Ges f Urol 28. Tg. Springer, Berlin Heidelberg New York, S 407

Bandhauer K (1977) Die Röntgenologie des Genitaltraktes. Verhandl Ber d Dtsch Ges f Urol 28. Tag. Springer, Berlin Heidelberg New York, S 404

Belfield WT (1913) Vasotomy-radiography of the seminal duct. J Am Med Ass 61:1867–1869

Comhaire F, Kunnen M (1976) Selective retrograde venography of the internal spermatic vein: A conclusive approach to the diagnosis of varicocele. Andrologia 8:1, 11

Coolsead B: zit. b. Blandy JB (1976) Male infertility and impotence. In: Scientific foundations of urology, vol II. Williams DI, Chisholm GD (eds) William Heinemann Med books, London

Hedinger Chr (1972) Pathologische Anatomie der Fertilitätsstörungen des Mannes. Urol A 11:201

Klosterhalfen H (1977) Operative Therapie der Verschluss-Azoospermie. Verhandl Ber d Dtsch Ges f Urol, 28. Tag. Springer, Berlin Heidelberg New York, S 422

Klotz, Luys: zit. b. Lindblom K, Romanus R (1962) Encyclopedia of urology V/1. Springer, Berlin Göttingen Heidelberg, S 447

Knöner M, Dathe G, Palm V (1974) Verbesserung der Ergebnisse der Varicocelenoperation durch praeoperative Serienphlebographien. Verhandl Ber d Dtsch Ges f Urol 25. Tg. Springer, Berlin Heidelberg New York, S 335

Lindblom K, Romanus R (1962) Encyclopedia of urology V/1, Springer, Berlin Göttingen Heidelberg

Völter D, Wurster J, Aeikens B, Schubert GE (1975) Andrologia 7:127

Winer JH (1975) The surgery of male infertility. In: Behrman SJ, Kistler RW (eds) Progress in infertility (sec ed) Little & Brown, Boston, p 723

Endocrine Evalution
of Male Fertility Disorders

B. Lunenfeld and M. Glezerman

With 2 Figures

A. Introduction

Normal reproductive processes of males depend endocrinologically on the
the presence of a normal responsive hypothalamus, pituitary gland, testes, and
accessory glands. These must be controlled by a balanced and coordinated
function of gonadotropin-releasing hormones, gonadotropic hormones, and testicular hormones and metabolites. The axis between hypothalamus and target
organ, the testes, is semiautonomous as its function is controlled by various
feedback mechanisms. However, dysfunction of other endocrine axes (adrenal,
thyroid, etc.) may influence its function and may interrupt the delicate interaction
between different components. Furthermore, extrinsic stimuli influence this system via cortical pathways. Any disruption in the delicately coordinated interaction between the integrated components of the hypothalamus-pituitary-testes
axis, which must operate within precise quantitative limits and accurate temporal
sequences, may lead to testicular dysfunction. Either the spermatogenic or the
steroidogenic compartment or both may be affected.

Advances in reproductive endocrinology have led to a better understanding
of the basic mechanisms regulating these processes and governing reproductive
function. This has furnished the impetus for transforming the field of male
infertility, at least as far as endocrinologic disturbances are concerned, from
a largely empirical approach to the firmer ground of a more rational basis.
Sensitive radio-ligand assays have been developed that allow accurate and specific measurement of gonadotropins and steroids in plasma. The gonadotropin-
releasing hormone has been synthesized and is available. Finally clomiphene
citrate and purified human gonadotropin preparations are powerful drugs for
diagnosis and treatment.

Armed with deeper knowledge about the physiologic basis of male reproductive endocrinology and with various compounds that act specifically at different
levels along the hypothalamus-pituitary-testes axis, we are now able to evaluate
this axis and to define the localization of dysfunction.

B. Hormone Base Levels

In rare instances clinical findings may necessitate the evaluation of adrenal
or thyroid function. These tests are not included in this presentation.

I. Testosterone

Measurement of testosterone is indicated if clinical symptoms of hypoandrogenization are present. These include physical characteristics such as sparse facial and body hair, female-type fat and muscle distribution, and eunuchoid body proportions. Furthermore, some cases of impotency will require measurement of testosterone. Since testosterone levels may show fluctuations up to 300% (Naftolin et al., 1973), serial samples should be evaluated. Testosterone exerts its effect on male secondary sex signs but also controls the function of the secondary sex glands (prostate, seminal vesicles, and excretory function of the epididymis). The functional capacity of these secondary sex glands may be evaluated by measuring specific markers for their activity (Glezerman et al., 1978). Carnitine and glyceryl phosphorylcholine (GPC) are mainly secreted by the epididymis, fructose is a typical marker for secretions deriving from the seminal vesicles, and acid phosphatase, inositol, and zinc are secreted mainly by the prostate gland. If biochemical analysis of the seminal fluid reveals reduced levels of any of these substances, estimation of testosterone is indicated to detect secondary insufficiency. Normal testosterone levels concomitant with reduced "markers" for secondary sex glands are an indication for the "HCG-seminal plasma test" (see below).

II. Prolactin

The identification (Lewis et al., 1971) and purification (Hwang et al., 1972) of prolactin and radioimmunologic methods to measure plasma levels (Sinha et al., 1973) have stimulated research on the role of this hormone in the reproductive process. However, its function is still poorly understood. An elevated prolactin level may be a symptom of hypothalamic insufficiency to secrete the prolactin-inhibiting factor (PIF). Various drugs increase plasma levels of prolactin (phenothiazine, reserpine, methyldopa, TSH), and elevated levels of this hormone may be an early sign of pituitary adenoma. Some investigators demonstrated correlations between prolactin levels and levels of gonadotropins in plasma (Krause, 1978) while others did not (Segal et al., 1976). Correlations between prolactin levels and spermatozoan concentration are equivocal (Segal et al., 1973; Fonzo et al., 1977). A striking correlation exists between elevated prolactin levels and impotency (Fonzo et al., 1977).

III. Follicle-Stimulating Hormone (FSH)

FSH levels usually show little fluctuation because of a slow metabolic clearance rate (Naftolin et al., 1972). The hypophyseal synthesis and secretion of FSH is stimulated by gonadotropin-releasing hormone (GNRH). Feedback control is exerted on the hypothalamus by testosterone or its metabolites (estrogen) by inhibition of GNRH secretion and by testicular inhibin, which modulates the responsiveness of the pituitary to GNRH stimulation. Measurement of FSH is indicated in all cases of aspermia, azoospermia, and in patients with severe oligospermia. Elevated FSH levels are invariably indicative of severe tubular damage. Testicular biopsy will only confirm primary tesicular failure and is thus of academic interest only. Normal or reduced levels of FSH do not exclude tubular damage. Adequate function of the steroidogenic testicular compartment with sufficient secretion of testosterone may reduce GNRH secretion to such a level as to mask an actual hypergonadotropic state. An exaggerated rise in FSH levels following stimulation by GNRH is of the same diagnostic value is primary elevated FSH levels (see below).

IV. Luteinizing Hormone (LH)

LH is secreted by the male pituitary gland with broad fluctuations; blood levels may vary by 900% within a 24-h period (SANTEN and BARDIN, 1973). If LH measurement is indicated, serial estimations should be performed to establish a base line. However, rather few indications exist for the estimation of LH. Reduced Leydig cell function, as expressed in low testosterone levels, is one indication. Since FSH levels are usually reduced concomitantly and since LH levels exhibit wide fluctuations, the estimation of the latter is usually of limited value. In rare cases of the so-called fertile eunuch syndrome (MAKLER et al., 1977), LH levels are reduced, and some cases of "male menopause" may exhibit low LH values while others show increased secretion of this hormone (LUNENFELD, ESHKOL and GLEZERMAN, see page 421 ff.).

C. Dynamic Tests

I. Clomiphene Citrate Test

Clomiphene citrate is an analog of chlorotrianisene and is structurally related to the potent synthetic estrogen diethylstilbestrol. The commercially available preparations are usually 1:1 mixtures of *cis*- and *trans*-clomiphene. The main body of existing evidence points to the hypothalamus and possibly the hypophysis as the main sites of action. It seems that clomiphene citrate exerts its action by competing with natural estrogens (derived from testosterone) at receptor sites. "Blinded" by clomiphene molecules occupying the estrogen receptor sites, the hypothalamus registers estrogen lack and acts upon it. Consequently, GNRH is produced and/or released into the portal system. Activation of the pituitary gland and secretion of FSH and LH follows. Thus, clomiphene citrate can be used to stimulate the hypothalamus and to evaluate its capacity to secrete GNRH. Ideally, GNRH levels should be measured following clomiphene stimulation. However, because only very minute amounts of GNRH are secreted into the general circulation, measurement of GNRH is rather difficult and restricted to date to experimental purposes only (JEFFCOATE et al.; NETT et al., 1973). In the presence of a responsive pituitary gland, the measurement of gonadotropin levels following clomiphene medication allows proper estimation of the functional state of the hypothalamus. In men, the dosage is 50 mg orally during a period of 7 days with daily estimation of gonadotropins, which should increase at least twofold.

II. GNRH Test

Synthetic GNRH is a decapeptide which has been shown to stimulate the pituitary gland to synthetize and secrete both FSH and LH (Eliasson and Lindholmer, 1972; Kastin et al., 1972; Glezerman et al., 1974). Thus, pituitary function can be estimated by means of the GNRH test. GNRH may be applied by all usual routes (Schally, 1976; Saito et al., 1977). The GNRH test is indicated in those cases in whom differential diagnosis between hypothalamic and pituitary failure is required, i.e., in cases of secondary testicular failure. Furthermore, normal or reduced FSH base levels in the presence of azoospermia or severe oligospermia require the GNRH test to detect masked hypergonadotropic hypogonadism. We administer 100 µg GNRH intramuscularly and measure FSH and LH levels twice prior to and at 15, 30, 90, and 120 min following injection. Results of the GNRH test are classified as follows:

Type 0: Neither FSH nor LH levels increase (pituitary failure)
Type I: FSH increase of less than twofold of the initial value and/or maximum FSH level not exceeding 3 mIU/ml
Type II: FSH increase less than threefold of the initial level and maximal level not exeeding 9 mIU/ml
Type III: FSH increase exceeding threefold of the basal level and/or maximal level exceeding 9 mIU/ml. This type of GNRH response is regarded as exaggerated and indicative of masked hypergonadotropic hypogonadism. (It is obligatory for each laboratory to establish its own normal values to make this test a useful tool for diagnosis. The above-mentioned absolute values should be regarded as binding for our laboratory only.)

III. Human Chorionic Gonadotropin (HCG) Test

Being biologically similar to LH, HCG stimulates development of Leydig cells and induces in these cells synthesis and secretion of testosterone. Thus, HCG can be used to evaluate the steroidogenic potential of the testes. HCG is administered IM in doses of 5000 IU for 3 weeks. The relative long biologic half-life of HCG allows spacing injections every 5 days and maintaining sufficient plasma levels (Lunenfeld et al., 1973). The test period of 3 weeks is necessary to stimulate the development of an adequate Leydig cell population. Rise of testosterone levels will point to a functional potential of Leydig cells. In patients in whom no testes can be palpated within the scrotum or the inguinal canal, this test will indicate the presence of ectopic testes, localization of which may then be attempted. Concomitantly with the serial measurement of testosterone, seminal markers may be measured during the HCG test. This so-called HCG-seminal plasma test (Lunenfeld and Glezerman, 1978) permits some conclusions on functional capacity of secondary sexual glands and allows differential diagnosis between primary and secondary failure.

Testosterone levels are measured concomitantly with seminal fluid levels of secondary sexual gland markers while Leydig cell function is stimulated by repeated HCG injections. Rising testosterone levels during HCG stimulation without an increase of "markers" point to a secretory defect, or if concomitant with azoospermia, to a mechanical block at the corresponding topographic level (Fig. 1). Normal increase of previously low levels of secretory products

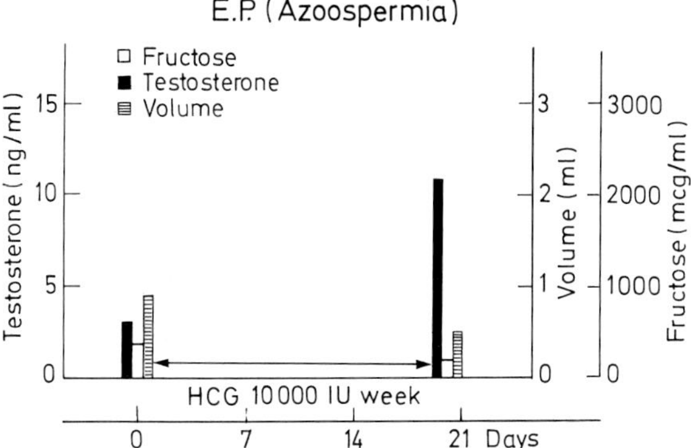

Fig. 1. The HCG-seminal plasma test: the effect of prolonged HCG stimulation on plasma testosterone and on seminal fluid volume and fructose concentration. Lack of increase of fructose levels in the presence of rising testosterone values point to dysfunction or agenesis of seminal vesicles

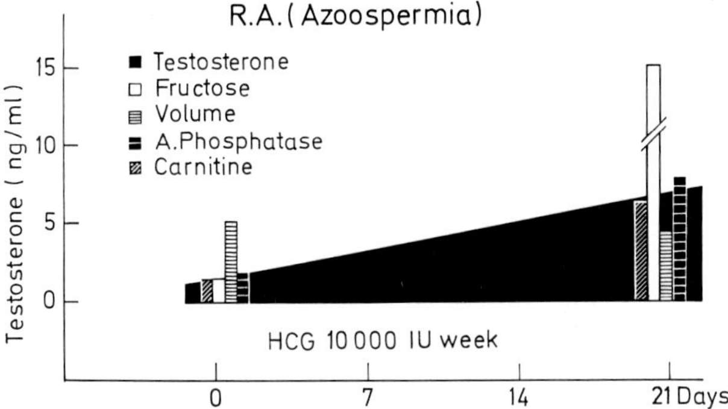

Fig. 2. The HCG-seminal plasma test: the effect of prolonged HCG stimulation on plasma testosterone, seminal values of fructose, acid phosphatase, and carnitine and seminal volume. Although seminal volume did not increase during HCG stimulation, all seminal marker values increased. This patient suffered from hypogonadotropic hypogonadism as reflected in low base levels of gonadotropins and testosterone. The HCG-seminal plasma test revealed potentially normal secondary sex glands

following the HCG medication (Fig. 2) point to relative androgen deficiency, which may be treated accordingly.

D. Usefulness of Hormonal Tests for Selection of Patients for Gonadotropin Therapy

We have evaluated retrospectively the usefulness of hormonal tests for selection of patients for gonadotropin therapy (LUNENFELD et al., 1979). Hormonal evaluation was started by measuring plasma FSH and prolactin levels in plasma.

Concomitantly, a testosterone estimation was performed since eunuchoidism may be masked by previous iatrogenic androgenization using either testosterone, mesterolone, or HCG. Elevated FSH values were considered to reflect treatment-resistant primary testicular failure. Cases of Klinefelter's syndrome were excluded after verification by cytogenetic studies. If normal a karyotype was found, focal tubular atrophy, Sertoli-cell-only syndrome, or maturation arrest were assumed, and patients were excluded from fertility restorative therapy. In patients who exhibited nonelevated FSH levels, a GNRH test was performed to detect masked relative hypergonadotropic hypogonadism. After exclusion of nonendocrine, genetic, and other causes for infertility, 37 patients remained who were scheduled for HMG/HCG therapy. All patients received daily IM injections of one ampul containing 75 IU FSH and 75 IU LH for at least 90 days. Every 5 days, every patient received IM in addition one ampulla of HCG containing 5000 IU. Venous blood was taken from all patients prior to therapy and assessed for FSH, LH, and testosterone by radioimmunoassay. All patients underwent a GNRH test prior to treatment.

We considered the appearance of sperm cells in the semen of a previously azoospermic male or a sperm count exceeding 10×10^6/ml semen in a previously severe oligospermic patient (less than 0.5×10^6 cells/ml semen) as a positive treatment result.

In 25 patients sufficient data were available for this retrospective evaluation: Of 25 patients who received HMG/HCG therapy, 17 had FSH levels less than 1.5 mIU/ml and 8 more than 1.5 mIU/ml (Table 1). The success rate in the former group was 70.6% (12 patients) and in the latter group 0%. In the 12 patients who showed improvement following HMG/HCG therapy the mean FSH level was 0.9 mIU/ml and in the 13 patients in whom gonadotropin therapy was ineffective it was 2.0 mIU/ml.

When relating treatment results to initial LH levels (Table 2), 10 of 12 patients with LH levels below 1.5 mIU/ml responded to therapy (83.3%) and only 2 of 13 men with LH levels above 1.5 mIU/ML (15.4%). The mean LH

Table 1. Correlation between basal FSH levels and response to HMG/HCG therapy

Basal FSH	< 1.5 mIU/ml	> 1.5 mIU/ml	Mean FSH (mIU/ml)
No. of cases	17	8	
Responsive to treatment	12 (70.6%)	0	0.9
Not responsive to treatment	5 (29.4%)	8 (100%)	2.0

Table 2. Correlation between basal LH levels and response to HMG/HCG therapy

Basal LH	< 1.5 mIU/ml	> 1.5 mIU/ml	Mean LH (mIU/ml)
No. of cases	12	13	
Responsive to treatment	10 (83.3%)	2 (15.4%)	1.0
Not responsive to treatment	2 (15.4%)	11 (84.6%)	2.9

Table 3. Correlation between basal testosterone levels and response to HMG/HCG therapy

Basal testosterone	< 4 ng/ml	> 4 ng/ml	Mean testosterone (ng/ml)
No. of cases	16	9	
Responsive to treatment	10 (62.5%)	2 (22.0%)	1.9
Not responsive to treatment	6 (37.5%)	7 (78.0%)	6.5

Table 4. Correlation between FSH pattern following GNRH administration (see text) and response to HMG/HCG treatment

FSH response to GNRH	Type 0/I	Type II/III
No. of cases	15	10
Responsive to treatment	12 (80.0%)	0
Not responsive to treatment	3 (20.0%)	10 (100%)

values were 1.0 mIU/ml for the responsive group and 2.9 for the nonresponsive group. Correlation between initial testosterone levels and therapy outcome showed the following (Table 3): 16 patients had initial testosterone levels of less than 4 ng/ml, and 9 patients had testosterone levels above this level. In the former group the success rate was 62.5% (ten males) and in the latter 22.2% (two males). The mean testosterone level in the responsive group was 1.95 ng/ml and in the latter 6.5 ng/ml.

Therapy results were related to outcome of the GNRH test (Table 4). Fifteen patients responded to the application of GNRH with a pattern described as type 0 and type I. Twelve of these (80%) showed ultimately a positive response to gonadotropin therapy. Seven patients exhibited type II and type III responses to GNRH. None of these responded to treatment with HMG/HCG.

By relating treatment results to the combination of all four parameters measured (i.e., basal levels for FSH, LH, testosterone, and FSH response to GNRH), the following results were obtained (Table 5): low gonadotropin and testosterone levels concomitant with type 0 or type I response to GNRH were followed by a positive treatment response in nine patients. Low gonadotropin levels concomitant with normal basal testosterone levels and a type 0/I pattern after GNRH administration were observed in the two patients in whom HMG/HCG therapy was successful.

In two patients basal testosterone levels and FSH levels were low, the GNRH pattern was type 0/I, but basal LH levels were in the "normal" range. One of these two patients responded favorably to gonadotropin therapy. In no other constellation of initial gonadotropin, testosterone, and FSH pattern following GNRH administration was gonadotropin therapy effective.

Evaluation of testosterone and gonadotropin levels and response to GNRH stimulation are used to evaluate the endocrine status of infertile males. This retrospective study indicates that such an evaluation may assist in selecting patients for gonadotropin therapy who have a fair chance of success. Absolute

Table 5. FSH pattern following GNRH administration (see text), basal FSH, LH, and testosterone levels related to response to HMG/HCG treatment

No. of cases	Pos. response to treatment	FSH response to GNRH	Basal testosterone	Basal LH	Basal FSH
9	9	Type 0/I	↓	↓	↓
2	2	Type 0/I	Normal	↓	↓
2	0	Type II/III	Normal	↓	↓
2	1	Type 0/I	↓	Normal	↓
2	0	Type I/III	↓	Normal	↓
1	0	Type 0/I	↓	Normal	Normal
2	0	Type II/III	↓	Normal	Normal
1	0	Type 0/I	Normal	Normal	Normal
4	0	Type II/III	Normal	Normal	Normal
25	12				

levels of hormone in plasma may fluctuate from laboratory to laboratory on account of differences in assay procedures. Thus, each laboratory has to establish its own values and criteria to make hormonal evaluation a powerful tool in the fertility survey of the infertile male patient.

References

Eliasson R, Lindholmer Ch (1972) Distribution and properties of spermatozoa in different fractions of split ejaculate. Fertil Steril 23:252

Fonzo D, Sivieri R, Gallone G, Andriolo S, Angeli A, Ceresa F (1977) Effect of a prolactin inhibitor on libido, sexual potency and sex hormones in men with mild hyperprolactin-emia, oligospermia and/or impotence. Acta Endocrinol [Suppl 212] (Kbh) 85:142

Glezerman M, Lunenfeld B, Insler V (1978) Male infertility. In: Lunenfeld B, Insler V Diagnosis and treatment of functional infertility. Grosse, Berlin (1978) p 114

Glezerman M, Birnboim N, Lunenfeld B, Kosary IA, Shaked R (1974) GnRH in a test to evaluate the effectiveness of intervention on the pituitary gland. Isr J Med Sci 10:797

Hwang P. Guyda H, Friesen HG (1972) Purification of human prolactin. J Biol Chem 247:1955

Jeffcoate SL, Fraser HM, Gunn, A, Holland DT (1973) RIA of LHRF. J Endocrinol (Kbh) 57:189

Kastin AJ, Schally AV, Gual C, Arimura A (1972) Release of LH and FSH after administration of synthetic LH releasing hormone. J Clin Endocrinol Metab 34:753

Krause W, Prolaktinspiegel im Serum bei Patienten mit Störungen der Spermatogenese. Hautarzt 29:77

Lewis, UJ, Singh RNP, Sinha YN, Laan WP van der (1971) Electrophoretic evidence of human prolactin. J Clin Endocrinol Metab 33:153

Lunenfeld B, Kohen F, Eshkol A, Beer R, Zuckerman Z, Birnboim N, Glezerman M (1973) Evaluation of male infertility by dynamic tests. In: James VHT, Serio M, Martini L (eds) The endocrine function of the human testis, vol I. Academic Press, New York London, p 561

Lunenfeld B, Glezerman M (1978) Grundschema zur Auswertung von Behandlungen ver-schiedener Formen männlicher Infertilität. In: Senge Th, Neumann F, Schenck B (eds) Physiologie und Pathophysiologie der Hodenfunktion. Thieme, Stuttgart, p 142

Lunenfeld B, Olchovsky D, Tadir Y, Glezerman M (1979) Treatment of male infertility with human gonadotropins: Selection of cases, management and results. Andrologia 11:331

Makler A, Glezerman M, Lunenfeld B (1977) The fertile eunuch-syndrome – an isolated Leydig cell failure? Andrologia 9:163

Naftolin F, Yen SSC, Tsai CC (1972) Rapid cycling of plasma gonadotropins in normal men as demonstrated by frequent sampling. Nature 236:92

Naftolin F, Judd HL, Yen SSC (1973) Pulsatile patterns of gonadotropins and testosterone in man: The effects of clomiphene with and without testosterone. J Clin Endocrinol Metab 36:285

Nett M, Akbar AM, Nisweder GD (1973) A RIA for GnRH in serum. J Clin Endocrinol Metab 36:880

Saito M, Kumasaki T, Yaoi Y, Nishi N, Arimura A, Coy DH, Schally AV (1977) Stimulation of LH and FSH by (D-Leu^6, Des-Gly^{10}-NH$_2$)-LHRH Ethylamide after subcutaneous, intravaginal and intrarectal administration to women. Fertil Steril 28:240

Santen RJ, Bardin CW (1973) Episodic luteinizing hormone secretion in man. Pulse analysis, clinical interpretation, physiologic mechanisms. J Clin Invest 52:2617

Schally AV (1976) Orally active analogs of luteinizing hormone releasing hormone. Fertil Steril 27:740

Segal S, Polishuk WZ, Ben-David M (1976) Hyperprolactinemic male infertility. Fertil Steril 27:1425

Sinha YN, Selby FW, Lewis UJ, Laan WP van der (1973) A homologuous radioimmunoassay for human prolactin. J Clin Endocrinol Metab 36:509

Neurology of Male Fertility Disorders

F. Scharfetter

With 1 Figure

Normal genital function is regulated by a complex interplay of the somatic and autonomic nervous systems in which sympathetic and parasympathetic activity is regulated by spinal reflex, under the influence of supraspinal (i.e., cerebral), cortical, and subcortical factors and subject to the hormonal environment. Just as the local autonomic ganglia in the periphery are subordinated to spinal centers, so the activity of the latter depends on the influence of cerebral centers. It is the very extent of these interconnections, and the variety of reciprocal activity in which they are involved, that presents the numerous opportunities for disorders of their functions. As an aid to understanding disturbances of genital function, and to interpreting them in the sense of a localized diagnosis, a broad picture is given below of the basic anatomy and physiology.

A. Anatomic and Physiologic Basis

Just as the pelvic organs bladder, genitalia, and rectum lie in the closest anatomic proximity, so they have a common innervation. Somatic and autonomic, efferent and afferent pathways cannot be separated out of the matted tangle of fibers, the anatomy of which is so unclear in the fresh specimen. In addition to this, the sympathetic and parasympathetic are not purely antagonistic in action, but rather coordinated in a complex fashion (reciprocal innervation; coordination of autonomic reflexes by intraspinal pathways, e.g. the coordination of secretory and vasodilator activity, von Bruecke, 1937; Gagel, 1953).

I. Spinal Centers Involved in Genital Function

The parasympathetic innervation of the pelvic organs is from a center in the sacral segments S2–4, most pronounced in S-3 and S-4. From preganglionic cells, which on cross section of the cord are seen to be localized in the lateral angle between anterior and posterior horns, efferent pathways arise between S-2 and S-4, leaving the cord with the anterior roots. They unite with the dorsal roots of the same segment to form the nervi erigentes (nervi pelvici).

The sacral segments S3–5 and the first coccygeal segment are termed the conus terminalis: this lies at the vertebral level L1–2. The lumbar segments L4–5 and the first sacral segments S-1 and S-2 are sometimes also known as the epiconus.

The sympathetic innervation of the pelvic organs arises from the lateral horn of the lumbar spinal segments L2–4. Efferent fibers travel with the anterior roots as Nn. mesenterici to the inferior mesenteric ganglion to form the hypogastric nerves.

II. Peripheral Innervation of the Genitalia

The parasympathetic nervi erigentes and the sympathetic hypogastric nerves form together with the somatic pudendal nerves from sacral segments S3–4 a plexus innervating the pelvic organs, and this may be subdivided into the seminal vesical plexus, the hemorrhoidal plexus, the deferent plexus, the spermatic plexus, and the prostatic and cavernous plexuses. In these plexuses, somatic motor fibers ramify with vaso- und visceromotor pathways arising in the spinal cord and with afferent pathways subserving sensation in the viscera, skin, and mucosae. These networks of nerve fibers lie on the surface of the organs and within the wall of the latter make connections with the local intramural nervous structures that give the viscera their intrinsic activity, which is thus in a limited way independent of the central nervous system. The integument of the penis is supplied by the dorsal nerve of the penis, which is a branch of the pudendal nerve.

III. Genital Function: Erection, Emission and Ejaculation, Orgasm

As a precondition for successful coitus, the genital functions of erection, emission, and ejaculation need to be intact and to follow in an ordered sequence. The normal composite reflex requires both the centrifugal pathways in the spinal cord transmitting psychogenic excitation and the centripetal pathways of external and proprioceptive sensation from the genital area. The latter involves activity of the sympathetic hypogastric nerves, the parasympathetic nervi erigentes, and the somatic pudendal nerves, which act in concert, here just as in the bladder and rectum. This coordination is not purely antagonistic. It is true that activity of the hypogastric nerves increases sphincter tone and that activity of the pelvic autonomics reduces vasomotor tone, but it is also the case that the pelvic autonomics reduce sphincter tone in a form of reciprocal innervation mediated by intraspinal reflexes. The afferent limb of the reflex arc lies in the nervi erigentes and pudendal nerves, probably also to some extent in the hypogastric nerves (VON BRUECKE, 1937). The sympathetic efferent limb runs in the hypogastric nerves, the parasympathetic efferents in the nervi erigentes, and the somatic in the pudendal nerves. In contrast to the innervation of bladder and rectum, the genital reflex sequence cannot be initiated voluntarily. However, the reflexes are facilitated by a variety of general and special sensory stimuli and psychological associations.

1. Erection

Vasodilator impulses arising in the parasympathetic center of the sacral cord S 2–5 and mediated by the nervi erigentes bring about an increased engorgement with blood of the corpora cavernosa. This change in volume is followed by an alteration of consistency due to obstruction of the venous drainage. The latter is brought about both by tonic contraction of the transversus perinei and bulbo- and ischiocavernosus muscles, and by the fact that the enlarging erectile tissue compresses the veins running deep to the tunica albuginea. The reduction of vasomotor tone in erection follows both from inhibition of vasoconstrictor enters (lumbar spinal segments) and from the stimulation of vasodilator centers in the sacral cord, which make connection with the vasomotor centers of the medulla and with the subcortical and cortical structures of the brain via the lateral columns of the cord. Contraction of the transversus perinei, bulbo- and ischiocavernosus muscles, tonic in erection, clonic in ejaculation, is controlled by centers in the anterior horn of the third and fourth sacral segment. The upper motor neurone, which is capable of bringing about voluntary contraction of these muscles runs in the lateral column of the cord.

2. Emission

By stimulating contractility of the smooth muscle, sympathetic impulses arising in the lumbar segments L 2–4 increase peristalsis in the seminal vesicles and vas deferens, allowing the secretions to enter the posterior urethra: this constitutes emission. Simultaneously, there is contraction of the internal sphincter of the bladder, thus preventing the semen awaiting ejaculation from refluxing into the bladder.

3. Ejaculation

The proprioceptive sensation of emission, together with external stimuli from the genital region, is relayed by afferents of the somatic pudendal nerves, and possibly also by autonomic pathways, to the sacral spinal center of genital function. These impulses now trigger the ejaculatory reflex, the efferent pathway of which runs in the pudendal nerves to the bulbo- and ischiocavernosus muscles where clonic contractions bring about ejaculation. It is supposed that the erection "center" lies at a slightly higher level than that for ejaculation,the former being at S 1–3 and the latter at S 3–4 (BING, 1948; FOERSTER, 1936, p. 62).

4. Orgasm

The orgasm is a complex reflex, affecting the entire person, in response to visceral and somatic proprioceptive and somatic exteroceptive afferent impulses from urethra and skin, which are conducted by autonomic and somatic nerves and then by intraspinal synapses. Supranuclear impulses influence the process, which is synchronized with and integrated into the climax. The sensation of orgasm is conducted centripetally in the lateral columns of the spinal cord.

The gerneralization of autonomic excitation in the orgasm and its relaxation in the climax alters the entire neurological – and thus the affective – state of the organism.

5. Synopsis: Sexual Function and Spinal Segments

Mediation of the erection and ejaculation reflexes is in the sacral cord. Emission reflex is relayed in the lumbar cord.

Erection

Parasympathetic centers in the sacral cord at S-2–S-4, possibly S1–3. This corresponds to vertebral level L1–2. Afferent proprio- and exteroceptive impulses via the pudendal nerves: efferent impulses via the nervi erigentes to the corpora cavernosa and via the pudendal nerves to the bulbo- and ischiocavernosus muscles.

Emission

Lumbar sympathetic centers in segments L2–4. These correspond to vertebral level D10–12. Afferent pathways in the pudendal nerves to the sacral cord-intraspinal synapses – efferent pathways in the hypogastric nerves.

Ejaculation

Parasympathetic centers in the sacral cord at S3–5, possibly S3–4. Afferent and efferent pathways in the pudendal nerves to the bulbo- and ischiocavernosus and transversus perinei muscles.

IV. Centripetal Spinal Pathways of Genital Function

The afferent autonomic pathway in the spinal cord (the connection between spinal autonomic centers and the supraordinate cerebral centers) is believed to lie in the anterolateral bundle of the spinothalamic tract. Centripetal conduction of impulses originating in the genital region may be considered to be bilateral, as is known to be the case for the anal region and the viscera, the pathways being part crossed, part uncrossed. All pleasurable or unpleasurable sensations, including those of libido and orgasm, involve conduction via the anterolateral bundle. The tactile sensations involved in sexual activity are conducted by the dorsal columns of the spinal cord, the funiculus gracilis and the funiculus cuneatus.

V. Centrifugal Spinal Pathways of Genital Function

The efferent pathways to the spinal centers probably lie in the lateral columns of the spinal cord, in close proximity to the pyramidal tract. The efferent pathways are also part crossed, part uncrossed (Foerster, 1936).

Spinal reflex activity in organisms of later phylogenetic derivation can no longer be explained at the segmental level of the simple reflex arc. On the contrary, such reflex activity is also conditioned by numerous exteroceptive, autonomic, and psychological influences. It depends on the balance of activity in the somatic and autonomic systems as well as on the balance within the autonomic system between sympathetic and parasympathetic activity, these being under the control both of hypothalamic activity and hormonal factors on the one hand and emotional tensions on the other.

VI. Pathways Connecting Spinal Centers

The intrinsic network or "elementary apparatus" of the spinal cord carries out the correlation of impulses entering via millions of synapses. In this way, the excitation originating at various receptors is coordinated into a reaction. Spinal activity is then integrated by the brain, which thus determines individual behavior.

VII. Genital Function and the Brain

So far only one center has been demonstrated in the brain that has an effect on gonadal maturation and is involved in the stimulation of sexual activity: the ventromedial area of the tuber cinereum in the floor of the hypothalamus immediately posterior to the infundibulum, which represents the connection to the adenohypophysis, whence hormonal control of sexuality originates. Hypothalamus and pituitary lie in close anatomic and functional association in the hypothalamic-pituitary axis (SPATZ, cited by ORTHNER, 1955; STUTTE, 1955). The hypothalamus receives impulses from the cerebral cortex (sensory impressions and association) and from the subcortical structure of the limbic system (subconscious sensations and the basic psychological condition). Whether sexuality is influenced by the lateral field of the tuber cinereum, by the mammillary bodies or by the region of the pineal is not yet known (ORTHNER, 1955).

B. Neurologic Disturbances of Genital Function

I. Spinal Transections and Their Significance for the Function of the Genital Organs

1. General Considerations on Spinal Transection: the Phase of Spinal Areflexia and the Phase of Increased Reflex Activity

Incomplete or complete acute spinal transection is followed immediately by the phase of spinal shock: complete paralysis and areflexia distal to the effective transverse lesion. This phase is followed by one of increased reflexivity, which may persist, if there is no further deterioration (cicatrization, circulatory disturbances, infection). If the interruption of conduction is gradual, the cord has time to adapt itself to intrinsic activity. The phase of spinal shock is then absent, and a neurobiologic picture develops that is similar to the secondary phase seen following acute transection, i.e., one of enhanced reflex activity.

This is true of spinal concussion (mechanical damage to the cord without histo-logic evidence of tissue damage), but also of cord compression secondary to spinal fracture, neoplasm, or abscess and equally for vascular and inflammatory transverse lesions.

The first phase of spinal areflexia (1–3 weeks) is similar in all acute transec-tions irrespective of level from cervical to sacral: it is the state of spinal shock. The neurologic picture comprises flaccid paralysis of the musculature and ab-sence of any sensation from parts of the body related to the cord distal to the damaged segments: there is absence of tendon jerk and skin reflexes and the autonomic functions are paralysed, with retention of feces and urine, with paradoxical dribbling from a full bladder due to reflex detrusor contraction mediated by an intramural arc. There may be paralytic ileus and vasomotor paralysis with the formation of dependent edema and engorgement of the penis through filling of the corpora cavernosa (Foerster, 1936, page 221).

During this first phase the prognosis following spinal transection is uncertain. Continuation of this state of spinal areflexia for more than the first few days or weeks signifies a poor prognosis. The sooner this condition starts to regress, the more likely is a satisfactory degree of recovery.

The second phase of enhanced spinal reflex activity commences after 3–4 weeks, in the case of incomplete transection after hours or days. The increase in reflexivity is a consequence of the loss of inhibitory cerebral efferent impulses.

The neurologic picture is characterized by reappearance and spastic enhance-ment of the tendon jerks and by synergistic reflexes in the legs, which may progress to flexor spasm.

Interruption of cerebral autonomic efferent impulses in supralumbar spinal lesions is followed by a state of hyperexcitability of spinal autonomic reflexes with enhanced viscerovisceral reflexes. Spinal automatism comes to govern void-ing of urine and defecation: emptying takes place as an autonomic reflex to a given state of distension. This automatism may be exaggerated to the point of spasticity so that reflex voiding occurs after ever decreasing intervals not only in response to the stimulus of bladder distention but also following the slightest tactile stimulus to the anogenital region and the legs. This effect is frequently subject to reflex synergism bringing about a mass reflex. (Synergy with the flexor reflex: the legs are flexed with a jerk at the hip and knee, the feet and toes are extended. The knees are drawn up to the chest and firmly adducted.)

Erection and ejaculation, almost invariably absent during the first phase, reappear in the second. Occasionally, an enhancement of reflex excitability becomes equally apparant in genital function so that mere touching not only of the genitalia but of the hypogastrium, perineum, or even the abdominal wall or legs may led to erection, ejaculation, or only to clonic contraction of the perineal musculature. If this mass reflex involves the legs and abdominal and spinal musculature, it is referred to as a coitus reflex (Riddoch, cited by Foerster, 1936, page 221). Incidentally, intrathecal neostigmine (Prostigmin) enhances the genital reflexes (Guttmann, 1971).

In the second phase, lesions of the lumbosacral cord become distinct from supralumbar lesions in that the former include direct damage to the autonomic centers for bladder, rectum, and genitalia. In higher lesions, it is only the efferent and afferent spinal pathways that are interrupted.

2. Destruction of the Lumbar Sympathetic Centers (L 2–4)

The destruction of the lumbar sympathetic centers (L 2–4) providing innervation to the vas deferens and the seminal vesicles interrupts the reflex arc involved in emission. Therefore ejaculation is also absent. If on the other hand the conus of the cord is preserved intact, erection may persist, and indeed persistent reflex dilatation of the corpora cavernosa may bring about priapism.

3. Destruction of the Sacral Parasympathetic Centers (S 2–4)

Lesions of the conus (S 3–cocc. 1) lead to the most severe disturbances of bladder, rectal and genital function. In such cases, the motor innervation of the lower limb and the tendon reflexes may be preserved, for the segmental innervation of the leg does not reach below S-2 for the majority of the foot musculature, only flexor digitorum longus and flexor hallucis longus and brevis receive a small contribution to their motor nuclei from S-3; the ankle jerk is mediated by the segments L-5–S-2. Sensory loss occurs over an area corresponding to the seat of riding breeches, so-called saddle anesthesia – S 3–5. Damage to the conus may also be differentiated from higher cord lesions by the fact that interruption of all afferent impulses, both exteroceptive and proprioceptive, removes all spinal reflex control of bladder, rectal, or genital function. For this reason, erection and ejaculation are absent. Only the intrinsic ganglia of the bladder wall remain intact, but these are not usually capable of bringing about complete automatic emptying, so the resulting picture is one of retention with paradoxical dribbling overflow.

Incomplete lesions of the conus (small hemorrhages, contusions, foci of multiple sclerosis) lead to partial (dissociated) impairment of sexual function (FOERSTER, 1936, p. 63 and 223), which may be explained on the basis of the anatomic relationship between the individual centers involved in each aspect of genital function: erection "center" S 1–3, ejaculation "center" S 3–4. Thus, ejaculation may be absent when erection is still possible. Efflux of semen without erection is sometimes termed pollutio flaccida.

Dissociated disturbances of genital function may also occur in the epiconus syndrome, which may be brought about by destruction of the lower two lumbar and upper two sacral segments. In contrast to the conus syndrome, the epiconus syndrome is characterized by extensive motor deficit in the lower limbs (paralysis of the foot and toe extensors and flexors, abduction and adduction of the foot, paralysis of knee flexors and extensors, hip extensors, rotators and abductors) and by absence of the patellar and achilles tendon reflexes. Sensory loss is found in the buttocks and in the legs in the distribution L-4–S-2. Bladder and rectum function reflexly, but are not under voluntary control. In the complete epiconus syndrome, the genital reflexes of erection (S 1–3) and ejaculation are absent (the latter due to absent emission as a result of interruption of intraspinal pathways betwwen sacral and lumbar cord). On the other hand, pollutio flaccida may be brought about by centrifugal corticospinal activity (psychological stimuli).

4. Cauda Equina Lesions

Upper and lower cauda equina lesions (distal to vertebral level L1/2) lead to complete paralysis of bladder, rectal, and genital function due to loss of afferent and efferent pathways in the parasympathetic nervi erigentes and the somatic pudendal nerves. As it lies within the nerve root bundle of the cauda equina, the conus medularis itself is often involved in higher lesions. For this reason, a pure conus syndrome is rare and is only to be found as a result of highly circumscribed lesions, contusions, intramedullary foci of demyelination, neoplasms, or hemorrhages. If the conus is affected by an extramedullary lesion or by injury, the cauda equina is usually also involved as it becomes a distinct entity below the level of the third lumbar root pair (vertebral level D11/12) and then encloses the conus medullaris. The cauda equina therefore comprises all sacral and coccygeal as well as the lower three lumbar roots, which course down from their emergence from the cord to their point of exit through their corresponding intervertebral foramina. It may thus be seen how difficult it is to differentiate the high lying cauda equina lesion at the level of the second or third lumbar vertebra from a conus and cauda equina lesion at the level of the 12th thoracic or first lumbar vertebra. In such cases, the site of the lesion may only be revealed by special investigations.

5. Supralumbar Cord Lesions

Following transverse lesions to the cord above the level of the lumbar and sacral centers, reflex erection, emission, and ejaculation are preserved in the phase of returining and enhanced spinal reflexivity. Due to the interruption of afferent and efferent pathways, however, orgasm and psychogenic genital excitation remain absent. This is not only true of complete transection of the cord for it occurs quite frequently in partial interruption, e.g., following bilateral cordotomy (Foerster, 1936, page 222). Erection is then no longer brought about by psychological activity but only by stimulation of the genital region. For the same reason, spontaneous morning erection as a reflex to bladder distension may be preserved. As reflex ejaculation takes place without the sensation of orgasm, sexual intercourse ceases to give physical pleasure.

II. Peripheral Nerve Lesions and Genital Function

Unilateral damage to the pelvic plexus or individual peripheral nerve lesions leave bladder, rectal, and genital function intact. The differentiation of a plexus lesion from multiradicular damage (i.e., incomplete cauda equina lesions) on the basis of purely clinical neurology may be difficult or even impossible and may require special investigations (electromyography, radiology). In both cases, the initial symptom is frequently that of pain in the distribution of the affected nerves so that precise description of the pattern of radiation together with the objective findings of motor loss, sensory impairment, and alteration of reflexes may lead toward a differential diagnosis between lesions either of the cauda equina or of the more peripheral nerves. Because of the close proximity of the nerve roots, any lesion of a certain size affecting the cauda equina will tend to lead to bilateral symptoms, although this is by no means always the case.

The commonest causes of peripheral nerve lesions are neoplasms infiltrating the pelvic wall and sequelae of major pelvic surgery, especially abdominoperineal excision of the rectum with its associated removal of the perirectal tissues and the nerve plexuses therein.

Among the peripheral nerve disorders associated with disordered genital function, the various polyneuropathies are worthy of mention, e.g., diabetic and alcoholic neuropathies. Other autonomic functions are frequently affected at the same time; thus the bladder may be atonic, there may be vasomotor impairment with trophic abnormalities and edema, and there may be absence of sweating. In tabes dorsalis – a late manifestation of neurosyphilis following many years after primary infection – the afferent fibers in the dorsal roots and dorsal columns degenerate leading to early sacral sensory impairment, absence of tendon reflexes, and atonic bladder and impotence. Irritation of the sacral roots, which leads to the characteristic bladder and rectal crises of tabes (HILLER, 1953, page 384), may also bring about painful priapism and pollutiones flaccidae (FOERSTER, 1936, page 222).

III. Cerebral Causes of Impotence

The cerebral integration and control of genital function may be impaired by a wide variety of intracranial disorders. Focal disorders of which the localizing symptom is impotence should be differentiated from a generalized decrease in cerebral function due to diffuse affections of the entire brain, such as raised intracranial pressure, anoxia, multiple cerebral contusions, atherosclerosis, infectious and toxic effects, and dystrophies or degenerations. The psychological concomitants of hypothalamic disease (blunting of affect and loss of drive) commonly include diminution of libido. Stereotactic destruction of the tuber cinereum (in the floor of the hypothalamus anterior to the mammillary bodies and posterior to the infundibulum) brings about loss of sexual drive – a discovery in animal experimentation that has been applied in humans suffering certain perversions (ROEDER, 1966). Occasionally, lack of libido is the first sign of pituitary tumor. On the other hand, libido may remain unimpaired for many years in the presence of a pituitary tumor and even after its complete surgical removal.

For further reading on the central stimulation of sexual development (precocious puberty) and inhibition of sexual function (pituitary or hypothalamic infantilism, diencephaloretinal degeneration, Simmond's disease, etc.) see ORTHNER and STUTTE.

C. Neurologic Assessment

As the investigator cannot himself witness the sequence of genital function, his conclusions will depend quite fundamentally on a detailed and explicit history. A good history and neurologic examination with particular emphasis on the lumbosacral region will allow recognition both of the type of disorder and the site of the focus. Special investigations, such as X rays, lumbar puncture, and electromyogram, will supplement and underpin the diagnosis.

I. History

The interview with the patient will provide a first impression of his personality and general health. The investigator will hear of past or current illnesses, of medication, of operations and injuries, of familial disorders, of concomitant disturbances of bladder and rectal function and of abnormalities of the lower abdomen and legs. Once these things have been discussed, attention should turn to the sequence of events associated with genital function and to individual abnormalities of that sequence. To understand the patient's attitudes and to find a common language may make considerable demands on the physician.

Has the patient experienced normal sexual drive? What is his conception of normal libido? Is he impotent despite normal libido? Once these things have been clarified, inquiries should be made as to the nature of the abnormality, when it first occurred, and how exactly it developed.

Does the patient know the normal sequence of genital function or has he never experienced it? If he is properly informed, when did the abnormality first occur and under what circumstances? Does it only occur under certain psychological conditions?

Which of the individual physiological functions is disordered? Does the patient have a proper erection or only priapism (filling of the corpora cavernosa but not of the glans)? Does erection occur spontaneously in response to psychological stimuli, or only following genital stimulation? What of the ridigity and durability of erection? Is intromission possible? Does the ejaculatory reflex occur and when? Is this associated with a sensation of orgasm resolving both tension and desire?

Does ejaculation take place in the normal way, or is it retrograde into the bladder? Was there ejaculation without complete erection? Was the sexual act associated with unpleasant sensations or pain?

1. Interpretation of the History

If erection occurs both as a psychological reaction and as an exteroceptive reflex, one may assume that both the supranuclear pathways and the sacral autonomic center as well as the peripheral efferent parasympathetic and afferent somatic fibers are intact.

If only reflex erection occurs, a lesion of the supranuclear spinal pathways should be considered. If only psychogenic erection occurs, the sacral autonomic center and the centrifugal spinal pathways are intact, but the afferent peripheral somatic pathways are inadequate. If erection is completely absent without a history of trauma, illness or major pelvic surgery, one needs to consider a psychogenic disorder.

The ejaculatory reflex is more easily interfered with than that of erection. Reflex erection without ejaculation may occur in lesions of the centrifugal supranuclear pathways or of the intraspinal synapses due to absence of the reflex of emission. Psychogenic erection without ejaculation or with incomplete, dripping ejaculation occur as dissociated disorders due to focal lesions of the lumbosacral autonomic centers. Ejaculation without preceding erection may be a psychological disorder in the sense of premature ejaculation and also occurs following various lesions of the pelvic nerves (e.g., trauma to the nerves in major pelvic surgery) as a consequence of damage to the posterior roots in tabes dorsalis and in incomplete spinal cord injuries affecting the intraspinal synapses.

Retrograde ejaculation may be a consequence of trauma to the hypogastric nerves in major surgery or a result of local muscular damage at bladder neck surgery.

Absence of orgasm for organic reasons occurs in lesions of the peripheral or central afferent pathways. As the power of the reflex depends more on clonic contraction of pelvic musculature (pudendal nerves, FOERSTER, 1936, page 63) than on contraction of the seminal vesicles and vas deferens (hypogastric nerves), it is more likely to be impaired by lesions of the somatic pudendal nerves or the cauda equina than by those of the autonomic nerves. Peripheral causes are the various types of traumatic, iatrogenic, inflammatory, neoplastic, or polyneuropathic afflictions; central causes include foci of disease in the medulla and cordotomy (transection of the spinothalamic tract). Even after complete destruction of the conus with absence of erection and ejaculation, there may be a form of orgasmic sensation: a feeling of tension and excitement felt low in the lumbar region, which may resolve in pollutio flaccida (seen but not felt).

II. Neurologic Status

On order that nothing be overlooked, a complete systematic neurologic examination should always be carried out with testing of the special senses, motor and tendon reflex examination, sensory charting and annotation of skin reflexes, of tone and trophic changes, and if possible of autonomic reflexes (skin moisture, dermographism). At the same time, general examination of the patient may yield clues to endocrine or other medical disorders: hypopituitarism with polyglandular insufficiency, color, beard development, cushingism, myxedema, acromegaly, cachexia, cardiopulmonary insufficiency, asthma, etc.

Emphasis in neurologic examination should then be concentrated on examination of the spinal and peripheral innervation of the trunk, pelvis and legs: the musculature of the abdominal wall (Beevor's sign: in unilateral paralysis the umbilicus is displaced when the head is lifted; HILLER, 1953, p. 368), of the back, the buttocks, the pelvic floor, and the various parts of the lower limb. The external anal sphincter may be taken as representative of the pelvic floor musculature, and the tone and power of this muscle can be felt at rectal examination. Enhanced reflexes, spastitcity, clonus, and pathologic plantar responses indicate a supranuclear spinal lesion (upper motor neuron) while absence of reflexes and flaccid tone suggest a lower motor neuron lesion.

1. Important Intrinsic Reflexes Bearing on Neurologic Fertility Disorders, According to Segmental Level

Tendon reflexes are intrinsic reflexes, in which the same muscle is the site of stimulation and of effect. The afferent pathway lies in several lumbar or sacral dorsal roots; the reflex arc is monosynaptic and contained within a single spinal segment. Such intrinsic reflexes are inhibited by centrifugal activity in the pyramidal system. Thus, pyramidal lesions, whatever their localization, lead to enhancement of intrinsic reflexes. In assessing reflexes, pathologic significance should be assigned to the following: any lateralization due to diminution of a reflex on one side, enhancement of the reflex, extension of a reflexogenic area (e.g., patellar tendon reflex in response to stimulation of the tibial margin), and contralateral response or accompanying spinal automatism (reflex synergy, mass reflexes).

L 2–3: the adductor reflex is elicited by tapping the medial femoral condyle with the leg passively abducted against slight resistance. The response is adduction of the thigh unilaterally or, in this reflex quite normally, bilaterally.

L 2–4, mainly L 3–4: the patellar tendon reflex (quadriceps reflex), is brought about by tapping the patellar tendon with the leg somewhat flexed both at the knee and at the hip. The reflex response is contraction of the quadriceps muscle leading to extension of the knee joint.

S 1–2: biceps femoris reflex. This is elicited with the patient in the lateral position, with knees and hips flexed, by tapping the tendon of the muscle, which is steadied at the lateral margin of the popliteal fossa with a fingertip. The response is contraction of the muscle and flexion of the knee joint.

2. Chief Extrinsic Reflexes of Importance for the Neurologic Aspects of Fertility, According to Spinal Segments

In extrinsic reflexes, the site of stimulation may be the skin or mucous membrane, while the effector organ remains the muscle. The reflex arc is polysynaptic and involves several spinal segments. Extrinsic reflexes are enhanced by centrifugal activity of the pyramidal pathway. Diminution, rapid fatigability or absence of extrinsic reflexes is a fine indicator of pyramidal pathway lesions.

D 7–9, upper, D 8–10 middle, and D 10–12 lower abdominal wall reflexes: these are elicited by a rapid stroking of the abdominal skin from lateral to medial; the response is twitching of the abdominal wall with displacement of the navel. Of pathologic significance is absence of the reflex on one or either side or at one level. Absence of the reflex is not pathologic in the elderly, where the abdominal wall is slack, scarred, or obese, or where the environmental temperature is low.

L 1–2: the cremasteric reflex is triggered by stroking the skin of the medial aspect of the thigh, and the response is retraction either of the ipsilateral testis or of both. This reflex is inconstant, but unilateral absence is of significance for the level of a lesion.

S 3–4: bulbocavernosus reflex. This is a sexual reflex elicited by stimulation of the glans penis, and the response is a contraction of the bulbocavernosi muscles (and of the external anal sphincter, BORS and COMARR, 1971; LAPIDES and BABBIT, 1956) palpable in the perineum.

S 5: the anal reflex is the visible contraction of the external anal sphincter in response to perianal stimulation.

S 1–2: The plantar reflex. Stroking the sole of the foot normally leads to plantar flexion of the toes. The Babinski response is a pathologic plantar reflex resulting from pyramidal tract damage; stimulation of the lateral margin of the sole leads to extension of the great toe (hypertonic hyperextension or brief extensile twitching). This reflex is absent in complete transection with flaccid paralysis of the legs and also in selective loss of the extrapyramidal pathways.

L-5–S-5: Contraction of the external anal sphincter on coughing or deep inspiration is a reflex normally preventing incontinence. This reflex is dependent on innervation of the abdominal muscle by segments D-6–L-1 and on an intact intraspinal pathway down to S-5. Objective testing may be carried out either by manometry or electromyography (BORS and COMARR, 1971).

Sensory testing comprises tests of light touch, position, and vibration as well as pain and temperature senses. Vibration is normally perceived right down to the toes, numbers written on the skin are correctly interpreted as far down as the calves. By the demarcation of sensory disturbances, spinomedullary, radicular, or peripheral causation of abnormalities may often be more clearly differentiated than by their motor effects. The spinal segment, root, or peripheral nerve appropriate to any given sensory disturbance may be derived from neurologic sensory charts (Fig. 1).

III. Special Investigations

Depending on the particular problem in hand and after consideration of the differential diagnosis, neurologic examination will need to be complemented by special investigations involving a variety of techniques. General medical assessment will require basic hematologic and urine examinations, laboratory tests of renal and liver function, blood sugar estimation, tests for inflammatory conditions, and serologic screening.

Suspicion of a spinal disorder involving the cauda equina or spinal cord should be regarded as an indication for lumbar puncture without delay so that protein estimation, cell count, sugar and chloride estimation, electrophoresis, and colloid curves may be carried out on the CSF, as should syphilis serology. Equally, when any feature suggests a spinal level, plain X rays of the relevant segment of the spine should be ordered together, possibly with a myelogram, to visualize the spinal subarachnoid space. Whole body computer tomography to visualize a cross section of the entire trunk has proved to be helpful in differentiating spinal tumors from retroperitoneal tumors.

Simple electrical tests on muscles and nerves rapidly produce information as to the reaction of a muscle or nerve to faradic or galvanic stimulation.

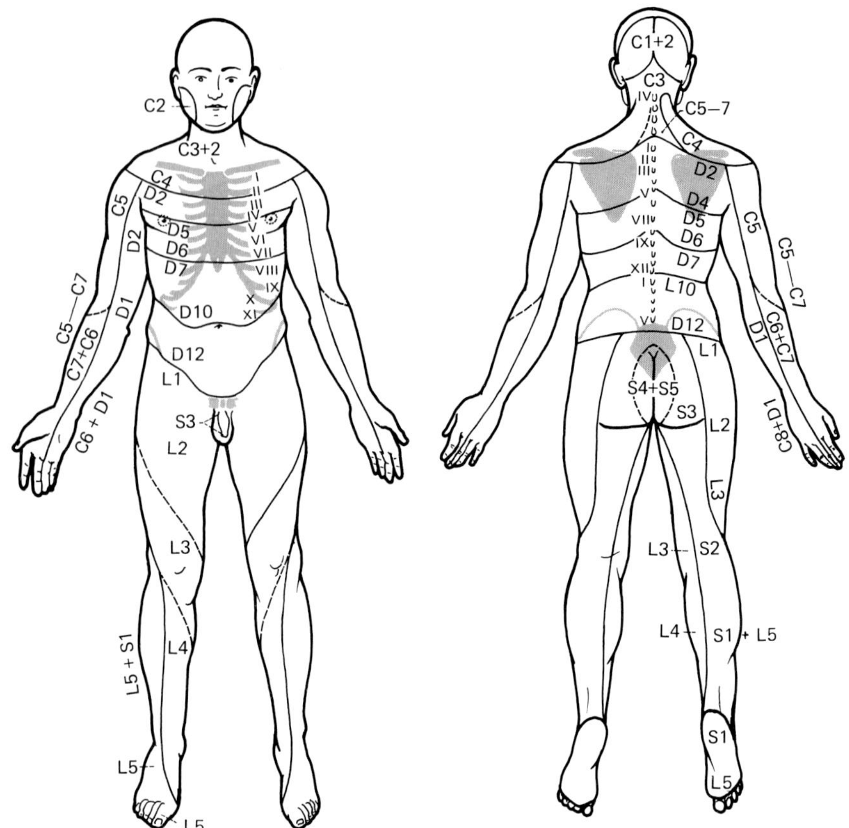

Fig. 1. Neurologic sensory charts

Electromyography is able to differentiate between myogenic and neurogenic paresis, to detect early stages of denervation, and to differentiate between paresis of nuclear or more peripheral site of origin, e.g., for the subject under discussion, the confirmation of a nuclear paralysis of the external anal sphincter (Taverner and Smiddy, 1959).

A series of urologic investigations should be mentioned along with neurologic techniques; estimation of bladder capacity, of urinary residual volume, of bladder tone and contractility, and measurement of sphincter tone. Minute changes of detrusor activity can be detected by detrusor electromyography.

D. Synopsis of Neurologic Disturbances of Potency

Normal coitus, presupposing the appropriate psychological attitude, requires that the genital functions of erection, emission, and ejaculation be intact. These are complex spinal reflexes involving both the somatic and sympathetic and parasympathetic autonomic nervous systems. These reflexes are easily impaired by psychological influences or by hormonal, neurologic, or local disease. In a systematic approach, we should differentiate between primary and secondary abnormalities, i.e., between those that were always present and those appearing subsequently. Various sensory impressions and acts of imagination frequently associated with copulation may become stimuli of "conditioned reflexes," which intervene in either a facilitatory or an inhibitory fashion in the sequence of sexual function.

I. Synopsis According to Functional Impairment

1. Absence of Libido

This may be primary or secondary, i.e., it may occur during or following an illness or as a psychogenic reaction to the emergence of a disorder of sexual function (MASTERS and JOHNSON, 1973).

Causes: general feeling of illness, depression, endocrine abnormality (pituitary, diencephalon, polyglandular insufficiency), intoxication (alcohol, drugs), metabolic disorders (diabetes, renal failure), and medication (sedatives, and hypotensives, anticonvulsants).

2. Total Impotence

Absence of erection and ejaculation as part of a cauda equina syndrome or following lesions in the region of the spinal genital center S2–5. Small foci in this region may lead to dissociated disorders of potency, usually abolition of ejaculation in the presence of erection.

3. Impotentia Generandi

Inability to procreate = sterility, not to be confused with infertility. Absence or inadequacy of erection, of emission, or or ejaculation including premature or retrograde ejaculation.

4. Impotentia Coeundi

Psychological or physical incapability of coitus due to absence or inadequacy of erection.

5. Erection

If both psychogenic and reflex erections take place, afferent and efferent peripheral and central pathways between genitalia and brain are intact. In approximately 90% of cases, the absence of erection is psychogenic (intra- or interpersonal).

6. Absence of Psychogenic Erection in the Presence of Reflex Erection

This occurs following interruption of the centrifugal spinal pathways above the spinal genital center S2–5 by transverse lesions of whatever etiology.

7. Absence of Psychogenic and Reflex Erections

Lesions of the spinal genital center S2–5 or of the nervi erigentes. Foci of demyelination in the sacral cord, lesions of the cauda equina affecting S2–5 or of the peripheral nerves and plexuses in the pelvis (operative damage, polyneuropathy of various causes, tabes).

8. Priapism (Semierection)

Priapism (Foerster, 1936, p. 220) appears in transection of the cord above the spinal genital center S2–5 due both to absence of centrifugal vasoconstrictor activity and to tonic contraction of the transversus perinei, bulbo-, and ischiocavernosus muscles – analogous to spasticity of the skeletal musculature. Priapism should be discerned from those cases where the penile volume is augmented simply by increased filling of the corpora cavernosa as a result of vasomotor paralysis in the spinal shock of fresh cord transections or of later stages of complete transection with maintained vasomotor paralysis. Priapism has also been observed in cases of sacral dorsal root irritation (Foerster, 1936, p. 222).

9. Ejaculation

This reflex is composed of a visceromotor component (emission) and of a somatic motor component (contraction of the transversus perinei, bulbo-, and ischiocavernosus muscles). In the second phase of spinal cord transection, most usually in complete cases, there is a hyperreflexia of ejaculation similar to the spasticity and hyperreflexia of skeletal musculature. Thus, the most insignificant stimuli may induce clonic twitching of the above-mentioned muscles or even ejaculation.

Ejaculation without preceding erection is usually a psychogenic functional disorder similar to premature ejaculation. Organic causes: lesions of the pelvic nerves following operative intervention, root damage in the cauda equina by tabes, intraspinal foci affecting intraspinal pathways.

10. Absence of Ejaculation or Disordered Ejaculation (Dripping) with or without Disturbance of Erection (Pollutio Flaccida)

Dissociated or partial impairment of potency by intraspinal foci affecting lumbar and sacral centers and their interconnections.

11. Absence of Ejaculation in the Presence of Reflex Erection

A lesion of the centrifugal spinal pathways above the level of the sacral autonomic center S2–4 in transverse lesions of various cause. The picture may also represent a dissociated disturbance of potency related to small foci in the spinal genital center S2–4 itself or following interruption of intraspinal pathways as high as L2–4.

12. Retrograde Ejaculation

Local muscular damage following bladder neck surgery or operative trauma to the pelvic nerves and plexuses.

13. Anorgasmia

Absence of the reaction of orgasm within an otherwise undisturbed sequence of sexual function. Psychogenic or resulting from organic disease: interruption of the afferent pathways of the lateral columns by multiple sclerosis, syringomyelia (Bors and Comar, 1971), bilateral cordotomy (transection of the spinothalamic tract for pain control).

II. Synopsis According to Localization in the Central or Peripheral Nervous System

1. Cerebral Lesions

Loss of libido due to hypothalamic lesions and to hormonal disorders resulting from pituitary tumor.

2. Supralumbar Spinal Transection

Loss of psychogenic erection in the presence of intact or enhanced reflex erection and ejaculation (analogous to enhanced reflexes of the skeletal musculature), filling of the corpora cavernosa or priapism (chiefly in incomplete transections with spastic contraction of the bulbo- and ischiocavernosus muscles and the transversus perinei). In the first phase of spinal transection, there is complete atonia and areflexia.

3. Lumbar Transection Involving the Sympathetic Genital Centers L 2–4

Absence of emission and therefore of ejaculation with intact clonic contraction of the transversus perinei, bulbo-, and ischiocavernosus muscles, which have their nuclei in the segments S 3–4. Small lumbar foci may lead to disturbance of ejaculation in the form of "dripping ejaculation."

4. Lesions of the Sacral Automic Center S 2–5

Total impotence or, in the case of small localized foci, possible dissociated impairment of potency (absence of ejaculation with intact erection), also pollutio flaccida and psychogenic orgasm.

a) Conus Syndrome (S 3–5 and Coccygeal Segment Cocc. 1)

Bladder disorders (flaccid atonic bladder, retention of urine, paradoxical dribbling), incontinence of feces, total impotence, possible dissociated disorder of potency, disordered sensation (perianogenital: saddle region), absent anal reflex (S-5) and bulbocavernosus reflex (S-3), paralysis of the external anal sphincter and of the perineal muscles (pudendal nerve S 3–4), and no paralyses or impairment of tendon reflexes in the legs (achilles tendon reflex: L-5–S-2, patellar tendon teflex L 2–4).

b) Epiconus Syndrome (L4–5 and S1–2)

Automatic voiding of bladder and rectum: reflex bladder, incontinence of feces, possible dissociated potency disturbance, absence of erection with preserved ejaculation, i.e., pollutio flaccida. Alternatively: absent ejaculation and presence of erection, loss of sensation in the distribution L-4–S-2, motor abnormalities in the legs, especially distally: paralysis of the dorsiflexors of foot and toes, of abduction and adduction of the foot, of the extensors and flexors of the knee and of the rotators and abductors of the hip. In addition, absence of ankle jerk (L-5–S-2) and possibly of the knee jerk (L2–4) and absence of any plantar reflex.

5. Cauda Equina Syndrome (Below Vertebral Level L1/2)

Flaccid atonic bladder with retention of urine and possible paradoxical dribbling, incontinence of feces, total impotence.

6. Peripheral Paralysis

Unilateral plexus damage will leave bladder, rectal, and genital function intact, while bilateral lesions will lead to the same picture as the cauda equina syndrome.

References

Bing R (1948) Kompendium der topischen Gehirn- und Rückenmarksdiagnostik. Schwabe, Basel

Bors E, Comarr AE (1971) Neurological urology. Karger, Basel

Bruecke ThE v (1937) Die Leistungen des normalen Rückenmarkes. Handbuch der Neurologie II. Springer, Berlin, S 138

Foerster O (1936) Symptomatologie der Erkrankungen des Rückenmarkes. Handbuch der Neurologie, Bd 5, Allgemeine Neurologie V, Rückenmark. Springer, Berlin, S 62

Gagel O (1953) Vegetatives System. Handbuch innere Medizin, Bd 5, Teil 1, Neurologie I. Springer, Berlin Göttingen Heidelberg

Guttmann L (1971) Prinzipien und Methoden in der Behandlung und Rehabilitation von Rückenmarksverletzten. Neurotraumatologie, Bd. II. Verletzungen der Wirbelsäule und des Rückenmarks. Urban & Schwarzenberg, München Berlin Wien

Hiller F (1953) Rückenmark. Handbuch innere Medizin, Bd 5, Teil 1, Neurologie I. Springer, Berlin Göttingen Heidelberg

Lapides J, Babbit JM (1956) Diagnostic value of bulbocavernosus reflex. JAMA 162:971–972

Masters WH, Johnson VE (1973) Impotenz und Anorgasmie. Zur Therapie funktioneller Sexualstörungen. Frankfurt/Main

Orthner H (1955) Anatomie und Physiologie der Steuerungsorgane und Anatomie und Physiologie der Sexualstörungen. Giese H (Hrsg) In: Die Sexualität des Menschen. Enke, Stuttgart

Roeder FD (1966) Stereotactic lesions of the tuber cinereum in sexual diviation. Confin Neurol 27:162–163

Stutte H (1955) Pubertas praecox. Giese H (Hrsg) In: Sexualität des Menschen. Enke, Stuttgart S 474–505

Taverner D, Smiddy FG (1959) An electromyographic study of the normal function of the external anal sphincter and pelvic diaphragm. Dis Colon Rectum 2:153–160

Immunologic Causes of Male Fertility Disorders

K. Bandhauer

A widespread realization that immunologic factors exert an influence on the fertility of the male followed mainly in the wake of publications by Rümke (1954) and Wilson (1954). Each author reported, independently of the other, on two patients who had remained childless and whose serum contained sperm-agglutinating antibodies, and thereby they stimulated intensive clinical research in this area. Landsteiner (1899), Metchnikoff (1900), and Metalnikof (1900), being the first workers to demonstrate antigenic properties in semen and testicular tissue, had already laid important foundations for the immunologic investigation of male fertility disorders. Similar studies were carried out by von Moxter (1900) and Farnum (1901) during the same period. Following these papers, the antigenic properties of the components of semen and of the male organs of reproduction became the object of extensive research.

A. Antigenicity

The first reports of antigenicity in semen did not differentiate between antigens in seminal fluid and those in the spermatozoa. By the experimental injection of human semen into animals, Hektoen and Manly (1923) were thus able to produce species- and semen-specific antihuman precipitins. At an early juncture animal experimentation also demonstrated a significant effect of immunologic factors on fertility. Guyer (1922) was able to produce partial or total sterility in rabbits and guinea pigs by passive immunization with sperm-specific antisera. In the experiments of Kennedy (1924), active immunization of experimental animals with autologous sperm led to degenerative change in the testes. By active immunization with testicular extracts Voisin et al. (1951, 1955) were able to produce aspermatogenesis.

Quite early on the species and organ specificity of antigens present in both human and various animal semen was the subject of numerous investigations (Hektoen and Manly, 1923; Weil et al., 1959; Bandhauer, 1966). Despite extensive species specificity, cross reactions between species were in some cases demonstrated, e.g., between the semen of bull and ram (Mudd and Mudd, 1929). Furthermore, Henle (1938) discovered a similarity in the antigenic properties of human and bovine semen.

The organ specificity of the antigens in human seminal fluid was found to be considerably less pronounced, to the extent that they showed cross reaction both with serum and with extracts of epididymis, seminal vesicles, and prostate. Stevens and Fost (1964) were able to detect an antigen common to human seminal fluid and human kidney extracts. Gabl (1963) and Grant (1963) used immunoelectrophoresis to demonstrate a cross reaction between proteins contained in seminal fluid and in saliva. The studies of Bandhauer (1966), on the other hand, did not reveal any antigens common to semen and testicular extract.

I. Blood Group Antigens in Seminal Fluid

Ever since the experiments of Landsteiner and Levine (1926), it has been well-known that blood group antigens may be found in human seminal fluid. However, this transfer of blood group antigens into seminal fluid only occurs in patients who are so-called secretors. According to Edwards et al. (1964), blood group antigens may also be found in the saliva of such people. A, B, O blood group antigens are also detectable in their spermatozoa, most probably adsorbed from the seminal fluid. The significance of these A, B, O antigens has not yet been determined with certainty. According to Weil (1961), there is no correlation between the antigens of the seminal fluid responsible for auto-sensitization and the blood group antigens. On the other hand, the spermatozoa of "secretors" are able to adsorb A, B, O antigens on their surface before they have come into contact with the secretions of the reproductive apparatus. Thus, Edwards et al. (1964) were able to demonstrate blood group antigens on the surface of spermatozoa recovered from spermatoceles and from the epididymis. However, Popivanov et al. (1969) believed that the main source of the blood group antigens carried on spermatozoa lies in prostatic secretion.

The clinical effects of blood group antigen carriage by spermatozoa has not yet been elucidated. Neither Solish (1969) nor Fernandez et al. (1972) were able to demonstrate immobilization, agglutination, or cytotoxic change in the semen following immunization with blood group antigens. Nevertheless, Ackermann (1967) and Solish (1969) have raised the possibility of metabolic impairment of spermatozoa by blood group antigens.

II. Antigenic Fractions of Seminal Fluid

Numerous studies of the antigenic fractions in seminal fluid have been published. By means of gel double-diffusion methods, Rao and Sadri (1959) were able to detect at least 16 different antigenic fractions in seminal fluid, many of which were however identical to antigens found in the serum. According to Goldberg (1973), the following antigenic fractions of semen correspond to those of the serum: albumin, α-globulin, β-globulin, γ-globulin, IgG, IgA, and IgM. Furthermore, the proteolytic enzymes of semen and spermatozoa, aminopeptidase, acid phosphatase, hyaluronidase, acrosomal protease, and lactic dehydrogenase-X (LDH-X) have antigenic activity, as do proteolytic enzyme inhibitors.

Those antigenic fractions specific to seminal fluid have been related to secretions of the glandular structures of the reproductive tract, both in human (Band-

HAUER, 1963, 1966; BANDHAUER et al., 1964) and animal semen (RAO and SADRI, 1960; HUNTER, 1969). By immunodiffusion it has been shown that there are two antigenic fractions whose lines of precipitation are closely approximated, corresponding to prostatic antigens (BANDHAUER, 1966; SHULMAN, 1971, 1972; SHULMAN and ORSINI, 1970) that four or five antigenic fractions are derived from the seminal vesicles, and that one fraction arises from the tail of the epididymis (BANDHAUER, 1966). On the other hand, testicular extracts have not been found to contain any precipitable antigens that can be shown to be identical with antigens in the seminal fluid (BANDHAUER, 1966). These results of gel double-diffusion investigations have been underpinned by absorption experiments. The work of HERRMANN and HERMANN (1969) and SHULMAN and BRONSON (1969) has revealed that seminal fluid contains both serum proteins and specific antigens produced in the glandular structures of the male reproductive tract. The serum proteins are albumin, transferrin, and immunoglobulin (IgG and IgA). These immunoglobulins are in all probability added to the seminal fluid in the prostate. Likewise, SEARCY et al. (1964) found between 8 and 13 antigenic components of seminal fluid not present in the serum.

The full range of antigens in the seminal fluid, or rather of the antigens secreted into seminal fluid by the glands of the reproductive pathway, have to date only partly been identified. Immunoelectrophoresis has allowed six fractions of human seminal fluid to be more closely characterized (BANDHAUER, 1966). The acid phosphatase of prostatic secretion probably represents an important antigenic fraction (FLOCKS et al., 1962). HEKMAN and RÜMKE (1969) were able to identify lactoferrin originating from the seminal vesicles as chief among those antigens of seminal fluid that become adsorbed onto the surface of spermatozoa. This "coating effect" had previously been described by WEIL (1960). It was long believed that such surface antigens of the spermatozoa, derived from the seminal fluid, played a major role in immunologic phenomena, particularly in sperm agglutination and sperm immobilization. Thus, it was considered that the glandular structures of the reproductive tract, or rather their secretions, played an essential part in the etiology of immunologic disturbances of fertility. In more recent years, there has been an increasing tendency to regard spermatic antigens of testicular origin as the agents in those immunologic reactions that are responsible for in- and subfertility (BOETTCHER et al., 1977).

III. Antigens of Spermatozoa

The antigenic properties of spermatozoa were originally attributed mainly to the "surface antigens," derived from the seminal fluid and adsorbed onto the surface of the spermatozoa. Thus, WEIL et al. (1960) found identical antigens in the seminal fluid and on the surface of spermatozoa. They believed in a so-called coating effect in which antigenic substances from the seminal fluid were deposited on the surface of spermatozoa in the seminal vesicles and prostate. In fact, this coating effect seems to commence in the epididymis (BANDHAUER, 1966). Identical antigenic fractions can be found in extracts of epididymis and on washed spermatozoa. According to a report by MANN (1964), it is also in the epididymis that the first enzymes (glycosidases) are deposited upon the sperms, so it is possible that these enzymes are themselves antigenic substances. Apart from the blood group antigens (A, B, O) already mentioned, the presence of leukocyte antigens (HLA) on the spermatozoa has been documented. The significance of these antigens for sub- or infertility in men or women has not yet been determined, although it does not seem to be great (Mumford et al., 1975; Jenning et al., 1976). Katsh and Katsh had previously (1965) demonstrated four antigenic fractions in epididymal spermatozoa: hyaluronidase, nucleic acid, polysaccharides, and a globulin fraction. The latter authors are sceptical of coating and believe these antigens to be sperm specific.

Barker and Amann (1969) demonstrated head and tail antigens as well as those common to the whole spermatozoon. Equally, Rümke and Hellinga (1959) found differing autoantigens in the head and tail. Kolk et al. (1974) documented an autoantigen related to the human sperm head nucleus.

Voisin and Toullet (1968) isolated three antigenic fractions from epididymal spermatozoa. By means of immunofluorescence and radioimmunoassay, it has been possible to detect H_2 antigens in the head and middle piece of mouse spermatozoa. In this connection, Voytiskova and Pokorna (1971) and Erickson (1971) have discussed the proposal that these too are so-called coating antigens. In 1973 Toullet et al. separated four autoantigens from the spermatozoa of guinea pigs. The most active antigen is a water-soluble glycoprotein localized on the acrosome. This is the only antigen to give rise to both sperm-agglutinating and sperm-immobilizing antibodies. Manarang-Pangan and Behrman (1971) were able to remove sperm-immobilizing antibodies from the serum of infertile women and vasectomized men by absorption with spermatozoa. No such effect could be demonstrated if seminal fluid was used in their place. On the other hand, sperm-agglutinating antibodies could be absorbed both by seminal fluid and by spermatozoa. This could be interpreted as indicating that sperm-immobilizing antibodies are generated by sperm-specific antigens. Similar studies have been undertaken by Menge (1967, 1970) whose results are practically the same.

Menge and Protzman (1967) recorded nine antigens in rabbit spermatozoa of which seven were also present in seminal fluid and two in serum. Two of these antigens seemed to be produced in the testes, and it is assumed that the antigens of spermatozoa play a more important immunizing role than those of seminal fluid and that they are therefore more important in the etiology of fertility disturbances. By an immunofluorescent technique, Hansen and Hjort (1971) found four sites with antigenic activity in human spermatozoa:
1. The tip of the acrosome
2. Equatorial segment
3. Postnuclear region
4. Principal piece of the tail

Two of these antigens would appear to be sperm specific, while the antigens of the postnuclear region and the acrosome are similar to antigens of seminal fluid and adrenal tissue. In animal experimentation, sperm-specific enzymes, such as lactic dehydrogenase-X (LDH-X) and hyaluronidase, have been shown to have auto- and isoantigenic properties. Their effects in man are not yet certain, although an isoantigenic effect in women has been ascribed to them by BOETTCHER et al. (1977). LERUM and GOLDBERG (1974) were also of the opinion that spermatic LDH was involved in the immunologic induction of fertility disturbances in the zona pellucida of the ovum. Such an effect of LDH on immunologic reactions is not however generally accepted (SPIELMANN et al., 1977).

To date the following auto- or isoantigens of the human spermatozoon have been identified chemically: LDH, the significance of which is contested, as already mentioned (BOETTCHER et al., 1977; KOLK et al., 1978), and furthermore a protamine (KOLK et al., 1974; KOLK and SAMUEL, 1975).

IV. Antigenic Properties of the Testes

LANDSTEINER (1899), METCHNIKOF (1900), and METALNIKOFF (1900) reported "spermatotoxic antibodies" in the serum of animals that had been sensitized with testicular extracts. These antibodies variously brought about either a loss or a reduction of sperm motility. VON MOXTER (1900) reported similar results after heterologous insemination, while VOISIN et al. (1951), DELAUNAY and VOISIN (1952), and FREUND et al. (1953) were able to induce aspermatogenesis by autologous or homologous sensitization using testicular extracts with or without the addition of Freund's adjuvant. In subsequent years, testicular antigens became the subject of numerous studies. RÜMKE reported the appearance of circulating antibodies without any detectable damage to the testicular parenchyma following repeated injection of testicular homogenates. By contrast, MANCINI et al. (1965) noted definite testicular damage following injections of testicular materials with Freund's adjuvant. The up-to-date results of investigations into the immune response in testicular tissue to testicular antigens have been reviewed by BEER and BILLINGHAM (1976), SCOTT and JONES (1977), and TUNG (1977). Typical lesions appear as early as 2–8 weeks after single injection or the administration of larger quantities of antigen with adjuvant and manifest themselves as interstitial edema, perivascular infiltrates of macrophages, accumulations of plasma cells and lymphocytes, and in cellular destruction in the region of the germinal epithelium, with concomitant azoospermia. According to the work of ISOJIMA and TIEN SUN LI (1968), the antigenic properties of testicular tissue depend on the state of maturation of the organ. While mature cells exhibit autoantigenic properties, immature cells are devoid of this quality, which suggests that under certain conditions the body is unable to tolerate the mature germ cell (spermatozoa).

To elucidate the nature of testicular antigens was the object of numerous studies, mainly involving animal experimentation (KATSH and KATSH, 1961; KIRKPATRIC and KATSH, 1964; BISHOP and CARLSON, 1965; MATURA and MOYER, 1967; SADRI et al., 1967; ALONSO et al., 1969; BISHOP, 1969; KATSH et al., 1972; EVREV et al., 1973; LUSTIG et al., 1973; DENDUCHIS et al., 1975; BANDHAUER, 1966). The following germ cell antigens are known to date: the enzyme sorbitol-dehydrogenase (1969), hyaluronidase, lactic dehydrogenase-X-isoenzyme (KATSH, 1960; EVREV et al., 1973; WELLERSON et al., 1974), a glucopeptide containing 13% hydrocarbon (KATSH et al., 1972), and a mucopolysaccharide (BROWN et al., 1965). It would appear that neither Sertoli nor Leydig cells

7. Cytotoxins: according to the studies of MANCINI et al. (1969), these antibodies bring about lytic changes in the acrosomes, spermatozoa, and spermatids. LE BOUTELIER et al. (1973) have described a specific antibody to T antigen, the latter being localized in the outer membrane of sperm acrosomes, and it is claimed that these are responsible for the lytic reaction.
8. Opsonizing antibodies: in the serum of guinea pigs sensitized with testicular homogenate and Freund's adjuvant, MAZZOLLI and BARRERA (1974) were able to detect opsonizing activity. Such an opsonizing effect of sperm antiserum depends on macrophages of the peritoneal cavity, which are able to absorb homologous or autologous spermatozoa. BARRERA et al. (1976) found a low titer opsonizing activity to be present in normal serum. This activity seems to be brought about by the IgG-2-globulin fraction.
9. Immunofluorescent antibodies: these antibodies play a part in allergic orchitis. TUNG et al. (1970) were thus able to record the passage of ^{125}I-labeled immune IgG into the channels of the rete testis and into the straight tubules, while MANCINI et al. (1974) report negative findings. These immunofluorescent antibodies probably correspond to antigens of the acrosome, explaining why spermatids and spermatozoa fluoresce, while spermatocytes, spermatogonia, and Sertoli cells do not.

II. Cellular Antibodies

Cellular immunity as expressed in the presence of cell-bound antibody and in delayed hypersensitivity has not yet been extensively investigated from the point of view of its role in male fertility disorders. It is nowadays generally regarded as certain that macrophages play an important part in the synthesis of specific antibodies in the lymphocytes (FISHMAN et al., 1973). Cellular antibodies may be detected either by the classic skin test or by macrophage migration. In allergic orchitis, skin testing will lead, 24–48 h after injection of small quantities of antigen, to a skin reaction consisting of proliferation of histiocytes and fibroblasts, edema, perivascular accumulation of round mononuclear cells, and hypertrophy of vascular endothelium. According to FREUND et al. (1953), this will lead after approximately 6 days to a granulomatous change that may persist for several months. The macrophage-migration-inhibition test described by GEORGE and VAUGHAN (1962) has the advantage over skin testing of being quantitative and capable of detecting delayed hypersensitivity earlier on (MAZZOLI, 1971). In the clinical context of male fertility disorders, however, these modalities of investigation have not yet been widely applied.

C. Diagnosis of Immunologic Fertility Disorders

Numerous tests of varying significance are available for the detection of antisperm antibodies, based mainly on their agglutinating, immobilizing, or spermatotoxic properties. Following the conference at Aarhus (Denmark) in 1974, a unified nomenclature of the various types of tests was proposed by ROSE et al. (1976) (Table 1). MUMFORD (1979) has reviewed the more important

Table 1. Tests for detection of antisperm antibodies

Earlier classification	New classification	
Agglutination methods		
1. KIBRICK K-B-M	Gelatin agglutination test	(GAT)

2. FRANKLIN-DUKES
   F & D
   F–D
	Tube-slide agglutination test	(TSAT)

3. MAT	Tray agglutination test	(TAT)
4. Capillary	Capillary tube agglutination test	(CTAT)
5. Slide	Slide agglutination test	(SAT)
Immobilization methods		
1. ISOJIMA	Sperm immobilization test	(SIT-I)
2. FJÄLLBRANT	Sperm immobilization test	(SIT-F)

methods available for the investigation of immunologic fertility disorders. The methods described below are taken from this work.

I. Sperm Agglutination Tests

The first such test was published in 1952 by KIBRICK et al., and it was by this method that in 1954 RÜMKE first demonstrated the presence of sperm-agglutinating antibodies in man. With various unimportant modifications, the principle of this test still underlies the most important methods for the detection of sperm-agglutinating antibodies and for the estimation of their titer.

1. Antisperm Antibodies Assay:
Gelatin Agglutination Test (GAT) (KIBRICK)

Method:

1. Heat inactivated serum samples diluted 1:4 or serially with Baker's buffer.
2. Fresh semen adjusted with Baker's buffer to 40×10^6 cells/ml and warmed to 37° C.
3. Mix warmed sperm suspension with an equal part of a 10% gelatin solution in Baker's buffer at 37° C.
4. 0.3 ml of each serum sample is warmed to 37° C in a serologic tube and mixed gently with 0.3 ml of sperm-gelatin mixture.
5. Each mixture is then transferred to a 3×30 mm tube.
6. Tubes are incubated at 37° C and results recorded at 1 h and again at 2 h.
7. Each run should include a known positive serum and a known negative serum control.

2. Microscopic Sperm Agglutination Test

The microscopic sperm agglutination test was used chiefly by FRANKLIN and DUKES (1974). The principle of this is the microscopic observation of agglutination of normal semen by admixture of the test serum. This test has been modified by Shulman (1971, 1972, 1974a) and has become known as the tube-slide test. This microsperm agglutination test has remained popular as a simple screening procedure because of the ease with which it is carried out.

Method

Fresh semen from a male of assured fertility and containing more than 60 million spermatozoa/ml, and of good motility is diluted with 0.9% NaCl solution or with Baker's solution to give a sperm concentration of approximately 40 million/ml. One drop of this dilute semen is mixed with one drop of the patient's serum on a microscope slide and incubated at room temperature. Agglutination is read at 5, 10, and 15 min. In reading this test, collections of spermatozoa around other cells, such as epithelial and white blood cells as well as crystals, should be carefully noted as this effect may mimic agglutination. In the microagglutination test, sperm motility is preserved.

This method is intrinsically inaccurate and subject to numerous sources of error; therefore, it should only be used as a screening test to be complemented on the slightest suspicion of sperm agglutination by the more sensitive method of Kibrick. On the other hand, the micromethod is suitable for differentiating various types of agglutination (head to head, tail to tail, or mixed). The method has been refined by the modification of Franklin and Dukes (1974).

Method

Fresh semen of at least 50% motility is diluted with Baker's solution to 50 million spermatozoa/ml; 0.05 ml of this dilute semen is mixed with 0.5 ml of serum that has been diluted in Baker's solution 1:4 and inactivated at 56° C for 30 min. This mixture is incubated at 37° C. After 0.5, 1, 2, and 3 h, one drop is examined under the microscope, and the motile sperms are counted in 12 fields. Notes should be taken of the following parameters: number of free spermatozoa, number of clumped spermatozoa, number of clumps, and the type of clumps – head to head, tail to tail, etc. The total number of clumped spermatozoa is expressed in ratio to the total number of all motile spermatozoa. If more than 20% of cells are clumped, the test is said to be positive. By serial dilution of the sera (1:8, 1:16, 1:32, etc.), the information value of the test can be extended.

Shulman et al. (1971, 1973, 1974) have also modified the test and renamed it the tube-slide agglutination test. They recommend carrying out both the tube-slide test and the GAT (Kibrick) test for the detection of agglutinating antibodies. Boettcher et al. (1977) have demonstrated that these methods detect a β-lipoprotein and not immunoglobulin.

A further microscopic test is the microagglutination test after Friberg (1974) – the tray agglutination test. This test is simple, but like all other agglutination tests, it requires fresh semen of good quality. Only positive agglutinations at a titer of greater than 1:32 should be regarded as positive agglutination tests.

II. Immobilization Tests

Sperm immobilization tests and sperm agglutination tests do not detect the same groups of antibodies and therefore are not interchangeable and should be performed independently of one another.

The method given by Isojima et al. (1968, 1972) is still valid. A similar method has been described by Fjällbrant (1965) but this has not gained such widespread acceptance as the Isojima test.

Method

1. Fresh semen diluted to 60×10^5 cells/ml in saline.
2. Heat-inactivated serum samples are diluted serially with saline.
3. Mix 0.025 ml of semen with 0.25 ml of serum and 0.05 ml of pretitered active complement (human, rabbit, or guinea pig serum).
4. In a duplicate tube, mix 0.025 ml of serum and 0.05 ml of heat-inactivated complement. This is to determine toxic effects by noncomplement dependent factors.
5. In each run, a saline, a known negative serum, and a known positive serum should be included as controls.
6. Incubate at 37° C for 60 min.
7. Examine sample under a microscope and visually determine the percentage of motile spermatozoa.

The test is considered positive when the loss of sperm motility is at least twice as great in the patient's serum as in the control serum.

III. Cytotoxin Tests

The procedure of HUSTED and HJORT (1975) and its modification by SUNG et al. (1977) have become the methods of choice for determination of cytotoxicity. This test is considerably more laborious than the agglutination or immobilization tests and should only be carried out in specialized laboratories.

Method, modified according to SUNG

1. Fresh semen, washed and adjusted to 10×10^6 sperm/ml in human complement in one tube and in inactivated complement in the other tube.
2. Heat-inactivated serum samples are diluted serially with Hank's basic salt solution (HBSS).
3. Mix 0.025 ml of serum with 0.05 ml of sperm complement.
4. Incubate at 37° C for 90 min.
5. Add 0.4 µc ^{3}H-actinomycin D (^{3}H-Act D) in 0.05 ml HBSS.
6. Incubate at 37° C for 60 min.
7. Harvest sperms onto glass filter paper using an automated harvester (MASH).
8. Quantitative ^{3}H-Act D uptake in each tube using a B-scintillation counter.
9. Specific binding index (SBI)

$$\frac{\text{Sample CPM} - \text{Negative control CPM}}{\text{Max. binding control CPM} - \text{Negative control CPM}} \times 100$$

The test is considered positive if the SBI is greater than 25%.

IV. Immunofluorescence

Immunofluorescence allows localization of antigens on the spermatozoa and in the testicular tissue and is an extremely sensitive method. Immunofluorescence does not, however, allow any statements to be made on the functional significance of loss of motility or agglutination tendency of the spermatozoa. The interpretation of the results may also present difficulties. The technique of HJORT and HANSEN (1971) is regarded as the standard method.

Method

1. Sperms are washed twice and adjusted to 10×10^6 cells/ml in saline.
2. Single drops are each spread on slides and dried under a fan for 30 min.
3. Fix slides for 30 min in absolute methanol phosphate buffered saline and rinse with PBS.
4. Place one drop of serum over the fixed cells. Incubate at room temperature for 1 h in a moist chamber.
5. Wash slides for 20 min in two changes of PBS.
6. In a similar way, the slides are incubated for 30 min with fluorescein isothiocyanate conjugated antisera and after repeated washing are mounted with 10% glycerol in PBS.
7. The test is read by examining the slides under a fluorescent microscope with ultraviolet illumination.

Indirect immunofluorescence detects antibodies to intracellular antigens, while other serologic procedures are sensitive to membrane-bound antigens.

Methods for the detection of cellular antibodies have not so far found any place in clinical andrologic practice and should therefore at the present time be considered to be of a more experimental nature. This is true not only of skin testing but also of the macrophage-migration-inhibition test of George and Vaughan (1962).

The diagnostic power of the tests available for the detection of humoral antibodies has been considered in a survey by the WHO. The data collected by Boettcher et al. (1977) allow the following provisional conclusions:

1. The comparability of the various tests is good if good test semen is available.
2. Sera, in which immobilizing and cytotoxic antibodies are present, usually also contain agglutinins.
3. All sera containing cytotoxic antibodies also exhibit sperm-immobilizing antibodies, while sera with sperm-immobilizing antibodies do not always contain cytotoxins.
4. Agglutinating antibodies in men generally show a tail-to-tail agglutination, while in women the configuration is head to head.
5. The Kibrick test and Friberg test are more sensitive than the immobilization test and the cytotoxic test.
6. The results for immunofluorescence vary markedly between laboratories. The interpretation of these tests is difficult.

D. Generation of Antibodies

It is beyond doubt that the humoral and cellular antisperm antibodies found in men are induced by autosensitization. Although this fact is well-known, the causes of such antosensitization and the points of emergence of antigen from the genital tract are far from being understood. Since some products of the male reproductive tract are only produced at the end of a period known as the adoptive phase, it is probable that the problems of "immune tolerance" play an important part in autosensitization of the male against sperm antigens. This is true, for example, of spermatozoa and some fraction of seminal fluid, which only become detectable after completion of puberty. Segal et al. (1961) made an immunologic study of the maturation processes in rat testicles. He found that with increasing age an increasing number of antigenic fractions could be found in testicular tissue extracts. According to the work of Isojima and Tien Shun Li (1968), the antigenic properties of testicular tissue are dependent on the stage of maturation of the organ. Mature germ cells possess autoantigenic properties absent from the immature. Equally, the tissue level of acid phosphatase increases, according, to GUTMAN and GUTMAN (1941), from approximately 1.5 units in the 4th year to over 500 units in adults. The circumstances that allow autoimmunization to take place, and the site in the male genital tract where autoantigens are liberated, have not yet been completely elucidated. RÜMKE and HELLINGA (1959) have given the first clues for solving this problem. They found circulating sperm autoantibodies in long-standing vasectomy subjects, and this was subsequently confirmed by PHADKE and PADUKONE (1964).

CRUICKSHANK and STUART-SMITH (1959) recorded antisperm antibodies in two patients with orchitis. These observations lead to a plethora of investigations, and since then almost every organ of the male reproductive tract has been considered as a possible portal of entry.

I. Testes as Portal of Entry for Sperm Autoantigens

GORDON et al. (1965) demonstrated that testicular biopsy was followed by a, usually temporary, drop in the sperm count, and they considered this to be an immunologic phenomenon dependent on the transfer of antigens into the blood stream. In both the subacute and chronic phase of mumps orchitis, ANDRADA et al. (1967) found positive sperm agglutinins and sperm-immobilizing antibodies as well as positive skin tests with the typical picture of delayed hypersensitivity. In a guinea pig experiment, MANCINI et al. (1974) were able to demonstrate "autoallergic orchitis" on the contralateral side following unilateral thermal or traumatic damage to a testis. Skin testing for delayed hypersensitivity was also positive, while circulating antibodies could not be detected. Following unilateral controlled experimental testicular trauma, focal lesions appeared in the contralateral testis showing cell shrinkage and cell lysis accompanied by collections of round mononuclear cells. Attention has already been drawn elsewhere to the possible connection between these experimental findings and the clinical observation of at least temporary disturbance of testicular function following severe unilateral testicular trauma or following torsion with proven testicular necrosis.

II. Epididymis as Portal of Entry for Sperm Autoantigens

There can be no doubt that the epididymis plays a significant role in the absorption of autoantigenic material, as evidenced by the recurrent demonstration of sperm-agglutinating antibodies in the serum of patients with acute or chronic indurating epididymitis (BANDHAUER, 1966; HAENSCH, 1969). Ever since the studies of VON LANZ (1926), the epididymis, and particularly its tail, has been well-known as a storage organ for spermatozoa. The period of storage, or rather the transit time, of spermatozoa in the epididymis has been investigated in animal experiments and amounts, e.g., in the rat, to 12–16 days (RISLEY, 1963; MACMILLAN and HARISSON, 1955). This long stay of the spermatozoa in the epididymis appears to be essential to their maturation. Thus, BLANDAU and Rumery (1961) found in animal experimentation that spermatozoa from the head of the epididymis had a reduced fertilization capacity in comparison to those from the tail. Redenz (1924) took the view that the secretions of the epididymis exercised an especially important influence on the maturation of spermatozoa and that this involved the close association of a lipoprotein fraction with the spermatozoa (lipoprotein coating).

The processes by which components of spermatozoa and fractions of seminal fluid, which have not been ejaculated, are degraded and reabsorbed from the epididymis are the subject of a much greater degree of debate than are the other functions of this organ. From experiments on dogs and rats, it became apparent that raised intratubular pressure in the epididymis is a factor capable of initiating the release of spermatozoa without the necessity for infection as an additional agent (Mullaney, 1962). More recent reports have considerably broadened the extent of our knowledge on this subject: the electron-microscopic studies of Burgos (1959) revealed absorption of colloidal mercuric sulfide, thorotrast, hemoglobin, and ^{59}Fe-citrate from the rete testis and efferent ducts. In the rete testis, reabsorbtion takes place both via the intercellular spaces and through a system of channels in the epithelial cell cytoplasm. Macrophages lying beneath the basement membrane were responsible for the removal of the absorbed substances. In the bull, Amann and Almquist (1962) found the epididymis to have a reabsorbtive capacity for spermatozoa of approximately 57%. These authors look on the tail of the epididymis as the principal site of reabsorbtion. As a result of his electron-microscopic studies of human epididymis, Horstmann (1965) subsequently drew attention to the possibility of reabsorbtive processes in this organ. The surface morphology of columnar cells in the epididymal duct epithelium and the presence of vesicles in these cells were both in favor of such an assumption. The same author was also able to demonstrate secretion in the duct of the epididymis. Holstein (1965) has drawn attention to the relationship between testicular function and the function of the epididymal epithelium. He investigated epithelial changes in the efferent ducts and in the duct of the epididymis in rabbits and was able to show transition of the cells into a "resting state" following castration.

A certain light is thrown upon reabsorbtion ratios of pathologic magnitude by the observations of numerous other authors (Oberndorfer, 1931; Capers, 1962; Glassy and Mostofi, 1956; Friedman and Garske, 1949). Thus, complete spermatozoa were to be found in the lymphatics in cases of so-called granulomatous epididymis (Bandhauer, 1966). In cases of obstructive azoospermia, Phadke and Phadke (1961) were able to demonstrate mononuclear and multinuclear "spermiophages" in large numbers. Histologically demonstrable, nonspecific sperm granulomas have been attributed to invasion by spermatozoa. Zettergren (1958) therefore coined the expression "spermiostatic granulomatous epididymitis." In obstruction of the vas and in granulomatous epididymitides, the presence of spermatozoa has been demonstrated interstitially, in the lymphatics, and even in blood vessels by Glassy and Mostofi (1956) and by Rümke (1972). Bandhauer (1966) has been able to observe spermiophages and collections of spermatozoa outside the lumen of the epididymis in cases of chronic relapsing epididymitis.

III. Sperm Autoantigens Entering via the Seminal Vesicles and the Prostate

These glandular organs of the male reproductive tract are considered together as routes of entry for sperm autoantigens because of the utter lack of any experimental studies that might allow them to be considered separately. Furthermore, there is clinical evidence for a relationship between inflammatory conditions of the prostate and seminal vesicles on the one hand and circulating sperm autoantibodies on the other. The largest such clinical series has been studied by FJÄLBRANT and OBRANT (1968). They found that in 16 of 43 patients (37%) vesiculoprostatitis correlated with the presence of sperm agglutinins in the serum. Circulating sperm antibodies have also been detected in patients with prostatic abscess or acute vesiculoprostatitis as well as following transurethral prostatectomy (BANDHAUER, 1966). A possible common significance for the prostate and seminal vesicles in the formation of sperm autoantibodies is also suggested by the studies of SHULMAN et al. (1966), as a common autoantigen was detectable in both organs.

E. Vasectomy and Sperm Antibodies

Since the first investigations of possible routes of entry for sperm antigens and of the causes of autoimmunization, there has also been some discussion of the relationship between ligation or division of the vas and the presence of detectable circulating sperm antibodies. As early as 1959, RÜMKE and HELLINGA had reported cases of obstructive azoospermia with sperm autoantibodies, particularly circulating sperm agglutinins. At that time, they drew attention to the possibility that pathologic conditions in the epididymis might lead to the reabsorption of autoantigenic material. Other authors have also reported a relatively high incidence of sperm antibodies in men who had undergone vasectomy (PHADKE and PADUKONE, 1964; ANSBACHER et al. 1972; SHULMAN, 1972). Autosensitization is not however, inevitable following division or ligation of the vas. The extensive study by ANSBACHER et al. (1972) revealed that 15 of 27 men (55.5%) had sperm-agglutinating antibodies 1 year following vasectomy; 40.7% of the same group of patients had raised sperm-immobilizing antibodies. SHULMAN (1972) has reported similar figures for his series. In a study of 60 patients, VAN LIS et al. (1974) first detected sperm agglutination 6–9 months following surgery.

In contrast, FYÄLLBRANT (1968a, b) was unable to substantiate any increase in sperm antibodies following vasectomy. In the author's own studies (BANDHAUER and OBERMAYER, 1977) on 56 vasectomy patients, sperm-agglutinating antibodies were detectable at a titer greater than 1:32 in 9 patients, and there were sperm-immobilizing antibodies in 4 patients. There was, however, a significant correlation with the presence of inflammatory change at the distal ligature, where the features of sperm granuloma were impressive. With the regression of these inflammatory changes (on average after 3 months), the antibodies became undetectable.

The possibility of autoimmunization against antigenic fractions of endogenous semen following vasectomy is ever present. However, it would seem that abnormal processes of reabsorption, probably caused by infective processes in the region of the epididymis or of the ligature, are a necessary cofactor. Clinical effects of such autoimmunization following vasectomy have not yet been convincingly demonstrated.

I. Clinical Significance of Sperm Antibodies for Male Fertility

There is no definitive data on the clinical relevance of sperm antibodies to sub- or infertility in man. In a study of 2015 male partners in infertile unions, Rümke and Hellinga (1959) found sperm-agglutinating antibodies at a titer of greater than 1:32 to be present in approximately 3%. However, the demonstration of sperm agglutinins is not necessarily equatable to infertility. Rümke et al. (1973) were able to show that 30 of a group of 137 patients with positive sperm-agglutinating antibodies had fathered a child. My own series (Bandhauer, 1966) showed the presence of sperm-agglutinating antibodies in about 3.5% of infertile patients, and it should be noted that in the vast majority of cases there was good evidence either in the history or on clinical examination of inflammatory illness of the genital tract, particularly of the epididymis. However, these studies still do not allow an exact relationship between agglutinins and fertility disorders to be established. The extensive work of Fjällbrant (1968a, b), which resulted in the finding that approximately 7% of husbands in childless marriages carry sperm antibodies, has equally failed to clarify this question. Fjällbrant did, however, draw attention to the reduced ability of spermatozoa to penetrate mucus in the presence of sperm antibodies. Similar studies by Manarang-Pangan and Behrman (1971) and by Boettcher (1975) produced almost identical results. Kremer and Jager (1976) found the cause of this reduced penetration to be an alteration in the type of movement exhibited by spermatozoa (shaking phenomenon). These workers elaborated a laboratory test for spermatic mucus penetrating power (sperm cervical mucus contact test, SCMC test). From a series of such tests, Kremer et al. (1978) came to the conclusion that SCMC test positivity was always associated with the presence of sperm-agglutinating antibodies in the serum of either the husband or the wife. In a study employing the Kibrick test, the Isojima test, and the indirect immunofluorescent method of Hjort and Hansen (1971), Hendry et al. (1978) demonstrated positive agglutination and immobilization in 8.5% of sub- or infertile men. On the other hand, there was no correlation with the immunofluorescent studies.

In his animal experimentation, Tyler (1945a, b) was able to alter sperm-agglutinating antisera by photooxidization in such a way that sperm agglutination was eliminated, but the fertility of the spermatozoa remained nonetheless impaired. In a series of 591 men who had been immunologically investigated because of the infertility of their marriage, Hendry et al. (1977) found 50 patients (8.5%) with sperm antibody titers of greater than 1:32. Twenty-seven of these patients appear to have had a normal seminal analysis. However, in 21 of 22 cases, mucus penetration testing suggested the spermatozoa of these patients were not able to penetrate normal cervical mucus. Despite these observations, it is still not possible at this time to make any valid numerical statement about the clinical significance of sperm antibodies for infertility.

The same is true for female carriers of antibodies. NAKABAYASHI et al. (1961) were unable to establish an unequivocal connection between the infertility of women and the presence of sperm-agglutinating antibodies in their serum. By a globulin-coating technique, COHEN and GREGSON (1978) found a significant effect of antibodies in the female on spermatozoa, both in animal experiments and in man. With full regard for this and much other mainly experimental evidence, HANCOCK (1978) still came to the conclusion that the effects of female sperm antibodies on fertility are not yet definable.

F. Treatment of Immunologic Fertility Disorders in Men

As yet no form of treatment for immunologic disorders of male fertility has been shown to be effective. In localized inflammatory change of the genital tract that may be regarded as a site of abnormal reabsorption of sperm antigens (chronic relapsing unilateral epididymitis, infected epididymal cysts, sperm granulomata at the distal vasectomy site), surgical intervention may lead to a waning of the antibody titer (BANDHAUER, 1966).

Beside this therapeutic attack on the apparent cause, which has a limited clinical application, the following therapeutic possibilities have been the subject of discussion:

1. *Artificial insemination with the husband's semen:* BARWIN (1974) achieved 13 pregnancies by this method in 18 childless couples who had a poor "postcoital test." By using centrifuged semen (split ejaculate: AMELAR and HOTCHKISS, 1965), DAVID (1975) achieved a pregnancy rate of approximately 33%. USHERWOOD (1976, 1978) used "washed spermatozoa" for artificial insemination if circulating sperm antibodies were detectable at a titer of greater than 1:32. In 22 patients whose sperm agglutination titer was 1:32, 7 pregnancies were induced by this method. Two pregnancies were achieved among four patients with sperm autoagglutination. Similar or poorer results were achieved by SCHRAM (1976), DIXON et al. (1976), STEIMAN and TAYLOR (1977), and others. SHULMAN (1978) employed artificial insemination with semen that had been ejaculated directly into 20 ml of albumin solution – apparently in the hope of influencing the antigen-antibody reaction. No results have been made available to date.

2. *Immunosupressive therapy:* RÜMKE and HELLINGA (1959) attempted without success to reduce the antibody titer by prolonged treatment with cortisone. We have had similar experiences in our own clinical trial using 40 mg of prednisolone daily over 3–4 weeks (BANDHAUER, 1966). However, BASSILLI and EL-ALFI (1970) found that a regimen of prednisone 40 mg daily for

Fjällbrant B (1968a) Sperm agglutinins in sterile and fertile men. Acta Obstet Gynecol Scand 47:89

Fjällbrant B (1968b) Studies on sera from men with sperm antibodies. Acta Obstet Gynecol Scand 48:131

Fjällbrant B (1968c) Spermatobodies and sterility in men. Acta Obstet Gynecol Scand [Suppl 4] 47:

Fjällbrant B (1975) Autoimmune human sperm antibodies and age in males. J Reprod Fertil 43/1:145–148

Fjällbrant B, Obrant O (1968) Clinical and seminal findings in men with sperm antibodies. Acta Obstet Gynecol Scand 47:151

Flocks RH, Bandhauer K, Patel Ch, Begley BJ (1962) Studies on spermagglutinating antibodies in antihuman prostate sera. J Urol 87:475–478

Franklin RR, Dukes CD (1974) Antispermatozoal antibody and unexplained infertility. Am J Obstet Gynecol 89:6

Freund J, Lipton MM, Thompson GE (1953) Aspermatogenesis in guinea pig induced by testicular tissue and adjuvant. J Exp Med 97:711

Freund J, Lipton MM, Thompson GE (1954) Impairment of spermatogenesis in the rat after cutaneous injection of testicular suspension with complete adjuvants. Proc Soc Exp Biol Med 87:408–411

Freund J, Thompson GE, Lipton MM (1955) Aspermatogenesis, anaphylaxis and cutaneous sensitization induced in the guinea pig by homologous testicular extract. J Exp Med 101:591–604

Friberg J (1974) A simple and sensitive micro-method for demonstration of sperm-agglutinating activity in serum from infertile men and women. Acta Obstet Gynecol Scand [Suppl] 36:21

Friedman NB, Garske GL (1949) Inflammatory reactions involving sperm and the seminiferous tubules: extravasation spermatic granulomas and granulomatous orchitis. J Urol 62:363

Gabl F (1963) Protides of the biological fluids. Peeters H (ed) vol 10. Elsevier, Amsterdam London New York, p 230

George M, Vaughan JH (1962) "In vitro" cell migration as a model for delayed hypersensitivity. Proc Soc Exp Biol Med 111:514

Glassy EJ, Mostofi FK (1956) Spermatic granulomas of the epididymis. Am J Clin Pathol 26:1303

Goldberg E (1973) Infertility in female rabbits immunized with lactate dehydrogenase X. Science 181:458–459

Gordon DL, Barr AB, Herrigel JE, Paulsen CA (1965) J Ferti Steril 16:4, 522

Grant GH, Everall PH (1963) Protides of the biological fluids. Peeters H (ed) vol 10. Elsevier, Amsterdam London New York, p 237

Gutman AB, Gutman EB (1941) Quantitative relations of a prostatic component (acid phosphatase) of human seminal fluid. Endocrinology 28:115

Guyer MF (1922) Studies of cytolysins. III. Experiments with spermatotoxins. J Exp Zool 35:207–223

Hafez ESE (1975) Agglutination patterns and plasmalemma of human spermatozoa as viewed by scanning electron microscopy. Int J Fertil 20/4:209–219

Hancock RJT (1978) Sperm antigens and sperm immunogenicity. In: Cohen J, Hendry WF (eds) Spermatozoa antibodies and infertility. Blackwell, Oxford London Edinbourgh Melbourne, pp 1–9

Hansen KB, Hjort T (1971) Immunofluorescent studies on human spermatozoa. II. Characterization of spermatozoal antigens and their occurrence in spermatozoa from the male partners of infertile couples. Clin Exp Immunol 9:21

Hekman A, Rümke P (1969) The antigens of human seminal plasma. Fertil Steril 20:312

Hektoen, L, Manly LS (1923) Specific precipitin reaction of semen. J Infect Dis 32:167–171

Hendry WF, Morgan H, Stedronska J, Chamberlain GVP, Dewhurst J (1977) Cervical hostility and antisperm antibodies in the male. Lancet 2:357

Hendry WF, Morgan H, Stedronska J, Scammell G, Chamberlain GVP (1978) The clinical significance of antisperm antibodies in male subfertility: crossed hostility testing and prednisolone treatment. In: Cohen J, Hendry WF (eds) Spermatozoa antibodies and infertility. Blackwell, Oxford London Edinbourgh Melbourne, pp 129–137

Henle W (1938) The specificity of some mammalian spermatozoa. J Immunol 34:325–336

Haensch R (1969) Fluorescenzimmunologische Spermienautoantikörperbefunde bei männlichen Fertilitätsstörungen. Arch Gynaekol 208:91

Herrmann WP, Hermann G (1969) Immunoelectrophoretic and chromatographic demonstration of IgG, IgA and fragments of γ-globulin in the human seminal fluid. Int J Fertil 14:211

Hjort T, Hansen KB (1971) Immunofluorescent studies on human spermatozoa. I. The detection of different spermatozoal antibodies and their occurrence in normal and infertile woman. Clin Exp Immunol 8:9

Hjort T, Brogaard Hansen K (1971) Immunofluorescent studies on human spermatozoa. I. The detection of different spermatozoal antibodies and their occurrence in normal and infertile women. Clin Exp Immunol 8:9

Holstein AF (1965) Neue Ergebn d Androl. Schirren C (ed) Springer, Berlin Heidelberg New York

Horstmann E (1965) Neue Ergebn d Androl. Schirren C (ed) Springer, Berlin Heidelberg New York

Hunter AG (1969) Differentiation of rabbit sperm antigens from those of seminal plasma. J Reprod Fertil 20:143

Husted S, Hjort T (1975) Sperm antibodies in serum and seminal plasma. Int J Fertil 20:97

Isojima S (1973) Antibodies against spermatozoa found in women and corresponding antigens in human semen. Proc Ist Inter Cong on Immunology in Obstetrics and Gynecology. Centaro A, Carretti N, Addison GM (eds). Int Congr Series No 281. Excerpta Medica, Amsterdam

Isojima S, Li TS (1968) Stepwise appearance of sperm specific antigens in rats and their disappearance after fertilization. Fertil Steril 19:999

Isojima S, Li TS, Ashitaka Y (1968) Immunological analysis of sperm immobilizing factor found in sera of women with unexplained infertility. Am J Obstet Gynecol 101:677

Isojima S, Tsuchiya K, Koyama K, Tanaka C, Naka O, Adachi H (1972) Further studies on sperm-immobilizing antibody found in sera of unexplained cases of sterility in women. Am J Obstet Gynecol 112:199

Jenning PB, McCarthy MK, Plymate SR, Wetthaufer JN (1976) Prevalence of circulating H L-A lymphocytotoxic antibodies in men after vasectomy. Fertil Steril 26:53

Katsh S (1960) The anaphylactogenicity of testicular hyaluronidase and a species difference in testicular hyaluronidase demonstrated by isolated organ anaphylaxis. Int Arch Allergy 17:70–79

Katsh S, Katsh GF (1961) Antigenicity of spermatozoa. Fertil Steril 12:522

Katsh S, Katsh GF (1965) Perspectives in immunological control for reproduction; past, present and future. Pacific Med Surg 73:28

Katsh S, Aguirre AR, Leaver FW, Katsh GF (1972) Purification and partial characterization of aspermatogenic antigen. Fertil Steril 9:644

Kennedy WP (1924) The production of spermatoxins. Q J Exp Physiol 14:279–283

Kirkpatrick CH, Katsh S (1964) Aminoacid content of antispermatogenic antigen. Nature 201:197

Kolk AHJ, Samuel T (1975) Isolation, chemical and immunological characterization of two strongly basic nuclear proteins from human spermatozoa. Biochim Biophys Acta 393:307–319

Kolk AHJ, Samuel T, Rümke P (1974) Autoantigens of human spermatozoa. I. Solubilization of a new auto-antigen detected on swollen spermheads. J Clin Exp Immunol 16:63

Kolk AHJ, Kuyk L van, Boettcher B (1978) Isolation of human lactate dehydrogenase-X by affinity chromatography. Biochem J (in press)

Kremer J, Jager S (1976) The sperm-cervical mucus contact test. A preliminary report. Fertil Steril 27:335–340

Kremer J, Jager S, Kuiken J, Slochteren-Draaisma Tiny van (1978) Recent advances in diagnosis and treatment of infertility due to antisperm antibodies. In: Cohen J, Hendry WF (eds) Spermatozoa antibodies and infertility. Blackwell, Oxford London Edinbourgh Melbourne, pp 117–127

Krieg H (1970) Immunology of reproduction. In: Gibian H, Plotz EJ (eds) Mammalian reproduction. Springer, Berlin Heidelberg New York, pp 286–314

Landsteiner K (1899) Zur Kenntnis der spezifisch auf Blutkörperchen wirkenden Sera. Zentralbl Bakteriol 25:546–549

Landsteiner K, Levine P (1926) On group specific substances in human spermatozoa. J Immunol 12:415–418

Lanz T von (1926) Ueber Bau und Funktion der Nebenhoden und seine Abhängigkeit von der Keimdrüse. Z Anat Entwickl-Gesch 80:177–282

Le Boutelier P, Toulet F, Voisin GA (1973) Etude ultrastructurale des lésions specifiquement induites par l'auto-anticorps anti-auto-antigene T sur les spermatozoides épididymaires de cobaye. C R Acad Sci (Paris) 276:509

Lerum JE, Goldberg E (1974) Immunological impairment of pregnancy in mice by lactate dehydrogenase-X. Biol Reprod 11:108

Lis JMJ van, Wagenaar J, Soer JR (1974) Sperm-agglutinating activity in serum of vasectomized men. Androl 6:2, 129

Lustig L, Denduchis B, Gonzalez N, Mancini RE (1973) Chemical and immunologic study of rat seminiferous tubule wall structures. Acta Physiol Lat Am 23:101

Lustig L, Denduchis B, Gonzalez N, Mancini RE (1976) Immuno-histochemical study of rat seminiferous tubule wall structures. Int J Fertil

MacMillan EW, Harrison RG (1955) The rate of passage of radiopaque medium along the ductus epididymidis of the rat. Stud Fertil 7:35–40

Manarang-Pangan S, Behrman SJ (1971) Spermatotoxicity of immune sera in humaninfertility. Fertil Steril 22:145–151

Mancini RE (1974) Immunologic and testicular response to a damage induced in the contralateral gland. In: Mancini RE, Martini L (eds) Male fertility and sterility. Academic Press, New York

Mancini RE (1976) Immunologic aspects of testicular function, vol. 9. Springer, Berlin Heidelberg New York

Mancini RE, Martini L (eds) Male fertility and sterility, vol. 5 Academic Press, London New York San Francisco

Mancini RE, Fainboim I, Alonso A (1974) Effect of homologous antisperm serum intratesticularly injected in guinea pigs. J Allergy Clin Immunol 54:69

Mancini RE, Scacciati JM, Bueno MP (1976) Immunobiological properties of antisera against glycoproteins from human seminal plasma. Int J Fertil (in press)

Mancini RE, Monastirsky R, Fernández Collazo E, Seiguer AC, Alonso A (1969) Cytotoxic action of antispermatic antibodies upon homologous germinal cells "in vitro". Fertil Steril 20:779

Mancini RE, Alonso A, Saraceni A, Bachmann AE, Lavieri JC, Nemibrovsky M (1965) Immunological and testicular response in man sensitized with human testicular homogenate. J Clin Endocrinol 25:859

Mann T (1964) The biochemistry of semen and of the male reproductive tract. Methuen, London and Wiley, New York

Maruta H, Moyer DL (1967) Immunological studies of the antigens of guinea pig semen. Fertil Steril 18:649

Mazzolli A (1971) Demonstration "in vitro" of delayed hypersensitivity in experimental allergic orchitis in guinea pigs. J Reprod Fertil 26:161

Mazzolli A, Barrera C (1974) A method for detecting cytophilic activity in a homologous system. J Immunol Methods 4:41

Menge AC (1967) Induced infertility in cattle by iso-immunization. J Reprod Fertil 13:445

Menge AC, Protzman WP (1967) Origin of the antigens in rabbit semen which induce antifertility antibodies. J Reprod Fertil 13:31

Menge AC, Burkons DM, Friedlaender GE (1972) Occurrence of embryo mortality in rabbits iso-immunized against semen. Int J Fertil 17:93

Metalnikoff S (1900) Études sur la spermotoxine. Ann Inst Pasteur 14:577–589

Metchinikoff EL (1900) L'influence de l'organisme lex toxines. Sur la spermotoxine et l'antispermotoxine. Ann Inst Pasteur 14:1–12

Mettler L, Tinneberg H, Birke R, Semm K (1979) Fertilitätsreduktion durch zelluläre Immunreaktion gegen Spermatozoen-Antigene. Andrologia 11(2):143–152

Moxter von (1900) Ueber ein specifisches Immunserum gegen Spermatozoën. Dtsch Med Wochenschr 26:61–64

Mudd S, Mudd EBH (1929) The specificity of mammalian spermatozoa with especial reference to electrophoresis as a means of serological differentiation. J Immunol 17:39–52

Mullaney J (1962) Granulomatous lesions associated with spermatozoal invasion of the interstitial tissues of the epididymis. Br J Urol 34:351–353

Mumford DM (1979) Immunity and male infertility. Invest Urol 16:4, 255

Mumford DM, Gordon HL, Ansbacher R, Sung JS, Rosen RD, Farrow S (1975) Incidence of lymphocytotoxins in vasectomy patients – a preliminary report. In: Sciaria JS, Markland C, Seidel JJ (eds) Control of male fertility. Harper and Row, 1975, p 196

Nakabayashi NT, Tyler ET, Tyler A (1961) Immunologic aspects of human infertility. Fertil Steril 12:544–550

Nieschlag E, Klaus-Henning U, Schwedes U, Kley HK, Schöffling K, Krüskemper HL (1973) Alterations in testicular morphology and function in rabbits following active immunization with testosterone. Endocrinology 92:1142

Oberndorfer S (1931) Handb. d. spez. path. Anat. u. Histol. Henke F, Lubarsch O (Hrsg), Bd VI/3. Springer, Berlin

Orsini F, Shulman S (1971) The antigens and autoantigens of the seminal vesicle. I. Imunochemical studies on guinea pig vesicular fluid. J Exp Med 134:120

Ouchterlony O (1949) Antigen-antibody reactions in gels. Acta Pathol Microbiol Scand 26:507

Phadke AM, Phadke GM (1961) Occurrence of macrophage cells in the semen and in the epididymis in cases of male infertility. J Reprod Fertil 2:400

Phadke AM, Padukone K (1964) Presence and significance of autoantibodies against spermatozoa in the blood of men with obstructed vas deferens. J Reprod Fertil 7:163

Popivanov R, Sturkalev I, Evrev T, Nakov L, Zhivcov S, Kirov K, Russev L, Boulanov I (1969) Proper and acquired blood group antigens in human testis cells and spermatozoa. In: Bratanov K (ed) Immunology of spermatozoa and fertilization. Bulgarian Academic Science Press, Sofia

Rao SS, Sadri KK (1959) Immunological studies with human semen and cervical mucus. Proc Sixth Int Conf Planned Parenthood, New Dehli, 1959, pp 313–318

Rao SS, Sadri KK (1960) The antigenic composition of buffalo semen. J Comp Pathol Therap 70:1–9

Redenz E (1924) Versuch einer biologischen Morphologie des Nebenhodens. Arch Mikr Anat 103:593–628

Risley PL (1963) Physiology of the male accessory organs. In: Hartman CG (ed) Mechanisms concerned with conception, vol 88. Pergamon Press, Oxford London New York Paris, pp 73–134

Rose NR, Hjort T, Rümke P, Harper MJK, Vyazov O (1976) Techniques for detection of iso- and auto-antibodies to human spermatozoa. Clin Exp Immunol 23:175–199

Rümke Ph (1954) The presence of sperm antibodies in the serum of two patients with oligozoospermia. Vox Sang 4:135–140

Rümke Ph (1959b) Auto-antibodies against spermatozoa in sterile men. 1st Int Symp Immunopathology, Basel, 1958. Schwabe, Basel, pp 145–153

Rümke P (1972) Autoantibody formation against spermatozoa caused by extravasation of spermatozoa into the interstitium of the epididymis of aged men. Int J Fertil 17:86

Rümke P, (1974) Antigens of semen and auto-immunity against spermatozoa in infertile men. In: Male fertility and sterility. Mancini RE, Martini L (eds) Academic Press, New York

Rümke Ph, Hellinga G (1959) Autoantibodies against spermatozoa in sterile men. Am J Clin Path 32:357–363

Rümke P, Amstel M van, Messer EN, Bezemer PD (1973) Prognosis of men with auto-spermagglutinins in the serum and the unsuccessful treatment with testosterone. Proc IInd Inter Symp on Immunology of Reproduction. Bratanov K, Edwards RG, Vulchanov VH, Dikov V, Somlev B (eds). Bulgarian Academy of Sciences Press 1973 p 339

Sadri KK, Shethye TA, Rao SS (1967) Immunological and biological studies with antiserum to mouse testis extract. Indian J Exp Biol 5:122

Schoysman R (1970) Treatment of male infertility due to auto-agglutinating antibodies. Proc VI. World Congr on Fertility and Sterility, Tel Aviv. Academic Press, New York, pp 112

Schram JD (1976) Retrograde ejaculation: a new approach to therapy. Fertil Steril 27:1216–1218

Scott JS, Jones WR (eds) (1977) Immunology of Human Reproduction. Academic Press, London, p 476

Searcy RL, Craig RG, Bergquist LM (1964) Immunochemical properties of normal and pathological seminal plasma. Fertil Steril 15:1

Segal S, Tyler ET, Rao S, Rümke Ph, Nakabayashi N (1961) Immunologic factors in infertility. In: Tyler ET (ed) Sterility. McGraw-Hill, New York, pp 386–399

Shulman S (1971) Immunity and infertility. A review. Contraception 4:135–154

Shulman S (1972) Immunologic barriers to fertility. Obstet Gynecol Surv 27:553

Shulman S (1974a) Sterilization, antibodies, and autoimmunity. In: Advances in voluntary sterilization. Proceedings of the Second International Conference, Geneva, 1973. Schima M, Lubell I, Davis JE, Connell E (eds) Excerpta Medica, Amsterdam, pp 86–95

Shulman S (1974b) Sperm antibodies as a cause of problems in infertility and in vasectomy. In: Immunology in obstetrics and gynaecology. Proceedings of the First International Congress, Padua, 1973. Centaro A, Caretti N (eds) Excerpta Medica, Amsterdam, pp 41–51

Shulman S (1978) Future prospects. In: Cohen J, Hendry WF (eds) Spermatozoa antibodies and infertility. Blackwell, Oxford London Edinburgh Melbourne, 88, pp 147–159

Shulman S, Ahmen S, Yantorno C, Soanes WA, Gonder MJ, Witebsky E (1966) Studies on organ specificity. XVI. Urogenital tissues and autoantibodies. Immunology 10:99

Shulman S, Bronson P (1969) Immunochemical studies on human seminal plasma. II. The major antigens and their fractionation. J Reprod Fertil 18:481

Shulman S, Orsini F (1970) The antigens of seminal vesicles and seminal plasma. Fertil Steril 21:794

Shulman S, Ahmed U (1971) Prostate antigens and antibodies. Proc Soc Exp Biol 137:97

Shulman S, Hekman A (1971) Antibodies to spermatozoa. I. A new macroscopic agglutination technique for their detection. Clin Exp Immunol 9:137

Shulman S, Hekman A, Pann C (1971) Antibodies to spermatozoa. II. Spermagglutination techniques for guinea pigs and human cells. J Reprod Fertil 27:31

Shulman S, Freidman MR (1975) Antibodies to spermatozoa v. Antibody activity in human cervical mucus. Am J Obstet Gynecol 122/1:101–105

Shulman S, Harlin B, Davis P, Reyniak JV (1978) Immune infertility and new approaches to treatment. Fertil Steril 29:309

Solish GI (1969) Distribution of ABO isohemagglutinins among fertile and infertile women. J Reprod Fertil 18:459

Spielman H, Eibs HG, Mentzel C, Nagel D (1977) Studies on the binding of antibody against mouse lactate dehydrogenase (Isoenzym X) by preimplantation of mouse embryos. J Reprod Fertil 50:47

Steiman RP, Taylor ML (1977) Artificial insemination homologous and its role in the management of infertility. Fertil Steril 28:146–150

Stevens KM, Fost CA, (1964) Sperm and antibody formation in rabbits following immunisation with sperm and semen. Proc Soc Exp Biol 117:125

Stevens VC (1975) Fertility control through active immunization using placenta proteins. Acta Endocrinol [Suppl I94] (Kbh) 78:357–375

Sung JS, Shizuya H, Black DD, Mumford DMA (1977) Radiomicroassay or cytotoxic antibody to human spermatozoa. Clin Exp Immunol 27:469

Toullet F, Voisin GA, Nemirovsky M (1973) Immunohistochemical localisation of the Guinea pig spermatozoal autoantigens. Immunology 24:635

Tung KSK (1977) The nature of antigens and pathogenetic mechanisms in autoimmunity to sperm. In: Edidin, Johnson (eds) Immunobiology of gametes. University Press, Cambridge, pp 157–185

Tung KSK, Alexander NJ (1977) Autoimmune reactions in the testis. In: Johnson AD, Gomes WR (eds) The testis, Advances in physiology, biochemistry, and function IV. Academic Press, New York, p 637

Tung KSK, Unanue ER, Dixon FJ (1970) The immunopathology of experimental allergic orchitis. Am J Pathol 60:313

Tyler A (1945a) Conversion of agglutinins and precipitins into "univalent" (non-agglutinating or non-precipitating) antibodies by photodynamic irradiation of rabbit antisera vs. pneumococci, sheep-red-cells and sea urchin sperm. J Immunol 51:157–172

Tyler A (1945b) Anaphylactic properties of photo-oxidized rabbit-antisera (vs. sheep-erythrocytes and pneumococci) and horse-antiserum (vs. diphtherial toxin) containing "univalent" antibodies. J Immunol 51:329–337

Usherwood M Mcd (1978) Sperm washing and artificial insemination. In: Cohen J, Hendry WF (eds) Spermatozoa antibodies and infertility. Blackwell, Oxford London Edinbourgh Melbourne

Usherwood M McD, Halim A, Evans PR (1976) Artificial insemination (A.I.H.) for sperm antibodies and oligozoospermia. Br J Urol 48:499–503

Voisin G, Delaunay A, Barber M (1951) Sur les lésions testiculaires provoquées chez le cobaye par iso- et autosensibilisation. Ann Inst Pasteur 81:48–63

Voisin G, Delaunay A (1955) Sur les lésions testiculaires observées chez des animaux soumis à des injections de substances adjuvantes, seules ou mélangées avec des extraits de tissus homologues. Ann Inst Pasteur 89:307–317

Voisin GA, Toullet F (1968) Etude sur l'orchite aspermatogenetique auto-immune et les autoantigénes des spermatozoides chez le cobaye. Ann Inst Pasteur (Paris) 114:727

Voytisková M, Pokorná Z (1971) Cellular antigens of mouse spermatozoa as possible markers of gene action. In: Proc Intern Symp on Genetics of the Spermatozoa. Beatty RA, Gluecksohn-Waelsch S (eds). Bogtrykkeriet Forum, Copenhagen, p 160

Vulchanov VH (1969) Testicular damage and autoantibody formation in guinea pigs immunized with homologous seminal vesicular fluid. In: Edwards RG (ed) Immunology and reproduction. International Planned Parenthood Federation, London, p 136

Weil AJ (1960) Immunological differentiation of epididymal and seminal spermatozoa of the rabbit. Science 131:1040–1041

Weil AJ (1961) Antigens of the adenexal glands of the male genital tract. Fertil Steril 12:538–543

Weil AJ, Wilson L, Finkler AE (1959) Immunological test for semen on female genitalia as evidence of intercourse. J Forensic Sci 4:372–377

Weil AJ, Rodenburg JM (1960) Immunological differentiation of human testicular (spermatocele) and seminal spermatozoa. Proc Soc Exp Biol Med 105:43–45

Wellerson R, Wagstaff P, Asculai F, Hudson Marie, Kupferberg AB (1974) Induction of a spermatogenesis in guinea pigs through immunization with lactate dehydrogenase-X-isozyme. Internat J Fertil 19:65

Wilson L (1954) Sperm agglutinins in human semen, blood. Proc Soc Ep Biol Med 85:652–655

Zettergren L (1958) Epididymitis spermiostatica granulomatosa. Acta Chir Scand 114:150

Treatment of Male Infertility

M. Glezerman and B. Lunenfeld

A. Hormonal Treatment of Male Infertility

Hormonal evaluation of the infertile male includes measurement of protein hormones and steroid hormones. In addition, dynamic tests have been designed that permit one to assess the function of various compartments along the hypothalamus-pituitary-testis axis (Lunenfeld et al., 1973; Glezerman and Lunenfeld, 1975). Based on the patient's history, thorough physical examination, and intelligent evaluation of seminal samples, the hormonal profile of the patient may indicate possible management of his infertility problem.

Basically, hormonal treatment is substitutional insofar as it is aimed at mimicking the function of specific compartments of the hypothalamus-gonad axis. We shall thus follow this axis and present the hormonal therapy, beginning with the hypothalamic-releasing hormone, followed by gonadotropins and androgens. Since the endocrine axis is controlled by feedback exerted upon hypothalamus and pituitary, drugs that act on the feedback mechanism system, such as antiestrogens, will be described. Finally, various hormonal compounds that have been used in cases of male infertility will be mentioned.

I. Gonadotropin-Releasing Hormone (GnRH)

Pulsatile therapy with GnRH should logically be the treatment of choice in hypothalamic failure. To date, however, contradictory results regarding treatment with GnRH have been reported (Zarate et al., 1973; Hann, 1975; Aparacio et al. 1976). No standardized treatment schemes have yet been established. Furthermore, the commercially available synthetic GnRH possesses a very short biologic half-life (4–9 min), and pulsatile daily applications are required. Attention was also shifted toward the development of more potent analogs (Saito et al., 1977) with longer biologic half-life. Schally et al. (1976) have summarized the state of the art regarding newly developed analogs of GnRH. Until sufficient clinical studies are available, one must continue to rely on gonadotropin therapy in cases of hypothalamic failure.

II. Human Gonadotropins

1. Human Chorionic Gonadotropin (HCG)

Treatment with HCG is based on the realization that this hormone, like the luteinizing hormone (LH), is able to induce the development of Leydig cells from precursor cells and to stimulate synthesis and release of testosterone from these cells. Consequently, local concentration of testosterone increases and levels of testosterone 50- to 100-fold higher than in the peripheral circulation are achieved. These are necessary for the spermatogenic function of the testes (Steinberger, 1977). Therapy with HCG is indicated in cases in whom endogene androgenization is desirable. Whether or not HCG exerts a direct effect on spermatogenesis is not certain. It has been postulated (Burgos and Vitale-Carpe, 1969) that LH and HCG may play a role in the release of spermatozoa from the cytoplasmic invaginations of Sertoli cells. The long biologic half-life of intramuscularly administred HCG (11–30 h) permits injection intervals of 5 days to secure effective blood levels. A rare side-effect is transient nipple tenderness; gynecomastia has been reported.

In cryptorchid children, HCG has been employed with considerable success. Usually, the hormone is injected IM twice weekly for 5 weeks in dosages between 250 and 1500 IU, according to the patient's age (Morger, 1968; Weissbach and Ibach, 1975). HCG is regarded to be the treatment of choice in patients suffering from the "fertile eunuch syndrome." This is an entity that is characterized by eunuchoid features associated with normal or inferior sized testes and presence of normal spermatogenesis despite absence or scarcity of Leydig cells (Pasqualini and Burr, 1955; Makler et al., 1977). Reduced spermatozoan concentration as well as asthenospermia and teratospermia have been treated with HCG although hormonal evaluation does not permit the identification of a distinct group of patients in whom this mode of treatment could be based on a scientific rationale. However, when causal therapy is not available, HCG treatment may be considered; the results obtained seem to be promising. Misurale et al. (1969) noted significant improvement of motility when administrating 2500 IU HCG every 5 days for approximately 3 months. The pregnancy rate achieved in the wives of his patients was 35%. Chehval (1978) treated 75 normogonadotropic infertile males with HCG and observed an increase in the spermatozoan concentration or motility in 70%. The pregnancy rate was 45%. Glezerman et al. (1980) treated 18 patients with idiopathic oligo-, astheno-, teratospermia with HCG and noted significant amelioration of seminal parameters in 10. Five patients reported pregnancies. We administer HCG IM every 5 days (5000 IU) for at least 90 days.

2. Human Menopausal Gonadotropin (HMG/HCG Therapy)

Induction of spermatogenesis requires follicle-stimulating hormone (FSH) and LH (Lunenfeld and Weisselberg, 1972). Commercially available preparations contain both hormones. However, the LH content is usually not sufficient for adequate stimulation of Leydig cells and HCG has to be administered in addition. In eunuchoid patients, i.e., in patients with very low gonadotropin activity, maturation of Leydig cells has to be induced prior to HMG/HCG therapy by a treatment course with HCG for at least 4 weeks (SMITH et al., 1974). Therapy with HCG is then continued in addition to HMG therapy and may be monitored by sporadic testosterone estimations. Injections of 5000 IU HCG every 5 days will usually suffice to maintain a testosterone level of at least 5 ng/ml. HMG/HCG therapy is a typical substitutional therapy, and duration of treatment courses is thus conditioned by the length of the spermatogenic cycle. HELLER and CLERMONT (1964) have demonstrated the spermatogenic cycle to be 74 ± 6 days. Thus, like other treatment schemes designed to induce or enhance spermatogenesis, gonadotropin therapy should be continued for at least 90 days and results evaluated only after this period. Generally, we administer 75 IU FSH and 75 IU LH during the first treatment course in daily IM injections. As stated before, patients continue concomitantly with HCG medication. Spermatogenic activity is assessed by monthly seminal analyses, the last of which is performed some days before termination of medication. If treatment was not successful in terms of increasing sperm concentration, the HMG dosage is augmented up to 300 IU FSH and 300 IU LH daily (four ampuls), and care is taken that medication is not interrupted. If satisfactory seminal results are achieved or pregnancy has ensued in the female partner, therapy is continued with HCG alone.

In one hypogonadotropic-hypogonad-eunuchoid patient we induced complete spermatogenesis following these treatment principles and then continued treatment with HCG. Within 2 years during which sexual life was satisfactory and repeated seminal analyses showed normospermia the patient fathered two children.

Neither the dosage nor interval of HMG injections mentioned should be considered rigid terms of reference. SHERINS et al. (1977) were able to induce complete spermatogenesis in hypophysectomized males with 10–30% of the conventional HMG dosis. LYTTON and KASE (1966) AND SCHWARZSTEIN (1974) reported satisfactory results of HMG therapy with thrice weekly injections.

GLEZERMAN et al. (1978) have summarized treatment results obtained with HMG/HCG therapy. As expected, hypophysectomized patients are ideally suited for gonadotropin therapy, since in these cases hypogonadism is directly related to pituitary failure. In 20 of 20 males complete spermatogenesis could be restored.

Hypogonadotropic hypogonadism either of hypothalamic or pituitary origin is also a definite indication for HMG/HCG therapy. In 27 of 33 such patients complete spermatogenesis could be induced. In non-eunuchoid azoospermic men (excluding Sertoli-cell-only syndrome), gonadotropin therapy is less effective, but still 60 of 123 patients exhibited complete spermatogenesis following HMG/HCG therapy. In oligospermic patients the value of this treatment seems rather doubtful. Of 275 patients with severe oligospermia (less than 10 million sperm cells per milliliter), 74 exhibited sperm counts of more than 30 million per milliliter following therapy and only 20 (7.3%) reported pregnancies.

We preselect patients for gonadotropin therapy by hormonal evaluation including GnRH tests. In patients in whom base levels of gonadotropins are low and GnRH application results in an increase plasma of FSH below twice the base level, the maximal plasma value (in our laboratory) not exceeding

3 mIU/ml, success rates may be anticipated as high as 80% (Lunenfeld et al. 1979).

III. Prolactin Inhibitors

Prolactin is secreted by the pituitary gland of primates (Friesen et al., 1972). Following the identification (Lewis et al., 1971) and the purification of this hormone (Hwang et al., 1972), radioimmunologic methods have been developed to measure plasma levels of prolactin (Sinha et al., 1973). Increased prolactin levels have been shown to appear following application of certain compounds (phenothiazines, reserpine, methyldopa, thyroid-stimulating hormone) and may be an early sign of pituitary tumors. The secretion of prolactin is controlled by hypothalamic prolactin-inhibiting factor (PIF). Thus, hypothalamic insufficiency as expressed in inadequate GnRH secretion may also result in reduced release of PIF and consequently in increased release of prolactin from the pituitary. Some investigators demonstrated correlations between prolactin levels and levels of plasma gonadotropins (Krause, 1978) while others did not (Segal et al., 1976). Correlations between prolactin levels and sperm concentration were equally equivocal (Segal et al., 1976; Fonzo et al., 1977). In most cases, elevated prolactin levels have been associated with impotency, although testosterone levels do not seem to be influenced by the elevation of prolactin (Fonzo et al., 1977). Promising results with drugs inhibiting the secretion of prolactin in anovulatory women have prompted investigators to employ prolactin inhibition in male infertility (Thorner and Besser, 1978). Bromoergocryptine (B) has been used as a potent prolactin inhibitor (1–7.5 mg/day p.o.). Saidi et al. (1977) treated eight oligospermic males with sperm concentrations between 1 and 8.4 million cells per milliliter with 2.5 mg B per day for 7 weeks. In all patients sperm concentration increased five to tenfold with three reported pregnancies. Montanari and Volpe (1978) presented the case report of a normoprolactinemic male suffering from primary sterility of 7 years' duration. Although initial levels of plasma gonadotropins and steroids were in the normal range, administration of 5 mg B per day for 10 weeks was associated with an increase in sperm concentration from 15 million/ml to 85 million/ml and sperm motility increased from 30% to 80%. Consequently, his female partner became pregnant.

Physiologic and pathophysiologic functions of prolactin in the reproductive process of the male are still only poorly understood. Increased prolactin levels require meticulous screening for pituitary tumors, including tomography of the sella turcica and examination of visual fields. Negative results in a patient suffering from either impotency or disturbed spermatogenetic function indicate treatment with prolactin-inhibiting compounds. Although only few clinical trials are available to date, this method of management is certainly promising.

IV. Androgens

Androgens and their metabolites (estrogen, dihydrotestosterone) promote and maintain the development of secondary sex characteristics, exert metabolic and psychic effects, stimulate the development and function of accessory sexual glands, inhibit hypothalamic GnRH secretion, and are crucial for spermatogenesis. These manifold actions of testicular steroids have prevailed upon many investigators to employ androgens for treatment of patients with spermatogenic failure, steroidogenic failure of the testes, for suppression of GnRH, and consequently as a contraceptive agent in males.

1. Androgen Replacement Therapy

In patients with primary testicular failure involving both the spermatogenic and the steroidogenic function of the testes (anorchism, certain cases of Klinefelter's syndrome, patients with hypogonadotropic hypogonadism in whom procreation can be neglected, etc.), androgen replacement therapy is the most effective means to ensure the development and maintenance of secondary sexual characteristics. Orally administered testosterone is rapidly metabolized by the liver and may be associated with cholestatic jaundice (GARDNER and PRINGLE, 1961). Treatment with 17α substituted testosterone, developed to increase the serum half-life of orally administered testosterone has been associated with development of hepatocellular carcinoma (JOHNSON et al., 1972). Thus, if oral testosterone therapy is indicated, preference should be given to compounds that are either not metabolized by the liver due to the fact that they do not convert to estrogen (like mesterolone) or to testosterone undecanoate in arachis oil, which is absorbed by lymph vessels and thus bypasses the hepatic portal system (NIESCHLAG et al., 1975). Still, orally administered testosterone requires multiple daily applications. Long-term androgen substitution therapy seems to be much easier if long-acting depot preparations are employed. Firstly, multiple daily ingestion of tablets will keep the patient continuously conscious of his dependence of hormonal substitution. Since androgen replacement is a long-term therapy, this may present a heavy strain on the patient's psychic state. Secondly, if long-acting compounds are administered, e.g., monthly injections of testosterone enanthate or proprionate, patients will be more motivated to return periodically to the physician's office, and the mandatory prostatic control is more easily secured. Thirdly, absolute amounts of testosterone are smaller if the parenteral route is selected. We usually initiate treatment with bimonthly injections of 250 mg testosterone proprionate until desired results are achieved. The interval between injections is then broadened according to the patient's subjective perception of its effect. Usually, long-acting therapy requires one injection every 4–6 weeks, the interval being titrated by the patients themselves. The patient is invited for check-ups three times a year.

FRICK and BARTSCH (1976) have suggested implanting polydimethylsiloxane capsules filled with dry crystalline testosterone subcutaneously in the submammillary region. Therapeutic doses of the hormone are released for 13 months. These authors have used this method in over 300 patients and have been impressed by the results obtained. We agree with the authors that constancy of hormonal supply, relative low amounts of required hormone, and rarity of side-effects promise to make implantation of testosterone-containing capsules an ideal solution for long-term substitution problems.

2. Androgens as Contraceptive Agents

A combination of androgens with progestins seems to be superior to employment of androgen alone (Frick, 1973). However, high doses of exogenous testosterone will arrest spermatogenesis in most cases. Since it is not predictable whether or not spermatogenic function of the testes will return to pretreatment levels and since rather high testosterone levels are required for prolonged periods and complete suppression of spermatogenesis is not always achieved, single-agent contraception using testosterone does not seem to be a very reliable tool. Discussion of various aspects of medical contraception in the male is beyond the scope of this presentation.

3. Androgens as Spermatogenetic Agents

The observation that testosterone maintains spermatogenesis in the hypophysectomized rat (Walsh et al., 1934) has prevailed upon many investigators to employ testosterone for use in male infertility. However, it has been shown that testosterone is not effective for maintaining spermatogenesis in man and fails to induce spermatogenesis in hypogonadotropic men (Paulsen et al., 1970). Steinberger et al. (1974) have pointed out that intratesticular levels of testosterone required to induce spermatogenesis in man are approximately 50–100 times higher than the concentration of this steroid in the peripheral circulation. The very high doses required to produce adequate peripheral levels of testosterone will result in the suppression of spermatogenesis secondary to inhibition of GnRH and consequently of pituitary gonadotropins. Furthermore, these high doses may produce systemic side-effects as described above. The principle that testosterone administered in high doses suppresses sperm concentration with subsequent increase of sperm count to higher levels than those present before treatment was described for the first time by Heller (1950) and has been employed as a therapeutic mode in oligozoospermic patients. This treatment scheme has been named "rebound therapy" and has been employed by different authors. Schill (1979) summarized clinical results that support the testosterone rebound therapy. Others (Joel, 1960; Schirren, 1961; Amelar, 1977; Walsh and Amelar, 1977) do not recommend rebound therapy due to the occurrence of permanently reduced sperm counts in patients treated with this method. We found this treatment rather disappointing because it functioned much better in normospermic males than in those who require treatment.

We feel that testosterone should not be used to treat male infertility. Patients in whom androgenization is required to stimulate function of accessory glands, to enhance motility of sperm cells, or to increase sperm count seem to benefit more from endogenous androgenization as achieved by HCG therapy. If the oral route is preferred, we administer an androgen that cannot be metabolized to estrogen and thus does not exert negative feedback on the hypothalamic or pituitary level (in therapeutic doses). Such an androgen is mesterolone. This is an orally effective androgen derivative with a methyl group at carbon 1. The drug exhibits little if any hepatotoxicity (Giarola, 1974). While some authors (Schellen, 1970; Mauss, 1974; Schirren, 1977) have reported that treatment with mesterolone is effective in idiopathic oligo- and/or asthenospermia, others (SOMAZZI et al., 1973) have failed to observe significant effects. GLEZERMAN et al. (1979) observed significant amelioration of seminal parameters in 40% of 56 patients. The pregnancy rate in this group was 32.1%.

V. Antiestrogens

1. Clomiphene Citrate

Clomiphene citrate, a derivative of chlortrianisene, is structurally related to the synthetic estrogen diethylstilbestrol. The commercially available preparations are usually 1:1 mixtures of *cis-* and *trans*-clomiphene. Clomiphene citrate is an antiestrogen insofar as it competes with estrogen receptors at the hypothalamic level and thus neutralizes the negative feedback exerted upon the hypothalamus. Consequently, GnRH is secreted and pituitary gonadotropins are released. Clomiphene citrate would thus be indicated in cases of feedback failures and in cases in which endogenous gonadotropin secretion is desirable. Unfortunately, treatment results with clomiphene citrate have not been very encouraging. This may be due to the fact that in certain unpredictable cases clomiphene citrate directly exerts a damaging effect upon the seminiferous tubules. HELLER et al. (1969) reported tubular shrinkage and hyalinization following this therapy. In hypogonadotropic hypogonadism no positive results with clomiphene citrate have ever been reported despite increases in gonadotropin levels.

As empiric treatment and in default of causal therapy, clomiphene citrate may be used. However, the daily doses should not exceed 50 mg since higher doses have been shown to suppress spermatogenesis (HELLER et al., 1969).

2. Tamoxifen

Tamoxifen is chemically related to clomiphene citrate. Like clomiphene citrate, tamoxifen competes with estrogen for hypothalamic receptors and similarly neutralizes the negative feedback exerted by estrogen. The hypothalamus consequently releases more GnRH, and the pituitary gland secretes more gonadotropins. Direct effects of this drug on the gonads seem to be negligible (COMHAIRE, 1976). Few clinical studies concerning tamoxifen are available to date: COMHAIRE (1976) treated 15 oligospermic males and 5 normal volunteers with this drug, administering 20 mg per day (p.o.) for periods of 3 or more months. In all cases plasma levels of testosterone increased by some 200%. In 13 of 15 men sperm concentration increased significantly, while motility and morphology did not change. Three patients reported pregnancies. On the other hand, WILLIS et al. (1977) could not observe any significant increase in sperm concentration in nine patients treated with tamoxifen (10 mg daily p.o.) for 6 months. Further studies are required to establish the usefulness of tamoxifen in the treatment of male infertility.

VI. Various Hormonal Compounds

To review the various reports on treatment of male infertility with thyroid hormones, corticosteroids etc. would be of historical rather that practical value.

feine inhibits cyclic nucleotide phosphodiesterase, thus preventing the degradation of cyclic nucleotides that in turn may stimulate sperm metabolism.

Schill et al. (1974) observed enhancement of sperm motility after adding kallikrein to semen samples of most asthenospermic males studied. (Parenteral treatment with kallikrein for 7 weeks increased motility of sperm cells by over 100% in 21 of 57 patients studied [Schill, 1975b].) Haesungsharern and Chulavtnatal (1973) reported that caffeine, theophylline, and aminophylline stimulated the motility of human spermatozoa in vitro, the percentage of motile sperm cells increased severalfold, and the mean motility rate was accelerated twofold; Johnsen et al. (1974) confirmed these findings. Doughtery et al. (1976), however, could not confirm these reports and questioned the quality of enhanced motility produced by in vitro treatment.

Asthenospermia is a major cause for male infertility. It seems justified to employ any method of treatment to overcome this problem. In vitro vitalization by means of substances such as kallikrein or caffeine is certainly one way of management worth a trial if confronted with asthenospermia resistant to systemic treatment.

IV. Antibiotic Treatment

Acute or chronic infections of secondary sex glands may result in morphologic changes of sperm cells, may impair prostatic and seminal vesicle function, or may even lead to occlusion of the excretory and ejaculative ducts (Arya et al., 1973). In these cases antibiotic therapy may be beneficial. It has been demonstrated that doxycycline (Oosterlink et al., 1976) and trimethoprim-sulfamethoxazole (Gnarpe and Friberg, 1976) achieve high concentrations in the fluids of the seminal vesicle and the prostate gland. These drugs are thus of value in the treatment of fertility problems due to infections of secondary sex glands. If indicated we administer twice daily 100 mg doxycycline for 1 week followed by a treatment course of four tablets trimethoprim-sulfamethoxazole (80/400 mg) daily for 3 weeks.

V. Various Compounds

Vitamin E has been employed in the treatment of male infertility (Bartak, V., 1974) following the realization of its physiologic role in lower species. Treatment results have been disappointing. Arginine has been used sporadically. Treatment results are controversial (Giarola, 1971; Jungling and Bunge, 1976; Keller and Polakoski, 1975).

There is almost no pharmaceutical group that has not been tried in the treatment of male infertility. It is beyond the framework of this presentation to review the various studies that were conducted to justify or to reject various compounds as therapeutic agents. Until a major breakthrough occurs in the treatment of the infertile male, more studies will appear evaluating different drugs that will be accepted by some investigators and rejected by others.

References

Amelar RD (1977) Medical management of male infertility. In: Cockett ATK, Urry RL (eds) Male infertility. Grune & Stratton, New York San Francisco London, p 239

Amelar RD, Dubin L (1977) Special problems in management. In: Amelar RD, Dubin L, Walsh PC (eds) Male Infertility. Saunders, Philadelphia London Toronto, p 191

Aparacio NJ, Schwarzstein L, Turner EA, Turner D, Mancini R, Schally AV (1976) Treatment of idiopathic normogonadotrophic oligoasthenospermia with synthetic luteinizing hormone releasing hormone. Fertil Steril 27:549

Arya OP (1973) Bull WHO 49:587

Bartak V (1974) Behandlungsverfahren bei männlicher Infertilität. Z. Hautkr. 49:889

Bunge RG, Sherman JK (1954) Liquefication of human semen by alpha-amylase. Fertil Steril 5:353

Burgos MH, Vitale-Carpe R (1969) Gonadotropic control of spermiation. In: Gual C (ed) Progress in endocrinology. Excerpta Medica Amsterdam, p 1030

Chehval MJ (1978) Chorionic gonadotrophins in the treatment of the subfertile male. Fertil Steril 29:233

Comhaire F (1976) Treatment of oligospermia with Tamoxiphen. Int J Fertil 21:232

Dmowski WP, Gaynor L, Lawrence M, Rao R, Scommegny A (1979) Artificial insemination homologuous with oligospermic semen separated on albumin columns. Fertil Steril 31:58

Doughtery KA, Cockett ATK, Urry RL (1976) Caffeine, Theophylline and human sperm motility. Fertil Steril 27:541

Fonzo D, Sivieri R, Gallone G, Andriolo S, Angeli A, Ceresa F (1977) Effect of a prolactin inhibitor on libido, sexual potency and sex hormones in men with mild hyperprolactinemia, oligospermia and/or impotence. Acta Endocrinol [Suppl] (Kbh) 85:142

Frick J (1973) Control of spermatogenesis in men by combined administration of progestin and androgen. Contraception 8:105

Frick J, Bartsch G (1976) Reversible inhibition of spermatogenesis by various steroidal compounds. In: Hafez ESE (ed) Human semen and fertility regulation in man. Mosby, St Louis, p 533

Friesen H, Belanger C, Guyda H, Hwang P (1972) The synthesis and secretion of placental lactogen and pituitary prolactin. In: Wolstenholme GEW, Knight J (eds) Lactogenic hormones. Churchill Livingstone, Edinburgh London, p 82

Gardner FH, Pringle JC (1961) Androgens and erythropoiesis. I. Preliminary clinical observations. Arch Int Med 107:846

Giarola A (1971) Klinisch-experimentelle Aspekte der Therapie der sekretorischen Sterilität des Mannes. Andrologie 3:35

Giarola A (1974) Effect of mesterolone on the spermatogenesis of infertile patients. In: Mancini RE, Martini L (eds) Male infertility and sterility. Academic Press, New York, p 479

Glezerman M, Lunenfeld B (1975) Erfolgschancen und Grenzen einer Hormontherapie bei männlichen Fertilitätsstörungen. Akt Derm 1:95

Glezerman M, Lunenfeld B, Insler V (1978) Male infertility. In: Lunenfeld B, Insler V (eds) Diagnosis and treatment of functional infertility. Grosse, Berlin, p 114

Glezerman M, Brook I, Potashnik G, Ben-Aderet N, Insler V (1980) Fertility pattern and reported pregnancies in 333 patients referred to male infertility clinics. Proceedings of V° ESCO, Venice. Salvadori B, Semm K, Vadora E (eds) Edizioni Internazionali, Rome p 495

Gnarpe H, Friberg J (1976) The penetration of trimethoprim into seminal fluid and serum. Scand J Infect Dis [Suppl] 8:50

Haesungsharern A, Chulavatnatal M (1973) Stimulation of human spermatozoal motility by caffeine. Fertil Steril 24:662

Hann J (1975) Gonadotropin releasing hormone therapy in males with hypogonadotropic hypogonadism and in boys with maldescended testes. Acta Endocrinol [Suppl 199] (Kbh) 80:266

Hehn S (1975) Einfluß von Rhodanid auf die Motilität menschlicher Spermatozoen nach verschiedenen Einwirkungszeiten und in verschiedener Konzentration. Andrologia 7:255

Heller CG, Clermont Y (1964) Kinetics of the germinal epithelium in man. Rec Prog Horm Res 20:545

Heller CG, Rowley MJ, Heller GV (1969) Clomiphene citrate: A correlation of its effects on sperm concentration and morphology. Total gonadotrophins, ICSH, estrogen and testosterone excretion and testicular cytology in normal men. J Clin Endocrinol Metab 29:638

Heller CG, Nelson WO, Hill IB, Henderson E, Maddock WO, Jungck EC, Paulsen CA, Mortimore CE (eds) (1950) Improvement in spermatogenesis following depression of the human testes with testosterone. Fertil Steril 1:415

Hwang P, Guyda H, Friesen HG (1972) Purification of human prolactin. J Biol Chem 247:1955

Insler V, Bernstein D, Glezerman M (1977) Diagnosis and classification of the cervical factor of infertility. In: Insler V, Bettendorf G (eds) The uterine cervix in reproduction. Thieme, Stuttgart, p 253

Israel S (1969) C-17 ketosteroid excretion in extreme endurance effort. Endokrinologie 54:277

Joel ChA (1960) The spermiogenetic rebound phenomenon and its clinical significance. Fertil Steril 11:384

Johnsen O, Eliasson R, Abdel Kader MM (1974) Effects of caffeine on the motility and metabolism of human spermatozoa. Andrologia 6:53

Johnson FL, Feagler JR, Lerner KG (1972) Association of androgenic-anabolic steroid therapy with development of hepatocellular carcinoma. Lancet 2:1213

Jungling ML, Bunge RG (1976) The treatment of spermatogenetic arrest with Arginine. Fertil Steril 27:282

Keller DW, Polakoski KL (1975) L-Arginine stimulation of human sperm motility in vitro. Biol Reprod 13:154

Krause W (1978) Prolaktinspiegel im Serum bei Patienten mit Störungen der Spermatogenese. Hautarzt 29:77

Lewis UJ, Singh RNP, Sinha YN, Laan WP van der (1971) Electrophoretic evidence for human prolactin. J Clin Endocrinol 33:153

Lunenfeld B, Weisselberg R (1972) The use of gonadotrophins in the induction of spermatogenesis. In: Prunty FIG, Gordina-Hill H (eds) Modern trends in endocrinology. Butterworths, London, p 412

Lunenfeld B, Kohen F, Eshkol A, Beer R, Zuckermann Z, Birnboim N, Glezerman M (1973) Evaluation of male infertility by dynamic tests. In: James VHT, Serio M (eds) Endocrine function of the human testis. Academic Press, London, p 561

Lunenfeld B, Olchovsky D, Tadir Y, Glezerman M (1979) Treatment of male infertility with human gonadotrophins: Selection of cases, management and results. Andrologia 11:331

Lytton B, Kase N (1966) Effects of human menopausal gonadotropins on a eunuchoidal male. N Engl J Med 274:1061

Makler A, Glezerman M, Lunenfeld B (1977) The fertile eunuch syndrome – an isolated Leydig cell failure? Andrologia 9:163

Mauss J (1974) Ergebnisse der Behandlung von Fertilitätsstörungen des Mannes mit Mesterolone oder einem Placebo. Arzneim Forsch 24:1338

Misurale F, Cagnazzo G, Storace A (1969) Asthenospermia and its treatment with hCG. Fertil Steril 20:650

Montanari GD, Volpe A (1978) Bromocriptine treatment for oligospermia and asthenospermia with normal prolactin. Lancet I 8056:160

Morger R (1968) Behandlung des Hodenhochstandes. Therapiewoche 18:2202

Nieschlag E, Mauss J, Coert A, Kicovic P (1975) Plasma androgen levels in men after oral administration of testosterone or testosterone undecanoate. Acta Endocrinol (Kbh) 79:366

Oosterlinck W, Wallijn E, Wyndale JJ (1978) The concentration of doxyxycline in human prostate gland and its importance in the treatment of prostatitis. Int J Androl (Suppl) 1:162

Pasqualini RA, Burr G (1955) Hypoandrogenic syndrome with spermatogenesis. Fertil Steril 6:144

Paulsen CA, Espeland DH, Michals EL (1970) Effects of hCG, HMG, HLH and HGH administration on testicular function. In: Rosenberg E, Paulsen CA (eds) The human testis. Plenum Press, New York, p 547

Paulson JD, Polakoski KL (1978) The removal of extraneous material from the ejaculate. Int J Androl [Suppl 1] 1:163

Saidi KR, Wenn V, Sharif F, (1977) Bromocriptine for male infertility. Lancet 8005:250

Saito M, Kumasaki T, Yaoi Y, Nishi N, Arimura A, Coy DH, Schally AV (1977) Stimulation of LH and FSH by (D-Leu^6, Des-Gly^{10}-NH$_2$)-LHRH Ethylamide after subcutaeous, intravaginal and intrarectal administration to women. Fertil Steril 28:240

Schally AV (1976) Clinical application of synthetic hypothalamic releasing hormones. In: Ebling FJG, Henderson IW (eds) Biological and clinical aspects of reproduction. Excerpta Medica, Amsterdam Oxford p 238

Schellen TMC (1970) Results with mesterolone in the treatment of disturbances of spermatogenesis. Andrologia 2:1

Schill WB (1975a) Caffein and Kallikrein-induced stimulation of human sperm motility. A comparative study. Andrologia 7:229

Schill WB (1975b) Erste Ergebnisse einer parenteralen Behandlung von männlichen Fertilitätsstörungen mit Kallikrein: Oligozoospermie. Hautarzt 26:541

Schill WB (1979) Recent progress in pharmacological therapy of male subfertility – a review. Andrologia 11:77

Schill WB, Braun-Falco O, Haberland GL (1974) The possible role of kinins in sperm motility. Int J Fertil 19:163

Schirren C (1961) Fertilitätsstörungen des Mannes. Diagnostik, Biochemie des Spermaplasma. Hormontherapie. Enke, Stuttgart

Schirren C (1977) Einführung in die Andrologie. Wissenschaftliche Buchgesellschaft, Darmstadt

Schoenfeld C, Amelar RD, Dubin L (1975) Stimulation of ejaculated spermatozoa by caffeine. Fertil Steril 26:158

Schwarzstein L (1974) HMG in the treatment of oligospermic patients. In: Mancini RE, Martini L (eds) Fertility and sterility. Academic Press, London, p 567

Segal S, Polishuk W, Ben-David M (1976) Hyperprolactinemic male infertility. Fertil Steril 27:1425

Sherins RJ, Winters SJ, Wachslicht H (1977) Physiologic studies of the role of FSH in stimulation of spermatogenesis in the hypogonadotrophic male. Symposion on: Recent progress in andrology. L'Aquila, Italy, April 21–23, 1977 (Abstract)

Shulman S, Harlin B, Davis P, Reyniak JV (1978) Immune infertility and new approaches to treatment. Fertil Steril 29:309

Sillo-Seidl G (1963) Int J Fertil 8:517

Sinha YN, Selby FW, Lewis UJ, Laan PW van der (1973) A homologuous radioimmunoassay for human prolactin. J Clin Endocrinol Metab 36:509

Smith KD, Fischer M, Steinberger E (1974) Clinical and laboratory findings during gonadotropin therapy of post pubertal hypogonadotropic hypogonadism. Andrologia 6:147

Somazzi S, Goor W, Ott F (1973) The efficacy of various treatments in oligospermia. Dermatologia 147/1:37

Steinberger E (1976) Medical treatment of male infertility. Andrologia [Suppl 1] 8:77

Steinberger E (1977) Male reproductive physiology. In: Cockett ATK, Urry RL (eds) Male infertility. Grune & Stratton, New York San Francisco London, p 1

Steinberger E, Smith KD, Tcholakian RK, Chowdhury M, Steinberger A, Fischer M, Paulsen CA (1974) Steroidogenesis in human testes. In: Mancini RE, Martini L (eds) Male fertility and sterility. Academic Press, London, p 149

Thorner MO, Besser GM (1978) Bromocriptine treatment of hyperprolactinemic hypogonadism. Acta Endocrinol [Suppl] (Kbh) 88:131

Urry RL (1977) Stress and infertility. In: Cockett ATK, Urry RL (eds) Male infertility. Grune & Stratton, New York San Francisco London, p 145

Walsh EL, Cuyler WK, McCullagh DR (1934) Physiologic maintenance of male sex glands: Effect of androlin on hypophysectomized rats. Am J Physiol 107:508

Walsh PC, Amelar RD (1977) Medical management of male infertility. In: Amelar RD, Dubin L, Walsh PC (eds) Male infertility. Saunders, Philadelphia London Toronto, p 179

Weissbach L, Ibach B (1975) Neue Aspekte zur Bedeutung und Behandlung von Hodendescensusstörungen. Klin Pediatr 187:289

Willis KJ, London RD, Bevis MA, Butt WR, Lynch SS, Holder G (1977) Hormonal effects of tamoxiphen in oligospermic men. J Endocrinol 73:171

Zarate A, Valdes-Vallina F, Gonzales A, Perez-Ubierna C, Canales ES, Schally AV (1973) Therapeutic effect of synthetic LHRH in male infertility due to idopathic azoospermia and oligospermia. Fertil Steril 24:485

Operative Therapy of Male Infertility

J. Frick

With 11 Figures

A. Varicocele

In spite of a very extensive literature the etiology of the impaired spermiogenesis with varicocele still remains unexplained. In view of the anatomic changes, a causal relationship with a hemodynamic disturbance in the venous drainage system of the testis, especially of the left spermatic vein, seems to be a logical possibility. The retarded outflow from the affected spermatic vein and a reflux from the left renal vein into the left spermatic vein has been repeatedly demonstrated by phlebography.

MacLeod (1965) has alluded to the possibility of a toxic impairment of the germinal epithelium through a repeated invasion of the left spermatic vein by suprarenal hormones and their metabolites as a consequence of the reflux from the renal vein. However, neither anatomic studies nor the detection of suprarenal hormones in the spermatic vein have ever supported this hypothesis of testicular damage arising from the adrenal gland.

Although the mechanism by which a varicocele might result in infertility has not been properly clarified, there are a great many reports that have indicated the possibility of such an interrelationship (Tulloch, 1952; Charney, 1962; Hanley and Harrison, 1962; Brown et al., 1968; Amelar and Dubin, 1973). It has been reported that in a normal population a varicocele can be found in about 10% of men (Johnson et al., 1970). On the other hand, a varicocele can be found in 30% of men in whom fertility is impaired (Amelar and Dubin, 1973) (Table 1). The great majority of men with varicocele nevertheless show only little change in seminal plasma. However, in a certain percentage of men with varicocele, this syndrome is associated with reduced fertility and with abnormalities in the seminal plasma.

In 1965, MacLeod defined certain characteristics of sterile men with varicocele; specifically, amorphous sperm and forms of immature germinal cells are present. Furthermore, oligospermia may also be found.

Our own experience and the results obtained by other authors have shown that an improvement in the semen quality follows ligature of the spermatic vein in approximately 50%–80% of patients. The reasons for the absence of any improvement in approximately 20%–50% of patients after the varicocele operation, and especially for the slow recovery of fertility in the cases that do show an improvement in the semen quality, are still largely unknown.

Table 1. Diagnosis of varicocele in various authors' series of patients with impaired fertility

Author	No. of patients	Diagnosis of varicocele (%)
Dubin and Amelar, 1971	1294	39.0
Hendry et al., 1973	152	21.0
Stewart and Montie, 1973	130	36.9
Johnson, 1975	120	31.7
Greenberg et al., 1979	425	37.4

Table 2. Data reported by various authors on improvement in quality of semen and pregnancy rates following surgical correction of varicocele

Authors	Number of patients	Improvement of the semen quality (%)	Pregnancy rate (%)
Tulloch, 1952	30	66	30
Charney, 1962	36	64	39
Hanley and Harrison, 1962	60	70	30
Scott and Young, 1962	166	39	31
Dubin and Hotchkiss, 1969	88	68	26
Charney and Baum, 1968	104	61	24
Brown et al., 1968	185	55	43
Dubin and Amelar, 1970	111	81	48
Glezerman et al., 1976	51	42–53	26

According to Lunenfeld and Glezerman (1978), patients with varicocele are affected by a normogonadotropic dysspermatogenesis. The term normogonadotropic dysspermatogenesis indicates subnormal or defective functioning of the testis at normal gonadotrophin levels and normal testosterone levels with inconspicuous masculine habitus in cases where endocrine, metabolic, and immunologic disturbances have been eliminated. The hypofunctioning of the tubuli can manifest itself in the entire OTA syndrome (oligo- terato- and asthenozoospermia) or as any combination of these symptoms.

If a patient with impaired fertility has a varicocele, surgical treatment is definitely advisable. Ligature of the vena spermatica results in an improvement of the semen quality within a year in approximately 60% of cases (Table 2).

It should also be pointed out that a symptomatic varicocele, which usually becomes apparent quickly in mature males, should lead one to suspect a local outflow disturbance in the vena spermatica. On the left the vena spermatica leads at right angles into the renal vein, while on the right it passes diagonally under the kidney and directly into the inferior vena cava. A large kidney tumor can also cause a symptomatic varicocele on the right through compression or through a tumor thrombus in the renal vein on the left, or in the inferior vena cava; this type, however, in contrast to the idiopathic form, drains only slowly or not at all when the testis is raised and positioned horizontally.

Before a discussion of the individual surgical techniques, it should be mentioned that the obliteration of the varicose complexes in the region of the pampiniform plexus by the injection of sclerosing substances has not proved successful. Furthermore, the detrimental consequences of a perivascular infiltration, probably with concomitant testicular atrophy in a high percentage of cases, must be pointed out. For this reason methods of this kind must be strictly ruled out.

I. Methods of Treatment

Only the current methods for the operative treatment of varicocele will be described in this Chapter. Several techniques that are still occasionally mentioned in the literature are of only historical interest. This category includes direct excision of the pampiniform plexus in the scrotal region; many have had unfortunate experiences with this method and have therefore given it up. The so-called suspension methods have also been largely given up and thus also belong in this category. In any case one would be well advised not to use suspension methods involving a pedicle flap from the testicle coat in this procedure (Tossadas, Borona), since there is the possibility that when the testis is no longer incased in the spermatic fascia (tunica vaginalis), it will be exposed to other influences that can cause dyszoospermia.

Three of the surgical procedures now most frequently used for curative treatment of varicocele are described below.

1. The Ivanissevich Technique

The skin incision is made parallel to the inguinal ligament and the external aponeurosis is then incised fiber by fiber and the spermatic cord examined; this is observed up to the point under the transverse muscle. In this region the individual branches of the spermatic vein will be examined, which at this level usually consist of two to three fairly thick venous funicles. These venous funicles are held in clamps, transected and doubly ligated (Figs. 1 and 2). Care must be taken that the spermatic artery and the vas deferens are not damaged. The wound is closed in layers. To be sure of avoiding injury of the vas deferens, ligature of the venous branches should be carried out as high up as possible, i.e., after the branching off of the spermatic cord from the funiculus on the posterior inguinal ring.

2. Palomo Technique

After a suprainguinal incision in the same direction as the fissure of the skin, the external aponeurosis is opened fiber by fiber above the inner inguinal ring at the approximate level of the anterior superior iliac spine, and the internal and transversal musculature pressed apart with a blunt instrument as for a lateral paraperitoneal gridiron incision. The spermatic vessels that constantly cling to the peritoneal cylinder displaced towards the center at this point are retroperitoneally laid bare. At this level the spermatic vein usually consists of one very thick or of two relatively thick venous cords, which can be severed

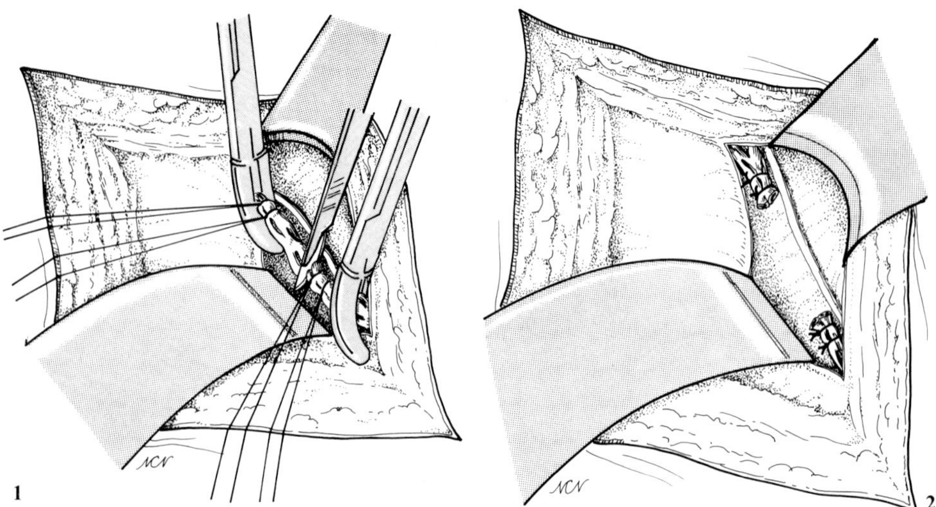

Fig. 1. Schematic drawing of the exposed left spermatic vein. The vena spermatica has already been ligated and 2–3 cm of the vessel is to be resected

Fig. 2. After ligation and resection of 2–3 cm of the left spermatic vein. No drainage of the retroperitoneum is used. The wound will be closed in layers

from the distinctly pulsating artery. It is important always to resect a piece 3 cm long between catgut ligatures in each case; in our opinion the state of the artery must be monitored constantly, since otherwise the danger of testicular atrophy is relatively high. In Palomo's original method high ligature of the spermatic artery is carried out simultaneously. Whether this method can be used in all cases without detrimental consequences is really doubtful, however. The danger injuring the vas deferens is practically nonexistent at this level. The wound is closed in layers, and we feel that if the region of the wound is really dry no wound drainage is necessary.

3. High Ligature of the Vena Spermatica

High ligature of the spermatic vein is the method that is now used most frequently. With the patient in a dorsal position a left-sided gridiron incision is made in the mesogastrium after blunt separation of the individual muscle layers; the peritoneal cylinder is displaced medially and the spermatic vein sought in approximately the middle third of the ureter. Usually at this level the vein is a vessel the thickness of a pencil or there are two relatively thick veins. These are then put in clamps and severed; 3–4 cm is resected from the spermatic vein or veins and the veins ligated bilaminarly. If the operation area is dry drainage of the retroperitoneum is not necessary. The would is then sutured in layers. The spermatic vein or veins must always be very carefully separated from the artery and the artery must not be ligated (with it or them) as it was in Palomo's original method. Furthermore, care must always be taken not to injure the ureter at this level.

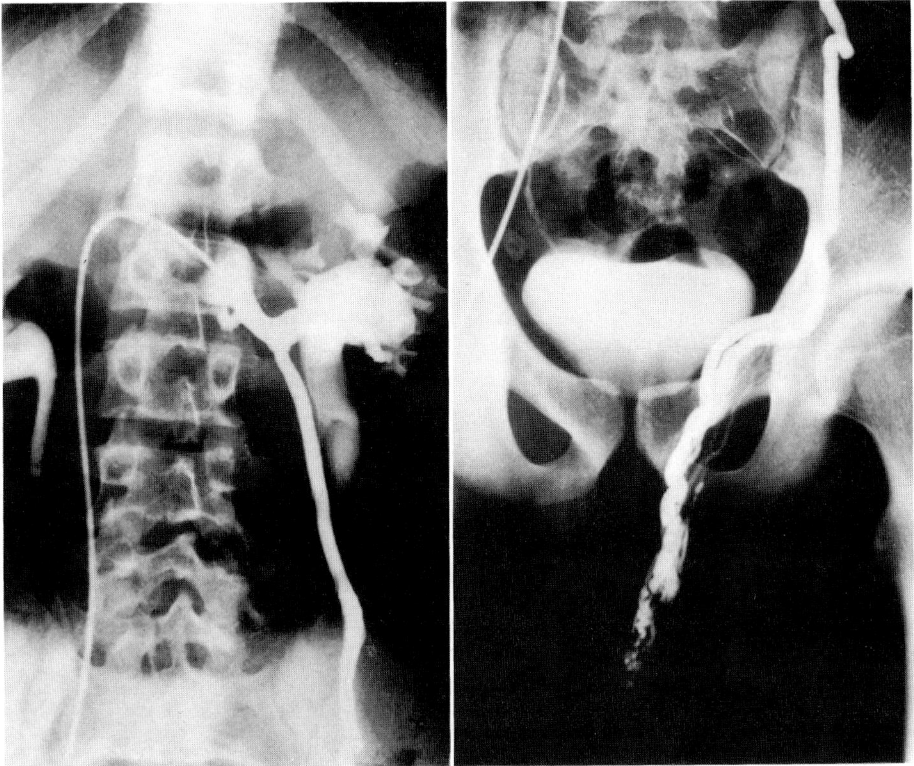

Fig. 3. Retrograde filling of the left spermatic vein in a 19-year-old man with varicocele: this X-ray shows a very thick left vena spermatica and dilatation of the left collecting system and the left ureter down to the point where the left spermatic vein and the ureter cross

Fig. 4. X-ray of the lower portion of the left spermatic vein, revealing a large varicocele

This has now become the method of choice since various other techniques for ligation of the pampiniform plexus in the inguinoscrotal region have resulted in more postoperative complications, such as hematomas, thromboses, and atrophy of the testes.

II. Complications

It should also be mentioned here that after surgery a certain percentage of varicocele patients always relapse and come back. In most of these cases it is found that not all of the branches of the spermatic vein complex have been ligated, especially if a high ligation of the spermatic vein was carried out. At this juncture, before further surgical steps are taken it is essential in all such cases to carry out selective retrograde angiography of the left vena spermatica through the left renal vein (Figs. 3 and 4).

Table 3. Incidence of hydrocele formation after surgical correction of varicocele

Author	Number of patients	Hydrocele	%
SCOTT and YOUNG, 1962	22	13	5.9
CHARNEY, 1962	36	1	2.8
DUBIN and AMELAR, 1975	504	17	3.4
WALLIYN and DESMET, 1979	114	9	7.0

A further complication that can arise, especially after PALOMO's technique or modifications of PALOMO's technique (i.e., when the spermatic vein and artery have been ligated and severed), is the formation of a hydrocele (Table 3).

B. Vas–Epididymis Anastomosis

I. Indications

The indication for vas–epididymis anastomosis is occlusion of the efferent spermatic ducts in the region of the epididymal canal. The occlusion is almost always in the region of the epididymal tail. If there is complete obstruction of the epididymal canal this change causes an azoospermia.

It is repeatedly and erroneously assumed that the finding of sperm in the ejaculated seminal fluid can be taken as an indication that the entire genital tract is functioning normally. This concept, however, can often be misleading, since very fine lesions in the region of the epididymis can cause decisive changes in the quality of the semen, even when there is no complete obstruction of the epididymis.

II. Etiology

1. Congenital Anomalies

Many congenital anomalies have been described as causes of such occlusions. The most frequent, however, are abnormal position of the epididymal head and extremely extensive atrophy of the middle section and tail of the epididymis, complete obliteration of the epididymal canal, loop formations of the vas deferens, and complete absence of the vas deferens. These malformations may have an historical developmental basis since the epididymal head is of testicular origin, whereas the distal part of the epididymis and of the vas deferens develop from the bud of the mesonephric duct. The most frequent type of malformation is that where the testes are normal in size, consistency, and morphology and the epididymal head is also normally formed, while the middle part of the epididymis and the epididymal tail are extremely immature, hypoplastic, or completely absent. It is also relatively common for these malformations to be associated with other disturbances in the urogenital tract.

2. Infections

Up to about the middle of the 1950s, gonorrhea was one of the main causes of obstruction of the epididymal duct. In the meantime, however, this has changed. Gonorrhea is now responsible for less than 20% of cases of epididymal occlusion. In gonorrheal infections it is mainly the distal part of the epididymis that is is affected, whereas the epididymal head remains intact. When an epididymal lesion is present the vas deferens can also be affected, either at one point or along the entire length, which makes an operative intervention very difficult or impossible. Naturally, inflammatory changes of the vas deferens with an epididymal inflammation and their sequelae can alsobe caused by commonplace urinary tract infections and inflammatory changes in the region of the posterior urethra.

Tuberculosis of the genital tract can be associated with complete destruction of the epididymis, including the epididymal head. In this situation a surgical stop-gap operation is impossible.

3. Cystic Changes

There can also be cystic changes in the epididymis. If these cystic changes occur outside the head of the epididymis surgical intervention is possible. In the distal genital tract malformations, obstructions, and atrophy can occur in the region of the accessory glands of the male genital system as congenital phenomena or as a result of inflammation. These conditions are generally not amenable to surgical therapy.

4. Trauma

After an earlier injury it is quite common to find extended cicatrical funicles instead of an epididymis. In the case of such lesions the testis is usually also injured. If such a disturbance occurs it is impossible to undertake any curative treatment.

III. Diagnosis

In the case of a patient with complete obstruction in the region of the epididymis, the testes are of normal size and consistency. The head of the epididymis is very often sightly enlarged, sometimes somewhat firm, but never painful. The vas deferens can be readily felt on both sides. If a hard nodule is felt in the region of the nearby epididymis this is certainly not normal, but it is not sufficient to justify the conclusion that obstruction of the epididymis is present. These patients also show a perfectly normal endocrinologic picture. Sperm analysis reveals azoospermia with normal levels of fructose, acid phosphatase, and citric acid in the seminal plasma, but an absence of carnitine (Table 4). When these clinical findings and laboratory results have been recorded a testicular biopsy is advisable; in a large percentage of the cases this reveals a normal histologic picture, i.e., spermiogenesis is fully maintained.

Table 4. Results obtained with use of marker substances in the seminal fluid as indicators of the localization of anatomic disturbances in the genital tract. Lunenfeld and Glezermann, 1978

Localization of the anatomic disturbance	Carnitine	Fructose	Acid phosphatase
Prostate	+	+	−
Seminal vesicle	+	−	+
Epididymis	−	+	+

IV. Surgical Technique

The operative procedures currently followed most frequently are the following:

1. *The vas is transected* and an end-to-side anastomosis is carried out between the vas deferens and the head of the epididymis.
2. *The vas and the epididymis are opened* and the vas, which usually forms a kink, is lowered into the epididymal head, which is then closed over the sunken structures (Hanley, 1955).
3. *A side-to-side anastomosis* is carried out between the vas deferens and the epididymal head; a latero-lateral (side-to-side) anastomosis is carried out without changing the relative positions of the anatomic structures (Bayle, 1950, 1953, 1958).

It should be mentioned that the best results of surgery recently have been achieved when magnifying spectacles giving up to a tenfold magnification or an operating microscope with up to 40-fold magnification have been used, if necessary. The patient lies on his back during the operation, which is carried out under a general anesthetic. The external genitalia are carefully washed and the exposure of the surgical field should be such that access to the scrotum and to the lower part of the inguinal canal is unobstructed. The operating theater should have X-ray facilities in case a radiograph seems necessary, but an anastomosis that promises to be successful can be carried out without an X-ray.

Since with purely scrotal incisions wound disturbances are frequent, we prefer an incision in the region of the scrotal root towards the groin, which also allows free access to the more distant distal part of the vas deferens. After the incision, the testis is mobilized and exteriorized, the testicular coats are incised and turned back, and the epididymis is carefully examined. The mobilization of the vas deferens and the exposure of the epididymis should be done as carefully as possible, so as not to disturb the blood supply. In addition, care should be taken that the vas is on no account completely stripped of surrounding fascia. Only the region of the vas deferens that will be used for the anastomosis (some 12–15 mm) is exposed. Similarly the epididymal area is examined at exactly the intended site of the anastomosis. During exposure of the vas deferens and the epididymis the surgical field should be constantly moistened by the assistants with a fluid mixture of 5% glucose, 5000 units heparin, and 200 mg hydrocortisone. The vas deferens is next incised on the side facing the epididymis for a length of approximately 12 mm with a sharp-pointed knife until the lumen is reached. To make sure that the incision extends to the opening of the lumen the vas is carefully explored in both proximal and distal directions with a very fine probe. During the incision the vas deferens should be held between the fingers and should not be irritated with a forceps.

To check whether the vas deferens is really open in the distal direction up to the posterior urethra, a contrast medium can be used to make a subsequent roentgen picture of the vas deferens possible; this is not absolutely necessary, however, since the patency can be checked by the injection of sodium chloride solution. If an X-ray of the vas deferens is required, a completely water-soluble contrast medium that does not cause irritation of the mucosa and is quickly absorbed should be used.

Should a second obstruction be detected in the vas deferens, this occlusion should be located by the insertion of a nylon thread. If it is located relatively far distally in the vas deferens it will definitely be impossible to carry out a satisfactory anastomosis between the vas deferens and the epididymis.

The incision in the epididymis should be made as far distally as possible for two reasons:

1. If the first operation is unsuccessful, another anastomosis can be performed further proximally.
2. The sperm in a more deeply located anastomosis have a better chance to mature because of their longer stay in the epididymis. The more proximally located anastomosis is certainly easier technically, but possibly has the one disadvantage that in this area the sperm present are not completely mature, whereas if it is possible to locate the anstomosis further distally between the vas deferens and the epididymis any sperm found after the opening of the epididymis may be of a better quality.

When the location of the epididymal incision has been definitely decided, the epididymis is held between the thumb and the index finger and an incision approximately 12 mm long is made. A very sharp, pointed scalpel should be used. Immediately after the incision is made a blood-tinged yellowish mixture usually gushes out. Several specimens should be removed at once and placed on a sterilized glass slide. These should be examined immediately under a microscope to determine whether any sperm at all are present, the quality of any sperm found, and whether or not they are mobile. If very mobile sperm are found in the epididymal specimens, there will of course be a better chance of restoring fertility. However, if the sperm found in the specimens are sluggish or more or less immobile, an anastomosis between the vas deferens and the epididymis should still be attempted.

After this swab has been taken, the incision of the epididymis should by sprayed several times with a salt solution to allow an assessment of the quality of the opened epididymal tubules. In a healthy epididymis with no obstruction the tubules normally appear to be relatively wide. If there is slight bleeding on the edges of the incision these small vessels should not be coagulated. It is better to wait a while, and carefully press the vessels together for a short time with wet swabs until the bleeding stops more or less spontaneously.

The anastomosis we have carried out almost exclusively is a side-to-side anastomosis between the vas deferens and the epididymis. First of all the corner

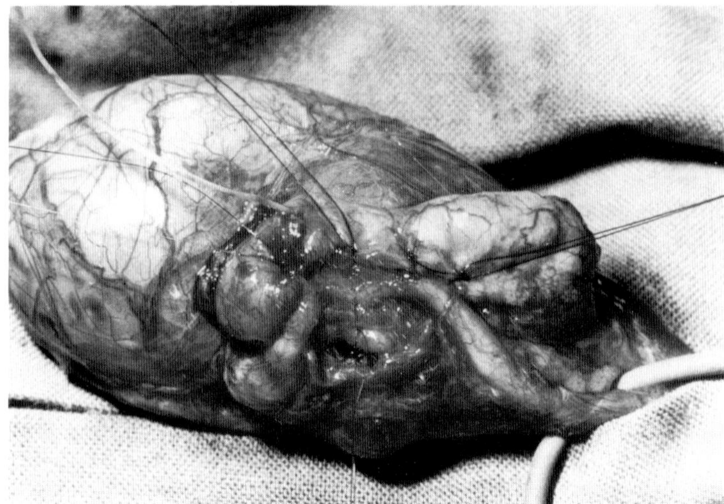

Fig. 5. Final situation with Frick method of vas–epididymis anastomosis: side-to-side anastomosis, 2-0 Pehafil thread as a splint, individual sutures with 6-0 atraumatic Mersilen

stitches are made. The suture thread we use is 6- to 9-ply 0 Mersilen. If a 9-0 suture thread is used, the anastomosis is possible virtually only with the aid of magnifying spectacles or under surgical microscope. We have always used a 2-0 Pehafil thread as a splint (Fig. 5). This splint is pushed forward distally approximately 10 cm into the vas deferens and brought out through the epididymal head. Furthermore, after retropositioning of the testis following the anastomosis, the splint is drawn out through the scrotum, from where it may be removed within 6–8 days.

Individual stitches are used for the anastomosis; the stitches are made at intervals of approximately 2 mm and all the layers of the vas deferens, namely, the adventitia, the muscularis, and the mucosa, are sutured separately. It should also be mentioned that the stitches should be made with as little trauma to the tissues as possible. After completion of the anastomosis, the testis is carefully repositioned in the scrotum, and if a splint has been applied its proximal end is brought out through the scrotal incision so that the splint can be removed 6–8 days after the operation. The wound should then be closed with 2-0 catgut.

V. Postoperative Care

Our patients are hospitalized for a week. Each patient must rest as much as possible and is not allowed out of bed. After leaving hospital he should continue to rest as much as possible for another 5–7 days. During the first postoperative week an antibiotic therapy with ampicillin and tetracycline is given. Most patients feel only minimal pan. The danger of infection is also minimal.

The first postoperative semen analysis is carried out 2 months after the operation. If after this period there is still no satisfactory ejaculation, this does

Table 5. Patency of anastomoses and numbers of pregnancies reported by various authors following vas– epdidymis anastomosis.

Author	No. of operations	No. of patiencies	No. of pregnancies
Bayle, 1969	178	130	89
Dell'Adami and Sidoti 1969			
Cognat, 1970	56	–	5
Johnson, 1975	5	1	∅
Pomerol, 1976	43	18	4
Schoysman, 1976	72	38	10

not necessarily indicate that the operation has been a failure, since in many cases positive ejaculation findings have not been recorded until 6–8 months after the operation. We are, however, of the opinion that azoospermia 1 year after the operation means that the procedure must be considered unsuccessful. Hormone therapy has never been successful in these cases.

It should be pointed out in concluding this Section that one should decide on one of the afore-mentioned methods and then employ this method as precisely as possible, with the aid of all microsurgical equipment necessary. It would certainly be a mistake to change methods frequently on the basis of bad experience.

Table 5 summarizes the results obtained with vas-epidiymal anastomoses by different authors.

C. Artificial Spermatocele

Congenital malformations of the epididymis and the vas deferens can naturally attain considerable degrees of severity. In the case of an extremely extensive or total aplasia of the vas deferens, surgical correction of the malformation is extremely difficult. In such cases various authors have attempted to construct an artificial spermatocele.

In 1955, Hanley became the first to attempt the construction of such a reservoir; it was made of amniotic tissue and a pregnancy was achieved.

In 1968, Schoysman attempted the creation of a sperm reservoir through a venous transplant, and he subsequently applied this technique in 52 patients. After a few functional initial successes, the most frequent sequel was nonetheless obliteration of the artificial spermatocele. Schoysman himself and other authors ceased to use this method several years ago.

Other methods have also given little promise of success. In six patients with duct aplasia the tunica vaginalis was superimposed on the opened-up epididymis. In other patients a small indwelling catheter was inserted in the sac thus created for the production of sperm. These two procedures, both with and without cortisone injections, have also yielded no satisfactory results (Schoysman, 1974). Moreover, in eight patients an alloplastic spiral was inserted

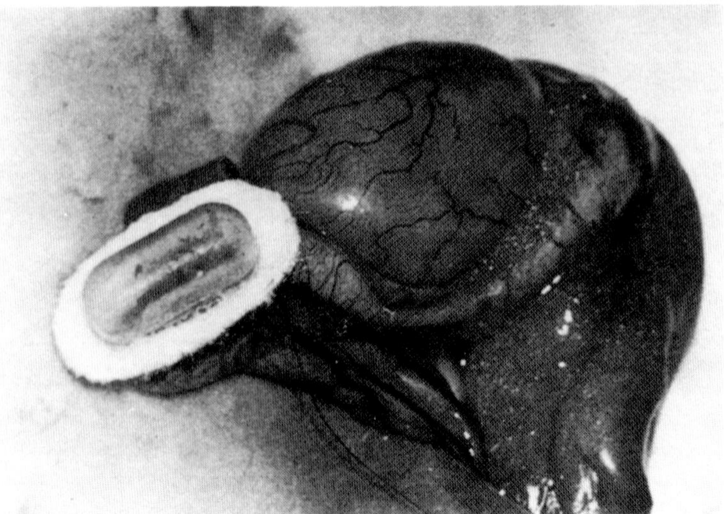

Fig. 6. The alloplastic prosthesis on the tail of the epididymis. (WAGENKNECHT et al. 1975)

in the spermatocele created by the superimposition of the tunica albuginea. The result was obliteration of the spermatocele in five cases, while in one patient 15% mobile sperm could be extracted in fluid sampled by puncture (SCHOYSMAN, 1974). In 1975, WAGENKNECHT et al. reported on animal experimentation directed at the development of an artificial spermatocele. It was shown that in rats a sperm reservoir made of an alloplastic material (silicone rubber) could be implanted on the epididymal head or tail. The morphology and motility of sperm tapped from these prostheses at different times after the operation declined with time elapsing between surgery and extraction increased with increasingly distal attachment of the prosthesis on the epididymis. With respect to the application of the alloplastic spermatocele (Fig. 6) in men there are still too few uniform results available to allow a conclusive opinion as to the absolute value of this method of operation.

D. Vas–Vas Anastomosis

Since vasectomy at present is the surest method of the male fertility control and since severance of the vasa has already been carried out on many million men around the world as a method of fertility control, the question of reanastomosis is now put to us with increasing frequency. The number of patients who desire restoration of their fertility after an earlier vasectomy grows larger from year to year. The indications for a vas–vas anastomosis are remarriage, death of children, change of mind, and correction of psychological ill effects.

I. Problems

There are two problems that must be discussed before reanastomosis of the vasa deferentia is undertaken, namely reversibility and the occurrence of sperm-immobilizing and sperm-agglutinating antibodies after vasectomy.

1. Reversibility

It is certainly possible to reunite the severed stumps of the spermatic ducts, and the patency rate after such an operation is at least 80%–85%. However the pregnancy rate after reanastomosis is considerably lower, possibly due to autoimmunization of the patients against their own sperm.

2. Frequency of Sperm-Immobilizing and Sperm-Agglutinating Antibodies After Vasectomy

The data concerning the frequency of the occurrence of sperm-immobilizing and sperm-agglutinating antibodies vary widely, from a few percent to about half the patients who have undergone a sterilization operation, and scarcely anything is stated about the extent of the antibody titers. How much these antibodies can be assumed to be implicated in the lowered fertility following reanastomosis of the vasa deferentia is also still an unanswered question.

In recent years a number of methods for reanastomosis of the vas deferens and modifications in the technique have been proposed. The most recent empirical results indicate that anastomosis of the spermatic duct can be carried out with the aid of microsurgical techniques and magnifying spectacles and, if possible, an operating microscope in such a way that a virtually 100% patency rate can be achieved.

One of the most important questions about the success rate after vasovasostomy in the past was that of sperm-immobilizing and sperm-agglutinating antibodies, their titers, and their relevance to restoration of fertility.

II. Immunologic Considerations

In 1964, Phadke and Padukone and later Rümke (1968) found that agglutinating antibodies were present in the serum of vasectomized men. In 1971, Ansbacher discovered that 6 months after vasectomy sperm-immobilizing antibodies and sperm-agglutinating antibodies were present in the serum of 33% and 54% of men, respectively. However, he noted that 2% of fertile men also have these antibodies. The high 70% "success" rate for vas reanastomosis, associated with a low 25% pregnancy rate, led him to speculate that an autoimmune response to sperm, triggered by vasectomy, was responsible for the discrepancy. Some problems with these in vitro assays are that the titers were generally low, between 1:2 and 1:32 (these could represent background activity rather than a specific antibody), and previous HL-A sensitization to the sperm donor with different HL-A antigens was not ruled out.

HALIM and ANTONIOU (1973) tested the serum of 100 men before and 6 weeks after vasectomy for the presence of sperm-agglutinating antibodies. They found that 2% had positive titers before vasectomy and 6% following vasectomy, a much smaller rise than found by other authors. Furthermore, spermatoxic antibodies had only increased from 1% before to 2% after vasectomy. They concluded that a low background level of antibody activity against sperm – not incompatible with fertility – exists in a low percentage of all men.

Studies on sperm antibody formation after vasectomy were also performed by ALEXANDER et al. (1974). Serum from rhesus monkeys was measured for sperm-agglutinating and sperm-immobilizing antibodies at 2 weeks and 6 months after vasectomy. At 2 weeks they found high titers (average, 1:760) of both immobilizing and agglutinating antibodies. However, by 6 months most titers had returned to low levels. More to the point, ALEXANDER and WILSON (1974) found no correlation between the fertility of vasectomized rhesus monkeys and their antibody levels. OWEN (1976) noted the same findings in human subjects.

Therefore, serious questions remain unanswered: What is the in vivo effect of antisperm antibodies? They have been measured solely by in vitro techniques. It is a weakly syngeneic system, and results of in vitro assays may not have physiologic importance. Sperm used for testing come from random donors, and so the antibodies measured must be specific for a general antigen found in human sperm (and yet not present in cells other than sperm). Obviously, allogeneic HL-A antigens could cause false-positive reactions in HL-A-sensitized patients' sera and yet would be of no clinical significance.

The results of many experiments in animals show that immunization with sperm may or may not lead to high levels of circulating antisperm antibodies (depending on the species or the investigator): but fertility at least is not impaired by this procedure unless sperm are injected with FREUND's adjuvant. These investigators (ANSBACHER, 1971) found that a low level of antisperm activity exists in many animals that are normally fertile. These studies led HULKA and DAVIS (1972) to entertain serious doubts of the importance of autoimmunity in preventing successful results of vasovasostomy.

PHADKE and PHADKE (1967), in their large series of vasovasostomies performed by conventional techniques, showed that fertility (i.e., pregnancy of the patients' wives) was closely related to sperm count and sperm quality of the ejaculate, but not to sperm antibody levels. Their results were among the best reported, with a 55% pregnancy rate and an 83% incidence of sperm in the ejaculate. They used a simple nylon splint with 6-0 arterial silk and three stitches through the seromuscular layer only. It is difficult to understand why they obtained better results than others with this technique; yet the fact remains that the good results correlated with good postoperative sperm counts and did not correlate with sperm antibody titers.

III. Technique

Numerous procedures for vasovasostomy have been reported (O'CONOR, 1948; CAMERON, 1945; MASSEY and NATION, 1949; DORSEY 1953; FREIBERG and LEPSKY, 1939; ROLAND, 1961; SCHMIDT, 1956, 1959a, b, 1961; LEE, 1970;

PARDANANI et al. 1973; ROWLAND et al., 1977; SILBER, 1977c), and a few of them are discussed in some detail below.

1. Schoysman Technique (1976)

The operation (SCHMIDT et al., 1976) is performed in the hospital operating room with the patient lightly anesthetized. Under these circumstances the surroundings are more sterile and the distraction of having the patient move or possibly complain of pain is avoided. The patient may be discharged on recovery from the anesthetic, since further hospitalization is unnecessary. The following technique may be used in both straight and convoluted vasa.

The site of an earlier previous vasectomy can usually be palpated as a thickening or a defect in the vas. A preoperative semen specimen is always tested for sperm, since not all men who have undergone vasectomy become, or stay, sterile. The scrotum is incised between visible vessels and the subcutaneous fascia is spread apart. The vas is grasped above and below the point of obstruction with Allis clamps, and the fascia is incised longitudinally until the scarred ends are exposed. At this point, it is not unusual to see a spermatic granuloma of the testicular end of the vas as a golden yellow or yellowish brown nodule (SCHMIDT and MORRIS, 1973). It must be resected. Histologic examination often reveals vasitis nodosa, a variant of granuloma (CIVANTOS et al. 1972).

The upper (or distal in terms of flow) vas is cut transversely through the scarred end until the lumen is visible. To prove its patency saline solution is injected. If the saline solution is easily admitted, this fact alone proves patency.

The testicular vas is then transected until the lumen is exposed; this lumen is usually much wider than the one at the other end. The vas (never the epididymis) is carefully stripped to secure spermatic fluid. This fluid may be either clear or creamy white in appearance. When obtained, it is easily examined. It is highly variable in content, but either its presence in a good quantity or the presence of sperm heads proves patency of the epididymis and vas up to that point. Any spillage of spermatic fluid should be carefully sponged and flushed away. When there is no fluid, the tunica vaginalis should be opened and the epididymis inspected for evidence of obstruction.

Unless there is evidence of a granuloma, the scarred ends of the vas are not resected, because the blood supply may be impaired. The fascia is stripped back from the fresh end of the vas for 3 mm to prevent it from becoming interposed in the anastomosis. This fascia is next approximated with a nonabsorbable suture (4-0 nylon) so that the ends of the vas lie together easily. The vas is then grasped on each side with modified Bonney clamps, which permit precise opposite rotation without twisting (SCHMIDT, 1975a, b, c). Its ends are now anastomosed by means of a fine nonabsorbable monofilament (never twisted) suture (preferably Ethicon 8718-H, a 6-0 polypropylene suture with needles at both ends). Starting at the most posterior point, sutures are placed into the lumen and out through the wall of the vas at 90° or 120° intervals and are held until all are in place. A nylon suture probe in the upper lumen will help to mark it until the first suture is placed, but the lumen on the testicular side is easily seen. Use of the operating microscope at magnifications of 10–16 times will facilitate placement of the sutures and will help to avoid interlocking them. The posterior suture is tied first, followed by the others. Reinforcing sutures can then be added if necessary, but they should not enter the lumen. Abutment of the thick walls of the vas makes this anastomosis leakproof (SCHMIDT 1974b, c). The fascia and skin are closed. A suspensory is worn for several weeks and sexual intercourse can be resumed after the tenth postoperative day.

Patency, as shown by sperm in the ejaculate, will be secured in 80%–90% of cases. Only 50% of these men's wives will become pregnant, however, and discrepancy is usually caused by the marked reduction in sperm quality below the "normal." Numbers, motility, and morphology of sperm are often subnormal and sometimes sperm does not appear for weeks after surgery, probably because changes in the epididymis often occur after vasectomy. The lumen of the epididymal tubule dilates, as does the vas, at the expense of the interstitial tissue. This dilatation becomes irreversible and the epididymis is less able to take sperm to the vas. With such an adynamic epididymis sperm transport takes longer and many sperm are phagocytosed en route; others are overage when they reach the vas and thus are less capable of fertilizing an ovum. Little is known about semen in men with an adynamic epididymis.

2. Schmidt Techniques

Several techniques have been presented by Schmidt. In a convoluted vas a nylon splint (No. 00) is placed in the distal part for a distance of 5–10 mm, while the other end of the splint is inserted into the proximal vas for a distance of 2 cm. It is then stabbed through the wall of the vas and through the skin by using a hypodermic needle. The anastomosis is then secured with three or four individual sutures of 6-0 monofilament nylon (Fig. 7, Fig. 8).

Another promising method uses a permanent endosplint. This endosplint is tapered, and the larger diameter is placed in the proximal end of the vas without external fixation. The larger diameter prevents it from moving distally. The endosplint is made of Silastic. The ends of the vas are approximated over the splint with 6-0 or even 9-0 monofilament nylon. For all these methods the sutures have to be positioned with care and therefore magnification is necessary: either a visor-type magnifier (magnification $4 \times$) or an operating microscope (magnification up to $20 \times$) should be used. The scrotal incision is closed with subcutaneous and cutaneous sutures of chromic catgut. A suspensory is always applied.

3. Silber Technique

According to the literature the Silber method shows the best results.

A scrotal incision is made, and the vas deferens is exposed above and below the area of the previous ligation. The scar between the two free ends is excised, and the two open ends of the vas are then pulled into the field of a Zeiss operating microscope.

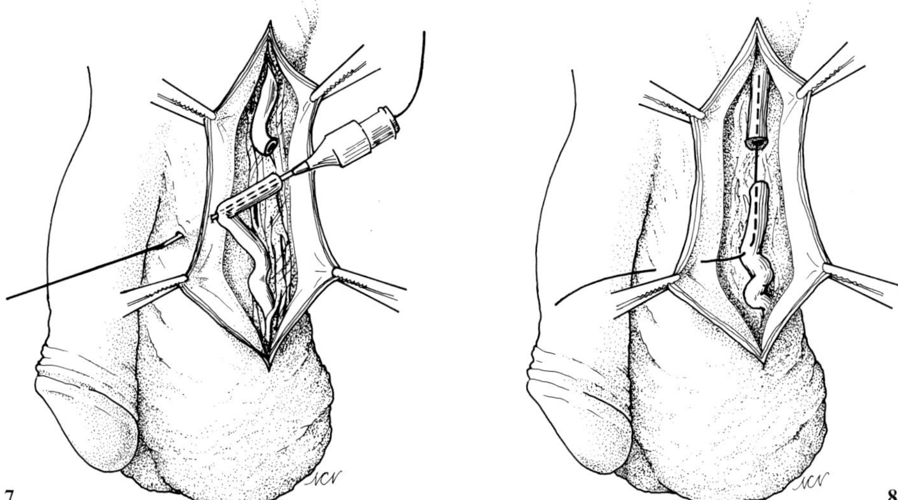

Fig. 7. Placement of the nylon splint through a hypodermic needle into the epididymal stump of the vas deferens

Fig. 8. Situation when the splint is placed in both stumps of the vas deferens before the interrupted sutures with 6-0 monofilament nylon are performed for approximation of the stumps

Under magnification ($\times 10$) the two ends of the vas are inspected after excising beyond the scar to ascertain that the lumen is open (Fig. 9 a). Magnification is increased to about 24 times and a finely polished No. 3 or No. 4 jeweler's forceps is used to dilate the narrower distal part of the lumen (diameter 0.3–0.5 mm). To make suturing easier, No. 9-0 monofilament nylon sutures on a tiny cutting needle and a mosified Barraquer needle holder are used to establish a separate mucosal anastomosis with four to six individual sutures. It might appear at first that a suture through the entire thickness of the vas muscularis and into the lumen would be easier to accomplish. However, such an approach precludes a precise junction of the mucosal lining of the two cut ends, leads to sperm leakage and subsequent stricture, and makes the placement of subsequent stitches in the lumen more difficult. Without a perfect, nonstrictured anastosmis, adequate numbers of sperm cannot be transferred to the semen at the time of ejaculation. In addition, a strictured anastomosis with partial obstruction suppresses normal spermatogenesis.

The muscularis is then joined separately with eight to ten 9-0 nylon sutures. This layer insures a leakproof anastomosis and will allow normal peristalsis during intercourse.

4. Frick Technique

We perform vas–vas anastomosis by means of a simplified end-to-end anastomosis. The operation is always carried out under a general anesthetic and under strict sterile operating theater conditions. With the patient in a dorsal

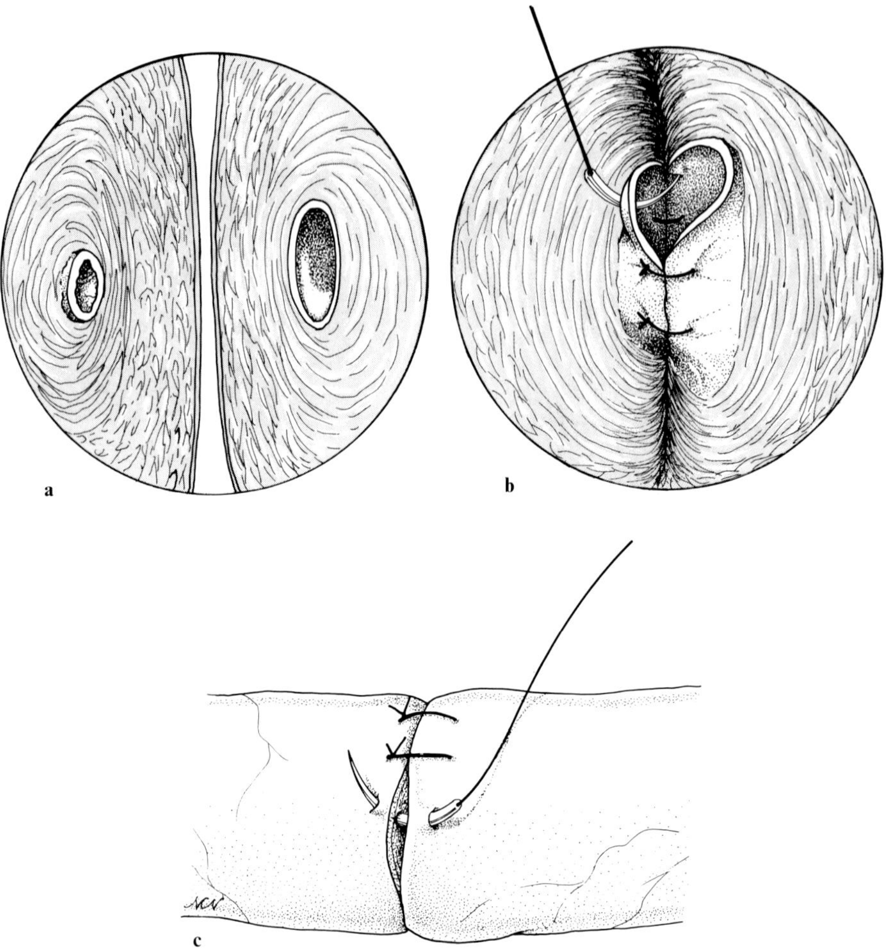

Fig. 9a–c. Schematic drawing illustrating S.J. Silber's method for vasovasostomy:
a The stumps of the vas deferens are prepared for the anastomosis, the patency is tested.
b Anastomosis of the mucosa. c Second-layer suture of the muscularis and adventitia

position, the genital area is aseptically washed and the scrotum uncovered and
then incised over the palpable stumps of the vas deferens. The stumps are
then exposed with strict attention to asepsis, special care being taken to see
that the blood supply is not disturbed. Usually a difference can be seen in
the diameter of the proximal and distal parts of the vas, since the proximal
part is usually about a third as wide again as the distal part. As a splint
we use either a 2-ply 0 nylon thread or a 2-ply 0 plain catgut. The splint
is pushed about 2–3 cm into the distal part of the vas and about 2 cm into
the proximal part of the vas (Fig. 10), where it is stabbed through the wall
of the vas and, after completion of the anastomosis, passed through the scrotal
skin and sutured above the scrotal skin so that it can easily be removed after

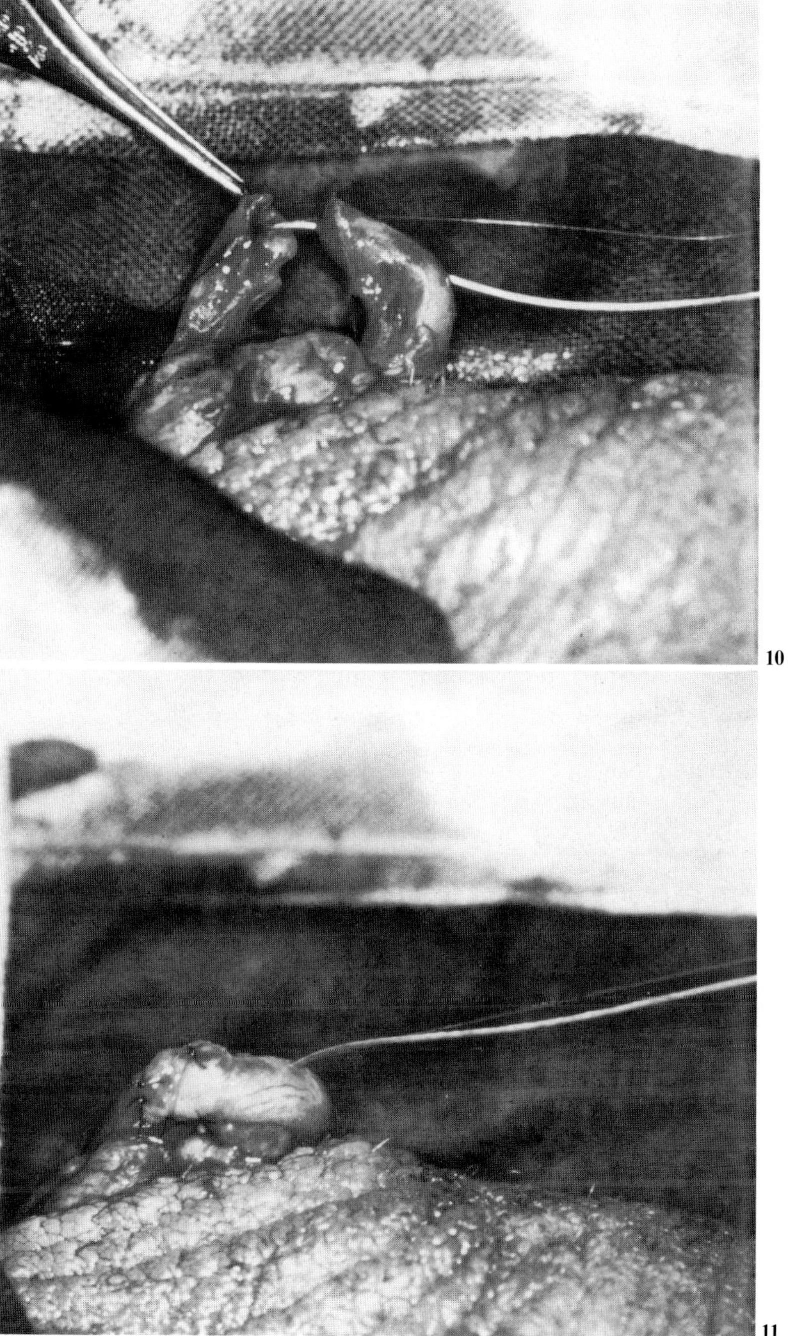

Fig. 10. Method of vasovasostomy used by Frick for the past few years: in a 33-year-old man a reanastomosis is performed 4 years after vasectomy. Both stumps of the left vas deferens are mobilized and a 2-0 Pehafil splint is inserted

Fig. 11. The anastomosis in the same patient is finished after five individual sutures have been made through the vas wall with 6-0 atraumatic Mersilen

a week. The operation is always performed with the aid of magnifying spectacles
($\times$ 6–8 magnification). The anastomosis itself is carried out with 6-0 atraumatic
Mersilen; specifically, an average of four individual sutures are applied, every
effort being made to match the two ends with complete precision. The individual
stitches are taken through the adventitia and the muscularis. After completion
of the anastomosis the vas is retroposed and the scrotal skin closed with 2-0
chromic catgut. The patient wears a suspensory bandage. He is hospitalized
for a week and receives antibiotic treatment with either ampicillin or tetracycline
(Fig. 11).

IV. Complications

In all the methods mentioned the direct postoperative complication rate
is very low. Healing difficulties, infections, and hematoma are extremely rare.

In surgery on such small structures as the spermatic cord it can easily
happen that the two ends are not fitted together exactly in an end-to-end anastomosis. The quality of the adaptation can definitely be considerably improved
by a splint, and it should once again be pointed out that the use of magnifying
spectacles or an operating microscope is invaluable for this operation, as the
results obtained by Silber prove; with the aid of an operating microscope he
was able to carry out a two-layered suture with precision.

To avoid performing the anastomosis under undue tension, which would
cause it to come apart, it is essential to apply sutures in the fascia surrounding
the vas to hold the ends of the vas deferens together once they are in approximately the desired position.

In addition it should be pointed out that in the case of imperfect positioning
of the ends the anastomosis will most probably not be impermeable: this means
that leakage could occur in the area of the anastomosis, with concomitant
extravasation of the sperm in the region surrounding the anastomosis, which
is likely to result in the formation of a spermatic granuloma. In this case
the spermatic granuloma may give rise to inflammation and possibly to renewed
obstruction of the vas deferens.

Spermatic granulomas also often form in the region of the epididymis. Spermatic granulomas in this area can lead to obstruction of the epididymal duct
and thereby prevent the sperm from flowing from the epididymis into the vas.

If azoospermia persists up to 6 months after the operation, the results will
not change and a second operation is advisable. It will be practically impossible
to open the old anastomosis, so that it is very probably much more reasonable
to remove the old anastomosis and to perform a new one under optimal operative
conditions.

V. Results

Table 6 shows the results obtained with vas–vas anastomosis by various
authors. According to the observations of Silber there are five very important
factors that influence the restoration of fertility after vas–vas anastomosis:

1. The use of a fine microscopic technique during the operation
2. The duration of obstruction of the vas deferens

Table 6. Summary of success rates and techniques reported by various authors for vas–vas anastomosis

Author	No. of cases	<10 years after vasectomy	>10 years after vasectomy	Patency (%)	Pregnancy rate (%)	Technique
O'Connor, 1948	420 (review)	–	–	45	–	Various methods: splinted and unsplinted
Phadke and Phadke, 1967	76	–	–	83	55	Nylon splint, 6.0 silk sutures, no microscope
Hulka and Davis, 1972	705 (review)	–	–	60	–	Various methods: splinted and un-splinted
Pardanani et al., 1974	20	3 months to 7 years	–	92	31	Splint of silicon rubber; 4–6 interrupted sutures with 6-0 or 7-0 arterial silk. Splint for 7 days, no microscope
Lee, 1975	156	–	–	81	35	Various techniques
Schmidt, 1975b	–	–	–	80–90	35	Unsplinted; 6-0 nylon through the vas wall, no microscopy
Amelar and Dubin, 1977	93	–	–	84	33	No splint, one-layer suture with 6-0 nylon
Rowland et al., 1977	14	4.8 ± 3.8 years	–	86	29	Plain catgut splint, 3–6 sutures of 5-0 or 6-0 Tevdek through vas wall without mucosa, no microscope
Silber, 1977b	80	–	–	∼100	71	Microscope technique, two-layer suture

3. The nature of the vasectomy
4. The region of the vas deferens at which the vasectomy was carried out
5. The presence or absence of a spermatic granuloma at the spot where the vasectomy was carried out. A spermatic granuloma prevents a pressure build-up in the proximal, i.e., nearby epididymal system, which would certainly occur otherwise. In general, the presence of a spermatic granuloma in the area of the vasectomy stump guarantees a good spermatic quality in the vas fluid at the time of a vas–vas anastomosis and the restoration of an excellent spermatic quality postoperatively.

If all these factors are favorable, vasectomy should be reversible for most patients. Until recently the presence of spermatic granulomas was considered a bad sign on the basis of earlier opinions, since it had always been assumed that these played an important part in the formation of antibodies and were therefore principally responsible for the reduced fertility following reanastomosis of the vas deferens.

References

Agger P (1971) Scrotal and testicular temperature: its relation to sperm count before and after operation for varicocele. Fertil Steril 22:28b

Agger P (1971) Plasma cortisol in the left spermatic vein in patients with varicocele. Fertil Steril 22:4

Ahlberg NE, Bartley O, Chidekel N, Fritjofsson A (1966) Phlebography in varicoceles. Acta Radiol 4:517

Alexander NJ (1977) Vasectomy and vasovasostomy in Rhesus monkeys: the effect of circulating antisperm antibodies on fertility. Fertil Steril 28:562

Alexander NJ, Wilson BJ, Patterson GD (1974) Vasectomy: Immunlogic effects in rhesus monkeys and men. Fertil Steril 25:149

Amelar RD, Dubin L (1973) Male infertility, current diagnoses and treatment. Urology 1:1

Amelar RD, Dubin L (1974) Importance of careful palpation of vas deferens. Urology 4:495

Amelar BD, Dubin L (1977) Male infertility. Saunders, Philadelphia London

Ansbacher R (1971) Spermagglutinating and sperm-immobilizing antibodies in vasectomized men. Fertil Steril 22:629

Ansbacher R (1973) Vasectomy: Sperm antibodies. Fertil Steril 24:788

Barker JF (1941) Anastomosis of the vas deferens. W Va Med J 37:22

Bayle H (1950) Male sterility. Latero-lateral vasepididymo-anastomosis in azoospermia by obliteration: statistics in ninety-five surgically explored cases. Urol Cut Rev 54:129

Bayle H (1953) Traitement chirurgical des obliteratious du canal déférent. Paper presented at the First World Congress on Fertility and Sterility New York 1953

Bayle H (1958) Traitement chirurgical de la sterilite masculine. La fonction spermatogenetique du testicule humain. Masson, Paris

Bayle H (1968) Traitement des azoospermies excretoires par l'anastomose epididymo – deferentielle latero laterale. Med Hyg Geneve 27:1365

Belker AM, Acland RD, Juhala CA (1977) Microsurgical two layer vasovasostomy: a word of caution. Presented at the Annual Meeting of the Southeastern Section of the American Urological Association, New Orleans, March 27–31, 1977

Belker AM, Acland RD, Sexter MS, Roberts TL (1978) Microsurgical two-layer vasovasostomy: laboratory use of vasectomized segments. Fertil Steril 29:38

Bennet WH (1889) Varicocele in particular in reference to it's radical cure. Lancet 1:261

Bernardi R (1967) Sur le traitement chirurgical du varicocéle. J Urol Nephrol (Paris) 73:609

Bradshaw LE (1976) Vasectomy reversibility – a status report. Population Rep Ser D(3): D41

Brown JS (1976) Varicolectomy in the subfertile male: A ten-year experience with 295 cases. Fertil Steril 27:1046

Brown SJ, Dubin L, Hotchkiss RW (1967) The varicocele as related to fertility. Fertil Steril 18:46

Brown SJ, MacLeod J, Hotchkiss RS (1968) Results of varicolectomy in subfertile men. Exhibit at American Fertility Society

Bunge RG (1968) Bilateral spontaneous recanalization of the ductus deferens. J Urol 100:762

Busse E (1950) Wiedervereinigung des Vas deferens nach chirurgischer Sterilisation. Dtsch Gesundh Wochenschr 5:330

Cameron CS (1945) Anastomosis of the vas deferens. JAMA 127:1119

Charney CW (1962) Effect of varicocele on fertility. Fertil Steril 13:47

Charney CW, Baum S (1968) Varicocele and infertility. JAMA 204:1165

Chavney CW, Gillenwater JY (1965) Congential absence of the vas deferens. J Urol 93:399

Civatos R, Lubin J, Rywlin AM (1972) Vasitis nodosa. Arch Pathol 94:355

Clarke BG (1966) Incidence of varicocele in normal men and among men of different ages. JAMA 198:1121

Clegg EJ (1970) The terminations of the left testicular and adrenal veins in man. Fertil Steril 21:36

Cognat M (1970) Traitement chirurgical de la stérilité masculine. Revue Lyonn Med 19: (No. spéc.) 51–53

Cohen MS, Plaine L, Brown JS (1975) The role of internal spermatic vein plasma catecholamine determinations in subfertile men with varicoceles. Fertil Steril 26:1243

Comhaire F, Vermeulen A (1974) Varicocele Sterility: cortisol and catecholamines. Fertil Steril 25:88

Coutinho EM, Melo JF (1976) Varicocele and impotence in men. 1st International Congress of Andrology, Barcelona, July 12–15, 1976

Davidson HA (1954) Treatment of male subfertility: testicular temperature and varicoceles. Practitioner 173:703

Dell'Adami G, Sidoti O (1969) L'anastomosi fra deferente ed epididymo. (Indicazioni, tecnica e risultati in 22 casi.) Monitore ostet ginec 40:541

Derrick F (1973) Vasovasostomy: results of questionnaire of members of the American Urological Association. J Uro 110:556

Donohue RE, Brown JS (1969) Blood gases and pH determinations in the internal spermatic veins of subfertile men with varicocele. Fertil Steril 20:365

Dorsey JW (1953) Anastomosis of the vas deferens to correct postvasectomy sterility. J Urol 70:515

Dorsey W (1957) Surgical correction of postvasectomy sterility. J Int Coll Surg 27:543

Dorsey JW (1973) Surgical correction of postvasectomy sterility. J Urol 110:554

Dubin L, Amelar RD (1970) Varicocele size and results of varicolectomy in selected subfertile men with varicocele. Fertil Steril 21:606

Dubin L, Amelar RD (1971) Etiologic factors in 1294 consecutive cases of male infertility. Fertil Steril 22:469

Dubin L, Amelar RD (1975) Varicolectomy as therapy in male infertility: A study of 504 cases. Fertil Steril 26:217

Dubin L, Hotchkiss RS (1969) Testis biopsy in subfertile men with varicocele. Fertil Steril 20:50

El Sadr AR, Mina E (1950) Anatomical and surgical aspects in the operative management of varicocele. Urol Cutan Rev 54:257

Esho JO, Ireland GW, Cass AS (1974) Recanalization following vasectomy. Urology 3:211

Etribi A, Girgis SM, Hefnaway H, Ibrahim AA (1967) Testicular changes in subfertile males with varicoceles. Fertil Steril 18:666

Fernandes M, Shah KN, Draper JW (1968) Vasovasostomy: improved microsurgical technique. J Urol 100:763

Fernando N, Leonard JM, Paulsen CA (1976) The role of varicocele in male fertility. Andrologia 8:1

Fogh-Andersen P, Nielsen NC, Rebbe H, Stakemann G (1975) The effect on fertility of ligation of the left spermatic vein in men without clinical signs of varicocele. Acta Obstet Gynecol Scand 54:29

Freiberg HB, Lepsky HO (1939) Restoration of continuity of the vas deferens. Eight years after vasectomy. J Urol 41:934

Frick J (1976) Therapeutische Probleme in der Andrologie. Subsidia Med 283:25

Frick J, Bandtlow K (1969) Die Angiographie der linken Vena spermatica. Fortschr Roentgenstr 111:241

Friend DS, Galle J, Silber SJ (1976) Fine structure of human sperm, vas deferens epithelium and testicular biopsy specimens at the time of vasectomy reversal. Anat Rec 184:584

Fritjofsson A, Akren C (1967) Studies on varicocele and subfertility. Scand J Urol Nephrol 1:55

Glezerman M, Rakowszczky M, Lunenfeld B, Beer R, Goldman B (1976) Varicocele in digospermic patients, pathophysiology and results after ligation and division of the internal spermatic vein. J Urol 115:562

Gösfay S (1959) Untersuchungen der Vena spermatica interna durch retrograde Phlebographie bei Kranken mit Varikokele. Z Urol 52:105

Greenberg StH (1977) Varicocele and male fertility. Fertil Steril 28:699

Greenberg SH, Lipshultz LI, Wein AJ (1979) Experience with 425 subfertile male patients. J Urol (in press)

Gunter D (1975) The Palomo operation for varicocele and its effects on fertility. Br J Urol 47:230

Halim A, Antonion D (1973) Autoantibodies to spermatozoa in relation to male fertility and vasectomy. Br J Urol 45:559

Hanley HS (1951) Reconstruction of vas deferens after operation for sterilization. Arch Middlesex Hosp 1:74

Hanley HG (1955) The surgery of male subfertility. Ann R Coll Surg 17:159

Hanley HG (1956) Surgical correction of errors of testicular temperature regulation. In: Proceedings of the Second World Congress of Fertility and Sterility. Tesauro A (ed) Naples, 1956, p 93

Hanley HG (1966) The results of the surgical treatment of varicocele. Proc R Soc Med 59:767

Hanley HG, Harrison RG (1962) Nature and surgical treatment of varicocele. Br J Surg 50:64

Hendry WF, Sommerville JF, Hall RR, Pugh RCB (1973) Investigation and treatment of the subfertile male. Br J Urol 45:684

Hodges RD, Hanley HG (1966) Epididymovasostomy: a microdissection study of two cases. Br J Urol 38:534

Hulka JF, Davis J (1972) Vasectomy and reversible vas-occlusion. Fertil Steril 23:683

Humphreys GA, Hotchkiss RS (1935) Vasoepididymal anastomosis. J Urol 42:815

Ibrahim AA, Awad HA, El-Haggar S, Mitawi BA (1977) Bilateral testicular biopsy in men with varicocele. Fertil Steril 28:663

Isojima S, Li TS, Ashitaka Y (1968) Immunologic analysis of sperm-immobilizing factor found in sera of women with unexplained sterility. Am J Obstet Gynecol 101:677

Ivanissevich C (1960) Left varicocele due to reflux: experience with 4470 operative cases in forty-two years. J Int Coll Surg 34:742

Ivanissevich C, Gregorini H (1918) Una nueva operacion para curar el varicocele. Semana Med 25:575

Javert LT, Clark RL (1944) A combined operation for varicocele and inguinal hernia. Surg Gynecol Obstet 79:644

Johnson DE, Pohl DR, Rivera-Correa H (1970) Varicocele: an innocuous condition? South Med J 63:34

Johnson W (1975) 120 infertile men. Br J Urol 47:230

Kar JK (1968) Surgical correction of post-vasectomy sterility. J Fam Welfare

Kelami A, Rohloff D, Preu K, Affeld K, Seppelt G (1976) Alloplastic reservoir on epididymis – an experimental study on minipigs and beagle dogs. Proc 1st Int Congr Andrology, Barcelona

Kibrick S, Belding DL, Merill B (1952) Methods for the detection of antibodies against mammalian spermatozoa. II. A gelatin agglutination test. Fertil Steril 3:430

Kiszka EF, Cowart GT (1960) Treatment of varicocele by high ligation. J Urol 83:713

Klosterhalfen H. Die operative Behandlung von Fertilitätsstörungen. In: Schirren C (ed) Neue Ergebnisse der Andrologie und Urologie. Springer, Berlin Heidelberg New York, pp 166–175

Klosterhalfen H, Wagenknecht LV (1972) Traitement chirurgical de l'infertilité de l'homme analyse de 442 cas. Kuss R, Auvert J (eds) Proc 66th Congr Franc Urol Masson Paris, pp 212–219

Koumans J, Steeno O, Heyns W, Michelson JP (1969) Dehydroepiandrosterone sulfate, androsterone sulfate and corticoids in spermatic vein blood of patients with left varicocele. Andrologia 1:87

Lane JW (1955) Radiographic studies in varicocele. US Armed Forces Med J 6:1589

Lassnig H, Frick J (1978) Left spermatic vein syndrome. Eur Urol 4:141–143

Lewis EL (1950) The Ivanissevitch operation. J Urol 63:165

Lee HY (1966) Studies on vasovasostomy. II. Anastomosis of vas deferens. Korean J Urol 7:1

Lee HY (1967) Studies on vasovasostomy III. A cumulative report of the anastomosis of vas deferens. J Korean Med Assoc 10:679

Lee HY (1969) Studies on vasovasostomy. IV. Surgical techniques and results of vasovasostomy. J Korean Med Assoc 12:815

Lee HY (1970) Studies on vasovasostomy. V. Effects of early ambulation on success rate and report of 85 vasovasostomies. J Korean Med Assoc 13:897

Lee HY (1972) Studies on vasovasostomy. Korean J Urol 13:1

Lee HY (1975) Technique and results of vasovasostomy. In: Sciarra JJ, Markland C, J (eds) Control of male fertility. Harper & Row, New York, p 68

Lindholmer C, Thulin L, Eliasson R (1973) Concentrations of cortisol and renin in the internal spermatic vein of men with varicocele. Andrologie 5:21

Lipshultz LJ, Corriere JN (1977) Progressive testicular atrophy in the varicocele patient. J Urol 117:175

Lunenfeld B, Glezerman M (1978) Grundschema zur Auswertung von Behandlungen verschiedener Formen männlicher Infertilität. In: Senge Th, Neumann F, Schenk B (Hrsg) Physiologie und Pathophysiologie der Hodenfunktion. Thieme, Stuttgart, p 142

Lykins LE, Witherington R (1977) Vasovasostomy. Urology 10:452

MacLeod J (1965) Seminal cytology in the presence of varicocele. Fertil Steril 16:735

MacLeod J (1969) Further observations on the role of varicocele in human male fertility. Fertil Steril 20:545

MacLeod J (1971) Recent advances concerning the role of varicocele in male infertility. Fertility disturbances in men and women. Jóél CA (ed). Karger, Basel, pp 268–277

Marberger M, Frick J (1973) Zur Ätiologie der Spermiogeneseschädigung bei der Varikokele: Untersuchungen über den Plasmatestosteronspiegel in der Vena Spermatica. Urol Int 28:377

Martin E, Carnett JB, Levi JV, Pennington ME (1902) The surgical treatment of sterility due to obstruction at the epididymis. University Pa Med Bull 15:2

Massey BD, Nation EF (1949) Vas deferens anastomosis, Report of 4 consecutive successful cases. J Urol 66:396

Mauritzen K (1952) Anastomosis operation on the vas. Acta Chir Scand 102:457

Mehta KC, Ramani PS (1970) A simple technique of reanastomosis after vasectomy. Br J Urol 42:340

Michelson L (1949) Congenital anomalies of the ductus deferens and epididymis. J Urol 61:384

Mobley DF (1974) Left spermatic vein cortisol in subfertile men with varicocele. Urology 3:461

Montie JE, Stewart BH, Levin HS (1973) Intravasal stents for vasovasostomy in canine subjects. Fertil Steril 24:877

Montie JE, Stewart BH (1974) Vasovasostomy: past, present and future. J Urol 112:111

Mori A (1963) Studies on vasovasostomy. J Jpn Fertil Steril 8:1

Nelson MT (1942) Anastomosis of vas deferens. A case record with details of repair. West J Surg 49:152

O'Conor VJ (1948) Anastomosis of vas deferens after purposeful division for sterility. JAMA 136:162

O'Conor VJ (1948) Anastomosis of vas deferens after purposeful division for sterility. J Urol 59:229

O'Conor VJ (1961) Surgical correction of male sterility. J Urol 85:352

Olson RO, Stone EP (1949) Varicocele, symptomatologic and surgical concepts. N Engl J Med 240:877

Oster J (1971) Varicocele in children and adolescents. Scand J Urol Nephrol 5:27

Owen ER (1977) Microsurgical vasovasostomy: a reliable vasectomy reversal. Aust NZJ Surg 47:305

Pai MC, Kumar BTS, Kaundinya C, Bhat HS (1973) Vasovasostomy. A clinical study with 10 years follow up. Fertil Steril 24:788

Palomo A (1949) Radical cure of varicocele by a new technique: preliminary report. J Urol 61:604

Pardanani DS, Kathari ML, Maheudrakar MN, Prodhan SA (1973) The use of a silicone rubber splint for post-vasectomy vas deferens anastomosis. Report of a new operative technique. Contraception 7:491

Pardanani DA, Kothari ML, Pradhan SA, Hahendraker MN (1974) Surgical restoration of vas continuity after vasectomy: further clinical evaluation of a new operative technique. Fertil Steril 25:319

Phadke GM (1961) Reanastomosis of the vas deferens. J Indian Med Assoc 36:386

Phadke AM, Padukone K (1964) Presence and significance of autoantibodies against spermatozoa in the blood of men with obstructed vas deferens. J Reprod Fertil 7:163

Phadke GM, Phadke AG (1967) Experiences in the reanastomosis of the vas deferens. J Urol 97:888

Pomerol JM (1976) Exploration and treatment of affections of the seminal duct and neighbouring glands. Post-Granduate Course. I. International Congress of Andrology, Barcelona, 2nd ed. 75, 1976. Editorial ECO, S.A.

Randall GR, Nanninga JB, O'Connor VJ (1977) Improved results in vasovastostomies using internal plain catgut stents. Urology 10:260

Rivington W (1873) Valves in renal veins. J Natl. Physiol 7:163

Robb WAT (1955) Operative treatment of varicocele. Br Med J 2:355

Roland SJ (1961) Splinted and non splinted vasovasostomy: a review of the literature and a report of nine new cases. Fertil Steril 12:191

Rosenbloom D (1956) Reversal of sterility due to vasectomy. Fertil Steril 7:540

Rowland RG, Nanninga JB, O'Conor VJ (1977) Results of vasovasostomy. Urology 10:260

Rümke Ph (1968) Sperm agglutinating autoantibodies in relation to male infertility. Proc R Soc Med 61:275

Rümke PH, Amstel N van, Nesser EN, Bezemer PD (1974) Prognosis of fertility of men with sperm agglutinins in the serum. Fertil Steril 25:393

Russell JK (1954) Varicocele in groups of fertile and subfertile men. Br Med J 1:1231

Schach H, Scheidt J, Mauss J (1973) Morphologische und klinische Untersuchungen bei Patienten mit Varikokelen. 15. Tagung der Vereinigung Norddeutscher Urologen. Lübeck-Travemünde, 1973

Schelor WC, Witherlington R (1975) Comparison of polypropylene and polyglycolic acid suture in experimental vasovasostomy: a preliminary report. Invest Urol 13:223

Schirren C, Klosterhalfen H (1966) Spermatogenese bei Varikokele. Z Hautkr 40:372

Schmidt SS (1956) Anastomosis of vas deferens. J Urol 75:300

Schmidt SS (1959a) Anastomosis of the vas deferens: an experimental study. II. Successes and failures in experimental anastomosis. J Urol 81:203

Schmidt SS (1959b) Anastomosis of the vas deferens: an experimental study. III. Dilatation of the vas following obstruction. J Urol 81:206

Schmidt SS (1961) Anastomosis of the vas deferens: an experimental study. IV. The use of fine Polyethylene tubing as a splint. J Urol 85:838

Schmidt SS (1975a) Principles of vasovasostomy. Contemp Surg 7:13

Schmidt SS (1975b) Vasaanastomosis: a return to simplicity. Br J Urol 47:309

Schmidt SS (1975c) Vasovasostomy: a review of principles. Contemp Surg 7:13

Schmidt SS Vas reanastomosis procedures. In: Richart RM, Prager DJ (eds) Human sterilization. Thomas, Springfield, Ill., pp 76–85

Schmidt SS, Morris RR (1973) Spermatic granuloma: the complication of vasectomy. Fertil Steril 24:941

Schmidt SS, Schoysman R, Stewart BH (1976) Surgical approaches to male infertility. In: Hafez ESE (ed) Human semen and fertility regulation in men. Mosby, St Louis, p 476

Schoenberg HW, Murphy JJ (1959) Technique of surgical correction of varicocele. Surg Gynecol Obstet 109:383

Schoysman R (1968) La creation d' une spmeratocèle arteficielle dans les agenesis du canal deferent. Bull Soc Belge Gynecol Obstet 38:307

Schoysman R (1974) Diskussion anläßlich der Workshop. Conference: Die Verschlußazoospermie – Ursachen, Diagnostik und Möglichkeiten der operativen Therapie. Hamburg 1974

Schoysman R (1976) Exploration and treatment of obstructions and infections in the seminal duct and accessory genital glands. Post-Graduate Course, I.: International Congress of Andrology, Barcelone, 2nd ed: 87, 1976. Editorial ECO, S.A.

Scott LS, Young D (1962) Varicocele: a study of its effects on human spermatogeneses and of the results produced by spermatic vein ligation. Fertil Steril 13:325

Silber SJ (1976) Microscopic technique for reversal of vasectomy. Surg Gynecol Obstet 143:630

Silber SJ (1977a) Intraabdominal microsurgery: inguinal reconstruction of vas deferens and testicular revascularization. Am Soc of Andrology, Palm Springs

Silber SJ (1977b) Microscopic vasectomy reversal. Fertil Steril 28:1191

Silber SJ (1977c) Perfect anatomical reconstruction of vas deferens with a new microscopic surgical technique. Fertil Steril 28:72

Silber SJ (1977d) Sperm granuloma and reversibility of vasectomy. Lancet 2:588

Silber SJ, Galle J, Friend D (1977) Microscopic vasovasostomy and spermatogenesis. J Urol 117:299

Steeno O, Koumans J, Moor P de (1976) Adrenal cortical hormones in the spermatic vein of 95 patients with left varicocele. Andrologia 8:101

Stephenson JD, O'Shaughnessy EJ (1968) Hypospermia and its relationship to varicocele and intrascrotal temperature. Fertil Steril 19:110

Stewart BH, Montie JE (1973) Male infertility: An optimistic report. J Urol 110:216

Swerdloff RS, Walsh PC (1975) Pituitary and gonadal hormones in patients with varicocele. Fertil Steril 26:1006

Tanaka HY, Takada MY (1968) Surgical correction of male sterility. Acta Urol Jpn 14:679

Tessler AN, Krahn HP (1966) Varicocele and testicular temperature. Fertil Steril 17:201

Trabucco A (1947) Vasepididymoanastomosis lateral intraepididymaria. Rev Argent Urol 17:488

Tulloch WS (1952) Consideration of Sterility. Infertility in the male. Edin Med J 59:24

Tulloch WS (1955) Varicocele in subfertility: results of treatment. Br Med J 2:356

Twyman EJ, Nelson CS (1938) Vas deferens anastomosis. Urol Cutan Rev 42:586

Uehling DT (1968) Fertility in men with varicocele. Int J Fertil 13:58

Urry RL, Thompson J, Cockett ATK (1976) Vasectomy and vasovasostomy. II. A comparison of two methods of vasovasostomy: sikastic versus chromic stens. Fertil Steril 27:945

Verstoppen GR, Steeno OP: Varicocele and the pathogenesis of the associated subfertility. Andrologia 9:133

Völter D (1972) Die idiopathische Varikokele aus andrologischer Sicht. Fortschr Med 90:683

Völter D, Wurster J, Aeikens J, Scubert GE (1975) Untersuchungen zur Struktur und Funktion der Vena Spermatica interna – Ein Beitrag zur Ätiologie der Varikikele. Andrologia 7:127

Vöske HD, Breitwieser P (1970) Ligatur der Vena Spermatica bei Subfertilität infolge Varikokele. Münch Med Wochenschr 2:1682

Wagenknecht LV, Holstein AF, Schirren C (1974) Verschlußazoospermie – Tierexperimentelle Untersuchungen an Ratten. Andrology Workshop Conference, Hamburg, September 1974

Wagenknecht LV, Holstein AF, Schirren C (1975) Tierexperimentelle Untersuchung zur Bildung einer künstlichen Spermatikele. Andrologia 7:273

Wagenknecht LV, Weitze KF, Hoppe LP, Krause D, Holstein AF, Schirren C (1976) Alloplastic spermatocele for treatment of male infertility. Proc 1st Int Congr Andrology, Barcelona, July 1976

Wagenknecht LV, Weitze KF, Hoppe LP, Krause D, Schirren, C, Peter KH, Rüsch R (1977) Further experiences with an alloplastic spermatocele: Experiments in bulls. Andrologia 9:179

Wallijn E, Desmet R (1979) Hydrocele; a frequently overlooked complication after high ligation of the spermatic vein in varicocele. (in press)

Weissbach L, (1975) Spermatological and histological findings in patients with varicocele. Urologe 14:277

Wilhelm SF (1937) Sterility in the male. Oxford loose leaf surgery. University Press, New York Oxford, p 746

Zorgniotti AW, MacLeod J (1973) Studies in temperature, human semen, quality and varicocele. Fertil Steril 24:854

Artificial Insemination and Semen Preservation

M. Glezerman

With 3 Figures

A. Artificial Homologous Insemination

Of the hundreds of millions of sperm cells that leave the male genital tract during intercourse and reach the vagina, only some will be successful enough to reach the female endocervix to be stored there for continuous release. Settlage et al. (1973) and Insler et al. (1979) reported the total sperm cell content in the endocervical storage space to be around 200000. The vast majority of spermatozoa are either spilled out from the vagina or destroyed there by its acidity and serve merely as cannon fodder to enable a tiny minority of cells to reach the endocervix as the first secure intermediate station on the perilous journey to the oviduct. Semen containing less than the normal amount of cells or containing a larger than usual amount of nonmotile or morphologically distorted cells will be at a disadvantage to provide the adequate "escort" for those cells destined to enter the uterus. Fertility will thus be impaired. It seems therefore logical to assist subnormal sperm by concentrating what little is offered as closely as possible to the external cervical os, or in some cases even beyond it directly into the uterine cavity. Artificial insemination has been used to compensate for poor seminal qualities with various results. Another indication for artificial insemination has been faulty delivery of semen into the vagina during intercourse due to impotency of either partner or due to anatomic malformations preventing proper intravaginal ejaculation. Actually, the first reported artificial insemination was done in the wife of a patient with severe hypospadias who constantly ejaculated "ante portas." John Hunter performed the procedure in 1790 by depositing the husband's sperm intravaginally with consequent conception. Today homologous insemination is an integral part in the armamentarium of the physician treating infertility, and a variety of indications and techniques have been defined.

I. Indications

The range of indications for artificial insemination, some of them mentioned in the introductory remarks, may be classified into female and male factors.

1. Female Indications

Displacements of the uterine cervix may prevent ascension of sperm cells and require artificial deposition of semen. Cervical mucus antibodies or cervical mucus of unfavorable physical properties (INSLER et al., 1977) may pose an impenetrable barrier to sperm cells and require artificial bypassing of this obstacle. In cases of female impotency (vaginismus), intravaginal insemination is usually rather successful as far as pregnancy rates are concerned. However, we feel that the treatment of infertility in couples in whom a potency problem exists should be postponed until this difficulty has been evaluated and treated properly.

2. Male Indications

In psychogenic male impotency with consequent deposition failure, semen can usually be obtained by masturbation and used for artificial insemination. However, as in the female, we feel that this bypassing of a central problem could bring more harm than benefit to the couple, and we prefer in these cases to postpone fertility treatment until the potency problem has been solved. In organic impotency, however, such as in paraplegic patients, in diabetics, etc., in whom causal treatment has been ineffective, artificial insemination may be performed. If ejaculatory difficulties exist, electrovibration may be useful to obtain semen (GLEZERMAN and LUNENFELD, 1976). Any malformation of the male genital tract that prevents semen from reaching the vaginal fornices during coitus and is resistant to treatment presents an indication for artificial insemination. Hypospadias has been mentioned and epispadias will similarly lead to seminal spilling outside the vagina during coitus. In cases of occlusion or agenesis of the ductus deferens, attempts have been made to produce artificial spermatoceles by means of transplanted veins (SCHOYSMAN 1973; COGNAT and GUILLARD, 1973) or by means of alloplastic material (WAGENKNECHT, 1976). These spermatoceles are then punctured and semen may be used for insemination. Results obtained by these methods are to date not yet at a scale allowing conclusions.

In rare cases semen may be ejaculated retrograde into the bladder instead of being propulsed antegrade via the urethra. This condition may be a sequela of bladder neck surgery or a complication of diabetes. Patients with retrograde ejaculation should receive alkalizing agents (sodium bicarbonate) prior to intercourse to neutralize the urinary pH; the postcoital urinary specimen, obtained as soon as possible following intercourse or masturbation, can then be centrifuged, washed with nutrient solutions, and used for artificial insemination (GLEZERMAN et al., 1976).

Subnormal semen may be treated in vitro to enhance motility (SCHILL, 1975), to separate motile and morphologically normal spermatozoa from abnormal forms and debris (PAULSON, 1978, DMOWSKY et al., 1979), and to be used subsequently for artificial insemination. If the seminal problem is mainly a reduced cell count, particularly concomitant with high seminal volume, the spermatozoan concentration may be enhanced by means of the so-called split ejaculate:

Roughly 30% of the ejaculate consists of prostatic gland secretions, spermatozoa, and epididymal fluids while the remaining 70% originates in the seminal vesicles. During the ejaculatory process, prostatic secretions and spermatozoa mixed with epididymal fluid are produced first. Subsequent emissions are composed mainly of secretions derived from the seminal vesicle. Consequently, the portion resulting from the first ejaculative contraction will contain the highest density of sperm cells (usually with a higher percentage of motile sperm cells than in the following spurts).

The husband may be instructed to perform a modified withdrawal technique during sexual intercourse in such a manner that only the first ejaculatory portion will enter the vagina. If this is not feasible, the husband is asked to masturbate into two different containers and the first portion may then be used for artificial insemination. Finally, semen stored at low temperatures for a variety of reasons will ultimately be used for artificial insemination.

II. Timing of Insemination

Before initiating artificial insemination, the average midcycle can be calculated from the observation of three basal body temperature charts. However, this preliminary observation period is not sufficient to be the sole basis for consequent therapy. The fertility status of the female partner has to be assessed thoroughly and the periovulatory period has to be identified as clearly as possible. The survey should include complete cycle evaluation with ovulation detection and timing by means of basal body temperature, progesterone levels, and observation of the cervical score (INSLER et al., 1972). The life span of the human ovum is believed to average 6–24 h, while motile human sperm cells have been observed in the cervical mucus for periods up to 205 h following intercourse. Thus, three inseminations per cycle at alternative days will usually suffice to "cover" the periovulatory period and ensure that sufficient sperm cells are available at the fertilization site when the ovum arrives.

Serial scoring of the cervical mucus, i.e., observation of its amount, spinnbarkeit, ferning, and the appearance of the external cervical os has been very useful as adjunctives in scheduling repeated inseminations.

III. Technique

Artificial insemination may be performed intravaginally, pericervically, intracervically and intrauterinely. Special insemination instruments such as cervical caps are available. Intravaginal insemination is easily performed with a plastic syringe, and the whole specimen may be used. This method does not require exposure of the cervix and may be performed by the couple themselves. The female partner is in Trendelenburg's position. If the procedure is performed by the couple at their home, the pelvis may be elevated slightly by means of a pillow. The position should be maintained for at least 20 min following insemination. Obviously, the intravaginal technique does not improve seminal qualities but does enable optimal delivery of the semen into the vagina. It is thus indicated in those cases involving faulty deposition. (Extreme care has to be taken not to inject air into the vagina and cervix since this could cause air embolism.)

If semen has to be treated in vitro, pericervical or intracervical insemination is indicated. Usually, both methods are used concomitantly. The patient is placed in Trendelenburg's position, and 0.2–0.5 ml are injected slowly to a depth of approximately 1 cm into the cervical canal by applying the blunt tip of a plastic syringe to the external os. The rest of the specimen is placed in the anterior vaginal fornix. The patient remains in the supine position for at least 20 min.

With the exception of the small amount of intracervically deposited semen, the major part of the specimen, usually subfertile and handicapped as such, is deposited in the vagina and will pour out immediately following insemination. Remaining spermatozoa will be inactivated rather quickly by vaginal acidity. Furthermore, all insemination techniques mentioned require that the patient remain supine for almost 0.5 h following insemination. This may tie up rooms in a busy practice. The cervical cap technique overcomes these drawbacks. A variety of caps have been designed. However, most systems do not provide close contact to the cervix, and dislocation of the cap may occur following placement. In addition, merely applying the cap to the cervix will protect only part of the semen from the vaginal environment while a more or less large part will still be spilled. The vacuum cap as developed by Fikentscher and Semm guarantees a close contact to the cervix and makes the sometimes tedious task of filling the adapted cap in situ with semen superfluous. This cap consists of a plastic hood available in two sizes and connected to a flexible plastic tubing which may be closed by a "roll-on" clamp (Fig. 1). Following exposure of the cervix by a speculum and cleansing of the vagina and cervix, the cap is placed on the portio using a grasping instrument. A vacuum is produced either by a commercially available small hand pump or simply by evacuating air by means of a 10-ml syringe. During this process the application to the cervix is controlled visually. The clamp is then closed and the semen-containing syringe attached. The clamp is now opened and the semen injected under vision. The speculum is withdrawn, and the patient may leave the table immediately. The cap remains in situ for 8–16 h. The patient is advised to open the clamp upon arising the next morning and to remove the cap by simply pulling the plastic tubing.

For some patients the production of an ejaculate on demand presents a serious problem. In these cases one should not exert further pressure on the patient but offer an alternative. This could be the vacuum cap. The instrument is fixed to the uterine cervix by the physician closely to the assumed ovulation (Semm et al., 1976). Within the next 16 h the male partner may in his homely surroundings fill semen into a syringe and complete the insemination procedure at a time convenient for the partners beyond the dictate of the physician's busy schedule (Fig. 1).

Intravaginal, intracervical, and pericervical insemination as well as cap inseminations are only useful if the female genital tract poses no obstacle to delivered semen. In couples in whom the cervical mucus of the female partner is scant or too viscid for sperm penetration, i.e., absolute or relative dysmucorrhea exists (Insler et al., 1977), or contains antisperm antibodies, bypassing of the cervix by intrauterine insemination is a reasonable tactic. However, intrauterine insemination is nonphysiologic in that spermatozoa are introduced into the uterine cavity together with seminal fluid (Asch et al., 1977). This may pose

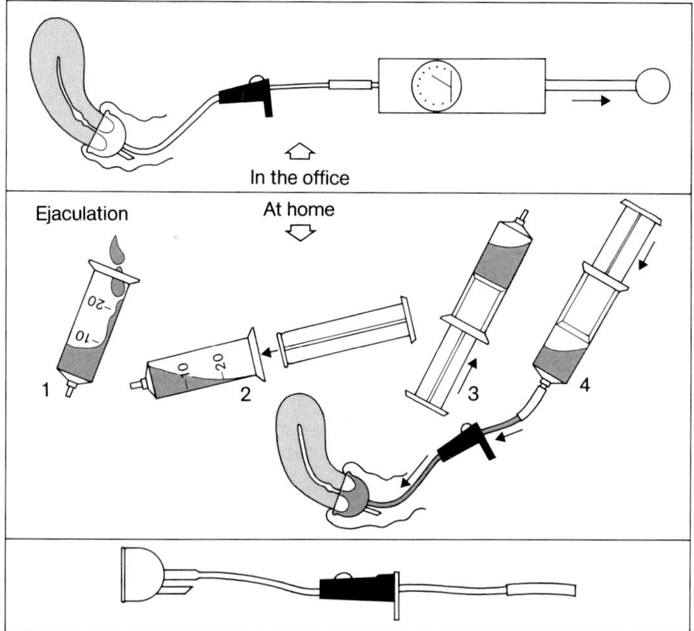

Fig. 1. Application of the vacuum cervical cap. The *upper part* of the figure shows the application of the cap to the uterine cervix and the production of a vacuum by a hand pump. The *middle part* shows the filling of a syringe with semen and the application of the syringe to the cap tubing. This procedure may be performed by the couple themselves in their home if for any reasons the husband cannot produce an ejaculate at a preset time. The *lower part* shows the vacuum cervical cap. (SEMM et al., 1976)

some unique problems. Firstly, uterine spermatozoa leave the female genital tract rather quickly via the uterine tubes and disappear in the peritoneal cavity, while no supply from the endocervical storage space replaces the loss. Thus, the chance element of whether spermatozoa will be able to meet a short-lived fresh ovum on their way through the oviduct is increased. More frequent insemination, i.e., daily, may compensate partially for this drawback.

Secondly, exclusion of the endocervix by intrauterine insemination also means to dispense with its bactericidal properties (POMMERENKE, 1946). The risk of infections may thus increase (RUSSEL, 1960). Meticulous cleansing of vagina and cervix by use of ample amounts of lactated Ringer's solution, for example, prior to insemination and strict sterile handling of the seminal specimen obtained in a sterile jar is of paramount importance. We advocate in addition prophylactic antibiotic treatment during the insemination period. Doxycycline 100 mg daily in a single dose answers to the requirement of good penetration into the secretions of the female genital tract and is thus suitable for this purpose.

Thirdly, intrauterine insemination with introduction of seminal fluid into the uterine cavity may lead to very painful uterine cramps due to the effect of the prostaglandin content of human semen (TAYLOR and KELLY, 1974). Most authors therefore advocate restriction of the inseminated volume to 0.3 ml (White and Glass, 1976). Prostaglandins are secreted by the seminal vesicles that contribute to the last ejaculatory spurts. Thus, the first ejaculatory portion, consisting mainly of epididymal and prostatic contributions, contains relatively few prostaglandins but a high concentration of spermatozoa. It is thus uniquely suited for intrauterine inseminations, and we have exclusively used the first split fraction for this purpose, injecting up to 0.8 ml per insemination.

IV. Results of Artificial Homologous Insemination

The success rate of homologous artificial insemination varies widely with its indications. Comparison of data are rather difficult if not impossible, since very often the attempt is made to treat multifactorial infertility by this method, equivocal indications are sometimes used, and data are often reported only incompletely. Controlled studies are almost nonexistent. The highest success rates are certainly observed in couples in whom normal sperm exists that cannot be delivered properly to the uterine cervix during intercourse. Pregnancy rates are reported as high as 86% (Barwin, 1974). Pregnancy rates reported for other indications vary largely with no apparent relation to the insemination technique used (Table 1), although split insemination seems to be somehow more successful (Table 2). If following six consecutive cycles no pregnancy ensues, the couple should be reevaluated.

B. Artificial Donor Insemination

Homologous artificial insemination is usually readily accepted by most couples, since it is regarded by husbands and wives as a mere supportive measure. On the other hand, the offer to perform donor insemination (AID) or the advice to adopt a child, even after the fertility status has been explained extensively, is often perceived by the male partner as a verdict, a disaster, and may induce a complex spectrum of emotional problems involving both partners. The realization of being irreversibly infertile leads almost invariably to an identity crisis in the male, crossed with guilt feelings toward the female partner. She may often produce guilt feelings for her part toward the husband for not sharing his reproductive failure, and it is not a rare phenomenon that previously ovulatory cycles turn subsequently to anovulatory ones (Beck, 1976). Hopes nourished for prolonged periods of time, during which exhaustive attempts with treatments have been tried and various doctors have been consulted, have to be abandoned, and the long avoided truth has to be faced. On the psychological level this is a process of mourning (Nijs and Rouffa, 1977). The couple has to come out of this crisis with a new self-definition without the biologic procreative dimension. The archaic connection between sexuality and procreation has to be untied. This identity crisis, involving both partners, has to be solved in a psychosocial vacuum without the support of family and friends. The physician who gave the verdict of irreversible infertility bears a heavy responsibility and has to provide help to enable the couple to come

Table 1. Homologous artificial insemination using whole semen: techniques, indications, and pregnancy rates

Authors	Year	Indications	No. of patients	Pregnancy rate (%)	Technique
WHITELAW	1950	Oligozoospermia	32	15.6	Cervical cap
KASCARELIS, COMNINOS	1959	Oligozoospermia	36	0	Intrauterine, intracervical
RUSSEL	1960	Oligozoospermia	34	5.8	Pericervical
HEUER	1971	Oligozoospermia	70	44.3	Cervical cap
BARWIN	1974	Oligozoospermia	20	55.0	Intrauterine
WHITE, GLASS	1976	Cervical factor	9	55.5	Intrauterine
WELLER	1976	Oligozoospermia	60	16.6	Pericervical
SPEICHINGER, MATTOX	1976	Oligozoospermia	24	8.3	Cervical cap
STEIMANN, TAYMOR	1977	Cervical factor impotency	28	35.7	Intracervical
NUNLEY et al.	1978	Oligozoospermia, retrograde ejacul.	53	24.5	Intracervical, cervical cap

Table 2. Homologous artificial insemination using the split fraction: techniques, indications, and pregnancy rates

Authors	Year	Indications	No. of patients	Pregnancy rate (%)	Technique
FARRIS, MURPHY	1960	Oligozoospermia	100	13.3	Intrauterine
AMELAR, HOTCHKISS	1965	Oligozoospermia	23	56.0	?
PEREZ-PALAEZ, COHEN	1965	Oligozoospermia	38	26.3	Intracervical, intrauterine
STEIMANN, TAYMOR	1977	Oligozoospermia	29	24.1	Intracervical
MOGHISSI et al.	1977	Oligozoospermia, retrograde ejac., deposition fail.	62	32.1	Intracervical
GLEZERMAN et al.	1978	Oligozoospermia	21	76.2	Intracervical, pericervical, autoinsemination
GLEZERMAN et al.	1982	Cervical factor	25	52.0	Intrauterine

through the painful process of adaptation to a new form of identity. Ideally, expert advice concerning AID is rendered by a team consisting of a gynecologist, an andrologist, and a psychologist. In Louvain, Belgium, an even more expanded panel includes a urologist and a moralist. However, in most centers it is the physician alone who bears the sole responsibility and will be happy enough to share it with a psychologist. It would be unwise to proceed to AID very soon after the husband has been confronted with his infertility. Adjustment of both partners takes time, and both AID and adoption should be discussed extensively leaving the choice to the couple. There may be questions regarding the legitimacy of a child born after AID, religious and ethic problems may arise, and the couple must be given enough information and time to overcome suspicions as to the other partners attitude toward the use of donor sperm. Parenthood is much more a psychosocial relationship toward the child and toward society than a biologic one. The myth of "blood and flesh" has to be uprooted, and a state of consiousness has to be achieved in which the donor, from the psychological point of view, does not exist. Donor semen should be then regarded as "material" from an anonymous testis, the donor being actually a "nonperson." For this purpose we restrict information given about the donor to an absolute minimum revealing only ethnic origin, negativity of familial and personal history of diseases, and stressing resemblance to the husband.

It is of paramount importance for the physician to assess the stability of the partnership. His responsibility also includes the child to be born. It is too large a burden to place on any child to save a marriage. Furthermore, an unstable marriage in which the desire for a child is more an expression of proof of one's self or a concession to social demands than a genuine wish for a child will not be salvaged by a baby, whether conceived naturally or by AID. On the other hand, stable marriages will remain so and be enriched when parenthood is added. Behrman (1968) reported that only 1 of 800 marriages with AID babies ended in divorce. Tekavic (1974) studied the destiny of couples after AID in comparison to childless couples and found the divorce rate to be almost 20 times higher in the latter group.

I. Indications for AID

The first artificial insemination using donor semen is reported to have taken place at the end of the nineteenth century. Gregoire and Mayer (1965) named a certain William Pancoast, a Philadelphian physician, and Amelar et al. (1977) give the credit to R.L. Dickinson. The most common indication is absolute male sterility, such as in cases of Klinefelter's syndrome, hypergonadotropic hypogonadism, and therapy-resistant azoospermia. Long-standing infertility in couples in whom any degree of oligo-, terato-, asthenospermia of the husband's semen remains therapy resistant is the next common indication (Taymor, 1978). Inheritable diseases in the husband's line (e.g., Tay-Sachs disease, juvenile diabetes, Hutchinson's chorea, etc.) are indications for AID. So are incompatibilities, such as concerning the Rh factor when the female partner is senisitized. Finally, in long-standing infertility with no apparent etiology when the female partner is approaching the end of her reproductive years, AID may be considered as a last measure.

II. Selection of Donors

Some patients offer a relative as donor to ensure "blood bondage." This choice should be definitely discouraged since serious emotional complications may ensue. The principle of the donor being a nonperson will be neutralized, positive or negative identification of either partner with the donor may result, and a theoretical possibility that the donor may one day claim the child, a very archaic fear, can hang like the sword of Damocles above the heads of the couples. It should be only the physician to whom the donor's identity is known. As trivial as this statement sounds, this is one of the basic pillars for AID. Consequently, one should avoid permitting a clerk to handle payments to the donor, a nurse to receive the specimen, etc. Although sometimes cumbersome, all technical procedures that demand contact with the donor should be the sole responsibility of the physician, thus ensuring maximal anonymity of the donor. Usually, patients request that the physical characteristics of the donor be matched to those of the husband. While the couple should be fully informed that matches of this kind in the human by no means guarantee resemblance and that the child may well inherit physical characteristics of a remote and unknown relative and not resemble either of the parents, attempts should be made to choose donors of the same ethnic origin, body proportions, and hair and eye color as those of the husband. If feasible, the same blood type as the husband's or at least the wife's should be present. The donor should be intelligent and fully aware about the use of his semen. Some authors insist on written consent (AMELAR et al., 1977; BECK, 1977). We make a point of employing only paid donors. If the motivation of an individual to donate semen is idealism, one should honor it but be aware of the fact that idealism is sometimes not a very constant feature. It is painful for a couple receiving AID to learn that a treatment program has to be interrupted due to a donor's sudden refusal to continue. If the basis of the "contract" with the donor is idealism connected with a clear-cut financial motivation on his part, the cooperation is usually far more reliable.

The first laboratory step in the evaluation of a potential donor is of course the semen evaluation (see page 203). At least two consecutive semen analyses should be present and demonstrate excellent qualities. A thorough physical examination should not reveal any pathologies, and an extensive familial and personal anamnesis should be negative. Basic laboratory tests should include complete blood pictures, blood typing, glucose tolerance test, urinary cultures, and chest X rays. Serologic tests for syphilis are advisable. There is a growing need to perform repeated tests for gonorrhea in potential and active donors. JENNINGS et al. (1977) demonstrated that semen contaminated with *Neisseria gonorrhea* collected in containers as used in AID does not lose viability in vitro in the time in which most specimens are used. For different countries specific tests should be performed to detect certain diseases especially common for the given area (e.g., sickle cell anemia for American blacks, etc.). In our country donors of European origin undergo enzymatic assays of serum or skin fibroblasts to ensure that they are not heterozygote carriers of Tay-Sachs disease, which occurs far more often in Jews of European origin than in non-Jews.

III. Technique of Insemination

The technique of insemination with donor's semen is essentially the same as with husband's sperm. A specific problem arises when the couple requires mixing the husband's sperm with that of the donor. A great advantage of this method is the positive doubt as to which spermatozoa eventually fertilized the ovum. Even in highly sophisticated couples we have often observed the phenomenon that the husband, while being fully aware of his irreversible infertility, discovers later features in his child that are interpreted by him as proof that his semen fertilized the ovum. On the other hand, adding husband's semen to the specimen provided by the donor will dilute it and may even have immobilizing and agglutinizing effects (Quinlivan and Sullivan, 1977a, b). We feel nevertheless that if preliminary tests for immobilization and agglutination in a mixed specimen are negative and postcoital tests following insemination with mixed sperm are good, one should perform inseminations with mixed semen. The husband will thus be given a better chance to overcome his identity crisis and to identify himself better with his role as a father. Furthermore, when the husband has to provide semen for each insemination and is thus involved actively in the therapeutic process, the abstraction of the donor's person is achieved more easily and the AID program is perceived by both partners as treatment for both. For the same purpose, we encourage sexual intercourse following inseminations in couples in whom mixing is not feasible. Excluded from this reasoning are obviously couples in whom the husband's procreation is not advisable (inheritable diseases in the husband, etc.).

IV. Results of AID

The results of artificial insemination using donor semen are excellent. Using fresh donor semen, more than 70% of treated women will eventually become pregnant, the specific technique playing no significant role (Table 3). An analysis of the cumulative distribution of pregnancies according to number of insemination cycles reveals that almost 53% of those women who will eventually be pregnant will do so within the first three treatment cycles and nearly 80% will be pregnant within the first six treatment cycles (Table 4). A fair chance for treatment success should thus be based on at least six ovulatory cycles following which the wife should be reevaluated and continuation of the AID program discussed with both partners.

Using thawed freeze-stored semen, pregnancy rates are lower. Evaluating 394 couples reported by four authors, the overall pregnancy rate was 51% (Table 5). The cumulative distribution of pregnancies relative to the number of insemination cycles using thawed freeze-stored semen, however, was similar to that when fresh semen was used (Table 6).

V. Legal Aspects of AID

Artificial insemination using donor semen raises legal questions as to the legitimacy of the child and to the child's rights in relation to the husband

Table 3. Pregnancy rates for artificial insemination using *fresh donor semen*

Authors	Year	No. of patients	Pregnancy rate (%)	Insemination method
BEHRMANN	1959	168	75.0	?
HAMAN	1959	399	76.0	Pericervical
MURPHY, TORRANO	1966	112	68.0	Intracervical
STEINBERGER	1973	48	73.0	Pericervical
WARNER	1974	320	72.0	Pericervical
WHITELAW	1974	1000	76.6	Cervical cap
CHONG, TAYMOR	1975	107	72.0	Intracervical + vaginal
GOSS	1975	113	79.6	Intracervical + vaginal
DIXON, BUTTRAM	1976	77	44.9	Pericervical
GLEZERMAN	1981	270	85.2	Pericervical
Total		2834	74.1	

Table 4. Cumulative distribution of pregnancy rates relative to number of insemination cycles for 1690 pregnancies following artificial insemination using *fresh donor semen*

Authors	Year	Pregnancies	Pregnancy rate following	
			Three cycles (%)	Six cycles (%)
BEHRMAN	1959	126	59,0	86.0
HAMAN	1959	303	67.0	87.0
MURPHY, TORRANO	1966	76	62.0	92.0
STEINBERGER, SMITH	1973	35	25.7	85.7
WHITELAW	1974	766	35.4	69.5
CHONG, TAYMOR	1975	77	73.0	95.0
DIXON, BUTTRAM	1976	77	72.1	95.0
GLEZERMAN	1981	230	69.5	86.5
Total		1690	53.0	78.8

Table 5. Pregnancy rates for artificial inseminations using *thawed freeze-stored donor semen*

Authors	Year	No. of patients	Pregnancy rate (%)	Insemination method
BEHRMAN, SAVADA	1966	28	42.9	?
STEINBERGER	1973	59	61.0	Pericervical
FRIEDMAN	1977	174	46.6	Intracervical + vaginal
MATTHEWS et al.	1979	133	54.0	Pericervical
Total		394	51.0	

Table 6. Cumulative distribution of pregnancy rates relative to number of insemination cycles for 129 pregnancies following artificial insemination using *thawed freeze-stored donor semen*

Authors	Year	Pregnancies	Pregnancy rate following	
			Three cycles (%)	Six cycles (%)
BEHRMAN, SAVADA	1966	12	66.6	97.2
STEINBERGER, SMITH	1973	36	46.8	83.3
FRIEDMAN	1977	81	58.0	85.0
Total		129	55.8	85.3

and to the donor, especially as far as inheritance rights and support claims are concerned. The state's courts and legislatures have generally ignored these issues, and only sporadically have the legal problems surrounding AID found their way into the courts. In Germany, at least until 1972, the law guaranteed to every individual the inviolable right to know the identity of his biologic father. Courts may thus require physicians who have performed AID to disclose the identity of the donor even decades after the insemination. From the legal point of view, the donor is then considered the biologic father, will have to support "his child" if necessary, and the child will be entitled to inherit from him just as hiw own legitimate children (HESS, 1972). On the other hand, if the donor should learn the identity of the child conceived by his sperm and this child should become wealthy, the donor may claim the right to be supported by or to inherit from "his" child. Thus, physicians who perform AID under these circumstances are extremely courageous. In the United States, the statutes of Georgia, Kansas, New York, North Carolina, Oklahoma, and Connecticut have established the legitimacy of the offspring resulting from AID. In other states, attempts are being made to clear the murky waters in regard to the legal aspects of AID. No court has stated that AID is illegal. For the time being, the physician performing AID should be well aware of the fact that husband, wife, child, and donor are all in a rather unsatisfactory position with regard to the law. The least one can do is to have both partners provide well-informed and written consent to the AID program.

Another important legal question is the birth certificate's validity concerning legitimacy. In many countries, birth certificates are documents stating fatherhood. In these cases, the physician who enters the name of the husband on the birth certificate, knowing that the baby has been born following AID, may be accused of falsifying records. AMELAR et al. (1977) reported on an English physician who has been charged with this offense and consequently jailed for 3 years. Actually, the real purpose of a birth certificate should be to establish citizenship and not paternity. In countries where this principle is not followed, it would be wise for the physician who has performed the successful insemination not to attend the birth of the baby (e.g., to sign a birth certificate).

Many legal aspects remain to be solved. It should be one of the goals of conscientious medicine to promote discussion and legislation to provide a sound basis from which help can be offered to desperate childless couples for whom other alternatives are closed.

C. Semen Preservation

Sperm storage is indicated whenever future availability of semen from a certain individual may be of importance but is questionable. When in 1866 MANTEGAZZA suggested for the first time the establishment of sperm banks, he had soldiers in mind who went to war and wanted to have their progeny guaranteed in case they would not return. The use of low temperatures for sperm storage was tempting ever since this idea was first proclaimed by SPALLANZANI almost a century earlier (1776). To date more than 1500 births have been reported worldwide that resulted from semen preserved by freezing (SHERMAN, 1977). Normal infants were born from semen stored for longer than 10 years (SHERMAN, 1973). It has been stressed (SHERMAN, 1977) that fewer abnormalities and abortions occurred in pregnancies after insemination with thawed frozen semen than in the normal population. Indications for semen storage are numerous:

1. The main indication for cryobanking today is probably the collection and preservation of donor semen. The main problem of artificial donor insemination, i.e., the coordination between donor and patient, may thus be solved, semen of the same donor can be used for further pregnancies, and availability of seminal specimens from a large group of donors facilitates matching. Frozen semen can be banked centrally and transported great distances, making artificial donor insemination more easily available. Comparing fresh and frozen semen for artificial insemination, the former is definitely more effective (STEINBERGER and SMITH, 1973). Following thawing, frozen semen exhibits reduced motility by some 20% with all freezing and thawing techniques used. Pregnancy rates achieved by thawed frozen semen are lower than with fresh semen. Still, the advantages of cryobanking should compensate for these drawbacks.
2. Men may want to store their semen before vasectomy or prostatectomy, in cases when radiation has to be applied for malignant disease and further fertility is jeopardized, and in situations in which their life is in danger and progeny is desired by the couple. However, patients should be informed that there is no method to predict how good a given semen sample will respond to cryoinjury (BECK and SILVERSTEIN, 1975). It is good practice to perform some freezing trials before cryobanking is offered to individuals for semen preservation.
3. Cryobanking may be of some value in storing, pooling, and concentrating oligospermic normokinetic semen for subsequent homologous insemination.
4. ALEXANDER and KAY (1977) have reported that cryobanking decreases the presence of certain surface antigens on spermatozoa. They stressed that cryobanking of semen may be useful if the female partner possesses high titers of antisperm antibodies.

The main handicap in freezing semen, as observed in early works, was poor spermatozoan motility after frozen semen had been thawed. In 1949, POLGE et al. suggested the addition of glycerol as a cryoprotective agent. Glycerol has since remained the basic agent for preventing cryoinjury, although a variety of other substances, such as egg yolk, glucose, sodium citrate, etc., have been added by different authors with various results. SHERMAN (1977) has pointed out that most semen samples are insensitive or only transitory sensitive to

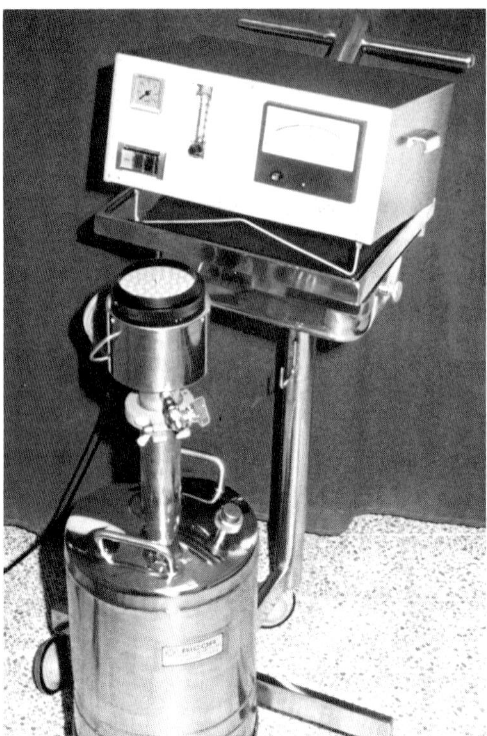

Fig. 2. Semiautomatic system for freezing and storage of semen in pellets (produced by Ricor Ltd., Ein Harod, Israel). A freezing chamber is connected to a pressurized liquid nitrogen container. Flow of refrigerant is manually controlled by a needle valve on the control panel enabling both rapid and slow freezing. The pellet freezing plate is interchangeable with a plate containing 12 slots to freeze straws. (Courtesy of Dr. BARKAY)

the osmotic changes introduced by the addition of glycerol prior to freezing, at least if stepwise addition of aliquots is employed. The mechanism by which glycerol protects spermatozoa from cryoinjury is only poorly understood. Probably salt buffering and membrane stabilization play a role, and glycerol may be important in modifying characteristics of ice formation (MERYMAN, 1966). Features of ice formation play an important role if procedures of freezing are evaluated. Very rapid freezing, as measured in degrees per second, is lethal to sperm cells. This is probably due to the fact that ultrarapid freezing reduces intracellular dehydration and favors formation of small and numerous nuclei of ice (SHERMAN, 1977). During lower rates of freezing, measured in degrees per minute ($1°$–$25°$ C), dehydration is greater and fewer, albeit larger ice crystals are formed. A very low storage temperature, i.e., $-196°$ C, seems to be better for sperm survival than dry ice temperature ($-75°$ to $-79°$ C) as far as recovery of motile cells is concerned. Thawing should be rapid according to MERYMAN (1966). SHERMAN (1963) and RUBIN et al. (1969), however, did not observe differences in motility or viability in semen samples thawed from $-75°$ C and from $-196°$ C at rates ranging $1°$–$60°$ C/min. SAWADA et al. (1967) even reported better oxygen consumption of sperm cells following slow thawing. Thus, it would be advisable for each sperm bank to experimentally evaluate different thawing procedures to reach their own conclusions. It appears that no agreement exists to date on the best method to freeze semen. Most centers use a rapid

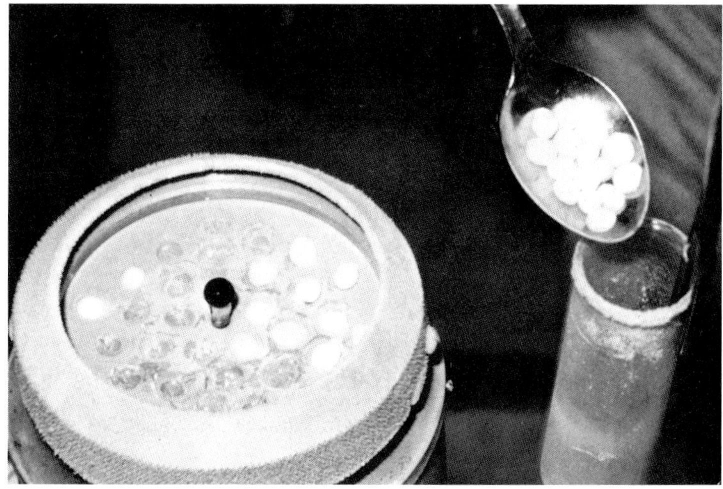

Fig. 3. Following freezing and pellet formation, these are removed with a spoon and transferred into a test tube containing liquid nitrogen. The test tube is then placed into the nitrogen container for storage. (Courtesy of Dr. BARKAY)

technique (PERLOFF et al., 1964). Plastic straws, vials, or glass ampuls containing the specimen are suspended over liquid nitrogen in such a manner that only vapor will contact the container. Within 15–30 min, a temperature of approximately $-80°$ C is achieved, and the semen containers are then submerged in liquid nitrogen for storage. This contact further reduces the temperature to $-196°$ C. BARKAY et al. (1974) and BARKAY and ZUCKERMAN (1978) have developed an apparatus that allows semiautomatic freezing of semen in pellet forms over vapor of nitrogen (Fig. 2). A mixture of semen with protective medium containing sodium nitrate, glycerol, egg yolk, and antibiotics is cooled to $5°$ C in a normal refrigerator and placed drop by drop into small impressions on a freezer plate. Vapor of liquid nitrogen tranforms these drops to pellets that are then removed and submerged in test tubes containing liquid nitrogen (Fig. 3). The test tubes are stored in a liquid nitrogen freezer at $-196°$ C.

The art of semen storage has made great progress in recent years. However, the medical community somehow still seems reluctant to accept the safety of frozen stored semen. Hopefully, large-scale studies of successful pregnancies will be available soon and may help to build confidence in this promising tool.

References

Alexander NJ, Kay R (1977) Antigenicity of frozen and fresh spermatozoa. Fertil Steril 28:1234

Amelar RD, Hotchkiss RS (1965) The split ejaculate: Its use in the management of male infertility. Fertil Steril 16:46

Amelar RD, Dubin L, Walsh PC (1977) Male infertility. Saunders, Philadelphia London Toronto

Asch RH, Balmaceda J, Pauerstein CJ (1977) Failure of seminal plasma to enter the uterus and oviducts of the rabbit following artificial insemination. Fertil Steril 28:671

Barkay J, Zuckerman H, Heiman M (1974) A new practical method of freezing and storing human sperm and a preliminary report on its use. Fertil Steril 25:399

Barkay J, Zuckerman H (1978) Further developed device for human sperm freezing by the twenty-minute method. Fertil Steril 29:304

Barwin BN (1974) Intrauterine insemination of husband's semen. J Reprod Fertil 36:101

Beck WW (1976) A critical look at the legal, ethical and technical aspects of artificial insemination. Fertil Steril 27:1

Beck WW (1977) Artificial insemination. In: Hafez ESE (ed) Techniques of human andrology. Elsevier/North Holland Biomedical Press, Amsterdam New York Oxford, p 421

Beck WW Silverstein I (1975) Variable motility recovery of spermatozoa following freeze preservation. Fertil Steril 26:863

Behrman SJ (1959) Artificial insemination. Fertil Steril 10:248

Behrman SJ (1968) Techniques of artificial insemination. In: Behrman SJ Kistner RW (eds) Progress in infertility. Little Brown, Boston, p 720

Behrman SJ, Sawada Y (1966) Heterologous and homologuous inseminations with human semen frozen and stored in a liquid nitrogen refrigerator. Fertil Steril 17:457

Bernstein D, Glezerman M, Insler V (1981) Intrauterine Insemination in infertility due to cervical factor. Isr. J Med Sci (in press)

Chong AP, Taymor ML (1975) Sixteen years experience with therapeutic donor insemination. Fertil Steril 26:791

Cognat M, Guillard M (1973) La spermatocele veineux pour aplasie congenitale du deferent. Caus d'echec et étude critique – A propos d'une statistique personelle de sept cas. Andrologie 5:37

Dixon RE, Buttram VC (1976) Artificial insemination using donor semen: A review of 171 cases. Fertil Steril 27:130

Dmowski WP, Gaynor L, Lawrence M, Rao R, Scommegna A (1979) Artificial insemination homologuous with oligospermic semen separated on albumin columns. Fertil Steril 31:58

Farris EJ, Murphy PD (1960) Characteristics of the two parts of the partioned ejaculate and the advantages of its use for intrauterine insemination. Fertil Steril 11:465

Friedman S (1977) Artificial donor insemination with frozen human semen. Fertil Steril 28:1230

Glezerman M (1981) 270 cases of artificial donor insemination. Management and Results. Fertil Steril 35:180

Glezerman M, Lunenfeld B (1976) Zur Therapie der männlichen Anorgasmie – ein Fallbericht. Aktuel Dermatol 2:167

Glezerman M, Lunenfeld B, Potashnik G, Oelsner G, Beer R (1976) Retrograde ejaculation: Pathophysiological aspects and report of two successfully treated cases. Fertil Steril 27:796

Glezermann M, Brook I, Potashnik G, Ben-Aderet N, Insler V (1980) Fertility pattern and reported pregnancies in 333 patients referred tro male infertility clinics. In: Proceedings of V.ESCO Venice. In: Fertility and Sterility. Salvadori B, Semm K, Vadora E (eds) Edizioni Internazionali. Rome p 495

Glezerman H, Bernstein D, Insler V (1982) Homologous intrauterine insemination as a treatment mode for infertility due to cervical factor. Fertil steril (in press)

Goss DA (1975) Current status of artificial insemination with donor semen. Am J Obstet Gynecol 122:246

Gregoire AT, Mayer RC (1965) The impregnators. Fertil Steril 16:130

Haman SJ (1959) Therapeutic donor insemination. Calif Med 90:130

Hess A (1972) Rechtsfragen der künstlichen Insemination. In: Deutscher Ärztekalender. Urban & Schwarzenberg, München Berlin Wien, p 670

Heuer D (1971) Die Portiokappe als therapeutische Möglichkeit bei Oligozoospermie des Mannes. In: Schirren C (ed) Fortschritte der Fertilitätsforschung, vol 2. Grosse, Berlin, p 128

Insler V, Melmed I, Eden E, Serr DM, Lunenfeld B (1972) The cervical score- a simple semiquantitative method for monitoring of the menstrual cycle. Int J Gynaecol Obstet 10:223

Insler V, Bernstein D, Glezerman M (1977) Diagnosis and classification of the cervical factor of infertility. In: Insler V, Bettendorf G (eds) The uterine cervix in reproduction. Thieme, Stuttgart, p 253

Insler V, Glezerman M, Zeidel L, Bernstein D, Misgav N (1980) Sperm storage in the human cervix – a quantitative study. Fertil Steril 33:288

Jennings RT, Dixon RE, Nettles JB (1977) The risks and prevention of Neisseria Gonorrhoeae transfer in fresh ejaculate donor insemination. Fertil Steril 28:554

Kaskarelis D, Comninos A (1959) Critical evaluation of homologuous artificial insemination. Int J Fertil 4:38

Mantegazza P (1866) Fisiologia sullo spermo umano. Rend Real Inst Lomb Sci Lett 3:183

Matthews CD, Broom TJ, Crawshaw KM, Hopkins RE, Kerin JFP, Svigos JM (1979) The influence of insemination timing and semen characteristics on the efficiency of a donor insemination program. Fertil Steril 31:45

Meryman HT (1966) Crybiology. Meryman HT (ed). Academic Press, New York

Moghissi KS, Gruber JS, Evans S, Yanez J (1977) Homologuous artificial insemination – a reappraisal. Am J Obstet Gynecol 129:909

Murphy DP, Torrano EF (1966) Donor insemination. A study of 112 women. Fertil Steril 17:273

Nijs P, Rouffa L (1977) AID couples: Psychological and psychopathological evaluation. Andrologia 7:187

Nunley WC, Kitchin JD, Thiajavajah S (1978) Homologuous insemination. Fertil Steril 30:510

Paulson JD, Polakoski KL (1978) The removal of extraneous material from the ejaculate. Int J Androl [Suppl] 1:163

Perez-Palaez M, Cohen MR (1965) Split ejaculate in homologuous insemination. Int J Fertil 10:25

Perloff WH, Steinberger E, Sherman JK (1964) Conception with human spermatozoa frozen by nitrogen vapor technique. Fertil Steril 15:501

Polge C, Smith AU, Parkes AS (1949) Revival of spermatozoa after vitrification and dehydration at low temperatures. Nature 164:666

Pommerenke WT (1946) Cycle changes in the physical and chemical properties of cervical mucus. Am J Obstet Gynecol 52:1023

Quinlivan WLG, Sullivan H (1977a) Spermatozoal antibodies in human seminal plasma as a cause for failed artificial donor insemination. Fertil Steril 28:1028

Quinlivan WLG, Sullivan H (1977b) The immunologic effect of husband's semen on donor spermatozoa during mixed insemination. Fertil Steril 28:448

Rubin SO, Andersson L, Bostrom K (1969) Deep freeze preservation of normal and pathologic human semen. Scand J Urol Nephrol 3:144

Russel JK (1960) Artificial insemination (husband) in the management of childlessness. Lancet II:1223

Sawada Y, Ackerman DR, Behrman SJ (1967) Motility and respiration of human spermatozoa after cooling to various low temperatures. Fertil Steril 18:775

Schill, WB (1975) Caffeine and kallikrein-induced stimulation of human sperm motility: A comparative study. Andrologia 7:229

Schoysmann R (1973) Commentaire sur la Revue par Cognat et Guillard. Andrologie 5:43

Semm K, Brandl E, Mettler L (1976) Vacuum insemination cap. In: Hafez, ESE (ed) Human semen and fertility regulation in men. Mosby, St Louis, p 439

Settlage DS, Motoshima M, Tredway R (1973) Sperm transport from the external cervical os to the fallopian tubes in women: A time and quantitation study. Fertil Steril 24:655

Sherman JK (1963) Improved methods of preservation of human spermatozoa by freezing and freeze-drying. Fertil Steril 14:49

Sherman JK (1973) Synopsis of the use of frozen human semen since 1964: State of the art of human semen banking. Fertil Steril 24:397

Sherman JK (1977) Cryopreservation of human semen. In: Hafez ESE (ed) Techniques of human andrology. Elsevier/North Holland Biomedical Press, Amsterdam New York Oxford, p 399

Spallanzani L (1776) Opuscoli di fisca. Animale e vegetabile. Opuscolo II. Osservazioni e sperienze intorno ai vermicelli spermatici dell'Uomo e degli animali. Moderna

Speichinger JP, Mattox JH (1976) Homologuous artificial insemination and oligospermia. Fertil Steril 27:135

Steiman RP, Taymor ML (1977) Artificial insemination homologuous and its role in the management of infertility. Fertil Steril 28:146

Steinberger E, Smith KD (1973) Artificial insemination with fresh or frozen semen. JAMA 223:778

Taylor PL, Kelly RW (1974) 19-OH E prostaglandins as the major prostaglandin of human semen. Nature 250:665

Taymor ML (1978) Infertility. Grune & Stratton, New York San Francisco London

Tekavcic K (1974) A study of couple's destiny after AID compared with childless couples. (Abstr.), 8th World Congress of Fertility and Sterility, Buenos Aires, 1974

Wagenknecht LV (1976) Modern trends of surgical treatment in male infertility: Alloplastic spermatocele in cases of excretory azoospermia. Eur Urol 2:37

Warner MP (1974) Artificial insemination, review after 32 years experience. NY State J Med 74:2358

Weller J (1976) Ergebnisse und Erfahrungen mit der artifiziellen Maritogenen Insemination als Möglichkeit der Behandlung steriler Ehen. Zentralbl Gynaekol 98:51

White RM, Glass RH (1976) Intrauterine insemination with husband's semen. Obstet Gynecol 47:119

Whitelaw MJ (1950) Use of the cervical cap to increase fertility in cases of oligospermia. Fertil Steril 1:33

Whitelaw MJ (1974) Observations on 1000 consecutive AID patients. (Abstr.), 8th World Congress on Fertility and Sterility, Buenos Aires, 1974

Male Contraception

J. Frick

With 17 Figures

A. Introduction

During the last 20 years research in the field of contraception, or the application of contraceptive methods, has been almost exclusively limited to the female reproductive tract. Only very recently has consideration been given to the question as to whether the male might also be included in the study of this problem.

There is now renewed interest in methods that involve the male, primarily by interfering with sperm production or development or by blocking the path of the sperm.

Male fertility control methods currently available are:

1. Coitus interruptus
2. Condom
3. Vasectomy.

Prospective new male fertility control methods under clinical investigation are:

1. Improved condoms
2. Improved vasectomy
3. Reversible vas occlusion
4. Pharmacologic male contraception.

It is envisaged that fertility control by these new methods will be achieved by way of

1. Control of the hypothalamus
2. Control of the pituitary gland
3. Negative feedback mechanism
4. Suppression of spermatogenesis
5. Maturation arrest of the sperm in the epididymis
6. Obstruction of sperm transport through the vas deferens
7. Manipulation of the biochemistry of the seminal fluid.

Work on direct influences on the hypothalamus and the pituitary gland through antireleasing hormones is certainly not yet sufficiently advanced for male contraceptive measures to be expected from it within the foreseeable future. For women, however, a method of this kind can perhaps be expected during the next few years. So far the retardation of glandular function, and especially of thyroid function, has been successful only in an indirect way.

The maturation process of the sperm in the epididymis and also the elimination and maintenance of sperm depend on the interaction of proteins, intact enzyme systems, and normal electrolyte conditions. No direct method of suppressing the maturation of the sperm locally in the individual segments of the epididymis has yet been worked out. Since, however, the epididymis (like the other subordinate glands of the male genital tract) is a target organ for certain steroids, especially the male and female sex hormones and the progestins, it is possible to influence the maturation process indirectly.

α-Chlorohydrin, for example, and certain alkalyzing substances that are used for medical tumor therapy also suppress on maturation. As we know from many experiments on animals, especially on rats, however, these drugs have a number of serious side effects, so that on the whole they cannot be used for this purpose.

According to current opinion, to achieve a suppression of fertility, azoospermia, i.e., complete arrest of spermiogenesis, is required. Extreme oligospermia of the seminal fluid has so far proved insufficient, even though we know that this greatly reduces the possibility of insemination.

On the basis of our present knowledge, the possibilities of contraceptive measures for men are still meager and are limited to two, or at the most three, points of the reproductive tract where action might be taken. These are:

1. The *suppression of spermiogenesis* through retardation of the pituitary gland or a direct effect on testicular function;
2. *Prevention of the flow of spermatic fluid* through the vas deferens.

With regard to 1, steroids, be they androgens, estrogens, or progestins, are capable of producing varied effects on the testicles. This depends upon the nature of the substances and the dosage. In brief, there are two possibilities of steroid action on spermatogenesis:

a) an improvement of spermatogenesis, e.g. in the case of subfertile patients through the administration of androgens and
b) suppression of spermiogenesis through the administration of estrogens or progestins.

In the following part of this chapter only a few branches of the whole problem can be discussed. Perhaps the near future will disclose to us new possibilities, e.g. through the influencing of partial functions of the hypothalamus and of the pituitary gland through the administration of subunits of an anti-releasing hormone. Up to the present however the combination of a progestin with testosterone has seemed to us be the ideal therapy. The progestin has the task of suppressing spermiogenesis. Since however through the solitary administration of this substance the function of the Leydig cells would also be suppressed and consequently the man who only gets progestins would forfeit his male behaviour to certain degree, the male gonadal hormone exogenously provided compensates for the loss of androgen, that is to say, libido and potency remain normal. The individual hormones can be administered orally, intramuscularly or in the form of subcutaneous implants.

B. The Need for Fertility Control

Whether one's perspective is limited to the personal effects of high fertility on individuals or its aggregate effects on nations and the world community, it seems evident that reduced fertility levels are a desirable, even urgent, objective. Some degree of decline in the birth rate would be expected as a consequence of social progress. But in many nations and subgroups within nations, high fertility itself retards social progress. If fertility could be reduced at the same time as other social developments were being pursued, this would have a multiplier effect on the overall process. In a direct attempt at reducing fertility levels, many nations have instituted national programs to educate individuals about the importance of fertility regulation for their own well-being and to give them greater access to existing contraceptive technology. Because the existing technology has many limitations, however, research is also under way in many countries, directed at new and improved techniques for fertility regulation.

It is important to recognize that these two approaches are entirely complementary and indeed, that both are necessary. A considerable decline in the birth rate would be expected to result from more vigorous family planning programs that distributed the current technology more efficiently throughout the world. At the same time, new methods, particularly those better adapted to mass application in nations lacking sufficient health resources, would make a great difference to the worldwide effort. At any level of motivation in fertility control, more effective and acceptable methods suitable for less costly and sophisticated delivery systems would increase the effectiveness of fertility control and the magnitude of the reduction in birth rate.

Current fertility control methods can conveniently be classified as conventional contraceptives (diaphragms, condoms, foams, creams, and so on), hormonal contraceptives, intrauterine devices (IUDs), and voluntary sterilization. Oral contraceptives and current IUDs are entirely the result of research on reproduction, which has also yielded important improvements in procedures.

These technological changes in the last 15 years have brought about a "contraceptive revolution" (RYDER and WESTOFF, 1971) in industrial nations with long histories of contraceptive practice, and were major stimulants for the initiation of family planning programs in developing nations in which fertility control was either minimal or dependent on folk methods.

There have been several attempts to induce infertility in men by taking advantage of the negative feedback regulation of gonadotropin release. The capacity of excess testosterone to lower plasma gonadotropin levels has been clearly established (LEE et al., 1972; SHERINS and LORIAUX, 1973), and the suppression of luteinizing hormone (LH) is more pronounced than that of follicle-stimulating hormone (FSH). Thus it was logical to expect that the administration of excess testosterone might suppress the release of LH, resulting in inhibition of spermatogenesis due to inadequate peritubular concentrations of testosterone. This expectation was borne out. The administration of testosterone proprionate daily or testosterone enanthate weekly resulted in infertility without suppression of libido or potency (HELLER et al., 1950a, b; MACLEOD, 1965; REDDY and RAO, 1972). Although the feasibility of this approach to fertility control has been demonstrated, it has not been actively pursued because the high dosage of testosterone required results in changes in lipoprotein metabolism and blood cell formation that might make long-term maintenance on this regime unsafe.

A synthetic derivative of ethynyl testosterone, danazol, appears to act directly upon the Leydig cells to suppress their steroidogenesis, and results in diminished sperm counts with no marked decrease in libido (SHERINS et al., 1971). Preliminary clinical trials have been carried out with danazol combined with small doses of testosterone, in the belief that they might act synergistically in the suppression of spermatogenesis. Sperm counts fell to infertile levels in 2 months, while normal libido was maintained (SKOGLUND and PAULSEN, 1973). The conclusion of SKOGLUND and PAULSEN that danazol plus some form of testosterone may prove to be a safe, effective contraceptive for men is not widely shared, but the principle underlying this approach is certainly deserving of further exploration.

Suppression of gonadotropins can also be achieved by administration of the female hormones, i.e., estrogens or progestogens. The administration of estrogens alone to men resulted in infertility but was accompanied by loss of both libido and potency, and was complicated by painful gynecomastia. Progestogens were also effective but had the same undesirable side effects (HELLER et al., 1959).

More promising results have been obtained in recent studies in which progestogens and testosterone have been used in various combinations in the hope of achieving synergism in gonadotropin suppression while avoiding both loss of libido and gynecomastia. Implants of Silastic capsules containing testosterone and others containing synthetic progestogens (norgestrienone or norethindrone) inhibited spermatogenesis for several months without depressing sexual drive or potency (COUTINHO and MELO, 1973; FRICK and BARTSCH, 1973; JOHANSSON and NYGREN, 1973). Fertility returned upon cessation of the medication.

C. Different Methods of Male Fertility Control

I. Coitus Interruptus

At least since biblical times, men have employed the technique of rapid withdrawal of the penis at the time of imminent ejaculation during coitus and deposition of the semen outside the vagina. In western and northern Europe during the Middle Ages and early modern times, when relatively late marriages co-existed with close and frequent contacts between unmarried adults and where pregnancy out of wedlock was strongly condemmed, coitus interruptus appears to have been the principal method for averting the consequences of premarital intercourse.

The lowest reported effectiveness rate, 23 pregnancies per 100 users per year, compares well with the lowest use–effectiveness rates of other contraceptive methods, with the exception of the most effective methods, the IUD and contraceptives containing steroid hormones. No effectiveness rates are available for the intermittent use of coitus interruptus as an adjunct to some other method, such as the diaphragm or temperature rhythm, although this practice is common.

Whether coitus interruptus can be practiced with complete effectiveness or not is uncertain, since it is known that even before ejaculation the penis frequently discharges a small amount of fluid, which may contain small numbers of sperm. It is certain that pregnancy can occur if withdrawal occurs too late and even part of the semen has been ejaculated into the vagina.

Accidental deposition of the semen on the external genitalia of the woman can also result in pregnancy if some of the seminal fluid finds its way into the vagina. Consequently, the margin for error is small, and the practice of coitus interruptus, especially on a routine basis, requires very high motivation on the part of both partners.

1. Side Effects

Historically, a wide variety of gynecologic, urologic, neurological, and psychiatric disorders have been attributed to the practice of coitus interruptus, but no objective data exist to justify these claims of side effects. MASTERS and JOHNSON have demonstrated that a progression of complex physiologic changes, from early excitation through plateau and orgasm to final resolution, occurs in the female during normal coitus, and these findings have led to new speculation that coitus interruptus might result in observable physiologic consequences in women if orgasm is prematurely abridged by this form of contraception on a regular basis. As with concerns that had been voiced earlier about consequences for male sexual performance or urologic function, thus far these speculations remain unstudied and undocumented. Of course, where there are preexisting sexual disorders, such as impotence or frigidity, a complex relationship between the etiology and maintenance of the disorder and the contraceptive method used by the couple is quite common. However, many couples practice this method for years without apparent ill effects or lack of sexual satisfaction for either partner.

The method requires no supplies and no particular preparation; it costs nothing.

The successful practice of coitus interruptus makes great demands on the self-control of the male; some men are physically or emotionally unable to use the method.

2. Extent of Use

Because of its simplicity and freedom from side effects, coitus interruptus remains an important contraceptive method in many countries. It was the primary contraceptive method used in Hungary according to surveys in 1965 and 1970: 62% and 53% of all users, respectively, used this method. In Teheran, 66% of survey respondents claimed some prior practice of fertility control, and for 52% of these the method used was coitus interruptus. In Great Britain and Wales, 20% of all contraceptive users rely on withdrawal, as determined by a 1970 national survey. In contrast, however, the use of coitus interruptus in the United States has been declining for several decades, and only 2% of those practicing contraception used this method exclusively by 1970. Its occasional practice as an adjunct to other methods, however, remains quite common.

In recent years, with increasing liberalization of sexual mores and practices, alternative techniques for achieving male orgasm and ejaculation outside the vagina appear to have become more common, at least in some developed countries. However, the prevalence with which these practices are applied for contraceptive purposes is unknown.

II. Condom

The condom, an elastic sheath that covers the penis during coitus, made its first appearance in England during the eighteenth century. Early condoms were made from the intestines of sheep and other animals. Rubber condoms were introduced in the latter part of the nineteenth century.

Modern condoms are available in a variety of shapes, colors, sizes, and materials, often with elaborate packaging. However, only two of these characteristics significantly influence the effectiveness of the condom: the thickness of its wall, and the material from which it is made; both of these features are related to the strength, and hence the effectiveness, of the condom, and to the physical sensations that the user and his partner experience.

Color, size, and shape, including shapes designed to increase friction during coitus, are believed to have primarily, and perhaps solely, a psychological impact. Most condoms are manufactured with a lubricating substance on the outer surface for purpose of facilitating coitus. All condoms are packed as tightly-rolled rings that have to be placed on the glans penis and then unrolled over the shaft of the erect penis prior to intromission at the time of coitus.

Most current condoms are manufactured from latex rubber, although condoms made from lamb intestines are also manufactured and sold, primarily in the United States. Condoms are available without prescription from pharmacies in almost every country in the world and, in many cases, from other commercial outlets and family planning clinics as well. In Japan, the country where condom use is the most extensive, visiting saleswomen offer condom products to housewives in their homes. Mail order condoms are popular in many countries. Skin condoms cost about twice as much as latex rubber condoms, but reportedly allow for greater sensitivity during intercourse. Previously, because of the inconvenience associated with washing and, especially, the potential for rupture of the latex, a new condom was used for each ejaculation. Recently, however, reuse of latex condoms has started to become more common in some parts of the world.

Most modern condoms meet national standards designed to minimize the possibility of rupture or leakage due to pinholes. The standards generally lay down requirements regarding the additives used in manufacture of the condoms; stipulations as to dimensions and wall thickness; and stated detection procedures and quality control standards for pinholes, overall strength, tensile strength, and aging. Standards vary widely from country to country. (Some countries have no standards at all, and a growing effort is under way to promote the universal adoption of a set of international standards established by the International Standardization Organization.) In general, however, most condoms manufactured today have a less than 1% chance of being defective, as judged by the standards employed. The quality control procedures and standards for skin condoms are not as rigorous as those for latex rubber condoms.

Exactly how these standards relate to the effectiveness of condoms when they are used for contraception is not known. If condoms are used correctly and consistently, so that all contraceptive failures are limited to those resulting from rupture of the device, almost complete effectiveness may be attained under conditions of general use by highly motivated couples. More commonly, however, use–effectiveness rates in studies of large populations have been in the range of 10–18 pregnancies per 100 couples per year. At least two studies have demonstrated that effectiveness is much higher among couples who plan to have no further children than among so-called spacing families. In one of these studies, it was also observed that among young women who have not yet had children, the condom is used with a much greater effectiveness (1 pregnancy per 100 couples per year) than among those with one or two children (5 pregnancies per 100 couples per year). In this study, which was conducted between 1968 and 1974 in Great Britain, neither social background nor age (for women below age 35) was found to affect the efficacy with which condoms were used.

1. Failure Rate

Pregnancy may result from a break or tear, estimated in one study to occur once in 150–300 instances of use. More commonly, contraceptive failures during condom use result from escape of the ejaculated semen from the condom if withdrawal of the penis is delayed until after detumesence. Most commonly of all, however, pregnancy is due to failure to use the device at each ejaculation. The risk of pregnancy associated with a single unprotected coitus, enjoyed at random during the menstrual cycle, is in the order of 2%–4%, which is higher than the risk of pregnancy observed in some studies during a full year of consistent use of the condom.

2. Side Effects

Side effects are extremely rare with the condom; an occasional individual may be sensitive to latex rubber or to the powder used for dusting the condom. Indeed, if sexual contact is never engaged in without the use of a condom, the transmission of venereal disease from one partner to another can be prevented.

Based on a low estimate of use–effectiveness, 13 pregnancies per 100 couples per year, the risk-to-benefit ratio associated with condom use in developed countries is about 0.6 deaths (all resulting from accidental pregnancies) per 10,000 births averted. Because of higher maternal mortality, the ratio would be higher in developing countries, approximately nine deaths (all maternal) per 10,000 births averted.

Condoms can be used by couples from all socioeconomic backgrounds and educational levels with moderately to very high use–effectiveness. They offer protection against infection with venereal disease and can be used in almost any situation where coitus is possible. The evidence immediately after intercourse of an intact contraceptive barrier gives reassurance. Because of their freedom from any pharmacologic mode of action, side effects are virtually nonexistent.

Condoms have received interest from family planning personnel in recent years. In India, for example, over 1 million condom users have been recruited in response to a multimillion dollar marketing and distribution program.

This 1 million represents 2.6% of all Indian couples practicing contraception. The extent of condom use in other developing countries varies widely from a few percent to 19% in Iran.

In developed countries, condom use makes up a very significant proportion of all contraceptive usage. In the United States, condom use has fallen off sharply following the introduction of oral contraceptives, but it still stands at 14%, about half the former level. Condom usage in Hungary is at the same level, but even higher proportions of couples who practice birth control use the condom in Sweden (38%) and Great Britain (28%). The condom has its highest degree of popularity in Japan, where an estimated 50%–60% of couples use this method.

III. Vasectomy

1. General Comments

Vasectomy or male sterilization has recently emerged as one of the simplest, most popular, and most readily available forms of voluntary family planning. In the Asian subcontinent the number of vasectomies has exceeded that of female sterilizations and/or IUD insertions for several years. It is estimated that 6 million vasectomies were performed in India alone in the years from 1968 through 1972. In Pakistan, Bangladesh, and Nepal, male sterilizations exceed female sterilizations. Men in Latin America and Arab countries are also showing considerable interest in the procedure whenever it is available.

Vasectomy has become increasingly popular in developed countries during the last few years. Spurred on by publicity on the hazards of various female methods of fertility control, family men throughout the world have discovered that this simple, single-occasion procedure can spare their wives the inconvenience of IUDs or daily pills, not to mention the more complicated female sterilization.

Vasectomy, performed on healthy, psychologically well-adjusted men, does not significantly affect male hormonal balance, sexual desire, capacity for erection, or ejaculation of semen. The operation involves the cutting or blocking of each vas deferens, the two tubes that carry sperm from the testes to the penis. Through a small incision in the scrotum, the surgeon cuts, ties, coagulates, and/or clips the vasa. Local anesthesia is commonly used. After resting briefly from the 10- to 15-min procedure, the patient walks out of the office, clinic, or mobile unit.

Vasectomy provides some advantages that no other birth control method can offer. It is:

Effective, as a single procedure that eliminates the need to buy and use contraceptives
Safe, involving only slight morbidity and almost no mortality
Simple, requiring minimal extra training for most physicians
Short, taking only 10–15 min
Convenient, since only local anesthesia is required
Inexpensive compared with female sterilization, which requires more extensive surgery and equipment
Culturally acceptable in many countries, expecially where the man makes the crucial decisions on sexual activity or reproduction
Culturally preferable in countries where women hesitate to go to a male doctor and female doctors and paramedics are scarce.

On the other hand, vasectomy also presents certain obvious disadvantages, for example:

Surgery is required
There are occasional complications, such as bleeding or infection
Vasectomy does not provide full protection until sperm already stored in the reproductive system are ejaculated (a matter of days, weeks or months)
It is not suitable for men who desire children at a future date, because in most cases it is not reversible
Psychological problems related to sexual behavior may be aggravated by any operation involving the male reproductive system
For men who equate masculinity with the ability to make a woman pregnant, vasectomy holds little appeal.

While vasectomy is increasing in popularity among couples who have all the children they want, current research on male fertility control is focusing on simpler techniques and reversibility. Among the new developments being tested are clips, electrocautery, plugs, valves, and chemicals.

Vasectomy, a simple procedure designed to block the passage of sperm through the vas deferens, was not understood until the nineteenth century and was not performed as a method of voluntary fertility control until the twentieth century. It is clearly different from castration, a form of sterilization that eliminates the production of male hormones through removal or impairment of the testes.

Traditionally, castration was performed on persons selected to serve as court eunuchs, in certain religious orders, or as punishment. There is no place for castration in modern voluntary fertility control programs. Some physicians even object to application of the term "sterilization" to vasectomy, because the testes and germ cells are left intact. "Vas occlusion" or "surgical birth control" have been suggested instead.

An early reference to vas occlusion was made by the English surgeon and anatomist JOHN HUNTER in 1775. While performing a dissection, HUNTER noted an obstructed vas deferens in the cadaver on which he was working. In 1830 HUNTER's student, Sir ASTLEY COOPER, began experimental work on vasectomy. Using dogs, he ligated the artery and vein of the spermatic cord on one side without touching the vas; on the opposite side, he ligated the vas itself. On the side where the artery and vein were obstructed, the testis became gangrenous. On the side where only the vas was obstructed, the tissue remained healthy and sperm survived in the ductal tract up to the point of ligation. The epididymis, or convoluted portion of the vas, gradually enlarged to accommodate the sperm.

In 1883 Felix Guyon, a French surgeon, concluded that blocking the vas caused atrophy of the prostate gland (cited by Yhaver and Ohri, 1960). This finding encouraged genitourinary surgeons of the 1890s to perform vasectomies concurrently with prostate operations to reduce the size of the gland and to avoid postoperative epididymitis. One of the first such operations is credited to Dr. H.G. Lennander of Uppsala, Sweden, who in 1897 published a report on his technique (cited by Popenoe, 1934). Some surgeons still perform vasectomies in conjunction with prostate operations. Although with the procedure currently used the prostate is not found to shrink significantly, the incidence of postoperative epididymitis is reduced.

Dr. Harry Sharp of Indiana (USA) (1909), reported performing a vasectomy in 1899 on a mentally ill patient whose complaint was excessive masturbation. The patient consented to the operation, believing it would relieve his obsession. The results, undoubtedly psychological, were favorable. In the next ten years, Sharp performed 456 voluntary vasectomies on both healthy and institutionalized men for the purpose of sterilization.

In the early twentieth century, vasectomies were sometimes carried out for eugenic reasons on criminals, the mentally ill, the retarded, or those with hereditary diseases. Paradoxically, even as its contraceptive effects were being documented, the operation was performed by Eugene Steinach, an Austrian exile, for the purpose of overall bodily rejuvenation. From his experiments on rats, Steinach determined that following ligation of the vas the sperm-producing tissue degenerated, while at the same time there was hypertrophy of the hormone-producing tissue, which, in turn, caused renewed germ cell production. This process was originally thought to counter the effects of aging. Later, Steinach's hypothesis was refuted, but doctors and scientists continued to advocate the operation for contraceptive purposes.

As national family planning programs were initiated in South Asia in the 1950s and 1960s, vasectomy filled the obvious need for a simple, inexpensive birth control technique that could be offered on a single-treatment basis. Moreover, vasectomy could be offered by male doctors to male volunteers. This factor, plus a system of remuneration or incentives for canvassers, physicians, and volunteers, stimulated large-scale vasectomy programs.

Meanwhile, in the United States and Europe vasectomy received a major boost when adverse publicity about oral contraceptives coincided with a feminist campaign to encourage greater male responsibility in reproduction. In the United States, the number of vasectomies performed annually jumped from a quarter of a million in 1969 to three-quarters of a million in 1970 and 1971, and is now leveling off at about half a million.

Although the number of vasectomies performed throughout the world fluctuates from year to year, depending on publicity, national budgets, or program guidelines, the simple procedure of vasectomy has clearly taken its place as a major technique in voluntary family planning.

At present vasectomy is probably the most reliable method of controlling male fertility, and on this account it is the most frequently applied. It is one of the birth control methods widely used in the United States, Korea, India, Pakistan, and China. At the same time, however, in a great many other countries it is either not allowed or is not applied in practice. Among these countries are Sweden, Great Britain, Turkey, Mexico, Egypt, a number of Latin-American countries and a great many African States. Restrictive legislation and the legal aspects of the use of sterilization as a contraceptive method are being changed and manipulated in many countries in such a way that the use of vasectomy for family planning is increasing very significantly on a worldwide scale.

In 1976 LEE reported that in recent years more than 20 million men had voluntarily agreed to undergo vasectomy for the purpose of birth control. In India alone 12.5 million men, and in the United States more than 4 million, had this operation. This figure for America accounts for about 13% of married men.

In spite of this already extensive experience with vasectomy, the desirability of sterilization for the purpose of family planning should be carefully examined in each case, above all in order to keep the number of patients who may wish to have a reversal operation as low as possible.

2. Factors to be Considered Before Vasectomy is Performed

In principle, conventional vasectomy can be performed in about 15 min and causes only insignificant discomforts and risks for the patient. As a small operation, this is usually or very often performed on an outpatient basis and under local anesthesia. Before the operation is carried out however, two problems should be carefully clarified, namely (a) the question of reversibility, and (b) the frequency of sperm-immobilizing and sperm-agglutinating antibodies following vasectomy.

a) Reversibility

There is a definite possibility of reuniting the severed stumps of the spermatic duct, and the permeability rate after such operations is between 80% and 85%. Silber has already carried out reoperation of the vasa deferentia in a large number of patients (300), using a special microsurgical technique with the help of an operational microscope and an improved suture technique in which first of all the mucosa is approximated and then in a second layer the muscularis and the adventitia; and if Silber's results are taken into account, a permeability rate of practically 100% can be expected. The pregnancy rate after reanastomosis is lower, however. The figures given up to now in the literature fluctuate between 30% and 60%. Nevertheless, here too a considerable increase has been attained with the most recent findings of SILBER (1977). He has achieved a pregnancy rate of approximately 71% after vas–vas anastomosis. Furthermore, SILBER has shed new light on the significance of the small sperm granulomas in the region of the proximal stump of the vas deferens following vasectomy. Previously it was always believed that these sperm granulomas were a fundamental cause of the augmented development of sperm-agglutinating and sperm-immobilizing antibodies. In his patients, Silber was able to show that there is no significant connection between the occurrence of small sperm granulomas and the percentage occurrence of any sperm antibodies. Silber believes, however, that the occurrence of small sperm granulomas brings about a pressure compensation in the region of the proximal genital tract, i.e., above all in the epididymis, and that in such patients the presence of sperm granulomas after vasectomy, observed at the time of the vas–vas anastomosis, shows that a considerably better sperm quality is present, which makes the chance of restored fertility following the reuniting of the spermatic cord considerably higher.

b) Frequency of Sperm-Immobilizing and Sperm-Agglutinating Antibodies After Vasectomy

The data concerning the frequency of sperm-immobilizing and sperm-agglutinating antibodies in the literature vary widely from a few percent to about 50% of patients who have undergone sterilization operations; pronouncements about the extent of antibody titers are rarely possible. However, it should be emphasized once again that there is no clear correlation between the presence of such antibodies and restored fertility following the reanatomosis of the vasa deferentia, and that it is not at all certain whether there is any connection at all between these two phenomena.

The fact that sperm antibodies can be present in the blood of vasectomized patients has raised the question as to whether vasectomy could not also be the cause of immunity diseases in some of these patients. Up to now a number of extensive and painstakingly controlled studies have not proved the presence of any such immunity disease. Such long-term prospective studies on monkeys and people will be continued.

3. Information to be Given to Patients and Preliminary Examinations

In our opinion vasoligation should not be performed in men whose families do not yet contain, say, two children, unless there are genuine medical reasons, such as hereditary diseases, the endangering of the life of the wife in case of pregnancy, etc. As to the question of vasectomy on juveniles for reasons of genitic indications, it is maintained that an interdisciplinary opinion should be obtained prior to the operation. Before the operation it is essential to talk to both the husband and the wife and explain to them the entire range of contraceptive methods, and to weigh the advantages and disadvantages of the individual techniques.

The patient should receive precise information about the operation: just what is to take place, how long it will last, possible side effects, how he should behave after the vasectomy, and the possibility of a reanastomosis. Furthermore, men planning to have vasectomies should be informed that sterilization has nothing to do with castration. These two terms are often confused. In the case of a carefully performed ligature of the spermatic duct there is no change at all in the libido or the patient's sexual behavior. This operation causes no disturbance in hormone production but merely stops the passage of sperm from the epididymis into the posterior urethra.

A preoperative sperm examination and postoperative semen analyses until azoospermia is established seem indispensable. The time between ligature of the spermatic duct and the absence of sperm in the accessory glands of the male genital apparatus varies; it can be as long as 10–12 weeks, even if the seminal vessels and the ampulla are irrigated with saline or some other substance during the operation.

4. Surgical Technique

Ligation of the spermatic duct is carried out under either a local anesthetic or a brief general anesthetic through two small scrotal incisions. The incisions should preferably be made near the scrotal root and the vas deferens should be mobilized as little as possible, so that the blood supply is not disturbed and so that in case a reanastomosis should be carried out later, conditions for this corrective surgery are favorable.

A section 1.5–2 cm in length is resected from each vas deferens. The stumps are sutured and ligated with a purse-string ligature of 3-0 atraumatic silk. The proximal stump is then coated with tunica vaginalis in order to prevent spontaneous reanastomosis as far as possible. The ligature of the stumps of the spermatic duct should be carefully tightened after the puncture so as not to cause necrosis on the vas deferens or necessitate cutting through of the ligature. If the formation of a necrosis on the proximal stump of the vas deferens or cutting through of the ligature is followed by an extravasation of sperm it is quite probable that a large sperm granuloma will develop at this point and that spontaneous reanastomosis will take place.

It has repeatedly been maintained that the different techniques for vasectomy are in approximately direct proportion to the number of surgeons carrying out such operations. From this it follows that there are many very different methods, with slight variations for the sterilization operation on men, all of which, however, have approximately the same rate of complications. Only the methods that run counter to the generally accepted principles of surgery and to nature involve, understandably, a considerably higher frequency of complications, which are often irreparable, i.e., restoration of fertility is rarely or never possible in such cases.

5. Complications

Complications can be divided into immediate postoperative complications and those that arise later on. Wound infections and hematoma formation are among the immediate postoperative complications. The formation of sperm granulomas and spontaneous reanastomosis are later complications, which arise up to 3 months following the operation.

There is already a great deal of information in the literature on complications in vasectomized patients. Wound infections occur in approximately 2.5% of patients, and hematoma arises in 0.4%–4.2%. Spontaneous reanastomosis occurs in less than 0.5% and when the technique described is followed precisely this percentage is considerably lower. Sperm granulomas have formed in approximately 2%–5.6% of patients subjected to this operation. The rates reported for all complications, serious and trivial, that occur in connection with vasectomy vary very widely, from less than one complication in 1000 operations up to 122 in 1000 operations. The average complication rate in some 25000 vasectomies is approximately 47 complications per 1000 operations. Hematoma forma-

Table 1. Plasma testosterone levels after vasectomy.
(Frick, 1978, unpublished)

No. of patients	Months after vasectomy	Mean T levels (ng/ml)
7	2	4.3
17	3	4.5
7	5–6	4.7

tion, infections, and epididymitis make up the vast majority of complications. The next most frequent complication is sperm granuloma, formating either shortly after the operation or a long time afterwards. Such cases are best treated on an outpatient basis.

6. Side Effects

As mentioned at the beginning, side effects are minimal, if not entirely negligible. In the case of a carefully performed severance of the spermatic duct, no change in the androgen production takes place, since the blood supply of the testis is not impaired. This should ensure normal male sexual behavior (Table 1). It is nevertheless possible, albeit very rarely, for men to develop a so-called sterilization neurosis following vasectomy and to complain of a loss of potency and libido and also of a change in male sexual behavior. The treatment of such a neurosis usually requires a great deal of empathy, tact, and understanding, and in many cases the interdisciplinary cooperation of an experienced psychotherapist.

In the first few postoperative weeks, in some 30%–40% of vasectomized patients there is swelling in the area of the epididymis and slight pain is caused by the congestion of the epididymis with spermatozoa, since there is no continuous drainage. This situation, however, is relatively quickly mitigated as soon as the supply and the catabolism mechanisms in the epididymis have adjusted.

In conclusion, it is maintained that vesectomy is a sure, simple, very effective, and also economical method, which provides constant protection after a single operation lasting some 15 min. Even though failure rates and side effects of varying intensity after vasectomy are repeatedly reported, on the basis of his own experience and results and of painstakingly prepared result analyses in the literature, the author maintains that the complication rates, when there is exact observance of surgical details and most meticulous performance of the operation, with all necessary precautions, can be kept as low as possible. In any case, so far, vasectomy still constitutes the safest method of family planning so far as men are concerned.

IV. New Concepts in Vas Occlusion and Vasectomy

An alternative approach that has been intensively pursued is the development of valves, clips, or plugs that can be used for reversible occlusion of the vasa

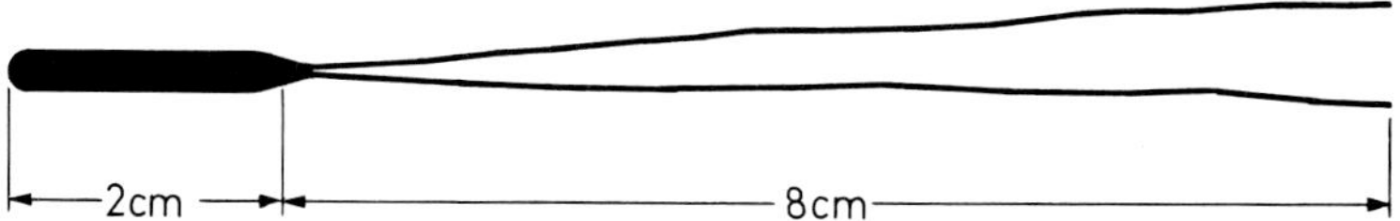

Fig. 1. Measurements of the nylon thread (no. 5, 3, or 1) used by LEE for vas occlusion. Nylon 6-0 thread is used to keep the occluding thread in place

deferentia. Such devices would achieve sterility by blocking the passage of sperm through the vas deferens in the same manner as conventional vasectomy. Reversal would be accomplished by removal of the clip or plug or, with a valve device, by switching into the "open" mode. A wide variety of devices of these different kinds have been developed and tested, mainly in animals, but so far none has proven suitable.

Efforts have also been made recently to develop simple techniques for temporary ligature of the spermatic duct. We too have endeavored to develop such a method. Other research groups have attempted to achieve temporary occlusion of the vas deferens by the insertion of occluding threadlike material or by the interposition of small plastic tubes to immobilize the sperm during passage through the plastic material. Furthermore, temporary occlusion is being attempted by the use of plastic valves inserted into the vasa deferentia, which can be turned off and on. Nevertheless hardly any of these studies have so far progressed beyond the stage of animal testing.

A few of these newly developed methods of fertility control in the male are discussed below.

1. Occlusion by a Filament

For many years Lee inserted nylon- or silicone-covered silk thread into the vas to occlude it (Figs. 1 and 2). These filaments permit both insertion and removal of the intravasal thread (IVT) without cutting the vas.

a) Procedure for Insertion

The IVT is inserted as follows: a single medial incision is made in the scrotum and a 4-cm section of each vas is exposed. A needle with thread attached is inserted into the vas. While the central portion of the thread fully blocks the lumen of the vas, the filaments are tied externally round the vas, tightly enough to keep the IVT in place but not so tightly as to cut through.

b) Clinical Studies

Lee has conducted studies with IVTs in a total of 216 men. The device was placed in the vas under a local anesthetic; a single (3–4 cm) scrotal incision was used.

Semen specimens in 195 cases contained no sperm (or fewer than 7 million/ml) 24 days after the operation or following three ejaculations. In 21 cases sperm reappeared in the ejaculate in amounts of 30.7 million/ml approximately

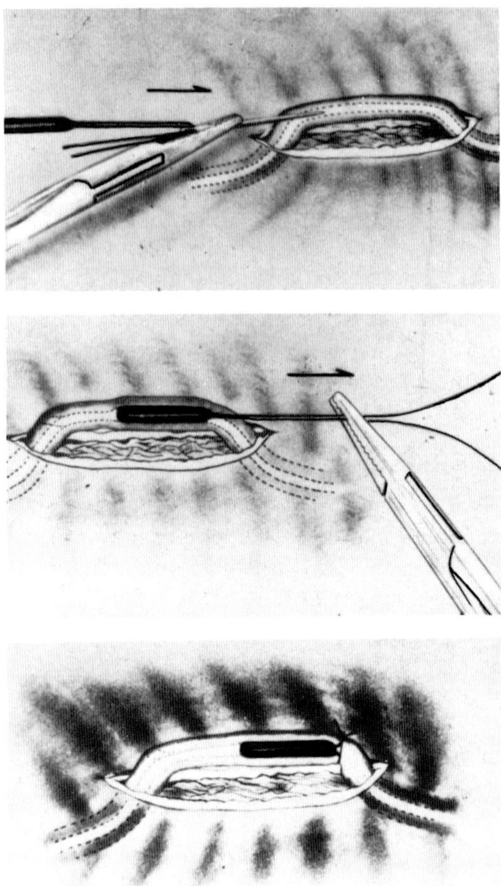

Fig. 2. The three different steps in insertion and fixation of the nylon thread

31 days after the previous azoospermic state. Six men whose ejaculates contained more than 60 million sperm/ml underwent further surgery. In four of these six cases, sperm had passed through the dilated lumen of the vas with the IVT in situ. It is possible that the vasal dilatation resulted from increased intravasal pressure caused by deposition or stasis of continued sperm production attributable to an imbalance between spermatogenesis and spermatolysis. In the other two cases, the distal end of the IVT had penetrated the vasal wall at one side and was almost protruding through the lumen. Thus, the IVT did not function as a plug in these cases. The normal course of the vas was found to be markedly distorted at the site of penetration; this might be attributable to extensive fibrotic contracture of surrounding tissues after insertion of the IVT. If it was close to the original aperture through which it had been inserted, the distal end of the IVT might erode and penetrate the vasal wall.

To reverse the procedure, the vas was exposed in the same manner as for insertion of the IVT. The thread was removed from the vas by cutting and pulling the filiform nylon thread with a pair of mosquito forceps.

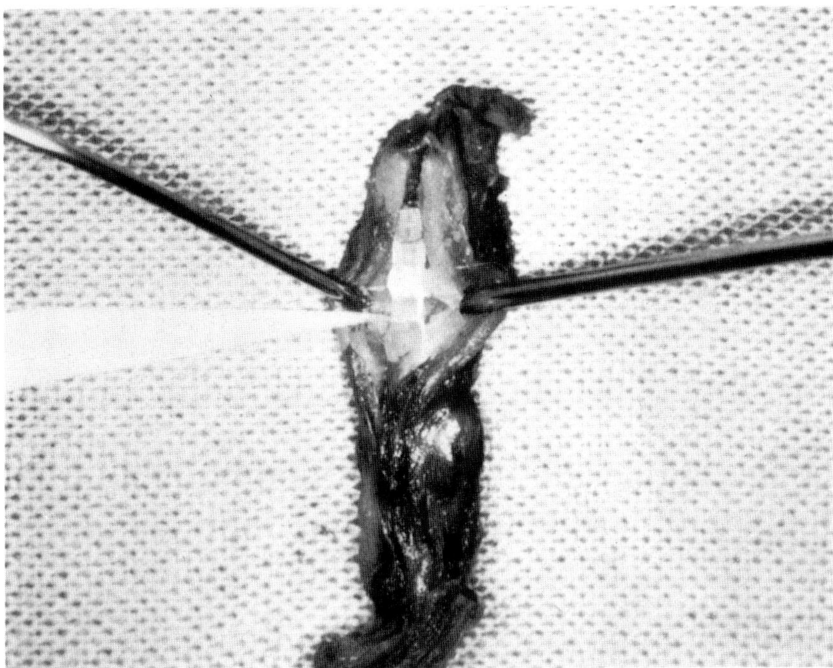

Fig. 3. Brodie's propylene device in the opened vas lumen of a rabbit 3 months after insertion (from present author's own experience)

Eight volunteers were studied as to reversibility about 5 months after the IVT had been inserted; their semen had been azoospermic about 1 month after the insertion. About 1 month after removal of the IVT, semen specimens from seven of the eight men contained an average count of 54 million viable sperm/ml. This indicates that vasal patency can be restored properly and satisfactorily. In the remaining case, marked vasal fibrosis was noted and the vas was divided accidentally during the surgery for removal of the IVT.

2. Reversible Intravasal Device (R-IVD)

A second method of occlusion, developed by Brodie in New York, is insertion into the vas of a bead-like strand of propylene 1 cm long (Fig. 3).

After administering a local anesthetic and incising the scrotum, the surgeon slits the exposed vas horizontally. The vas lumen is then dilated by a special probe scored at 1.5 mm. The propylene device is inserted 2–3 cm into the vas, beginning with the smallest bead, which is 0.7 mm in diameter, and ending with the largest bead, which has a diameter of approximately 1.4 mm. At this stage, the surgeon places Prolene ligatures between the third and fourth beads and then between the fourth and fifth beads to secure the device. The nonbeaded portion (approximately 1 cm) is then cut off, leaving the beaded portion (about 1 cm) inside the vas. The vas incision and then the scrotal incision are closed with Prolene ligatures.

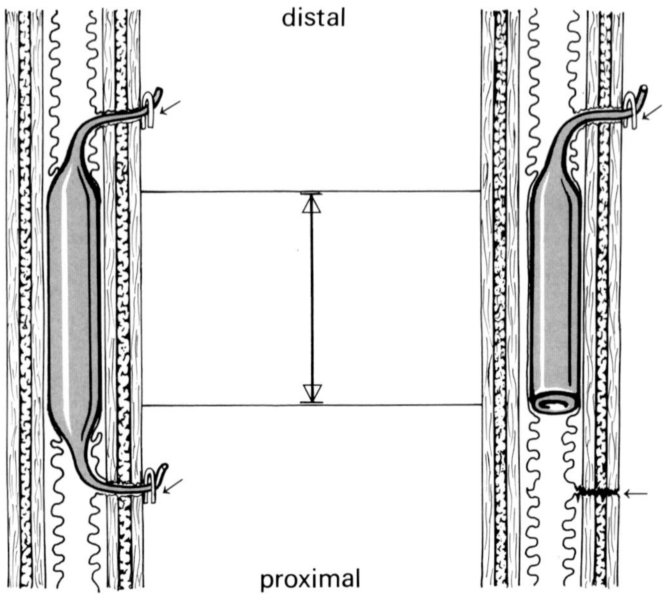

Fig. 4. Schematic drawing of plastic device used by Moon and Bunges for reversible vas occlusion in the lumen of the vas deferens, secured with silver clips (*small arrows*). *Long arrow* indicates point of insertion. The distal ends are at the top of the drawing

Thus far, the R-IVD has not proven sufficiently effective for general use. It has a 20% failure rate. In some experiments, the device has caused excessive scarring or eroded through the vas wall. Reversibility has also not been adequately tested. However, a modified R-IVD or similar device may hold promise.

3. Plugging of the Vas

Moon and Bunge have developed a method for temporary occlusion of the vas that is based on mechanical obstruction such as blockage of a portion of the vas with minimum damage. Fertility is restored on removal of the plugging material.

This technique was carried out in 13 adult male dogs; all the animals had been proved to be normospermic before surgery.

a) Technique

General anesthesia is applied before the scrotal skin is prepared. The ductus deferens is palpated through the right scrotal sac and brought to just below the skin surface by digital pressure. Two towel forceps are then applied around the vas.

A small incision is made over the ductus deferens between the two clips, and the tissue over the ductus is separated by blunt dissection. The ductus is isolated with as little impairment as possible of its vascular supply. When the distal portion of the exposed ductus is stretched digitally, a translucent

Table 2. Semen analyses in dogs after insertion and after removal of a vasal plugging device.[a] (NOON and BUNGE, 1972)

Dog no.	Weeks after insertion			Weeks after removal		
	2	3	4	2	3	4
1	−	−	−	+	+ +	+ +
2	−	−	−	+	+ +	+ +
3	−	−	−	+ +	+ +	+ +
4	−	−	−	+	+ +	+ +
5	−	−	−	+	+ +	+ +
6	−	−	−	+	+ +	+ +
7	−	−	−	+	+ +	+ +
8	−	−	−	+ +	+ +	+ +
9	−	−	−	+ +	+ +	+ +
10	+ +	+ +	+ +			
11	−	−	−	+ +	+ +	+ +
12	−	−	−	+ +	+ +	+ +
13	−	−	−	+ +	+ +	+ +

[a] +, less than 10 sperm in high-power field; + +, more than 10 sperm in high-power field; −, no sperm in high-power field.

whitish streak appears; this is the lumen. A straight needle carrying the device is inserted into the lumen. Both ends of the device, which are out side the ductus, are clamped with silver clips (Fig. 4). The clips prevent movement of the device in the vasal lumen and also act as markers for identification at the time of removal. The same procedure is applied to the left ductus deferens, and the incision is then closed.

b) Results

As shown in Table 2, consistent azoospermic conditions were obtained in 12 of the 13 dogs 2, 3, and 4 weeks after the insertion of devices. One case, in which azoospermia was not attained, was shown to have had an incomplete occlusion in the right ductus, with motile sperm beyond the occluded area. In addition, the occluded area was only 1 cm long. Complete occlusion in the left ductus was proved by the absence of sperm beyond the occluded area and was also demonstrated by the injection of indigo dye. The length of this occluded area was 3 cm. Therefore, it is apparent that nonocclusion of the right ductus was the cause of failure.

4. Reversible Intravasal Occlusive Device (RIOD)

A reversible intravasal device has been developed by Free (Fig. 5) and tested in animal studies with guinea-pigs, rabbits, and rhesus monkeys. The reversible intravasal occlusive device (RIOD) is easily and cheaply produced. It can be inserted in the vas with a minimum of disturbance to blood, nerve, lymph, and muscle continuity, it permits tissue in-growth, and it is flexible. Pore sizes of 20–150 are obtained in the surface of ethylene vinyl acetate tubing by generat-

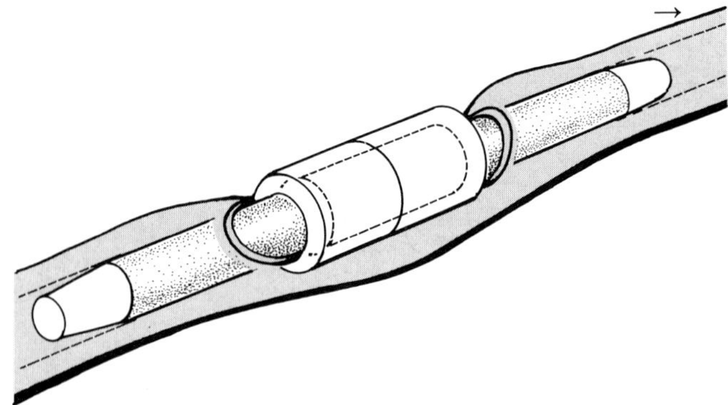

Fig. 5. Schematic drawing of the RIOD (Free) in place in the vas deferens (*arrow*)

ing bubbles during the molding process, and these are subsequently broken open by means of abrasives. More recent versions of the RIOD have used polyurethane in place of ethylene vinyl acetate; these have an outside diameter of 0.8–1.0 mm and an inside diameter of 0.5–0.7 mm. Normal sperm counts have been achieved in rabbits with this device installed in the open mode. The RIOD is reversed through surgical intervention by replacement of each blocking plug with a patent insert (Free, 1975).

Initial testing of this device in human beings has already started, but it is too early to say anything about effectiveness, side effects, or safety.

5. Spermatozoa Controller (SPACER)

Another flexible device system, the spermatozoa controller (SPACER), has been devloped by Brueschke. This system has been implanted in 60 dogs, which are ejaculated weekly. The success rate is said to be very high.

The body of the device is fabricated entirely of medical-grade silicone rubber, and is specially molded to incorporate a mechanism for reversible occlusion of the path of sperm (Fig. 6). The valve mechanism consists of a stainless steel shuttle stem that occludes the lumen of the device when it is depressed into the valve body. Two flanges are attached at each end of the body of the device, and these are reinforced with Dacron mesh to act as suture rings. Material for tissue in-growth (Dacron velour) is also applied to these rings and makes direct contact with the cross-sectional area of the transected vas. The in-growth surface thus provided has proved to be highly effective, and sperm leakage has never been observed. Flexible polot tubes (0.6 mm outside diameter, 0.3 mm inside diameter) of silicone rubber extend 4 mm beyond the flanges and are inserted into the exposed lumen at the transected end of the vas without removal of the epithelium. Four simple individual sutures are used to attach the vas end to the suture ring. Sutureless implant techniques have been studied, and one method employing a barbed clamp has been used successfully to attach the device to the vas end.

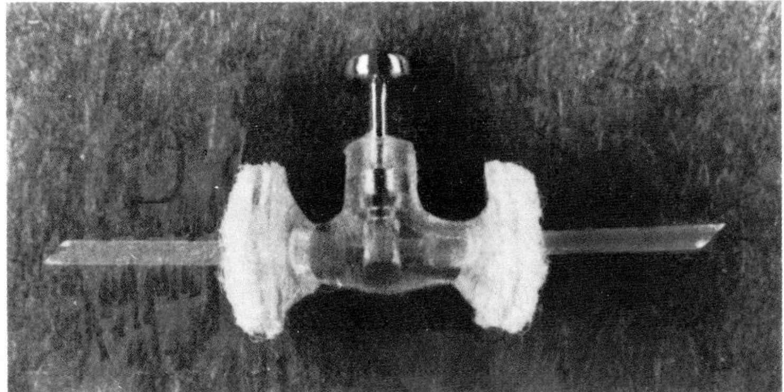

Fig. 6. BRUESCHKE's spermatozoa controller system (SPACER)

Table 3. Sperm counts in human ejaculates (10^6/ml) following a single injection in each vas deferens of 0.25 ml 90% ethanol and 3.6% formaldehyde. (COFFEY and FREEMAN, 1975)

Patient	Weeks after single injection									
	0	4	8	12	16	20	24	28	32	39
D.D.	28			0		0			0	0
K.H.	40	0	0		0	0		0		
R.K.	45	<1		<1	<1		0	0		
R.W.	64	15		20	<1	0	0	0		
W.H.	40	70		65	67					
H.M.	160	25		0	0					
J.R.	60	<1		<1	0					
H.P.	54	1.5		0						

6. Injection of Sclerosing Chemicals

Even greater simplification of the vasectomy procedure would be achieved if surgical opening of the scrotum to locate the vas deferens could be avoided. Both animal and clinical studies have been conducted by COFFEY and FREEMAN (1975) to evaluate a procedure for direct injection of a sclerosing chemical into the wall and lumen of the vas deferens through the scrotum. In the human studies a local anesthetic injection precedes injection of the sclerosing agent, but no incision or sutures are required. A solution of formaldehyde in ethanol has been tested for its ability to cause permanent occlusion of the vas deferens by this technique, and it has been effective in the limited number of cases studied so far (Table 3).

7. A Possible Reversible Vasectomy Procedure (Frick)

a) Technique

The basic idea of the technique suggested for reversible vasectomy is to form a loop of the vas deferens and to occlude the lumen by placing two

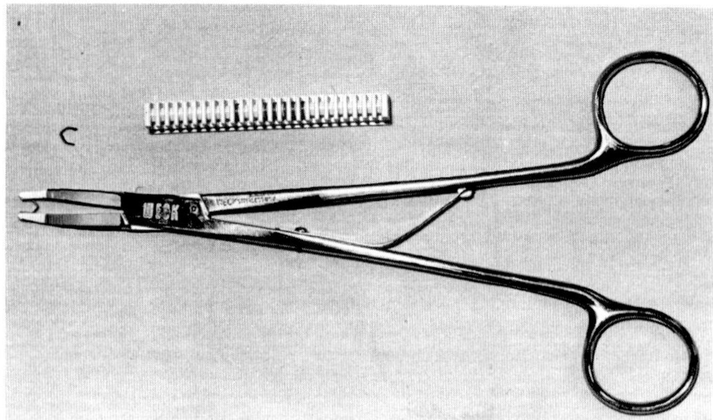

Fig. 7. The medium-size tantalum clips (Weck Company, Long Island, New York) and the clip holder

tantalum clips 3–4 mm below the loop of 2–3 mm apart (Fig. 7). This technique has been studied in rats, rabbits, and men in the reproductive age group and also in a group of men over 60 in whom prostatectomy was being performed. In animals, the effectiveness of the method was proven by vasograms after clip fixation and clip removal. In the younger men regular spermiograms were taken until azoospermia occurred 8–10 weeks after the operation. In the older age group, vasograms were also done after clip fixation to demonstrate the vas occlusion and the restored patency when the clips were removed after different periods.

A special clip holder (Fig. 7) was used to apply two tantalum clips (Weck Company, Long Island, New York), normally to the outside of the vas about 2–3 mm apart (Fig. 8); small clips were used for animals, and medium-size clips for humans. The scrotal incision was closed with one 3-0 chromatic catgut suture.

b) Results

In rats and rabbits, spermatocele formation at the site of the clips was frequently observed. In semen samples from regions above and below the site of occlusion there was separation of sperm heads from tails. Incomplete closure of one or both vasa was observed in 9 of 19 rats. Infections due to hematoma formation were also seen at the clip sites in about half the animals.

Mating tests were carried out in five rats after vas occlusion. There were no pregnancies in this group, whereas there were pregnancies in the control group. Three months after vas occlusion, the clips were removed. The animals were again placed with sexually mature female rats, and one pregnancy occurred.

In the older men, the vas occlusion was performed at the same time as suprapubic or transurethral prostatectomy. To determine the effectiveness and reversibility of the method and the damage caused by the clips, vasograms were performed at different intervals and histologic sections of the vas were studied.

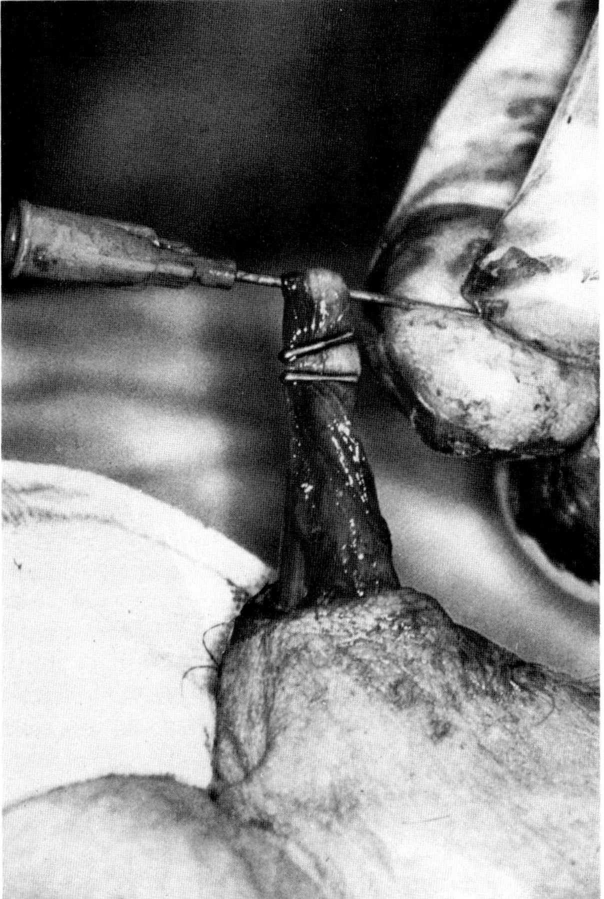

Fig. 8. Exposed human vas, formed into a loop and the clips in place

In the 36 younger men requesting vasectomy, this method of vas occlusion produced azoospermia in 80% between 3 and 8 weeks after surgery. None of these men has subsequently asked to have the clips removed.

The other 20%, in whom azoospermia was not attained, were vasectomized. Almost all these patients had developed sperm granulomas of different sizes, which may account for the failure of vas occlusion. In a few cases, it was found that the clips had opened slightly at the branches. This may have been due to postoperative edema. After a few weeks, any swelling of this kind would subside, leaving ill-fitting clips.

V. Pharmacologic Male Contraception

Ever since the development of oral contraceptives for women, there have ben efforts to identify suitable drugs for inhibition of fertility in the male.

The drugs known to suppress the production of sperm by the testis include a variety of antimetabolic agents and steroid hormones. The antimetabolic agents cannot be considered serious contraceptive possibilities due to their general systemic toxicity. At appropriate dose levels, estrogens, progestins, androgens, and antiandrogens block the production of sperm, probably by interfering with the availability of testosterone in the testis.

Estrogens are among the most potent agents for this purpose; but it is known that long-term administration of estrogens to men can cause breast enlargement, loss of libido, and an increase in thromboembolic disease. Nonetheless, limited clinical investigations are being conducted, in which these problems are minimized by using very low doses of estrogens in association with testosterone. The preliminary results of these clinical studies have been promising: suppression of sperm production has been achieved without evident side effects.

However, it is likely that the toxicity with long-term administration estrogens will discourage any vigorous development of this approach.

Progestins are less potent inhibitors of spermatogenesis than estrogens; but because there is no evidence linking them with an increased incidence of cardiovascular disease they have been much more widely tested in men. So far it has been established that sperm production can be suppressed with progestins supplemented by androgens while normal levels of plasma testosterone, are maintained, and that this procedure is readily reversible. Current research seeks to identify effective dosages of suitable combinations that can be administered as monthly injections or daily pills without an unacceptable level of side effects. One regimen of monthly injections of Depo-Provera and testosterone enanthate has yielded encouraging results.

Testosterone itself is known to inhibit sperm production in men if given in sufficiently high doses. Frequent IM injections are required, however, and there is concern about health hazards (cardiovascular problems in particular) over the long term with the high doses required. As a potential means of reducing the toxicity, some work has been done with orally active steroids that are less androgenic than testosterone. A common finding to date has been only partial effectiveness with the relatively high doses of the anabolic agents studied.

1. Steroidal Effects on Spermatogenesis

a) Orally Administered Steroids

The field of pharmacology of male reproduction is too large for everything to be summarized in one short paper. We shall attempt to condense some of our knowledge concerning steroidal compounds that affect the testis or its function.

In general, the steroidal compounds studied in the field of testicular function have been examined for their effects on fertility, testicular histology, endocrinology, and testicular biochemistry.

Most natural and synthetic androgenic compounds also act as inhibitors of pituitary gonadotropins, but they may also stimulate spermatogenesis in the absence of gonadotropic hormones.

As long ago as 1933, WALSH et al. found that spermatogenesis was maintained with crude preparations of androgens in hypophysectomized rats. Many other groups have confirmed that this occurs in rats, mice, monkeys, and fish.

Severe and extensive damage has been observed in the testes of several species following administration of estrogen (E), e.g., prevention of testicular descent, testicular atrophy, and inhibition of spermatogenesis.

All these effects of in vivo estrogen treatment on the testis can be explained by changes in gonadotropin levels. Estrogen and, with a similar mode of action, progestins can have a direct effect on the testicular function, but it is very difficult to differentiate between indirect and direct effects.

Steroidal compounds can produce different effects on spermatogenesis in men, depending on the nature of the compound and on the dosage regimen. There are two possible steroidal effects on spermatogenesis:

1. Improvement of the spermatogenesis, e.g., in subfertile men by administration of androgens
2. Inhibition of sperm production by the administration of E, estrogens, progesterone-like substances, or even high doses of testosterone (T).

At the beginning of this chapter it should be stated that we still do not have a practicable and ready method for male contraception by administration of one of the multiple steroids. There are many studies under way but the final outcome is not yet clear.

The data available so far strongly suggest that significant suppression of spermatogenesis can be induced with doses of 200 mg testosterone enanthate (TE) IM at weekly intervals, that 7–10 days might be an appropriate induction period, and that the necessary maintenance dose is in the order of 200 mg every 10–12 days to reduce the sperm count to highly depressed levels, bearing in mind that this does not include complete suppression of spermatogenesis.

Further, there is hardly any information on the relationship between the dosages of testosterone (T) used and the daily production rate; however, there is no doubt that information on the pharmokinetics of the androgens becoming increasingly important.

A second possibility being considered for male contraception is a combination of an E with T or of a progestogen with T. But the type combination and the appropriate dosage are still not clear. In these combinations the progestogen is intended to act as an inhibitor of sperm production, and the exogenous T to compensate for androgen loss – this normally causes decreased libido and potency – resulting from Leydig cell suppression.

b) Steroid Implants

In some of the regimens mentioned below, the T substitution was achieved by the insertion of Silastic implants filled with T. The pharmokinetic problems of these implants will be discussed in Section C.V.1.b)α).

α) Mode of Action of Implants

Steroids diffuse steadily through polydimethyl-siloxane (PDS) membranes (Silastic, Dow Corning Corp.) into various media at a relatively constant, low

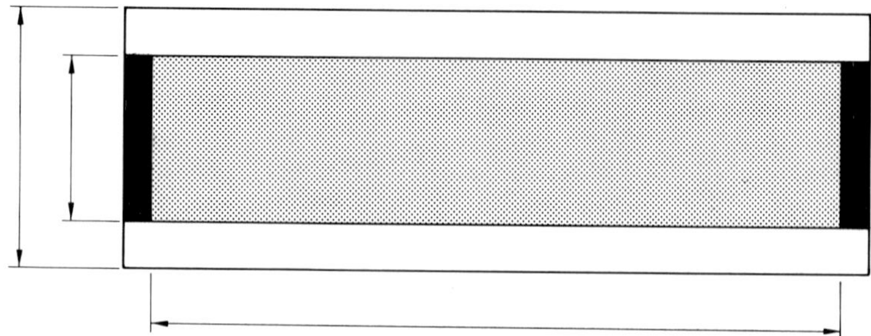

Fig. 9. Measurements of the standard Silastic capsule for subdermal implantation. *Vertical bars* represent 2.41 mm (*left*) and 1.58 mm, and *horizontal bar*, 20 mm. Surface area is 150 mm². □, Silastic tubing; ▣, steroid; ■, medical adhesive

rate. Subcutaneous implantation of PDS capsules filled with dry, crystalline hormone assures a good constancy of hormonal supply to the organism over fairly long periods. As this results in an optimal steadiness of hormone concentration at the site of action, the steroid is utilized more efficiently and its biologic effectiveness increased. The necessary dosage chosen for an attempted therapeutic effect can therefore be lower than with conventional administration. Above all, this therapy depends hardly at all on cooperation from the patient.

The pharmacokinetic principles of this mode of hormone administration have been well established in numerous in vitro and in vivo investigations, primarily by authors interested in long-term contraception in the female.

The releasing factor, i.e., the amount of steroid released from the capsule within a certain time, is in proportion to the surface area of the PDS capsule and in indirect proportion to its thickness. It is dependent on the molecular structure of the hormone administered, and therefore shows considerable differences among the various steroids.

To ensure comparable conditions, we use only one size of PDS capsule. Figure 9 gives the measurements of this standard capsule. Different dosage regimens are attained by varying the number of capsules implanted. A standard capsule of 20 mm length, with membrane thickness ~0.8 mm, and surface area about 150 mm² was used. Capsules filled with dry crystalline T (22–23 mg/capsule) have a release rate of 55 µg/capsule/24 h. The release rate of one testosterone proprionate capsule is 200 µg/24 h.

The usual implantation site is the right submammillary region (Fig. 10). There is well-developed subcutaneous tissue in this area, and a low level of mechanical irritation. In the case of accidental overdosage or change of therapy the capsules can easily be removed. A constant implantation site considerably facilitates retrieval of implanted capsules.

Table 4 gives the pharmacologic data for our standard PDS capsule and the two steroids we use most frequently, ethynylestradiol (E₂) (Merck Co., Darmstadt, FRG No. 3658) and T (Merck Co., Darmstadt, FRG Nr. 24615). The data were calculated from our results, all obtained in vivo in the human male in a gravimetric investigation of the contents of capsules that had been impanted for different periods. Identification of the contents of these retrieved

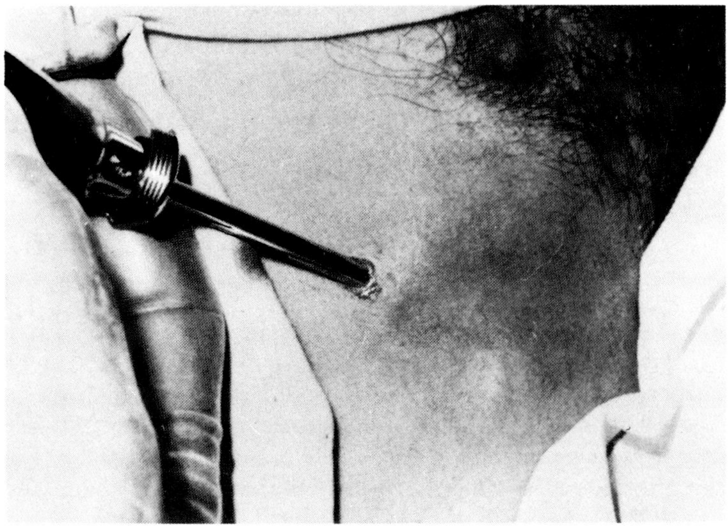

Fig. 10. Region most commonly used for implantation of Silastic implants: right sub-mammillary area

Table 4. Data relating to single standard Silastic capsules for implantation

Drug	Steroid content (mg)	Release rate (μg/24 h)	Duration of effect
Ethynylestradiol	22–23	45	17 months
Testosterone	21–23	70	13 months

capsules by thin-layer chromatography proves that the steroid remains unchanged in its chemical structure during implantation. Steady-state conditions and a relatively constant releasing factor are achieved with most steroids within the first 10 days after implantation, apparently after subsidence of local inflammatory and posttraumatic reactions.

In the last 9 years, we have implanted PDS capsules in about 500 patients, in many repeatedly. Only once have we seen local infection and a purulent discharge from a capsule. There have been no other undue side effects or complications. Patients who had previously had oral or parenteral long-term hormonal treatment considered this kind of hormone administration a definite alleviation of their therapeutic burden.

c) Other Pharmacologic Methods of Sperm Suppression

During the last decade a number of groups have tried to introduce methods of male contraception, and the relevant data will be summarized in the next section. This section, however, makes no pretence of completeness, and should be considered more as a cross-section of the studies pertaining to these problems.

Table 5. Effect of testosterone enanthate (TE) on sperm concentration during the first 6 months of drug administration. (PAULSEN et al., 1978)

Dosage	Oligospermia		Azoospermia	
TE 200 mg/week (I, II)	39/42	(93%)	20/42	(48%)
TE 200 mg/2 weeks (III)	13/20	(65%)	6/20	(30%)

α) Testosterone and Synthetic Analogs

PAULSEN et al. (1978) used TE as a possible male contraceptive. Three dosage regimens of TE were used for this purpose. Group I received 200 mg TE/week IM until azoospermia was achieved or 6 months had elapsed (whichever was earlier), then 200 mg TE/month. Group II received 200 mg TE/week until azoospermia was achieved or 6 months had passed, then 400 mg TE/month; and Group III received 200 mg TE every other week throughout the period of drug exposure.

Monthly physical examinations were performed on each volunteer throughout the study. In addition, monthly determinations of serum LH, FSH, and T levels, routine toxicology, urinalysis and lipid profiles, and bi-weekly seminal fluid analyses were performed during all phases of the study. Periodic serial sera sampling for determination of LH "spinking" patterns were performed in nine men.

Preliminary data indicate that TE administered at a dosage of 200 mg weekly induced severe oligospermia or azoospermia in 93% of the volunteers and the subsequent monthly "spacing" regimens of 200 mg or 400 mg may not be sufficient to maintain these low sperm concentration levels for an optimum period (PAULSEN et al., 1978).

Table 5 shows the effect of TE on sperm density in Groups I and II combined and in Group III during the first 6 months of drug administration. In Groups I and II, 39 of 42 men (93%) achieved pronounced oligospermia (sperm density < 5.0 million/ml). Of these 39 men, 20 (39%) achieved azoospermia. The regimen for Group III was less effective. Only 13 of these 20 men (65%) achieved pronounced oligospermia, and 6 of these 13, i.e., 30% of the total group, became azoospermic.

SWERDLOFF et al. (1978) have also been working with TE as a possible male contraceptive. They administered TE 39 adult men (aged 21–39) by IM injection. Of these, 17 men (Group A) received 200 mg TE/week over 16–20 weeks. In 16 of the 17, sperm counts were lowered to < 5 million/ml; 9 of the 17 became azoospermatic. Group B (22 men) received 200 mg TE every second week. In 10 of the 22 sperm density was > 5 million/ml at 16 weeks (5 of the 22 were azoospermatic). When those with a sperm density of > 5 million/ml were switched to weekly treatment (for a further 3–16 weeks), 9 of the 12 then had a sperm density of < 5 million/ml. Overall, 19 of the 22 men in Group B attained this level.

Plasma LH and FSH levels were decreased with both regimens. These effects were dose-related. Serum levels of T were higher than control values (64%)

Table 6. Sperm count after administration of 200 mg each week or every second week for different periods. (SWERDLOFF et al., 1978)

No. of patients	Rx	Duration of therapy (weeks)	Sperm count $< 5-10^6$/ml	Azoospermia
17	200 mg/wk	16	8	9
		17–20	8	9
22	200 mg/2 wk	16	10	5
		17–32	16	6

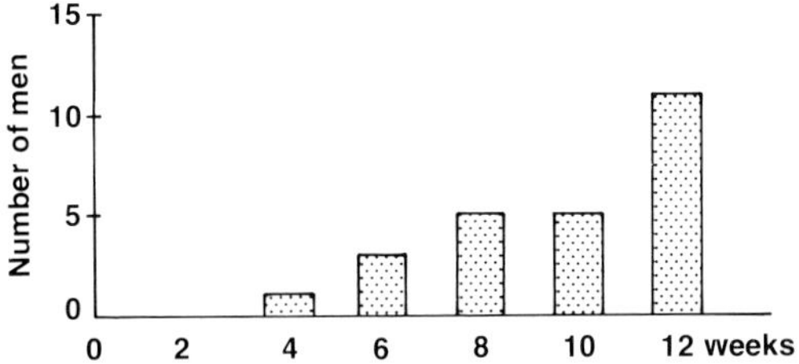

Fig. 11. Sperm density during weekly administration of 200 mg TE. The number of subjects with extreme oligospermia increases from the 4th to the 12th week of treatment. ▨, <1 million sperm per milliliter. (CUNNINGHAM et al., 1978 a)

in Group A, but basal levels were maintained in Group B. Decreasing the frequency of TE for 3 or 4 weeks resulted in a rebound of plasma LH and FSH levels above the baseline and increased sperm density. After discontinuation of the treatment, sperm density and hormone plasma values returned to normal.

Table 6 shows the sperm density in 39 patients treated with two different regimes of TE. In the group receiving 200 mg TE/week, 9 of 17 men showed azoospermia as little as 16 weeks after the treatment started. In the second group (200 mg TE every second week) only 5 of 22 were azoospermic after the initiation of therapy.

CUNNINGHAM et al. (1978a, b) have also used TE in a group of 20 healthy mean as a sperm suppressant. The treatment schedule was as follows: control period (10 weeks), induction/period (12 weeks), and maintenance period (30 weeks). Each individual received 200 mg TE/week IM during the induction period. After the induction period, 11 of the 20 had a sperm density of under 1 million/ml, but 3 of 20 had sperm counts of over >10 million/ml.

During the first 2 weeks of the induction period the plasma LH and FSH values were suppressed to very low or undetectable levels, but these levels rose again during the maintenance period, when the subjects received 200 mg TE by injection every 3 weeks. The mean sperm density remained suppressed, but only 25% of the treated men had sperm counts below 10 million/ml, and only one subject consistently had a sperm density below 1 million/ml after the 18th weeks of treatment.

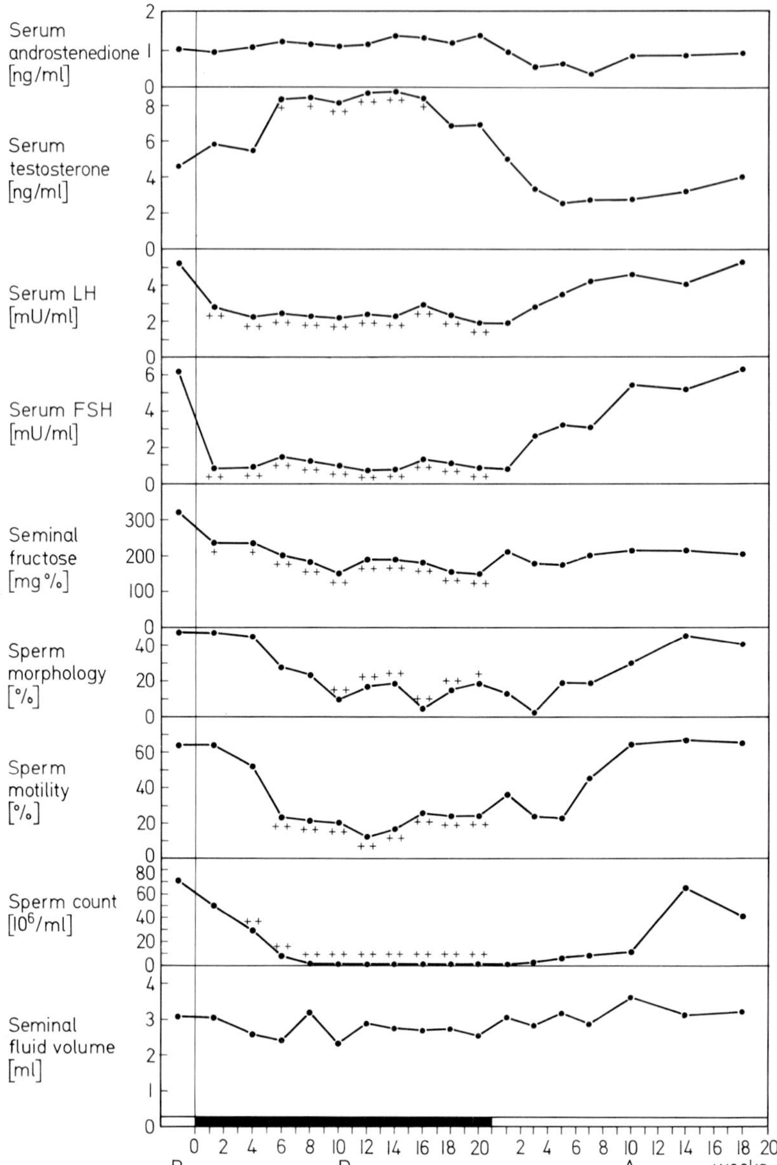

Fig. 12. Plasma levels of androstenedione, testosterone, LH, and FSH, and data on fructose, sperm morphology, motility, sperm density, and seminal fluid volume in seven healthy young men before (*B*), during (*D*), and after (*A*) treatment with 250 mg TE weekly over 20 weeks. ■, administration of TE; +, *P* < 0.05; + +, *P* < 0.01. (Mauss et al., 1978)

The authors conclude that

1. Weekly 200-mg injections of TE suppressed the concentrations of FSH and LH in serum to very low levels and induced azoospermia or pronounced oligospermia in most men, but the induction time varied and pronounced oligospermia had not been achieved in some men by the 12th week;
2. Suppressed concentrations of FSH and LH and severe oligospermia were not reliably maintained when 200 mg/TE was given every 3 weeks.

Figure 11 shows the sperm density during weekly administration of TE (200 mg/week). The number of men with pronounced oligospermia increased continuously from the 4th through the 12th week of treatment.

MAUSS and BÖRSCH (1978) treated seven healthy young men with TE for sperm suppression. The treatments schedule was 250 mg TE/week for 21 weeks.

Figure 12 summarizes the results obtained by these authors. The curves represent the mean values for plasma androstenedione, T, LH, FSH, seminal fructose, sperm morphology, sperm motility, sperm density, and seminal fluid volume.

STEINBERGER and SMITH (1978) have published several reports on their experiences on sperm suppression with TE. In one series (involving 21 healthy men) they gave the collected data of their findings on this subject. Only 16 of these 21 men ultimately ended the study. (One subject was excluded because of mild diabetes found during the screening period, and four men discontinued the treatment early in the study.)

The treatment schedule was as follows: During the induction phase: 200 mg TE twice a week for the first 2 weeks, then weekly for 2 weeks and then once every second week for 1 month. During the maintenance phase 200 mg TE was injected every third week. During the first phase the sperm density decreased to azoospermia of pronounced oligospermia ($< 100,000$/ml), gonadotropins became undetectable, and during the first month of treatment the plasma testosterone levels increased by 100% over the pretreatment mean concentrations. During the second phase (200 mg TE every 3 weeks) subjects showed a partial breakthrough of gonadotropins and sperm suppression. On the basis of these findings the time schedule of the 200-mg TE injections was changed insofar as the drug was then administered every second week. But this schedule also failed to maintain azoospermia or even pronounced oligospermia in a sufficiently high percentage of cases, so that 200 mg TE was then administered every 10–12 days (most probably and injection schedule that would no be appropriate for an adequate male contraceptive method). Finally, under this regimen all subjects treated in this way maintained azoospermia or extreme oligospermia ($< 100,000$/ml). LH plasma levels were undetectable again; FSH was markedly suppressed, and T stayed within the normal rage. Of the 16 individuals in this study, 7 were observed during the recovery period after treatment was stopped. The original sperm density was completely restored within several months.

In addition to all these well designed studies, similar attempts to suppress spermatogenesis by administering TE or T proprionate had already been made by REDDY, LEE, and others. The results obtained with regard to the inhibition of spermatogenesis were very uniform.

Table 7. Sperm density during administration of danazol (taken daily PO) and testosterone enanthate (given by IM injection once monthly). (Leonard and Paulsen, 1978)

Group	Drug combination	No. oligospermic/ No. in group	No. azoospermic/ No. in group
I	D 400 mg/day TE 200 mg/month	8/14	4/14
II	D 600 mg/day TE 200 mg/month	11/13	3/13
III	D 800 mg/day TE 200 mg/month	46/54	19/54

Leonard and Paulsen (1978) carried out a study of sperm suppression in 81 healthy young men, using danazol (D), a synthetic analog of ethynyl testosterone, plus TE.

Table 7 shows the patient sample involved, the drug combinations for the different groups of patients, and the appearance of oligospermia or azoospermia. Danazol was administered PO daily and TE was injected IM once every month.

On the basis of this study the authors conclude that the combination of D plus T is effective in inducing reversible oligospermia or azoospermia. The failure of some subjects to achieve oligospermia/azoospermia appears to be related to incomplete suppression of the hypothalamopituitary axis, as assessed by measurement of serum LH and FSH.

β) Progestogens and Progestogen–Androgen and Estrogen–Androgen Combinations

Hammerstein and his group and other authors initiated studies of sperm suppression in healthy young men with cyproterone acetate (CPA), a synthetic steroid with antiandrogenic activity. The drug is administered PO each day, the daily dose being either 10 mg or 20 mg.

High doses of CPA impair but do not abolish spermatogenesis, and it is uncertain to what extent even this partial effect is due to the antiandrogenic activity of the drug and to what extent it results from its known progestational activity. However, CPA in low doses may be effective as a male contraceptive agent because of a second pharmacologic action of the drug.

Sperm produced during treatment with the drug appear to be unable to penetrate the cervical mucus of women as normal sperm do. This effect may be a consequence of the reported inhibitory action of CPA on sperm maturation in the epididymis, a finding that remains controversial and must be confirmed. Clinical studies of CPA are still under way in several centers, and other antiandrogenic substances are being sythesized and tested to expand efforts based on this approach.

The E–T combination has already been extensively studied as a possible male contraceptive in animal trials (rats, rabbits, and monkeys): limited human studies have already been performed with a combination of E_2 and methyltestosterone.

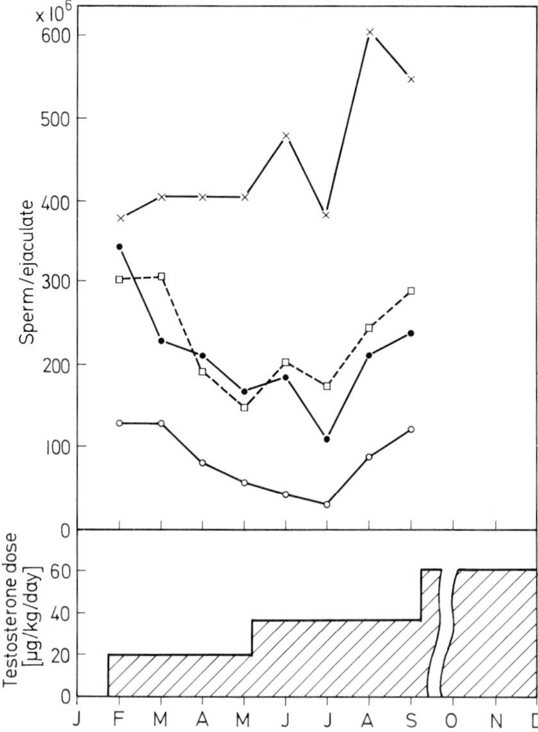

Fig. 13. Effect of testosterone and estradiol (*E*) (both drugs administered in SC Silastic implants) on spermatogenesis in rhesus monkeys, × — ×, controls; □----□, no E; ●——● 120 ng E/kg/day; ○——○, 240 ng E/kg/day. (Ewing, 1978)

Figure 13 demonstrates the effect of T and E – both administered in SC Silastic implants – on spermatogenesis in rhesus monkeys.

There is a marked seasonal increase in sperm production in control monkeys from June to September. Sperm production following this same seasonal trend can be seen in all four groups. It is obvious that T alone suppressed sperm production. However, the maximum sperm suppression occurred in monkeys receiving T plus 240 ng E/kg/day.

Briggs and Briggs published their preliminary results on an oral contraceptive for men in 1974. In five normal healthy men they had the following therapeutic schedule: Ethynylestradiol, 2 × 20 mg/day PO for 18 weeks and methyltestosterone 10 mg/day PO for 18 weeks. Azoospermia was reached in 8–10 weeks after treatment was commenced in all these cases, and was maintained for the remaining therapeutic period. No side effects were reported by the authors with this combination.

As this limited experience shows, complete suppression of spermatogenesis may be achieved with an E–T combination, and azoospermia or pronounced oligospermia can also be maintained. The question as to whether or not long-term administration of E to males for contraceptive purposes involves the hazard of causing cancer or cardiovascular disease has still not been definitively answered.

Since 1971, most studies on sperm suppression with progestins, alone or with androgens, have been performed by ICCR (International Committee for

Table 8. Progestins tested for capacity to suppress spermatogenesis in men.
(Schearer, 1978)

Progestin	In combination with	No. of major dosage regimens
Megestraol acetate	Without androgen With testosterone	3
Norethindrone	With testosterone	4
Norethandrolone	Without androgen With testosterone	2
d-Norgestrel	With testosterone	1
Norgestrienone	With testosterone	3
R 2323	Without androgen With testosterone With testosterone propionate	4
DMPA	Without androgen With testosterone With testosterone propionate With testosterone enanthate	8

Contraception Research). The studies demonstrate that when high doses of progestins were administered to men, sperm production was suppressed to very low levels in the majority of cases. But full suppression of sperm production in all men could not be achieved even when high doses of progestins were given alone or in combination with relatively high doses of an androgen.

Table 8 shows the seven progestins used in different regimens tested by ICCR for their capacity to inhibit spermatogenesis in men.

The following abbreviations have been used for steroids in this description of the regimens:

MA: megestrol acetate (17α-acetoxy-6-methyl-pregna-4,6-diene-3,20-dione acetate); NET: norethindrone (17β-hydroxy-17α-ethinyl-4-estren-3-one); NOR: norethandrolone (17α-ethyl-17-hydroxy-19-norandrost-4-en-3-one); d-NG: d-norgestrel (d-13β-ethyl-17α-ethynyl-17β-hydroxygon-4-en-3-one); R 2010: norgestrienone (17α-ethynyl-17β-hydroxy-estra-4,9,11-trien-3-one); R 2323 (17α-ethinyl-17β-hydroxy-18-methyl-4,9,11-estrien-3-one); DMPA: Depo-medroxyprogesterone acetate (17α-acetoxy-6-methyl-pregna-4-en-3,20-dione); T: testosterone (17β-hydroxyandrost-4-en-3-one); TE: testosterone enanthate; TP: testosterone propionate.

The data presented later represent a minor part of the work we have carried out on sperm suppression in recent years. Most of the results from the different studies have already been published in various articles. We shall concentrate here on the findings we have obtained with the combination of DMPA and TE given in monthly IM injections.

Group I contained two men, who received monthly injections of 150 mg DMPA and 100 mg TE.

One of the two subjects attained pronounced oligozoospermia, and the other azoospermia, within 8–12 weeks of the beginning of treatment. Each then main-

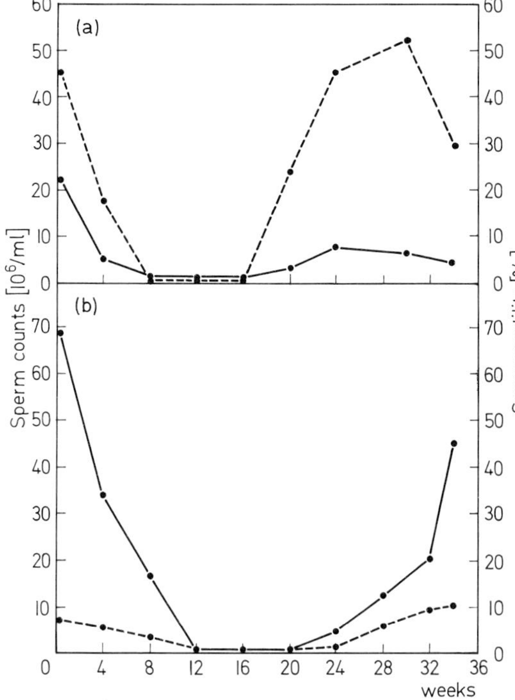

Fig. 14a, b. Effect of monthly injections of 150 mg DMPA and 100 mg TE on sperm density (10^6/ml) and motility (%) in two young men, one aged 32 (a) and the other 42 (b) years. (FRICK et al., 1977b)

tained his respective state for 2 months (Fig. 14). In the oligozoospermic subject, the depression in sperm count continued for at least 18 weeks after the last DMPA injection, although sperm motility had recovered fully during this time. In the azoospermic subject the reverse was true; spermatogenesis recovered before motility was restored.

Plasma LH, FSH, and T decreased during the first weeks of treatment (Fig. 15). FSH fluctuated during treatment, but LH and T began to rise even before the decline in MPA levels, which occurred before the cessation of injections. E_2 was unchanged during the injection period. In most instances, hormonal rebounds were observed following the end of the regimen, though plasma MPA concentrations to 0.9 ng/ml were measured 8 weeks after the last DMPA injection.

Except for a transient, slight decrease in libido in one subject, there were no changes in libido or sexual activity, or in the size, consistency or sensitivity of the breasts, testes or prostate. There were no changes in metabolic parameters or body weight.

Group II consisted of 12 men, 27–40 years old. Following initial injections of 1000 mg DMPA and 250 mg TE, they received monthly injections of 150 mg DMPA and 250 mg TE for 4–5 months.

Table 9 shows the data relating to sperm density in these 12 subjects during treatment with DMPA and TE.

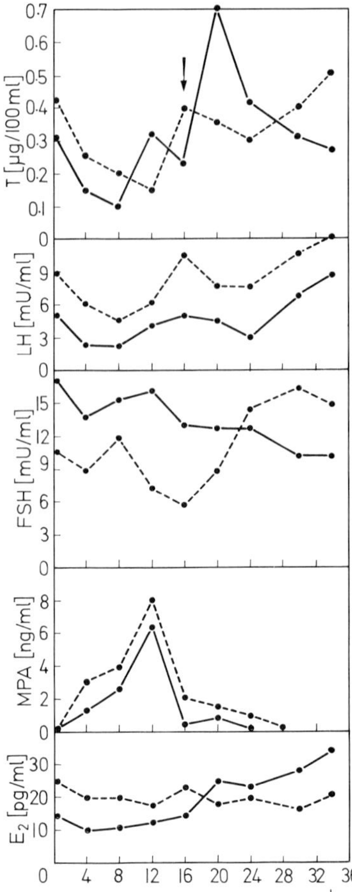

Fig. 15. Effect of monthly injections of 150 mg DMPA and 100 mg TE on plasma levels of T, LH, FSH, MPA and estradiol in two young men aged 32 (●——●) and 42 (●---●) years. ↓=discontinuation of treatment. (FRICK et al., 1977b)

Six of the 12 subjects achieved azoospermia. Four other subjects attained lowest sperm counts of <0.5 million/ml. Another reached a low of 4 million ml from a pretreatment level of 37 million/ml. Only one subject failed to respond with sharply reduced sperm production. He received 20 weeks of treatment.

Of the six azoospermic subjects, two did not maintain azoospermia during 4–6 weeks of further treatment. In the five oligozoospermic subjects (<10 million/ml), three did not maintain the lowest sperm count attained, despite 4–8 weeks of further treatment. Nevertheless, no subject showed complete recovery to pretreatment sperm levels during treatment.

Impairment or abolition of sperm motility was a common occurrence. However, the lowest level was not always maintained during treatment, and in some cases there was even a recovery to the pretreatment motility level. There was no consistent correlation between reductions in sperm concentration and reductions in motility.

Table 10 shows the mean plasma levels (with SE) of LH, FSH, T, E_2, and MPA in the same 12 subjects.

Table 9. Sperm density during treatment with DMPA (1000 initially, then 150 mg at monthly intervals) and testosterone enanthate (250 mg at monthly intervals)

After (weeks)	GE	DH	KW	KH	TU	RP	HJ	TR	OH	SL	BG	HR
Before treatment												
	24	16	13	16	13	76	14	19	12	67	37	9/15
2												
4		2	3	9	12	56	6	3	6	<0.5	36	35
6	0					<0.5						
8		0	0	0.01	<0.5		<0.5		1	6	56	15
12		0	0	0	0	0	<0.5	<0.5	<0.5	0.8	4	16
14	0											
16		0		0	0	7		0.4	1	<0.5	6	
18	0		<0.5									
20		0						0.3			6	17

Table 10. Plasma levels of LH, FSH, testosterone, ethynylestradiol and medroxyprogesterone acetate during the same treatment as in Table 9 (means $\pm$ SE)

After (weeks)	No.	Before treatment				
		LH (mIU/ml)	FSH (mIU/ml)	T (ng/ml)	E_2 (pg/ml)	MPA (ng/ml)
	12	7.6 ± 1.1	14.2 ± 3.0	5.6 ± 0.6	28.8 ± 2.6	0
4	11	4.4 ± 0.5	6.6 ± 1.6	2.3 ± 0.5	14.0 ± 1.9	8.2 ± 1.0
8	9	5.6 ± 0.8	8.5 ± 1.7	2.6 ± 0.5	12.4 ± 2.2	3.6 ± 0.6
12	9	10.0 ± 3.0	7.2 ± 1.3	2.5 ± 0.3	19.3 ± 0.3	3.4 ± 0.7
16	6	14.6 ± 5.4	6.8 ± 0.8	2.8 ± 0.8	19.8 ± 3.4	2.3 ± 0.3

LH. At 4 weeks after the initial DMPA injection, the LH mean was 58% of the pretreatment mean ($P < 0.02$). The LH decrease was not maintained during continued monthly treatment with the reduced DMPA dose; none of the subsequent means differed significantly from the pretreatment level.

FSH. At 4 weeks after the initial DMPA injection, the FSH mean was 46% of the pretreatment mean ($P < 0.05$). During continued monthly treatment with the reduced DMPA dose, mean FSH values remained below the pretreatment level ($P < 0.05$) except at the 8th week.

Testosterone. At 4 weeks after the initial DMPA injection, the mean T value was 41% of the pretreatment mean ($P < 0.001$). The T decrease was maintained during continued treatment at the reduced DMPA dose ($P < 0.01$, 0.001, and 0.02 at weeks 8, 12, and 16, respectively).

Estradiol. At 4 weeks after the initial DMPA injection, the E_2 mean was 49% of the pretreatment mean ($P < 0.001$). After 3 more months of treatment

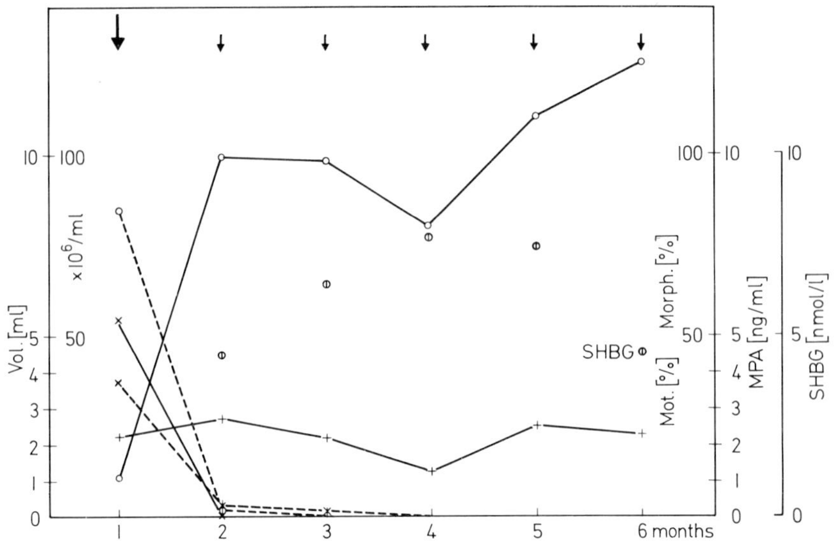

Fig. 16. Effect of 1000 mg MPA and 500 mg TE on day 0 (*large arrow*) followed by five monthly injections of 150 mg MPA and 500 mg TE (*small arrows*) on sperm density (o----o), sperm morphology (×——×), motility (×----×), and seminal fluid volume (+——+), and plasma levels of MPA and SHBG in four young men. (FRICK 1978, unpublished data)

at the reduced DMPA dose, the E_2 mean had risen to 69% of the pretreatment mean ($P < 0.10$).

Medroxyprogesterone Acetate. At 4 weeks after the initial DMPA injection, the mean blood level of MPA was 8.2 ± 1.0 ng/ml. At the reduced monthly DMPA dosage, MPA did not disappear completely in the 4 weeks following an injection. The MPA mean declined to 3.6 ± 0.6 ng/ml at 1 month after the first reduced DMPA dose, and then declined only slightly after the two subsequent monthly injections. Following the final injection, the duration of the presence of MPA in the blood varied widely. In one subject, MPA had disappeared by 12 weeks after the end of treatment, whereas another subject had detectable MPA after 18 weeks. No MPA was found after 20–24 weeks in the three subjects for whom such data were available.

Group III consisted of four healthy young men aged 34–53. The injection schedule was as follows: 1000 mg MPA and 500 mg TE on day O, followed by monthly injections of 150 mg MPA and 500 mg TE.

Figure 16 shows the mean values for sperm density, morphology, motility, and volume, and plasma and sex hormone-binding globulin (SHBG) in these four subjects over a period of 6 months. Extreme oligospermia and finally azoospermia was attained in 8–10 weeks after the treatment started in all subjects, and azoospermia was maintained for up to 6 months of treatment with not a single break-through. The volume of the ejaculate did not change throughout the observation period. From the second month of treatment the plasma MPA

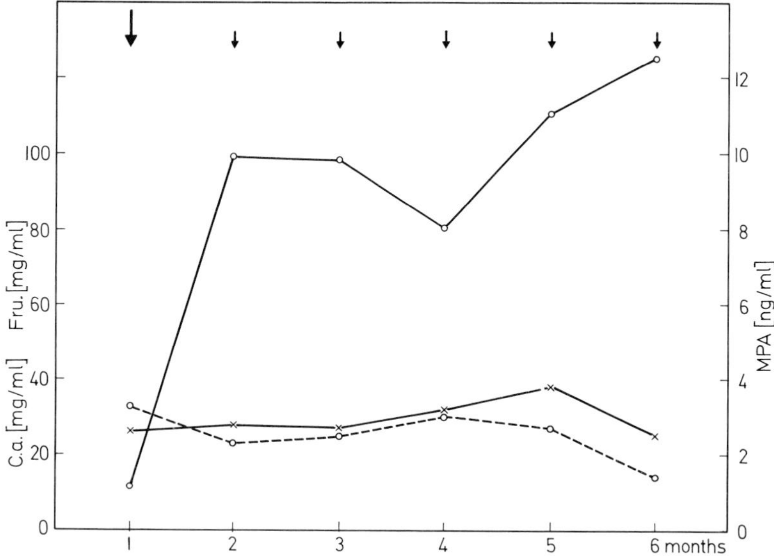

Fig. 17. Effect of 1000 mg MPA and 500 mg TE on day 0 (*large arrow*) followed by five monthly injections of 150 mg MPA and 500 mg TE (*small arrows*) on seminal plasma c.a. (o---o) and fru. (×——×) and on plasma levels of MPA (o——o) in four young men. (FRICK, 1978, unpublished data)

levels varied between 8.0 ng/ml and 12 ng/ml. The SHBG level showed a moderate increase from the third to the fifth month of treatment.

Figure 17 demonstrates the mean values of plasma MPA levels, citric acid (c.a.) and fructose (fru.) content of the seminal fluid in the same four subjects with the same treatment regimen over a period of 6 months. There was no significant change in the seminal plasma, c.a., or and fru. content during this observation period.

Table 11 summarizes the findings of the 25 studies carried out by the ICCR group on the effectiveness of different regimens in the suppression of sperm production.

Group IV contained four young men aged 25–35 years, who had prostatitis, and three men over 60 with benign prostatic hypertrophy. Three of the young men and all the older men each received four implants of megestrol acetate and three implants of T. One 25-year-old man of proven fertility received five implants of megestrol acetate and four implants of T.

In the young men, the effects of this treatment were monitored by regular spermiograms and determination of plasma T before and 6–8 weeks after implantation. In the older men, testicular biopsies and measurements of plasma were performed immediately before and 8 weeks after implantation.

In one of the young men, who was 35 years old, the treatment of four megestrol acetate implants and three T implants had no noticeable effect: ejaculate volume was 1.2 ml and 2.3 ml, sperm count was 87×10^6/ml and 62×10^6/,

Table 11. Summary of effectiveness of progestins tested in studies reported. Schearer (1978)

Progestin tested	Total numbers of subjects treated	Effectiveness of treatment in suppressing sperm counts (number of subjects who exhibited the indicated effect)				
		Effect unknown	No effect[b]	Slight to moderate suppression[b]	Oligo-spermia[b]	Azoo-spermia[b]
Megestrol acetate[a] (3 regimens)	25	15	0	0	6	4
Norethindrone[a] (4 regimens)	27	0	5[c]	9	6	7
Norethandrolone[a] (2 regimes)	8	0	0	8	0	0
d-Norgestrel[a] (1 regimen)	1	0	0	0	1	0
Norgestrienone[a] (3 regimens)	9	0	0	2	3	4
R 2323[a] (4 regimens)	42	1	2	0	7	32
DMPA (2 regimens)	12	2	0	2	3	5
DMPA + TE (6 regimens)	88	5	2	6	39	36

[a] Includes regimens involving androgen-releasing implants in combination with the progestin.
[b] See text for definitions.
[c] In some cases, it is not certain that subjects complied fully with the scheduled administration of treatment.

and sperm motility was 43% and 45% each before and 7 weeks after the start of treatment, respectively. Plasma T values remained constant in both groups (Table 12). The young man implanted with five capsules of megestrol acetate and four of T showed a decrease in sperm count from 23×10^6/ml before treatment to 8×10^6/ml after 6 weeks, to 5×10^6/ml after 8 weeks, and finally to complete azoospermia 11 weeks after implantation. This patient reported that libido and frequency of sexual intercourse remained unchanged throughout the treatment period. When examined 4 months after implantation of capsules the patient was still azoospermic. At this date all subdermal implants were removed and the spermiogram of the patient was taken again after 8 weeks. The semen analysis indicated a sperm count of 25×10^6/ml and a sperm motility of 45%. During the periods of treatment and recovery, the plasma T levels of the patients did not differ significantly from the pretreatment values (Patient 4, Table 12).

In Patient 1 of the older men there were no significant differences in the testicular biopsy before treatment and 7 weeks after implantation, although

Table 12. Effect of four megestrol acetate and three testosterone implants on plasma testosterone levels in men

	Number of patients	Plasma testosterone (ng/ml)	
		Before treatment	After treatment[a]
Young men	1	4.9	4.6
	2	3.0	3.0
	3	3.8	3.4
	4[b]	4.6	4.3
Older men (>60 years)	1	3.2	2.9
	2	3.7	3.5
	3	3.9	3.7

[a] 6–8 weeks.
[b] Five megestrol acetate implants and four testosterone implants.

there was some degree of desquamation and disorganization of the germinal epithelium.

All the progestins tested are capable of suppressing sperm production in men. Overall, of 189 men treated with progestins and followed up for long enough to observe the full effects of the treatment, a total of 153 (81%) exhibited sperm counts below 10 million/ml. Among men treated with regimens including either R 2323 or DMPA combined with TE, over 73% of those monitored (91 of 124 men) exhibited sperm counts of less than 1 million/ml at some time during treatment.

Some of the progestins tested were more effective than others in suppressing sperm production. Although differences in the dosage regimens and in the frequency of monitoring of sperm counts make exact comparisons impossible, R 2323 appears to be the most effective, and norethandrolone the least.

Not surprisingly, in view of the pharmacologically small doses involved, regimens based on androgen-releasing implants were not more effective than those with progestins alone. For the one progestin tested with and without pharmacologically significant doses of an androgen (DMPA), the combined regimens appeared to be only slightly more effective than those with the progestin alone. Even when large doses of the androgen were combined with this progestin, the treatment was not successful in producing azoospermia or near-azoospermia in more than about 75% of the men treated.

2. Side Effects in all Studies of Sperm Suppression Reviewed

a) Studies with TE only in Different Regimens

A very common finding was that hemoglobin and hematocrit values increased in most subjects during testosterone treatment. This upward trend appears to be dose-related.

Cholesterol, triglyceride, and the lipoproteins did not change significantly throughout the treatment period. Furthermore, glucose tolerance tests and Trijodthyomin-RIA (T_3), Thyroxin-RIA (T_4), and cortisol values indicate that they are normal during the treatment periods completed so far.

More than 50% of the subjects treated with different regimens of TE reported a mild degree of acne, about 10% had a slight increase in the hair growth on the chest, back, or lower abdomen, and approximately one-third noted a weight gain of 3%–7%.

Transient breast tenderness or some mild degree of breast swelling was reported in 10% of the subjects. However, hardly anyone complained of persistent changes in sexual behavior.

Most investigators found a decrease in testicular size in two-thirds of the subjects examined but these changes were reversible; testicular size reverted to control measurements during the recovery period.

It is surprising that the authors did not see, changes in prostatic size and consistency, even in those cases where relatively high doses of androgen were administered.

On the basis of these short-term studies we know that with carefully selected subjects the incidence of difficulties is minimal, but we have no information on long-term therapy or on what the relationship of treatment to clinical effects might be.

b) Studies with Estrogen and Testosterone in Combination

A full analysis of side effects during the administration of an E–T combination for sperm suppression is impossible: the available data are too few to allow any conclusions.

c) Studies with Progestins Alone or in Combination with Androgen

The main short-term side effects after treatment with progestins alone or a progestin-androgen combination in ICCR studies are demonstrated in Table 13.

The regimens tested varied considerably in the side effects they produced. This is particularly evident when the 25 regimens are divided into three groups:

Few side effects were noted for nine of the most effective regimens. Six of these involved DMPA alone or in combination with TE, and three norgestrienone. Among the 91 men who were treated with one of these regimens, side effects were limited to occasional, transient declines in libido in 21 men; moderate weight gain in many men; and two instances of reversible gynecomastia. Periodic analyses of blood samples from the 82 men who were treated with DMPA alone or in combination with androgen revealed no significant adverse metabolic changes.

In the studies of 12 other regimens entailing the treatment of 79 men, side effects were more pronounced. On the whole, these regimens produced decline in libido, weight gain, and gynecomastia more frequently or with greater intensity. Isolated cases of night sweats (presumably resulting from the thermogenic action of the progestin), painful erections, and occasional delays in reaching orgasm were also reported. Periodic blood samples were collected and analyzed for seven of these regimens; two regimens gave evidence of mild liver toxicity

Table 13. Summary of short-term side effects observed in studies. (SCHEARER, 1978)

	Side effect[a]								
	Transient decrease of libido	Weight gain	Night sweats	Gynecomastia or nipple pain	Elevated trans- aminases	Hepatic pain	Delayed orgasm	Pailful erection	Epididy- mitis
Megestrol acetate[b] (3 regimens)	×	n.m.	—	—	—[c]	—	—	—	—
Norethindrone[a] (4 regimens)	×	×	—	×	n.m.	—	—	—	—
Norethandrolone[a] (2 regimens)	×	×	—	—	—	—	—	—	—
d-Norgestrel[a] (1 regimen)	×	×	×	—	n.m.	—	—	—	—
Norgestrienone[a] (3 regimens)	×	×	—	—	n.m.	—	—	—	—
R 2323[a] (4 regimens)	×	×	×	×	×	×	×	—	×
DMPA (2 regimens)	×	×	—	×	—	—	—	—	—
DMPA+TE (6 regimens)	×	×	—	×	×[d]	—	—	×[e]	—

[a] ×, observed; —, not observed— n.m., not monitored.
[b] Includes regimens involving androgen-releasing implants in combination with the progestin.
[c] Monitored only for one regimen, i.e., 10–30 mg MA PO daily.
[d] Only observed in three men with highest dosages tested; see text.
[e] Only observed in one man at highest doses of TE tested (500 mg monthly).

Table 14. Frequency of decreased libido and gynecomastia observed in the studies. (Schearer, 1978)

Progestin tested	Proportion of subjects reporting decreased libido		Proportion of subjects reporting gynecomastia or nipple pain	
Megestrol acetate[a] (3 regimens)	17/25	(68%)	0/25	(0%)
Norethindrone[a] (4 regimens)	4/27	(15%)	3/27	(11%)
Norethandrolone[a] (2 regimens)	2/8	(25%)	0/8	(0%)
d-Norgestrel[a] (1 regimen)	1/1	–	0/1	–
Norgestrienone[a] (3 regimens)	1/9	(11%)	0/9	(0%)
R 2323[a] (4 regimens)	10/42	(24%)	3/42	(7%)
DMPA (2 regimens)	9/12	(75%)	1/12	(8%)
DMPA+TE (6 regimens)	10/88	(11%)	1/88	(1%)
Total	54/212	(25%)	8/212	(4%)

[a] Includes regimens involving androgen-releasing implants in combination with the progestin.

reflected in slight or moderate elevations in transaminase levels in three of the men who were treated with these regimens.

Four of the regimens tested produced numerous side effects, some of which were potential causes of serious medical sequelae. These four regimens all involved R 2323 in studies involving a total of 42 men. Most of the side effects noted with other progestins were observed. In addition, several men receiving these four regimens also experienced hepatic pain, nipple pain, and epididymitis.

Table 14 summarizes the frequency of decreased libido and gynecomastia.

As indicated in Table 14, apparent declines in libido were associated with the use of all the progestins. However, a high incidence of this side effect was reported for only two progestins, megestrol acetate (17/25 cases) and DMPA (9/12 cases). These were the only C_{21} steroids tested in these studies. However, when DMPA was combined with high doses of an androgen, the reported incidence of decline in libido was much lower (10/88 cases), suggesting that this side effect may be linked with suppression of T production. In nearly all instances, treatment was maintained in men who reported a decline in libido, and their libido returned spontaneously during the course of treatment. Recovery of normal libido also occurred in several cases where treatment was discontinued. Since the design of these studies did not include placebo treatments, the extent to which decreases in libido resulted from pharmacologic after action of the treatment is uncertain. It is likely that psychological reactions to the treatment were partially responsible.

As shown in Table 14, about 4% of the men who participated in these studies experienced gynecomastia. In all cases, the gynecomastia was fully reversed upon cessation of the treatment. The incidence of gynecomastia in the studies entailing the use of TE was far lower (1.1%) than in those with progestins alone (5.6%). No other changes in secondary sex characteristics and no indications of feminization as a result of the treatment were reported in these studies.

It might seem that we are well on the way to devising a medical treatment for reversible inhibition of spermatogenesis without undue side effects.

It also seems, however, that we do not yet know the optimal progestin–testosterone combination, or perhaps simply the optimal dosage regimen. From what we have seen in all these studies, relatively high doses of progestins are needed to achieve and maintain a complete arrest of spermatogenesis. Obviously careful investigations into what other changes may occur in men during long-term treatment with high doses of progestins are necessary.

There has not yet been any long-term follow-up of a large number of patients treated with the different progestins.

DMPA in connection with the right regimen of a well-tolerated T replacement therapy could perhaps be used as a short-term (e.g., for 1 year) male contraceptive technique.

D. New Aspects for the Future

An ideal fertility control method would be the prevention of sperm maturation. Sperm do not acquire the capacity of fertilize until their slow passage through the epididymis. The discovery that the epididymis requires an unusually high concentration of T suggested that an antitestosterone might interfere with its physiologic integrity. CPA is an antitestosterone, but as the clinical trials have already shown, the effect of this drug is not limited to the epididymis; it also causes an inhibition of spermatogenesis. α-Chlorohydrin is another drug that might exert an antifertility effect in the epididymis, but the compound may be too toxic for use in humans. However, an has recently been found that it is hoped will prove to be sufficiently free of toxicity for human trials.

Enthusiasm for the development of a posttesticular fertility control agent continues to run high, and the rapid progress of recent years in our understanding of epididymal functioning makes it likely that efforts in this direction will ultimately be successful.

The receptor chemistry and intracellular molecular biology of steroid hormones has been broadly elucidated in a remarkably short time. Specific cytoplasmic receptors in target cells carry the steroid (E or progesterone, and probably all biologically active steroids) to the nucleus, where a transcriptional activity brings about quantitative and qualitative changes in messenger RNA synthesis and alters the pattern of structural and secretory products of the cell, converting it from the nonstimulated to the stimulated state. Many steps in this sequence are now clearly worked out. Factors that play a role in the generation of cytoplasmic receptors, in the rate of receptor degeneration, in the binding of the steroid to the receptor, and in the binding of the steroid–receptor complex to chromatin have also been described. The synthesis of chemical substances that can block the normal steroid – receptor interaction has been reported, and clinical application of this principle or others mentioned may soon become feasible.

References

Adil E (1969) Pakistan's family planning programme. In: Sadik N, Anderson JK, Siddiqui KA, Ahmad B, Butt MN, Samad S, Sharih K (eds) Population control: Implications, trends and prospects. Pakistan Family Planning Programme, Islamabad, p 15

Alexander NJ (1972) Vasectomy: long term effects in the rhesus monkey. J Reprod Fertil 31:399

Altman M (1972) Place of vasectomy. Br Med J 1:311

Altman M (1972) Vasectomy in the Surgery. Br Med J 4:671

Alvarez F, Faundes A, Brache V, Leon P (1977) Attainment and maintenance of azoospermia with combined monthly injections of depot medroxyprogesterone acetate and testosterone enauthate. Contraception 15:635

Ansbacher R (1971) Spermagglutinating and spermimmobilizing antibodies in vasectomized men. Fertil Steril 22:629

Ansbacher R, Keung-Yeung K, Wurster JC (1972) Sperm antibodies in vasectomized men. Fertil Steril 23:610

Ansbacher R, Williams BS, Mumford DM (1975) Vas ligation: Sperm antibodies. In: Sciarra JJ, Markland C, Speidel JJ (eds) Control of male fertility. Harper & Row, New York, p 189

Bartke A, Steele RE, Musto N, Caldwell BV (1973) Fluctuations in plasma testosterone levels in adult male rats and mice. Endocrinology 92:1223

Benjamin KB (1972) Vasectomy as an office procedure. In: Leader L (ed) Foolproof birth control. Beacon Press, Boston, Mass, p 82

Bernstein GS (1974) Conventional methods of contraception: condom, diaphragm and vaginal foam. Clin Obstet Gynecol 17:21

Blandy J (1971) Male Sterilization. In: Smith AJ (ed) Contraception today. Family Planning Association, London, p 101

Bloomfield E (1972) Vasectomy and intravenous anesthesia in a health center. Gen Practitioner 209:76

Bottger P (1972) Vasectomy for sterilization. Selecta 14:1629

Boyce JMH (1973) Sperm counts after vasectomy. Lancet 1:492

Boyer JL, Preisig R, Zbinder G, De Kretser DM, Wang C, Paulsen CA (1976) Guidelines for assessment of potential hepatotoxic effects of synthetic androgens, anabolic agents and progestagens in their use in males as antifertility agents. Contraception 13:461

Bremner WJ, De Kretser DM (1977) The prospects for new, reversible male contraceptives. N Engl J Med 295:1111

Brenner PF, Bernstein GS, Roy S, Jecht EW, Mishell DR Jr (1975) Administration of norethrandrolone and testosterone as a contraceptive agent for men. Contraception 11:193

Brenner PF, Mishell DR Jr, Bernstein GS, Ortiz A (1977) Study of medroxyprogesterone acetate and testosterone enanthate as a male contraceptive. Contraception 15:679

Brenner PF, Brernstein GS, Mishell DR (1978) Combination of gestagen and androgen as a male contraceptive. In: Proceedings Hormonal Control of Male Fertility, DHEW Publication Na (NIH) 78–1097, p 247, 1978

Briggs M, Briggs M (1974) Oral contraception for men. Nature 252:585

Brodie N Reversible intravas device (Unpublished)

Brodsky SA (1973) Evaluation of a new instrument for sterilization by elective bilateral vasectomy. (Unpublished)

Brotherton J (1974) Effect of oral cyproterone acetate on urinary and serum FSH and LH levels in adult males being treated for hypersexuality. J Reprod Fertil 36:177

Brown S (1975) The effect of orally administered androgens on sperm motility. Fertil Steril 26:305

Brown-Woodman PDC, White JG (1975) Effect of α-chlorohydrin on cauda epididymis and spermatozoa of the rat and general physiological status. Contraception 11:69

Bruce PT (1972) Vasectomy, a survey of 98 men. Med J Aust 1:17

Bruce PT (1973) Vasectomy. Med J Aust 1:462

Buchanan JM (1971) Vasectomy. Br Med J 4:749

Brueschke EE, Wingfield JR, Burns M, Zanenveld LJD (1974a) Development of a reversible vas deferens occlusive device. II. Effect of bilateral and unilateral vasectomy on semen characteristics in the dog. Fertil Steril 25:673

Brueschke EE, Zanenveld LJD, Rodzen R, Berns D (1974b) Development of a reversible vas deferens occlusive device. III. Morphology of the human and dog vas deferens: a study with the scanning electron microscope. Fertil Steril 25:687

Brueschke EE, Burns M, Maness JH, Wingfield JR, Mayerhofer K, Zanenveld LJD (1974c) Development of a reversible vas deferens occlusive device. I. Anatomical size of the human and dog vas deferens. Fertil Steril 25:659

Brueschke EE, Zanenveld LJD (1975) Development and Evaluation of reversible vas occlusive devices. In: Sciarra JJ, Markland C, Speidel JJ (eds) Control of male fertility. Harper & Row, New York, pp 211–222

Brueschke EE, Zanenveld LJD, Free MJ, Wingfield JR (1976) Vas deferens contraceptive methodology. In: Hafez ESE (ed), The human semen and fertility regulation in the male. Mosby, St Louis

Carlson HE (1970) Vasectomy of election. South Med J 63:766–770

Chang CC, Kincl FA (1970) Sustained hormonal preparation. IV. Biologic effectiveness of steroid hormones. Fertil Steril 21:134

Charney CW (1956) Treatment of male infertility with large doses of testosterone. JAMA 160:98

Civantos F, Lubin J, Rywlin AM (1972) Vasitis nodosa. Arch Pathol 94:355

Coffey DS, Freeman C (1975) Vas injection: A new surgical procedure to induce sterility in human males. In: Sciarra JJ, Markland C, Speidel JJ (eds) Control of male fertility. Harper & Row, New York, pp 234–245

Cornes JS (1973) Sperm counts after vasectomy. Lancet 1:721

Coppola JA, Saldarini RJ (1974) A new orally active male antifertility agent. Contraception 9:459

Coutinho EM, Melo JF (1973) Successful inhibition of spermatogenesis in man without loss of libido: A potential new approach to male contraception. Contraception 8:207

Coyotupa J, Parlow AF, Abraham GE (1972) Simultaneous radioimmunoassay of plasma testosterone and dihydrotestosterone. Anal Letters 5:329

Crabo BG, Hunter AG (1974) Sperm maturation and epidiymal function. In: Sciarra JJ, Markland C, Speidel JJ (eds) Proceedings of a Workshop on Control of Male Fertility. San Francisco. Harper & Row, Hagerstown, pp 2–23

Craft J (1973) Irrigation of vasectomy and the onset of sterility. Br J Urol 45:441

Crosignani PG, Nakamura RM, Hovland DN, Mishell DR Jr (1970) A method of solid phase radioimmunoassay utilizing polyprophylene discs. J Clin Endocrinol Metab 30:153

Croxatto H, Diaz S, Vera R, Etchart M, Atria P (1969) Fertility control in women with a progestogen released in microquantities from subcutaneous capsules. Am J Obstet Gynecol 105:1135

Cummins JM, Orgebin-Crist MC (1974) Effects of the anti-androgen SK and F 7690 on the fertility of epididymal spermatozoa in the rabbit. Biol Reprod 11:56

Cunningham GR, Silverman VE, Kohler PO (1978a) Clinical Evaluation of testosterone enanthate for induction and maintenance of reversible azoospermia in man. In: Proceedings Hormonal Control of Male Fertility, DHEW Publication No (NIH) 78–1097, p 71, 1978a

Cunningham GR, Silverman V, Kohler PO (1978b) Gonadotropin suppression in normal males and males with primary hypogonadism: Evaluation of four andorogens. Int J Androl Suppl 2:720–731

Dalsimer JA, Piotrow PT, Dumm JJ (1973) Barrier methods: Condom – an old method meets a new social need. Population Reports, Series H No 1, December (1973)

De Kretser DM (1974) The regulation of male fertility: The state of the art and further possibilities. Contraception 9:561

Denniston GC (1972) Vasectomy technique. Population Dynamics, Seattle, Wash

Dixit VP, Lohiya NK, Agrawal M (1975) Effects of α-chlorohydrin on the testes and epididymes of dog in a preliminary study. Fertil Steril 26:781

Donald RA, Espiner EA, Cowles RJ, Fazackerley JE (1976) The effect of cyproterone acetate on the plasma gonadotropin response to LH-RH. Acta Endocrinol (Kbh) 81:680

Dumm JJ, Piotrow PT, Dalsimer JA (1974) Barrier methods: The modern condom – quality product for effective contraception. Population Reports. Series H, May, (1974)

Dzink PJ, Cook B (1966) Passage of steroids through silicone nibber. Endocrinology 78:208

Edqvist LE, Johansson EDB (1972) Radioimmunoassay of estrone and estradiol in human and bovine peripheral plasma. Acta Endocrinol (Kbh) 71:716

Eliasson R (1971) Standards for investigation of human semen. Andrologie 3:49

Ewing LL (1978) Effects of testosterone and estradiol, silastic implants, on spermatogenesis in rats and rhesus monkeys. In: Proceedings Hormonal Control of Male Fertility, DHEW Publication No (NIH) 78–1097, p 173, 1978

Farell CG, Joshua DE, Uren RF, Baird PJ, Perkins KW, Kronenberg H (1975) Androgen induced hepatoma. Lancet 1:430

Fiumara NJ (1971) Effectiveness of condoms in preventing V.D. N Engl J Med 285:972

Folkman J, Long DM (1964) The rise of silicone nibber as a carrier for prolonged drug therapy. J Surg Res 4:139

Free MJ (1974) Animal experiments with a reversible intravasal occlusive device (RIOD). (Abstract), International Congress of Physiological Science, New Delhi, 1974

Free MJ (1975) Development of a reversible intravasal occlusive device. In: Sciarra JJ, Markland C, Speidel JJ (eds) Control of male fertility. Harper & Row, New York, p 124

Free MJ, Duncan GW (1973) New technology for voluntary sterilization. Paper presented at the Symposium on Population and New Biology, London, England, September 25, 1973

Free MJ, Duncan GW (1974) New technology for voluntary sterilization. In: Benjamin BJ, Cos PR, Peel J (eds) Population and the new biology. Academic Press, London, p 65–82

Freeman C (1975) Preliminary human trial of a new male sterilization procedure: vas sclerosing. Fertil Steril 26:162

Freeman C, Coffey DS (1973a) Sterility in male animals induced by injection of chemical agents into the vas deferens. Fertil Steril 24:884

Freeman C, Coffey DS (1973b) Chemical induction of male sterility by injection of vasosclerosing agents. Fed Proc 32:310

Freund M, Davis JE (1969) Disappearance rate of spermatozoa from the ejaculate following vasectomy. Fertil Steril 20:163

Frick J (1973) Control of spermatogenesis in men by combined administration of progestin and androgen. Contraception 8:191

Frick J (1974) Effect of androgens and progestins on spermatogenesis. In: Mancini RE, Martini L (eds) Male fertility and sterility. Academic Press, New York, p 441

Frick J (1975a) A reversible method of vasectomy. Contraception 12:125

Frick J (1975b) Effect of steroids on spermatogenesis. In: Sciarra JJ, Markland C, Speidel JJ (eds) Control of male fertility. Harper & Row, New York, p 230

Frick J (1977a) Male contraception. Proceedings of the Vth International Congress of Endocrinology, Hamburg, July 18–24, 1976. James VHT (ed), vol 1. Excerpta Medica, Amsterdam Oxford, p 366

Frick J (1977b) Sterilisation beim Mann. oest Aerzteztg 32:1294

Frick J, Bartsch G (1973) Inhibition of spermatogenesis. In: Coutinho EM, Fuchs F (eds) Physiology and genetics of reproduction, part A. Plenum Press, New York, p 259

Frick J, Bartsch G (1974) Inhibition of spermatogenesis. In: Coutinho EM, Fuchs F (eds) Physiology and genetics of reproduction, part A. Plenum Press, New York, p 230

Frick J, Bartsch G, Jakse G (1977a) Radioimmunoassays of ethinyl-vorgestrienoue (R-2323) and medroxyprogesterone acetate (MPA) and their clinical applicability. Urol Res 5:55

Frick J, Bartsch G, Weiske WH (1977b) The effect of monthly depot medroxyprogesterone acetate and testosterone on human spermatogenesis. I. Uniform dosage levels. Contraception 15:649

Frick J, Bartsch G, Weiske WH (1977c) The effect of monthly depot medroxyprogesterone acetate and testosterone on human spermatogenesis. II. High initial dose.Contraception 15:669

Frick J, Bende T, Aulitzky H (1979) Possibilities of hormone administration through subcutaneous implants. (In press)

Fried JJ (ed) (1972) In: Vasectomy. Saturday Review Press, New York, p 25

Gersh J (1972) Vasectomy. Rocky Mt Med J 69:67

Giri K (1973) Sterilization and post-conception control of fertility in Nepal. Proceedings of the 1st Meeting of the IGCC Expert Group Working Committee on Sterilization and Abortion. Intergovernmental Coordinating Committee, p 34, 1973

Greenblatt RB, Dmowski WP, Mahesh VB, Scholer HFL (1971) Clinical studies with an antigonadotropin-danazol. Fertil Steril 22:102

Greene LF (1971) Bilateral partial vasectomy for elective sterilization. Am Fam Physician 4:73

Greep RO, Koblinsky MA, Jaffe FS (1976) Reproduction and human welfare: A challenge to research. MIT Press, Cambridge, Mass, London, Engl

Hackett RE, Waterhouse K (1973) Vasectomy reviewed. Am J Obstet Gynecol 116:438

Hammerstein J, Brotherton J (1978) Methods for evaluation of antifertility agents in the male. Int J Androl [Suppl] 2:659–680

Hanley HG (1973) Vasectomy – current male techniques. 2nd International Conference of Voluntary Sterilization, Geneva, Switzerland, February 25–March 1, 1973. Schima ME, Lubell J, Davis JE, Connell E (eds). Excerpta Medica, Amsterdam Oxford, pp 7–75

Heckel NM, Rosso WA, Kestle L (1951) Spermatogenic rebound phenomenon after administration of testosterone proprionate. J Clin Endocrinol 11:235

Heller CG, Nelson WO, Hill JB, Henderson E, Maddock O, Jung EC, Paulsen CA (1950a) Improvement in spermatogenesis following depression of the human testis with testosterone. Fertil Steril 1:145

Heller CG, Nelson WO, Hill JC, Henderson E, Maddock WO, Jung EC (1950b) The effect of testosterone administration upon the human testis. J Clin Endocrinol Metab 10:816

Heller CG, Laidlaw WM, Harvey HT, Nelson WO (1958) Effects of progestational compounds on the reproductive process of the human male. Ann NY Acad Sci 71:649

Heller CG, Moore DJ, Paulsen CA, Nelson WO, Laidlaw W (1959) Effects of progesterone and synthetic progestins on the reproductive physiology of normal men. Fed Proc. 18:1057

Heller CG, Lally MF, Rowley MJ (1966) Factors affecting the testicular function in man. In: Diczfalusy E, Kovarikova A (eds) Pharmacology of reproduction, vol 2. Pergamon, Oxford, pp 86–94

Heller CG, Morse HC, Su M, Rowley MJ (1970) The role of FSH, LH and endogenous testosterone during testicular suppression by exogenous testosterone in normal men. In: Weshub LP (ed) The human testis. Thomas, Springfield, Ill, p 249

Hiro M, Stanczyk FY, Goebelsmann U, Brenner PF, Lumkin ME, Mishell DR Jr (1975) Radioimmunoassay of serum medroxyprogesterone acetate (Provera) in women following oral and intravaginal administration. Steroids 26:373

Hobbs JJ (1972) Vasectomy in general practice. J Coll Gen Pract 11:583

Hotchkiss J, Atkinson LE, Knobil E (1971) Time course of serum estrogen and luteinizing hormone concentrations during the menstrual cycle of the rhesus monkey. Endocrinology 89:177

Hotchkiss RS (1944) Effects of massive doses of testosterone proprionate upon spermatogenesis. J Clin Endocrinol 4:117

Howard PJ, James LP (1973) Immunological implications of vasectomy. J Urol 109:76

Jackson H (1970) Antispermatogenic agents. Br Med Bull 26:79

Jhaver PS, Ohri BB (1960) The history of experimental and clinical work on vasectomy. J Int Coll Surg 33:482

Johansson EDB, Nygren KG (1973) Depression of plasma testosterone levels in men with norethindrone. Contraception 8:219

Kantor WM (1937) Beginnings of sterilization in America. J Hered 28:374

Ketchel MM (1978) Available clinical data concerning effects of androgen treatment of men on outcome of subsequent pregnancies. In: Proceedings Hormonal Control of Male Fertility, DHEW Publication No (NIH) 78–1097, p 341, 1978

Kincl FA, Benagino G, Angee J (1968) Sustained release hormonal preparations. I. Diffusion of various steroids through polymer membranes. Steroids 11:673

Koch VJ, Lorenz F, Danchl K, Ericsson R, Hasan SH, Keyerlink VD, Lübke K, Mehring M, Römmler A, Schwartz V, Hammerstein J (1976) Continuous oral low-dosage cyproterone acetate for fertility regulation in the male. A trend of analysis in 15 volunteers. Contraception 14:117

Krishnakumar S (1972) Kerala's pioneering experiment in massive vasectomy camps. Stud Fam Plann 3:177

Leader AJ, Axelrad SD, Frankowski R, Mumford SD (1974) Complications of 2,711 vasectomies. J Urol 111:365

Lee HY (1961) Clinical aspects on vasectomy. Korean J Urol 2:109

Lee HY (1966) Studies on vasectomy. III. Clinical studies on the influences of vasectomy. Korean J Urol 7:11

Lee HY (1966) Studies on vasectomy. V. Vasectomy through single incision and immediate sperm clearance method. New Med J 9:133

Lee HY (1967) Studies on vasectomy. IV. Experimental studies on biological, histologic and histochemical effects of vasectomy. J Korean Med Assoc 10:893

Lee HY (1972) Reversible vas occlusion by intravasal thread. In: Richart RM, Prager DJ (eds) Human sterilization. Thomas, Springfield, Ill, p 193

Lee HY (1973) Male new technique (current status of reversible vas occlusion). Paper presented at the 2nd International Conference on Voluntary Sterilization, Geneva, Switzerland, February 25 – March 1, 1973

Lee HY (1973) Studies on residual sperm in the distal ductal system following vasectomy. Korean J Urol 14:19

Lee HY (1975) Technique and results of vasectomy in Korea. In: Sciarra JJ, Markland C, Speidel JJ (eds) Control of male fertility. Harper & Row, New York, p 68

Lee LT (1976) Compulsary sterilization and human rights. Popul: 3(4):2–9

Lee PA, Jaffe RB, Midgley AP, Kohen F, Niswender D (1972) Regulation of human gonadotropins, Suppression of serum LH and FSH in adult males following exogeneous testosterone administration. J Clin Endocrinol Metab 35:636

Leiman G (1972) Depo-medroxyprogesterone acetate as a contraceptive agent: its effect on weight and blood pressure. Am J Obstet Gynecol 114:97

Leonard JM, Paulsen CA (1978) Contraceptive development studies for males: Oral and pareuteral steroid hormone administration. In: Proceedings Hormonal Control of Male Fertility. DHEW Publication No (NIH) 78–1097, p 223, 1978

Lipsett MB (1974) Endocrinology of the testis. Paper presented at the Workshop on Control of Male Fertility, San Francisco, Calif

MacLeod J (1965) Control of spermatogenesis. In: Austin CR, Perry JS (eds) Agents affecting fertility. Little, Brown & Co, Boston, p 93

MacLeod J (1974) Effects of environmental factors and of antispermatogenic compounds on the human testis as reflected in seminal cytology. In: Mancini RE, Martini L (eds) Male fertility and sterility. Academic Press, New York, p 123

Marshall S, Lyon RP (1972a) Variability of sperm disappearance from the ejaculate after vasectomy. J Urol 107:815

Marshall S, Lyon RP (1972) Transient reappearance of sperm after vasectomy. JAMA 219:1753

Matsumoto YS, Koizuma A, Nohara T (1972) Condom use in Japan. Stud Fam Plann 3:251

Mauss J, Börsch G, Richter E, Bormacher K (1974) Investigations on the use of testosterone enauthate as a male contraceptive agent: a preliminary report. Contraception 10:281

Mauss J, Börsch G, Bormacher K, Leyendecker G, Nocke W (1975) Effects of long-term testosterone enauthate administration on male reproductive function: clinical evaluation, serum FSH, LH, testosterone and seminal fluid analysis in normal men. Acta Endocrinol (KbHh) 78:373

Mauss J, Börsch G, Bormacher K, Richter E, Leyendecker G, Nocke W (1978) Seminal fluid analyses, serum FSH, LH and testosterone in seven males before, during and after 250 mg testosterone enauthate weekly over 21 weeks. In: Proceedings Hormonal Control of Male Fertility, DHEW Publication No (NIH) 78–1097, p 93, 1978

Means AR, Fakunding JL, Huckins C, Tindall DJ, Vitale R (1976) FSH, the sertoli cell and spermatogenesis. Recent Progr Horm Res 32:477

Means AR, Dedman JR, Tindall DJ, Welsh MJ (1978) Hormonal regulation of sertoli cells. Int J Androl [Suppl] 2:403–424

Menge AC, Fuller B (1975) Testis antigens of man and some other primates. Fertil Steril 26:473

Moltz L, Römmler A, Schwartz V, Hammerstein J (1978) Effects of cyproterone acetate on pituitary gonadotropin release and on androgen secretion before and after LH-RH double stimulation test in men. Int J Androl [Suppl] 2

Morgan R (1972) Vasectomy. Pennsylvania Med 75:38

Morse HC, Leach DR, Rowley M, Heller CG (1973a) Effect of cyproterone acetate on sperm concentration, seminal fluid volume, testicular cytology and levels of plasma and urinary LH, FSH and testosterone in normal men. J Reprod Fertil 32:365

Morse HC, Horike N, Rowley MJ, Heller CG (1973b) Testosterone concentrations in testes of normal men: Effects of testosterone proprionate administration. J Clin Endocrinol Metab 37:882

Moss WMA (1972) Sutureless technic for bilateral partial vasectomy. Fertil Steril 23:33

Nash HA (1975) Depo provera: A review. Contraception 12:377

Nash JL, Rich JD (1972) The sexual after-effects of vasectomy. Fertil Steril 23:715

Nelson WO, Papanelli DJ (1965) Chemical control of spermatogenesis. In: Austin CR, Perry JS (eds) Agents affecting fertility. Little, Brown, Boston, p 177–196

Neumann F, Berswordt-Wallrabe R (1966) Effects of the androgen antagonist cyproterone acetate on the testicular structure, spermatogenesis and accessory sexual glands of testosterone treated adult hypophysectomized rats. Endocrinology 35:363

Neumann F, Elger W (1966) Permanent changes in gonadal function and sexual behaviour as a result of early feminization of male rats by treatment with an androgenic steroid. Endokrinologie 50:209

Noon KH, Bunge RG (1972) Temporary occlusion of the ductus deferens. In: Richart RM, Prager DJ (eds) Human sterilization. Thomas, Springield, Ill, p 204

Patanelli DJ, Nelson WO (1964) A quantitative study of inhibition and recovery of spermtogenesis. Recent Prog Horm Res 20:491

Paul R, Williams RP, Cohen E (1974) Structure-activity studies with chlorohydrins as orally active male antifertility agents. Contraception 9:451

Paulsen CA, Leonard JM (1976) Clinical trials in reversible male contraception: I. Combination of danazol plus testosterone. In: Spilman CH, Lobl TJ, Kirton KT (eds) Regulatory mechanisms of male reproductive physiology. Elsevier Excerpta Medica, Amsterdam, p 197

Paulsen CA, Leonard JM, Everett CB, Ospina LF (1978) Male contraceptive development: Re-examination of testosterone enauthate as an effective single entity agent. In: Proceedings Hormonal Control of Male Fertility, DHEW Publication No 78–1097, p 17

Petry R, Mauss J, Rausch-Stroomann JG, Vermeulen A (1972) Reversible inhibition of spermatogenesis in men. Horm Metab Res 4:386

Pincus G (1965) The control of fertility. Academic Press, New York

Popenoe P (1934) The progress of eugenic sterilization. J Hered 25:19–26

Pugh RCB (1969) Spontaneous recanalization of the divided vas deferens. Br J Urol 41:340

Rajalakshami M, Prasad MRN (1975) Action of cyproterone acetate on the accessory organs of reproduction in prepubertal and sexually mature rats. Fertil Steril 26:137

Reddy PRK, Rao JM (1972) Reversible antifertility action of testosterone proprionate in humab males. Contraception 5:295

Redford MH, Duncau GW, Prager DJ (1974) The condom: Increasing utilization in the United States. San Francisco Press, San Francisco

Rodgers DA, Ziegler FJ (1974) Effects of surgical contraception on sexual behaviour. In: Schima ME, Lubell J, Davis JE, Connell E (eds) Advances in voluntary sterilization. American Elsevier, New York, p 161

Roy S, Chatterjee S, Prasad MRN, Poddar AK, Pandey DC (1976) Effects of cyproterone acetate on reproductive functions in normal human males. Contraception 14:403

Ryder N (1973) Contraceptive failure in the United States. Perspect Fam Plann 5:133

Ryder NB, Westoff CF (1971) Reproduction in the United States. Princeton University Press, Princeton

Sackler AM (1973) Gonadal effects of vasectomy and vasoligation. Science 179:293

Schearer BS (1978) The use of progestins and androgens as a male contraceptive. Int Androl [Suppl] 2:680–713

Schmidt SS (1970) Male sterilization. In: Calderone MS (ed) Manual of family planning and contraceptive practice. 2nd ed. Williams & Wilkins, Baltimore, p 417

Schmidt SS (1971) Technique of vasectomy. Br Med J 2:524

Schmidt SS (1971) Vasectomy. JAMA 216:522

Schmidt SS (1973a) Caution on vasectomy. Med World New 14:14

Schmidt SS (1973b) Prevention of failure in vasectomy. J Urol 109:296

Schmidt SS (1975) Complication of vas surgery. In: Sciarra JJ, Markland C, Speidel JJ (eds) Control of male fertility. Harper & Row, New York, p 78

Schooenees R, Schalch DS, Murphy GP (1971) The hormonal effects of anti-androgen (SH-714) treatment in man. Invest Urol 8:635

Schwallie PC, Assenco JR (1972) Contraceptive use-efficacy study utilizing medroxyprogesterone acetate administered as an injection one every six months. Contraception 6:315

Scott LS (1972) Voluntary vasectomy. Scott Med J 17:203

Segal SJ (1974) Male Contraception: a male chauvinistic plot? Sci Am 231:3

Segal SJ, Croxatto HB (1967) Single administration of hormones for long-term control of reproductive function. Presentation at the XXIII. Meeting of American Fertility Society, April 14–16, 1967, Wash. D.C.

Sharp HC (1909) Vasectomy as a means of preventing procreation in defectives. JAMA 53:1897–1902

Sherins RJ, Gandy HM, Thorsland TW, Paulsen CA (1971) Pituitany and testicular function studies: Experience with a new gonadal inhibitor (Danazol). J Clin Endocrinol 32:522

Sherins RJ, Loriaux DL (1973) Studies in the role of sex steroids in the feedback control of FSH concentrations in man. J Clin Endocrinol Metab 36:886

Silber S (1977) Sperm granuloma and reversibility of vasectomy. Lancet 17:588

Skoglund RD, Paulsen CA (1973) Danazol-testosterone combination. A potentially effective means for reversible male contraception, a preliminary report. Contraception 7:357

Smith KD, Chowdhury M, Tscholakian RK (1975) Endocrine effects of vasectomy in humans. In: Sciarra JJ, Markland C, Speidel JJ (eds) Control of male fertility. Harper & Row, New York, p 169

Sorcini G, Sciarra F, Silverio F, Fraioli F (1971) Further studies on plasma androgens and gonadotropins after cyproterone acetate. Folia Endocrinol (Roma) 24:196

Speidel JJ (1973) Male sterilization and its contribution to solution of population problems Urology 1:277

Steinach E (1940) Sex and life: forty years of biological and medical experiments. Viking Press, New York

Steinberger E (1971) Hormonal control of mammalian spermatogenesis. Physiol Rev 51:1

Steinberger E (1973) Recent advances in regulation of male fertility. Presented at the 9th Harold C. Mack Symposium Detroit, October 1973

Steinberger E (1976) Biological action of gonadotropins in the male. Pharmacol Ther [B] 2:771

Steinberger E, Chowdhury M (1977) The effects of testosterone proprionate and estradiol benzoate on the in vitro synthesis of FSH. Biol Reprod 16:403

Steinberger E, Root A, Fisher M, Smith KD (1973) The role of androgens in the initiation of spermatogenesis in man. J Clin Endocrinol 37:746

Steinberger E, Smith KD (1977a) Testosterone enanthate: a possible reversible male contraceptive. Contraception 16:261

Steinberger E, Smith KD (1977b) Effect of chronic administration of testosterone enauthate on sperm production and plasma testosterone, FSH and LH levels: A preliminary evaluation of a possible male contraceptive. Fertil Steril 28:1320

Steinberger E, Smith KD (1978) Suppression and recovery of sperm production subsequent to administration of testosterone enanthate. Morphologic and hormonal evaluation. In: Proceedings Hormonal Control of Male Fertility. DHEW Publication No (NIH) 78–1097, p 195, 1978

Steinberger E, Smith KD, Rodriguez-Rigau LJ (1978) Suppression and recovery of sperm production in men treated with testosterone enanthate for one year. A study of a possible reversible male contraceptive. Int J Androl Suppl 2:748–763

Stewart-Bentley M, Odell W, Horton R (1974) The feedback control of LH in normal adult men. J Clin Endocrinol 38:545

Swerdloff RS, Odell WD (1968) Feedback control of gonadotropin secretion. Lancet 2:683

Swerdloff RS, Palacios A, McClure RD, Campfield LA, Brosman StA (1978) Clinical evaluation of testosterone enanthate in the reversible suppression of spermatogenesis in the human male: Efficacy mechanism of action and adverse effects. In: Proceedings Hormonal Control of Male Fertility, DHEW Publication No (NIH) 78–1097, p 41, 1978

Tauber AS (1973) A long term experience with vasectomy. J Reprod Med 10:147

Tietze C (1960) The Condom as a Contraceptive. National Committee on Maternal Health, Inc, Publication No 5, New York

Tietze C, Gamble CJ (1944) The condom as a Contraceptive method in public health work. Hum Fertil 9:97

Tietze C, Lewit S (1968) Statistical evaluation of contraceptive methods: use-effectiveness and extended use-effectiveness. Demography 5:931

Tietze C, Lewit S (1974) Statistical evaluation of contraceptive methods. Clin Obstet Gynecol 17:121

Tindall DJ, Means AR (1976) Concerning the hormonal regulation of androgen binding protein in rat-testis. Endocrinology 99:809

Ulstein M (1972) Sperm Penetration of Cervical Mucus as Criterion of Male Fertility. Acta Obstet Gynecol Scand 51:335

Ulstein M, Nettu N, Leonard J, Paulsen CA (1975) Changes in sperm morphology in normal men treated with Danazol and testosterone. Contraception 12:437

Urquhart HD (1973) Immediate sterility after vasectomy. Br Med J 3:378

Vosbeck K, Keller PJ (1971) The influence of antiandrogens on the excretion of FSH, LH and 17-Ketosteroids in males. Horm Metab Res 3:273

Walsh EL, Cuyler WK, McCullagh DR (1933) Effect of testicular hormone on hypophysectomized rats. Proc Soc Exp Biol Med 30:848

Walsh PC, Swerdloff RS, Odell WD (1973) Feedback control of FSH in the male: Role of estrogen. Acta Endocrinol (Kbh) 74:449

Weiss F, Vallejos CF (1972) Vasectomy technic using an auto-suture. Int Surg 57:660

Wieland RG (1972) Pituitary gonadal function before and after vasectomy. Feril Steril 23:779

Wortman J, Piotrow PT (1973) Sterilization: Vasectomy old and new techniques. Population Reports, Series D, No 1, pp 20

Wortman J (1975) Sterilization: Vasectomy – what are the problems? Population Reports, Series D, No 2, pp 15. Dept Med Publ Affairs, George Washington University Medical Center, Washington

Impotence

K. Bandhauer

The following chapter is intended as a short appendix to "fertility disorders in the male". It aims at giving the urologist with an andrologic interest some idea of the wide variety of factors that may be responsible for impotence, insofar as this plays a part in evaluating the male fertility status. Since impotence and its normal opposite, potency, are separated by a broad spectrum of disorders of differing degree, an encyclopedic representation of all these problems would be far beyond the limited scope of this contribution to the handbook. However, the urologist quite frequently comes across problems of disordered potency and finds himself faced with the clinical task of excluding organic or provable endocrine causes. It may well be that to establish an overall opinion on such complex problems will in practice almost always require the consultation of a psychiatrist and possibly of an endocrinologist in the planning of diagnosis and treatment. It should be pointed out from the very beginning that long-standing impotence of organic cause may, in itself, have such a profound effect on the psyche of a man that removal of the morphological abnormality alone does not suffice to restore potency.

The childlessness of a marriage is more frequently due to the inability of the husband to cohabitate than is commonly supposed. If the concept of impotence is broadened to include disorders of erection and ejaculation and loss of libido, then disorders of the patient's potency may be found to account for approximately 10% of childless marriages (STEENO, 1971).

The causes of impotence are manifold, often overlap one another, and may not be rigorously separable. Despite this difficulty, a broad division into psychological, endocrine and organic (including iatrogenic) causes of impotence has remained of value.

Numerically, psychogenic causes represent the vast majority. Between 80% and 90% of cases of male impotence may be attributed to primary or secondary psychogenic disorders (BEHERI, 1966; COOPER, 1972), although in individual cases organic and endocrine causes may coexist. Thus, purely psychogenic factors were the cause of impotence in only 68% of the series described by GEBOES et al. (1975a, b). Organic causes of impotence manifest themselves as inadequacy of erection or absent ejaculation, usually in the presence of normal libido.

A. Abnormalities of Erection

Erection, i.e., rigid distention of the corpora cavernosa, requires unimpaired arterial supply, patency of vascular channels in the erectile tissue, venous drainage, and an intact nerve supply. The cerebral center of erection in the precentral gyrus and the lumbar erection center (L-2–L-4) are the origin of vasoconstrictor impulses travelling in the pudendal nerves and of vasodilator impulses transmitted by the nervi erigentes. Arterial filling of the coropora cavernosa is via the internal pudendal arteries, venous drainage by the deep dorsal veins; the latter together with the bulbourethral and urethral veins drain the corpus spongiosum. There is free communication of the venous drainage pathways with oneanother in the venous plexus of the urogenital diaphragm. Arterial, venous, and arteriovenous anastomoses contain muscular subendothelial cushions (Conti, 1952), which under neural control are able to open and close these pathways.

Erection results from maximal arterial supply while the venous drainage is shut down. In the nonerect penis, the arterioles are partly closed and the veins and arteriovenous anastomoses widely opened.

Although these anatomic and functional principles of the erectile mechanism are not yet completely and fully established (Blandy, 1976), they form a basis for the explanation of organic and iatrogenic abnormalities of erection.

I. Congenital Abnormalities of the Penis Interfering with Erection

The most frequent inborn malformation of the penis associated with abnormal erection is hypospadias. In most cases, the extent to which erection is disordered correlates with the degree of hypospadias (glandular, penile, scrotal, or perineal), but some cases of glandular hypospadias may be associated with the extensive development of chordae and therefore marked curvature of the erect penis. Occasionally, chordae are present without ectopia of the urethral meatus. Culp and McRoberts (1968) have reported 14 such cases where the urethra reached the tip of the glans, but was short, as was the corpus spongiosum.

The abnormality of erection due to fibrous chordae being present in place of the missing urethra is not the only way in which hypospadias may bring about impotence, for the "cosmetic" abnormality due to the flattening and broadening of the glans and the constriction-ring deformity of the prepuce may lead to further, psychogenic effects. Hypospadias is the manifestation of an at least temporary delay in development of hormonal origin and as such may be associated with permanent endocrine abnormality requiring corresponding investigation.

1. Epispadias

Similar forms of impotence result from epispadias, of which the glandular (balanitic) type is often overlooked. However, the penile and pubopenile forms are usually associated with such considerable incontinence that the obstacle to coitus is obvious.

2. Phimosis

"True" phimosis – a constricted prepuce that cannot be retracted over the glans – is a rather uncommon congenital affliction that should not be confused with preputial adhesions. In most civilized countries, true congenital phimosis is now generally diagnosed early and corrected in good time. Rather more common barriers to intercourse are represented by minor degrees of preputial narrowing, which only become apparent as constriction rings on erection when they lead to painful engorgement of the glans. Of similar frequency are acquired phimoses of inflammatory origin with calculus formation and ulceration (diabetes!). Such painful erection may lead to disorders of potency that can also have a considerable psychologic overlay. It is not infrequently that one comes across impotence caused by such minor degrees of preputial stenosis, and in such cases cure may be effected by simple measures.

II. Acquired Abnormalities of the Penis Associated with Impotence

1. Peyronie's Disease (Induratio Penis Plastica)

This affliction usually appears in middle life with a peak incidence between the 5th and 6th decade, although younger men may also be affected. It is characterized by a usually circumscribed fibrous infiltration of the intercavernous septum of the penis. These changes, which usually represent fibrous plaques, lead to pain or erection and a varying degree of curvature of the penis. No treatment is available that would be aimed at the cause of this disease, which frequently occurs in combination with diabetes mellitus and Dupuytren's contracture. There has been no general trend toward an improvement of the therapeutic outcome despite the multiplicity of treatments, which include operative excision of the plaque with or without penile prosthesis, radiotherapy, and medical treatment with cortisone, procarbazine, etc. Spontaneous regression of the fibrous plaque and improvement of erection without treatment have been recorded.

2. Abnormal Erection Following Priapism

Fibrous induration of the corpora cavernosa, in the wake of priapism that was not controlled at an early stage (6–8 h), is an extremely rare cause of impotence (WAGENKNECHT, 1974; HINMAN, 1960). The patient usually gives a clear history that will focus attention on this cause of his symptoms. As the priapism itself has often been brought about by pelvic tumors, leukemia, sickle cell anemia, or pelvic vein thrombosis, there is little place for further consideration of such erectile disorders among causes of male infertility since the primary illness will within a short time become of dominant severity.

3. Posttraumatic Change in the Penis

Fracture of the penis (injury to the erectile tissue with disruption of the tunica albuginea) with or without simultaneous urethral injury may lead to coital difficulties. Despite primary operative repair of the corpora cavernosa and urethra, ensuing cicatrization may lead to abnormal erection. A concomitant posttraumatic stricture of the urethra may also interfere with ejaculation so that the efflux of semen is greatly retarded.

4. Impotence Following Pelvic Fracture

Severe pelvic fractures may lead to irreversible loss of potency quite independently of any injury to the urethra. There is no particular mechanism of injury to the bony pelvis that could be made responsible for the ensuing impotence. We have seen cases of impotence following simple diastasis of the pubic symphysis and preservation of potency following the severest of pelvic injuries.

The pathogenesis of impotence following pelvic fracture has not been definitely elucidated. Thrombosis of the arterial supply to the corpora cavernosa and injury to the pudendal and pelvic parasympathetic nerves have been discussed as possible mechanisms.

Pelvic parasympathetic nerve damage may equally be the cause for the various degrees of impotence seen after surgery to sigmoid and rectum, especially radical tumor surgery (Blandy, 1976).

III. Vascular Causes of Impotence

The significance of vascular influences on erection has been known for a great deal of time, and as early as 1668 de Graaf drew attention to the improvement of erection that followed ligature of the venous drainage of the penis. In 1902 ligature of the dorsal vein of the penis was suggested by Wooten as a treatment for impotence. Lydston (1908) reported good results of treating impotence by ligation of all accessible penile veins. In 1938 Semans and Langworthy reported a significant correlation between aortic perfusion and erection and thus related the syndrome described by Lériche (1951) to impotence. Twenty impotent men reported by Casey (1979) had deep cavernous and superficial dorsal penile arterial obstruction. Atheromatous change in the penile arteries and in the internal pudendal artery were described as a cause of impotence by Ginestie and Romieu (1976). The relationship between diabetes mellitus and penile perfusion problems has also been established and indeed measured in the studies of Denis Abelson (1975), who used Doppler ultrasound to quantify the penile pulse.

Impotence caused by arteriovenous fistulas of the internal pudendal artery has been described by Zorniotti et al. (1979). Degrees of impotence brought about by vascular impairment may be susceptible to treatment by revascularization: anastomosis of the femoral and internal pudendal arteries by interposition of a vein graft (Michal et al., 1974), anastomosis of the inferior epigastric artery to the corpora cavernosa (Laveen, 1977; Ginestié and Romieu, 1976, 1977) or anastomosis of the inferior epigastric and superficial dorsal penile arteries have all led to some improvement.

IV. Diabetes Mellitus and Disorders of Erection

Between 35% and 59% of patients with clinically manifest diabetes suffer from some degree of impotence (Rubin and Babbot, 1958; Ellenberg, 1966, 1971; Cooper, 1972; Montenero and Donatone, 1962; Raush-Strooman et al., 1970; Faerman et al., 1974: Abelson, 1975).

Three possible ways should be considered in which diabetes may cause impotence:

1. Vascular disorders: these have been mentioned in the previous section.
2. Neurogenic disorders: impairment of potency is common as part of a picture of diabetic neuropathy (Sprague, 1963; Ellenberg, 1971). Faerman et al. (1974) studied the autonomic nerve fibers in the corpora cavernosa of five patients with diabetes, and in four of them they were able to demonstrate swelling, rupture, vacuolization, and variations in caliber of axons. These nerve fibers did not appear to be involved in inflammatory processes, and the arterioles of the corpora cavernosa were unremarkable. In particular, no superadded diabetic microangiopathy could be detected in these patients.
3. Endocrine disorders: the causal relationship of diabetes mellitus and endocrine disorders is uncertain, but the association of testicular insufficiency and diabetes mellitus is not infrequently observed (Faerman et al., 1974; Jadzinsky et al., 1969; Bataille, 1963). This hypogonadism may be just as much of vascular as of neurogenic or endocrine origin (pituitary disorders – panhypopituitarism).

The neurogenic disorders brought about by diabetes are not however limited to abnormalities of erection but also include retrograde ejaculation. Ellenberg and Weber (1966) described five diabetics with retrograde ejaculation; furthermore, they described this disorder as a presenting symptom of diabetes. Impotence ensued as a further sign of diabetic polyneuropathy. Retrograde ejaculation in the context of diabetes may be regarded as the result of diabetic neuropathy involving mainly the pelvic autonomic nervous system.

V. Drugs, Poisons, and Disorders of Erection

A series of drugs and medicaments are reputed to have a detrimental influence on potency. As well as chronic alcohol and nicotine abuse, mention is frequently made of lead, arsenic, aniline, and narcotics, such as morphine, heroine, cocaine, and LSD. The exact relationship between these substances and abnormal erection is not known. Psychogenic factors may well play a major part. In the case of alcohol, there is clearly a question of dosage: small quantities may have a stimulatory effect and are useful in suppressing the "anxiety of anticipation" in psychogenic impotence. Among those therapeutic substances known to have an unfavorable effect on erectile capacity, tranquillizers and antihypertensive agents of sympathomimetic action have pride of place. As far as the tranquillizers diazepam (Valium), chlordiazepoxide hydrochloride (Librium), and medazepam (Nobrium) are concerned, Joel (1975) was able to demonstrate a beneficial effect on the psychogenic impotence of patients whose hypospermia is simultaneously treated with testosterone.

VI. Blood Pressure and Impotence

The relationship between changes in blood pressure and varying degrees of impotence has been documented by Joel (1975). Among 4190 cases of impotence, he found 300 patients with abnormalities of blood pressure (28% hypertensives and 72% hypotensives). Using Hydergine, a combination of equal of dihydroergocornine, dihydroergocristine and dihydroergocryptine, good results have been achieved in the treatment of hypotensive disturbances of erection.

B. Abnormalities of Ejaculation

Normal ejaculation requires simultaneous contraction of the vas deferens, seminal vesicles and ampulla, and of the musculature of the posterior urethra and pelvic floor with a coordinated contraction of the bladder neck. As early as 1896 Langley and Anderson had demonstrated that contraction of the vas deferens and of the seminal vesicles was brought about by stimulation of the hypogastric nerve. Root and Bard (1947) were able to show that resection of the sympathetic chain below the diaphragm led to abnormalities of emission. Ejaculation may be looked on as a sympathetically mediated process, even if the fine detail of its neural control is not yet known. Furthermore, ejaculation is subject to central nervous system control (Siroky and Craen, 1979).

I. Premature Ejaculation

Early ejaculation is generally a psychogenic disturbance without organic cause. The same is true of delayed ejaculation and of anorgasmia, the latter being failure of orgasm to occur despite normal erection.

In this context, the delayed ejaculation should be mentioned that occurs in urethral stricture, a symptom often only elicited after most careful questioning. Absence of ejaculation with preservation of orgasm may be due to failure of emission or to retrograde ejaculation into the bladder.

II. Failure of Emission

The transport of semen into the posterior urethra is brought about by rhythmic contraction of the smooth musculature of the vas deferens, the seminal vesicles, and the ampulla and is mediated by sympathetic fibers in the hypogastric nerve. Interference with this nerve supply by lumbar sympathectomy, by ablation of sympathetic ganglia in retroperitoneal lymphadenectomy (e.g., in testicular tumors) and by sympatholytic drugs may all lead to interference of the transport of semen, which should not be confused with retrograde ejaculation. According to Whitelaw and Smithwick (1951), bilateral sympathectomy at the L-2 level interfered with emission in 38% of cases. Kedia et al. (1975) recorded that high retroperitoneal lymph node clearance led to loss of ejaculation in almost 100% of their patients. The author's own observations on six patients with absent ejaculation after bilateral retroperitoneal lymph node dissection revealed no case in which spermatozoa were present in the first fraction of urine passed after coitus that had included orgasm. Thus, absence of semen transport can be assumed in these cases. The frequency of interference with semen transport following retroperitoneal lymphadenectomy varies in individual studies between 4% and 100% and appears to be correlated with the extent of lymphadenectomy (unilateral, bilateral, etc.). Among 100 patients who had undergone bilateral sympathectomy for essential hypertension, POPPEN and LEMMON found only 41 ejaculating normally.

Pharmacologic sympathectomy by α-receptor blockade, guanethidine, and α-methyldopa, etc. may equally lead to the abolition of emission. BEETZ (1972) recorded an incidence of almost 8% of such loss of emission in patients on guanethidine therapy. For this reason, childless husbands should always have a careful drug history taken, all the more since α-receptor blockade is gaining ever increasing application.

III. Retrograde Ejaculation

Retrograde ejaculation, i.e., expulsion of semen into the bladder, presupposes morphological or functional incompetence of the bladder neck. The commonest morphological cause of retrograde ejaculation is prostatectomy with bladder neck resection, irrespective of whether the operation was carried out transurethrally or by any other route. There is a 70%–80% chance of retrograde ejaculation occurring after prostatectomy (BANDHAUER et al., 1977). However, it is reasonable to point out that the age group most affected in this way does not generally have a strong interest in procreation and is thus unlikely to play a major role in fertility clinics.

Of greater significance is retrograde ejaculation as a consequence of transurethral or open bladder neck resection in childhood. OCHSNER et al. (1970) studied 21 patients who had either Y-V-plasties or transurethral or open wedge resection of the bladder neck. In seven cases, retrograde ejaculation was present 10–20 years after surgery.

The functional competence of the bladder neck may be disturbed by lesions of the hypogastric nerves such as ensue from major surgery in the true pelvis, lymphadenectomy, and anterior spinal fusion. Sympatholytic medication, such as Phenoxybenzamine, guanethidine, α-methyldopa, may also lead to retrograde ejaculation. Diabetic neuropathy, described above, can also be interpreted as a cause of bladder neck incompetence.

Therapeutic trials of sympathomimetics (BERGEANT and STEWARD, 1974; STOCKAMP et al., 1974) have lead to the conclusion that 50 mg ephedrine or 100 mg phenylpropanolamine may correct retrograde ejaculation resulting from retroperitoneal lymphadenectomy. The therapeutic value of α-receptor agonists in the treatment of such retrograde ejaculation resulting from retroperitoneal lymphadenectomy is generally attributed to an increase in bladder neck tone leading to reduction in the reflux of semen into the bladder. These drugs remained ineffective, however, in the treatment of disorders of emission.

References

Abelson D (1975) Diagnostic value of the penile pulse and blood pressure: A Doppler study of impotence in diabetics. J Urol 113:636

Antonini FM, Petruzzi E (1970) Sexual disturbances in male diabetics. Excerp Méd Found ICS 209:97

Antoniou LD, Shalhoub RJ, Sudhakar T, Smith JC Jr (1977) Reversal of uremic impotence by zinc. Lancet 2:895

Bandhauer K, Grob HU, Keller U, Kreutz G (1977) Die transurethrale Prostatektomie – Ein Ausbildungsproblem. Akt Urol 8:173–179

Bartels H, Möller GU (1974) Komplikationen nach retroperitonealer Lymphknotenausräumung bei malignen Hodenteratomen. Urol A 13:75

Bataille JP (1963) Le testicule endocrine du diabetique impuissant. Diabete 11:283

Beetz D (1972) Das Abklingen der Spermiogrammveränderungen nach Beendigung der Applikation von Guanethidinsulfat. Andrologia 4:239

Beheri GE (1966) Surgical treatment of impotence. Plast Reconstr. Surg 38:2

Bergeant J, Stewart BH (1976) Correction of retrograde ejaculation by sympathomimetic medication. A preliminary report. Fertil Steril 26:208

Bergquist N (1954) The gonadal function in male diabetes. Acta Endocrinol [Suppl] (Kbh) 18:3–29

Blandy JP (1976) Male scientific foundations of urology. Williams DI, Chisholm GD (ed) vol II, p 187

Borelli S (1960) Die psychogenen Fertilitäts- und Sexualstörungen beim Manne. In: Handbuch der Haut- und Geschlechtskrankheiten. Jadassohn J (ed) VI/3. Fertilitätsstörungen beim Manne. Springer, Berlin Göttingen Heidelberg, p 641

Bors E, Comarr AE (1960) Neurological disturbances of sexual function with special reference to 529 patients with spinal cord injury. Urol Survey 10:191–222

Britt DB, Kemmerer WT, Robinson JR (1971) Penile blood flow determination by mercury strain gauge plethysmography. Invest Urol 8:673

Canning JR, Lloyd FA, Cottrell TLC (1963) Genital vascular insufficiency and impotence. Surg Forum 16:298

Casey William C (1979) Revascularization of corpus cavernosum for erectile failure. Urology 14:135

Charny CW (1941) In: Eagle E (ed) Diagnosis in sterility. Thomas, Springfield, Ill

Conti G (1952) L'érection du pénis humain et ses bases. Morphologica-Vascularies. Acta Anat (Basel) 14:217

Cooper, AJ (1972) The causes and management of impotence. Postgrad Med J 48:548

Culp OS, McRoberts JW (1968) Hypospadias. In: Encyclopedia of urology, vol VII/1. Springer, Berlin Heidelberg New York, p 307

De Graaf R (1668) Tractus de usa siphonis in anatomica. p 230

Dubin L, Amelar RD (1972) Sexual causes of male infertility. Fertil Steril 23:8

Ebbehoj G, Wagner G (1980) Abnormal drainage of the corpus cavernosum causing erectile dysfunction. Proc First International Conference on Corpus Cavernosum Revascularization. Thomas, Springfield, Ill (in press)

Ellenberg, M. (1970) Significance of diabetic neuropathy in impotence. Diabetes 19 (Suppl. 1): 384

Ellenberg M (1971) Impotence in diabetes: The neurologic factor. Ann Intern Med 75:213–219

Ellenberg M, Weber H (1966) Retrograde ejaculation in diabetic neuropathy. Ann Intern Med 65:1237–1246

Ellenberg M, Weber H (1967) The incipient, asymptomatic diabetic bladder. Diabetes 16:331–339

Faerman I, Maler M, Jadzinsky M, Fox D, Alvarez E, Zilverbarg J, Cibeira JB, Colinas R (1969) La vejiga neurogénica en los pacientes diabéticos. Rev Argent Urol 38:16

Faerman I, Maler M, Jadzinsky M, Alvarez E, Fox D, Zilverbarg J, Cibeira JB, Colinas R (1970) Vejiga neurogénica en dibéticos juveniles. Excerp Méd Found ICS 209:127

Faerman I, Vilar, O, Rivarola MA, Rosner JM, Jadzinsky MN, Fox D, Perez-Lloret A, Bernstein-Hahn, L, Saraceni D (1972) impotence and diabetes. Diabetes 21:23

Faerman J, Glocer L, Fox D, Jadzinsky MN, Rapaport M (1974) Impotence and diabetes: Histologic studies of autonomic nervous fibers of corpora cavernosa in impotent diabetic males. Diabetes 23:971

Fawcett DW, Burgos MH (1960) Studies on the fine structure of the mammalian testis. II. The human interstitial tissue. Am J Anat 107:245

Fitzpatrick TJ (1974) Venography of the deep dorsal venous and valvular systems. J Urol 111:518

Fitzpatrick T (1975a) The corpus cavernosum intercommunicating venous drainage system. J Urol 113:494

Fitzpatrick TJ, Cooper JF (1975b) A cavernosogram study of the valvular competence of the human deep dorsal vein. J Urol 113:497

Foglia VG, Borghelli FR, Chieri RA, Fernandez Collazo EL, Spindler I, Wesely O (1963) Sexual disturbances in the diabetic rat. Diabetes 12:231

Friedman D (1977) Psychoandrology. In: Money J, Musaph H (eds) Handbook of sexology, chap 65. Excerpta Medica, Amsterdam London New York, p 863

Gaskell P (1971) Importance of penile blood pressure in cases of impotence. CMAJ 105:1047

Geboes K, Steeno O, De Moor P (1975a) Sexual impotence in man. Andrologia 7:217

Geboes K, Steeno O, De Moor P (1975b) Primary anejaculation: Diagnosis and therapy. Fertil Steril 26:1018

Gee WF (1975) A history of surgical treatment of impotence. Urology 5:401

Ginestié JF, Romieu A (1976) Traitement des impuissances d'origine vascularie: La révascularisation des corps caverneux. J Urol Nephrol (Paris) 10:853

Ginestié JF, Romieu A (1977) Exploration radiologique de l'impuissance. Maloine, Paris

Gittes RF, Waters B (1979) Sexual impotence: The overlooked complication of a second renal transplant. J Urol 121:719

Guzman JM (1964) La vejiga neurogénica. Actas VIII Congreso Argentino Urologia, 541

Harrison RF, De Louvois J, Blades M, Hurley R (1975) Doxycycline treatment and human infertility. Lancet 1:No 7907, 605

Hinman F Jr (1960) Priapism: Reasons for failure of therapy. J Urol 83:420

Horstmann P (1950) The excretion of androgens in human diabetes mellitus. Acta Endocrinol (Kbh) 5:261–269

Jadzinsky M, Faerman I, Fox D, Varela J, Gonzalez Casco J, Schvartsman R (1969) Tratamiente hormonal de la impotencia sexual en hombres diabéticos. El Dia Méd 41:862

Jarvik ME, Brecher EM (1977) Drugs and sex inhibition and enhancement effects. In: Money J, Musaph H (eds) Handbook of sexology, chap 88. Excerpta Medica, Amsterdam London New York, p 1065

Jimenez JF, Conejero J, Llanazares G, Sole Balleus (1977) Impotence and diabetes mellitus. Eur Urol 3:78

Joel CA (1972) Zur Pathogenese, Diagnostik und Therapie der Impotentia coeundi mit besonderer Berücksichtigung der Diazepinderivate. Andrologia 4:7

Joel CA (1975) Male impotence. In: Behrman, SJ, Kistner RW (eds) Progress in infertility, 2nd edit. Little, Brown Boston, p 735

Johnson J (1968) Disorders of sexual potency in the male. Pergamon Press, New York

Karacan I (1969) A simple and inexpensive transducer for quantitative measurements of penile erection during sleep. Behav Rec Meth Instr 1:251–252

Karacan I (1970) Clinical value of nocturnal erection in the prognosis and diagnosis of impotence. Med Asp Human Sex 4:27–34

Kedia KR, Markland C, Fraley EE (1975) Sexual function following high retroperitoneal lymphadenectomy. J Urol 114:3, 237

Kent JR (1966) Gonadal function in impotent diabetic males. Diabetes 15:537

Kent JR (1969) Gonadal function in impotent diabetic males, In: Abstracts of the 26th Annual Meeting of the American Diabetes Association, San Francisco, p 537

Keye JD (1956) Hyperplasia of Leydig cells in chronic paraplegia. Neurology (Minneap) 6:68

Kimura Y, Adachi K, Kisaki N, Ise K (1975) On the transportation of spermatozoa in the vas deferens. Andrologia 7:55

Kinsey AC, Pomeroy WB, Martins CE (1948) Sexual behavior in the human male. Saunders, Philadelphia

Kirschner MA, Coffman GD (1968) Measurement of plasma testosterone and "delta-4"-androstenedione using electron capture gas-liquid chromatography. J Clin Endocrinol 28:1347–1355

Klebanow D, MacLeod J (1960) Semen quality and certain disturbances of reproduction in diabetic men. Fertil Steril 11:255–261

Langley JN, Anderson HK (1895–96) The inervation of the pelvic viscera and adjoining viscera. J Physiol (Lond) 19:85

Laveen H (1977) Revascularization of the penis. Presented at the Los Angeles Vascular Society

Learmouth JR (1931) A contribution of the neurophysiology of the urinary bladder in man. Brain 54:147–176

Lema BE, Foglia VG, Fernandez Collazo EL (1965) Lesiones histologicas testiculares en la rate diabetica. Rev Soc Argent Biol 41:197

Lériche R (1951) Les obliterations de terminaison de l'aorte. Etude Arteriographique. Langenbecks Arch Klin Chir (K6.BD) 270:85

Machleder HI (1978) Sexual dysfunction in aorto-iliac occlusive disease. Med Asp Human Sex 12:125

Malvar T, Baron T, Clark SS (1973) Assessment of potency with the Doppler flowmeter. Urology 2:396

Mancini R (1968) Testiculo Humano (Simposio). Panamericana, Buenos Aires, p 87

Michal V, Kramar R, Bartak V (1974) Femoro-pudendal bypass in the treatment of sexual impotence. J Cardiovasc Surg 15:356

Montenero P, Donatone E (1962) Diabète et activité sexuelle chez l'homme. Diabète 8:327–332

Newmann HF, Northup JD, Devlin J (1964) Mechanism of human penile erection. Invest Urol 1:350

Oakley WG: In Discussion of Strauss EB, ref 1950

Ochsner MG, Burns E, Henry HH (1970) Incidence of retrograde ejaculation following bladder neck revision as a child. J Urol 104:596

Paulson CA (1968) The testes. In: Williams RH (ed) Endocrinology. Saunders, Philadelphia, pp 405–458

Poppen JL, Lemmon Ch (1947) The surgical treatment of essential hypertension. J Am Med Ass 134:1

Raush-Strooman JG, Petry R, Mauss J, Hienz HA, Jakubowski HD, Senge T, Muller KM, Eckhardt B, Berthold K, Sauer H (1970) Studies of sexual function in diabetes. Excerp Med Found ICS 209:112

Rivarola MA, Saenz JM, Meyer WI, Jenkins ME, Migeon CJ (1966) Metabolic clearance rate of testosterone and androst-4-ono-3-17-dione under basal conditions, ACTH and HCG stimulation. Comparison with urinary production rate of testosterone. J Clin Endocrinol 26:1208

Roen PR (1965) Impotence. NY J Med 65:2576–2583

Root WS, Bard P (1947) The mediation of feline erection through symathetic pathways with some remarks on sexual behavior after deafferentation of the genitalia. Am J Physiol 150:80

Rubin A (1958b) The influence of diabetes mellitus in men upon reproduction. Am J Obstet Gynecol 76:25–29

Rubin A, Babbott D (1958a) Impotence and diabetes mellitus. JAMA 168:498–500

Schoffling K (1970) Diabetes mellitus and male gonadal function. Presented at VIIth Congress of International Federation of Diabetes, Buenos Aires, Argentina, August (1970)

Schoffling K, Federling K, Schmidt W, Pfeiffer EF (1967) Histometric investigation on the testicular tissue of rats with alloxan diabetes and Chinese hamster with spontaneous diabetes. Acta Endocr (Kbh) 54:335

Semans JH, Langworthy OR (1938) Observations on the neurophysiology of sexual function in the male cat. J Urol 40:836

Simpson SL (1949); (1966) Impotence. Med Soc Trans 64:279–291; Fertil Steril 17:429–438

Simpson SL (1950) Impotence. Br Med J 1:692–697

Siroky MB, Krane RJ (1979) Physiology of male sexual function. In: Krane RJ, Siroky MB (eds) Clinical neuro-urology. Little Brown, Boston, p 45

Sprague RG (1963) Impotence in male diabetics. Diabetes 12:559

Steeno O (1971) L'impuissance sexuelle chez l'homme. Ed Acco Leuven, 23

Stockamp K, Schreiter F, Altuein JE (1974) α-adrenergic drugs in retrograde ejaculation. Fertil Steril 25:9

Strauss EB (1949) Impotence. Med Soc Trans 64:291–299

Strauss EB (1950) Impotence from the psychiatric standpoint. Br Med J 1:697–703

Tordjman G, Thierree R, Michel JR (1977) Nouvelles acquisitions en pathologie vasculaire dans les dysfunctions érectiles de l'homme. Cah Sex Clin 3:19

Vilar O, Christian JJ (1967) Light and electron microscopy of adrenocorticotrophin-induced renal glomerular disease in mice. Lab Invest 17:645

Villanueva GA, Garcia G, Hernandez P, Cesarman E (1964) Diabetes e Impotencia sexual. Imagen histologica del testiculo y respuesta hormonal con gonadotrofina corionica. Rev Invest Clin 16:31

Wagenknecht LV (1974) Zur Aetiologie und Behandlung des Priapismus. Urol A 13:133

Whitelaw GP, Smithwick RH (1951) Some secondary effects of sympathectomy with particular reference to disturbance of sexual function. N Engl J Med 245:121

Wooten JS (1902) Ligation of the dorsal vein of the penis as a cure for atonic impotence. Tex Med J 18:325

Zilverbarg D, Cibeira JB, Colinas R (1970) Vejiga neurogenica en diabeticos juveniles. Excerp Méd Found ICS 209:127

Zorgniotti AW, Padula G, Rossi G (1979) Impotence caused by pudendal arteriovenous fistula. Urology 14:161

Functional Sexual Disorders in the Male

W. Pöldinger

Ninety percent of sexual disorders in men are functional and rightfully belong within the compass of psychosomatic disease. However, since 10%–20% of such complaints prove to have an organic cause (diabetes mellitus, circulatory abnormalities, etc.), full physical examination and endocrinologic screening are prerequisites in the management of impotence.

The ever increasing incidence of potency disorders in men is in probability related to the increasing liberalization of sexuality. This liberalization itself has brought not only advantages but also disadvantages for male sexuality. Increasing knowledge of and opportunity for sexuality may lead a man to look on his relationships as pressurizing him toward a high level of performance. It is under this very pressure that he may fail. This performance orientation on the one hand, and the fear of failure on the other, are the commonest causes of functional sexual disorders, where a fateful "chain reaction" may take place, with fear of a symptom leading to the symptom itself.

On the other hand, research and advance in sexual medicine have led to the emergence of new therapeutic modalities and strategies, a principal feature of which is their ability to bring about improvement and cure in a shorter period of time than was previously the case. Both behavior therapy and couple therapy, communication therapy, and focused short-term therapy should be mentioned among those types of psychotherapeutic treatment that have shown themselves to be of value in the management of functional disorders. MASTERS and JOHNSON (1973) did not use any of these terms, but their great achievement was to pioneer new strategies of treatment in this field. One great advance was the decision only to treat couples and that these should always be treated together. Indeed, in the original method of these authors, the patient-couple were to be treated by a male and female therapeutic pair. In Europe the method of MASTERS and JOHNSON (1973) has been adopted mainly in the simplified form involving a single therapist.

The individual types of functional sexual disturbance in men comprise disorders of libido (impotence of desire), disorders of erection (impotence of erection), disorders of ejaculation (impotence of ejaculation), in which premature ejaculation and delayed ejaculation should be differentiated, and finally emotional impotence (impotence of satisfaction).

Table 1 summarizes the various individual forms of therapy available for functional sexual disorders.

Table 1. The therapy of functional sexual disorders

Enlightenment	Discursive forms of therapy
Prohibition of intercourse	Communication therapy
Paradoxical intention	Focused analytical methods
Autogenic training	Psychoanalytical methods
Behavior therapy	Existential analysis
In vitro	Logotherapeutic methods
In vivo	

It should be emphasized that in any consultation for functional disorders of potency great importance attaches to sexual enlightenment. Although advances have been made in the sex education of children by comparison to earlier standards, there is frequently still considerable ignorance of the normal sequence of events at sexual intercourse and of normal sexual practices. It is therefore important in the first interview to find out the extent of the couples knowledge of the physiology and psychology of intercourse and to close those gaps that are thus revealed. In particular, it is important to give clear information as to the variability of normal intercourse, since many people live in fear that their minor deviations from the norm, e.g., of position, may represent some form of "perversion."

In many sexual disorders, it may be quite adequate simply to prohibit coitus for the duration of treatment. This leads to a disappearance of the fear of failure since there is thus virtually no expectation and no performance requirement from either partner. The couple may then be lying in bed one evening in a tender embrace, feel sexually stimulated, and start to bemoan their promise not to practice sexual intercourse. That frequently results in a protracted discussion of whether or not to break this stipulation, during which there may be increasing intimacies finally resulting in a psychological barrier being overcome. In this situation, the "enemy" is no longer the symptom but the physician who had imposed a ban on sexual intercourse. Thus, the greater part of the therapy will be complete when this couple appears for the next consultation and begins amid some embarrassment to confess their transgression.

Although it is really a behavior therapeutic method, mention should be made in connection with these simple methods of so-called' paradox intention, as devised by V.E. Frankl (1975) who was the founder of logotherapy. Paradox intention means that a person, who for example is afraid of blushing, instead of saying to himself before entering a room where there are other people: "I hope I am not going to blush," firmly resolves: "today I hope I shall blush as red as a beet." If he really succeeds in making this resolution, he is often pleasantly surprised at his inability to blush although this was precisely what he wanted. The same process may be applied to functional disorders such as impotence. The therapist has to persuade his male patient that at the next encounter, instead of continually thinking "I hope this doesn't turn out to be yet another failure," he must firmly resolve himself to say, for example: "having failed so often, why shouldn't I do so today" or "today I have decided to be impotent, and why the hell not!"

Since functional sexual disorders are, as a rule, related to fear, inward unrest, and tension, methods involving the practice of relaxation techniques are of particular value. In this context, the relaxation exercises of JACOBSON (1938) are worthy of mention – quite apart from autogenic training techniques. The former are a set of exercises involving vigorous muscular contractions with conscious attention to the ensuing muscle relaxation. JACOBSON has compiled an extremely extensive compendium of individual muscles that may be contracted and relaxed. The following is a simplified version: Eyelids tightly shut, mouth tightly shut, the head pressed down to the trunk, fists clenched, biceps tensed, elbows squeezed into the sides, contraction of abdominal muscles, contraction of pelvic floor, knees squeezed together, in the sitting position the toes pressed against the floor.

These relaxation exercises play an important role in so-called desensitization, one of the techniques of modern behavior therapy that finds a wide field of application in functional sexual disorders. Desensitization is a technique based on the concept that the symptoms arise for reasons that may be explained by learning theory. Classic conditioning, as described by PAVLOV (1955), plays some part in this process. This therapeutic attitude assumes that at some time sexual excitement coincided with the emergence of fear so that subsequently, whenever there is sexual excitement there is also fear – which then interferes extensively with the sequence of sexual events. The first step in desensitization, therefore, is to draw up with the patient a hierarchic list of his fears. For a man suffering from impotence, such a hierarchy might appear roughly as follows: firstly, the mere thought of sexuality brings about fear, followed by the concrete realization that coitus is to take place at a given time, then by the situation, the person, the preparatory activities, foreplay, and finally intromission. A crescendo fear of failure might develop throughout such a sequence. The next therapeutic step then is to teach the patient JACOBSON's relaxation exercises, and following such exercises the patient should be instructed to concentrate his imagination on the least significant stage in his hierarchy of fears. Once he becomes able to imagine this particular situation without fear, he can proceed to the next stage, i.e., to the consideration of the next most fearful situation. Should such stepwise progress come to a halt, repeated relaxation exercises should be carried out and the imaginary progression reversed by one stage. The advantage of this technique is that once the hierarchy of fears has been drawn up, and the patient has learned the relaxation exercises, he can practice the technique alone and without the presence of the therapist. At first this desensitization is only carried out in a mental context, i.e., in imaginary situations. The next step is to transfer the technique into the practical sphere, thus approximating the technique of MASTERS and JOHNSON. Their method aims at ridding the patient-couple of anxieties by continuous and repeated experiments interrupted by therapy sessions. The classic method of MASTERS and JOHNSON is reproduced in Table 2. The technique commences with each partner being examined individually and interviewed in depth about his degree of sexual knowledge, problems, and conflicts. Following this, the first communal session takes place in which those problems that lead to mutual difficulties in sexual encounters are discussed quite openly. This discussion provides an

Table 2. Therapy according to Masters and Johnson with
paired therapists

Separate interview and examination
Communal round table discussion
Enlightenment
Discussion of conflicts
Practical behavior modification by "sensate focus"
Ongoing round table progress monitoring

---

opportunity to make good any lack of sexual knowledge that may have been discovered in the previous interviews. Particular personal conflicts are grasped and discussed quite openly. This session is followed by practical instructions for the next cohabitation so that repeated step-by-step attempts by both patients to draw closer are continually interspersed with therapy sessions as progress-checks. In common with the principals of behavior therapy, the general intention is to proceed by very small steps, and relaxation exercises and autogenic training techniques may be included in the process. It is of particular importance that both patients should learn step by step to verbalize their feelings to each other during cohabitation. Thus, instructions might be given to the effect that the partner who initiates intimacies should break off after a short while so that the other partner is able to explain their experience of this approach, what was disagreeable about it, and what might have been preferable. This second partner will then assume a more active role in attempting to stimulate the other and this is followed once again after a short while by a further discussion, this time on the pleasant and unpleasant sensations and possible fears of the first partner. Thus, a graduated process is built up subject to both partners being instructed to break off the experiment for the day if one of them finds his or her fear of proceeding intolerable.

In addition, specific practical hints may be of particular importance in the dispersal of fear and anxiety. Thus, for example, an impotent man may be relieved of the compulsion to perform by the recommendation that coitus be carried out in a position in which the man lies supine and the woman sits astride him. Thus, the man will feel under less pressure, since most of the activity will eminate from the woman. This position, in which the man lies on his back and the woman sits astride his thighs, also plays an important in the "squeeze" technique described by Masters and Johnson for premature ejaculation. In this technique the man is instructed to remain as inactive as possible, while it is the woman's task to gently stimulate him by hand until he becomes aware that ejaculation is imminent and learns to tell her of this, in time for her to prevent ejaculation by pressure applied to the end of the penile shaft. The main object of the training it to teach the man to recognize impending ejaculation in time to reduce his level of sexual preoccupation. Once this has been successful several times in succession during the course of one cohabitation – and this will require the woman to wait each time she exerts pressure on the glans until excitation of the male organ has diminished – stimulation in following sessions may cease to be manual and may be carried out

Table 3. Analytical problems involved in functional sexual disturbances in the male

Impotence	*Fear of castration:* fear of retribution *Oedipal fixation:* incessant competition with imaginary rivals *Fear of aggressive components* of own sexuality
Premature Ejaculation	*Oedipal idealization* of women: wanting neither to injure, nor to give *Urethral fixation:* not wanting to give
Delayed Ejaculation	*Guilt feelings* preventing enjoyment *Not wanting to give* for fear of castration, for fear of loss of self in orgastic regression (fear of death)

by the woman sitting astride the man. He will remain in the supine position so that most of the activity comes from her and he is not subject to any specific pressures.

This technique of MASTERS and JOHNSON has found widespread application and represents a kind of combination of behavior therapy, conversation therapy, and communication therapy. Like classic behavior therapy, this technique concentrates on behavior, i.e., on a specific symptom, without investigating any possible subconscious conflicts and problems.

However, following successful treatment by the application of such behavioral concepts, it may be advantageous to focus some form of analytical therapy upon the subconscious origin of the anxieties in question, particularly if there is a tendency to recurrence. In this context, it should be emphasized that the controversy that has for so long existed between behavior therapists and psychotherapists has been far from fruitful, and in particular has yielded nothing to help patients. It is not, after all, the job of the physician to confirm in the course of treatment the validity of a particular preconceived opinion or theory, but rather, if one form of treatment fails, to develop alternative therapeutic strategies.

Whereas it was previously a common practice in the treatment of functional sexual disorders to undertake extensive psychoanalysis of the presenting patient without even speaking to his partner, couple-therapy on the one hand and focal and abbreviated forms of psychotherapy on the other have gained considerable ground. It is worth remembering that SIGMUND FREUD, who was fundamentally opposed to abbreviated forms of therapy, did indeed himself carry out such a treatment. In just three sessions he was able to cure Gustav Maler of impotence, following which the famous conversation took place in which Freud suggested to Maler that he should be analyzed. The latter retorted that he would have to decline, as he preferred to continue composing music.

Various analytical problems that frequently play an important part in functional sexual disorders in the male are listed in Table 3 (after BECKER, 1975). However, in view of the phenomenon of transference and reverse transference that may arise in the course of conversation with the patient, it is clearly important for the physician to acquire the requisite knowledge to carry out such analytical therapy, not only in theory, but also in his own emotional field. It has already been pointed out that Balint group sessions (BALINT et al.,

1973) are extremely suitable for this purpose. These are 2-hourly meetings of 8–12 interested practitioners, occurring at 14-day intervals over several years, under the guidance of an experienced psychotherapist or of a fellow physician with extensive psychotherapeutic experience – even if he is not a fully qualified specialist.

Finally, in the context of the psychotherapy of functional secual disorders, attention should be drawn to logo- and existential therapy since sexual problems are often related to questions concerning the meaning of life in general. We have already mentioned the paradoxical intention concept of the logotherapist V.E. FRANKL (1975).

Any discursive therapy of functional sexual disorders must also aim at breaking down taboos in the course of conversation and must provide opportunities for open discussion of the problems of sexuality, neither moralizing nor, at the same time, being unduly casual. It is of considerable importance to resolve the patient's performance-orientated attitude to the success of therapy itself. Thus, such therapy, and indeed any future psychotherapeutic intervention, can be looked on less and less in terms of performance or work capability and more and more in terms of capacity for life and for love. With special regard to matters of eroticism, it will be quite unavoidable to point out that quality is superior to quantity.

References

Balint M, Ornstein PH, Balint E (1973) Fokaltherapie, Suhrkamp, Frankfurt a.M.

Beck D (1974) Die Kurzpsychotherapie. Huber, Bern Stuttgart Vienna

Becker N (1975) Psychoanalytische Ansätze bei der Therapie sexueller Funktionsstörungen. In: Sigusch V, Therapie sexueller Störungen. Thieme, Stuttgart

Braeutigam W (1977) Sexualmedizin im Grundriss. Thieme, Stuttgart

Duss-von Werdt J, Hauser GA (1970) Das Buch von Liebe und Ehe. Walter, Olten Freiburg i.Br.

Frankl VE (1975) Theorie und Therapie der Neurosen. "Uni" paperback 457. Reinhart, Munich

Fromm E (1965) Die Kunst des Liebens. Ullstein Book No 258, 1965

Jacobson E (1938) Progressive relaxation. University of Chicago Press, Chicago

Jores A (1976) Die Psychosomatik der Sexualstörungen des Mannes. In: Praktische Psychosomatik. Huber, Bern Stuttgart Vienna

Kremser M (1975) Psychotherapie und Sexualstörungen. In: Strotzka H, Psychotherapie: Grundlagen, Verfahren und Indikationen. Urban & Schwarzenberg, Munich Vienna Berlin

Kockott G, Dittmar F (1972) Diagnose und Behandlung von Kohabitationsstörungen und Deviationen. Sexualmedizin 1:340–343, 386–389, 449–452

Kockott G, Dittmar F (1973) Verhaltenstherapie sexueller Störungen: Diagnostik und Behandlungsmethoden. Nervenarzt 44:173–183

Langen D (1973) Psychotherapie, 3. Aufl. Thieme, Stuttgart

Lazarus AA (1965) The treatment of a sexually inadaequate man. In: Ullman LP, Krasner L (eds) Case studies in behavior modification. Holt, Rinehart & Winston, New York

Luban-Plozza B, Poeldinger W (1977) Der psychosomatisch Kranke in der Praxis, 3. Aufl. Springer, Bern Heidelberg New York

Mandel KH (1969) Sexuelle Störungen. Lecture notes at the Psychological Institute Munich, 1969 (unpublished)

Mandel A, Mandel KH, Stadter E, Zimmer D (1971) Einübung in Partnerschaft durch Kommunikationstherapie und Verhaltenstherapie. Munich, Pfeiffer

Masters WH, Johnson VE (1970) Die sexuelle Reaktion. Rowohlt, Hamburg
Masters WH, Johnson VE (1973) Impotenz und Anorgasmie. Goverts Krüger Stahlberg, Frankfurt
Nikolowski W, Poeldinger W, Spechter HJ (1978) Kompendium der Kohabitations- und Fertilitätsstörungen. Karger, Basel
Pawlow I (1955) Ausgewählte Werke (Selected works). Akademie Verlag, Berlin
Poeldinger W (1977) Sexuelle Störungen aus psychosomatischer Sicht. Z Allgemeinmed 53:86–91
Poeldinger W (1978) Sexualmedizin in der Praxis. Sexualmedizin 7:399–402
Rogers CR (1972) Die nicht-direktive Therapie. Kindler,
Schirren C (1971) Praktische Andrologie. Brüder Hartmann, Berlin
Sigusch V (1975) Therapie sexueller Störungen. Thieme, Stuttgart
Watzlawick P, Beavin JH, Jackson DD (1969) Menschliche Kommunikationen, Formen, Störungen, Paradoxien. Huber, Bern Stuttgart Vienna

Male Climacteric?

B. Lunenfeld, A. Eshkol, and M. Glezerman

With 2 Figures

A. Introduction

With advancing age, some men complain about fatigability, decreasing productivity, lack of concentration, depressions, anxiety, sleep disturbances, hot flushes, sweating, tachycardia, constipation, and skin atrophy. These symptoms may occur as isolated complaints or in various combinations and are sometimes associated with decreasing potency or libido. Any association of some of these 12 symptoms, occurring randomly in men with advancing age, was called by Werner (1939) "male climacteric syndrome" assuming an endocrine origin as in women. This concept also led others to designate these symptoms "the male menopause." Since menopause means cessation of menses, the term male menopause should be avoided. There is no question today that the above symptoms may occur in men with advancing age; they may, however, occur as a neurasthenic symptom complex associated with aging and not always associated with a decrease of endocrine function of the testes. Kies (1974) attempted an analysis of configuration frequency for the above 12 symptoms in 5000 male patients aged 45–65 years. In his study only three combinations of two related symptoms occurred with a higher than expected frequency:
1. Sexual disturbance and sweating
2. Sexual disturbance and nervousness
3. Constipation and insomnia

Thus, it seems that although there is an increasing incidence of certain symptoms with advancing age, they cannot be classified as a single pathologic entity. We will try to differentiate between three clinical situations, which are commonly called male climacteric:
1. Aging: any combination of the above 12 symptoms without decrease of sexual potency or libido and not explained by an underlying pathologic cause
2. Male climacteric or male senescence: similar to the above, but combined with a decrease of sexual potency or libido, with no evidence of decreased endocrine function of the testes
3. Andropause: similar to male climacteric, associated, however, with a demonstrable decrease of androgenicity

Androgenicity is defined as an expression of two separate but associated parameters:

1. The availability of physiologically active androgen, which is influenced by (a) the secretion rate, (b) the metabolic disposal rate of androgens, and (c) the portion of free testosterone
2. The responsiveness of target cells

Thus, decreased androgenicity can arise as a result of any of the above parameters or a combination. The term andropause seems to us a suitable term to describe the clinical symptoms associated with decreased androgenicity.

The clinical entities outlined above should be identified and diagnosed taking particular care to rule out pathologic factors (e.g., cold nodule of the thyroid, hepatic and renal malfunction, circulation disturbances, diabetes, neuropathology, etc.), which are only too easily ignored since it is so tempting to classify the complaining aging male as suffering from male climacteric.

The events leading to aging and male climacteric as defined above and the treatment of the symptomatology of these two entities are beyond the scope of this chapter, and the reader is referred to specialized texts in geriatrics and psychosomatic medicine. In this chapter we will deal specifically with the third entity, namely, the andropause.

Since the 1930s, increasing attention has been paid by scientists to aging symptoms associated with a deficiency state resulting from age-related failure of the endocrine glands to secrete their hormones. Andropause is thus an overt hormone deficiency state of the gonads (and possibly adrenals). A fall in the excretion of 17-oxysteroids and testosterone glucuronide with advancing age as well as lower levels of testosterone in spermatic vein blood of old men as compared to young men has been described (Engle and Pincus, 1956; Hollander and Hollander, 1958; Morer-Fargas and Nowakosky, 1965).

As more sophisticated methods for the evaluation of pituitary-testicular function became available, a clearer picture evolved describing events that eventually may lead to the andropause. In 1976 Baker et al. made an important contribution by extensively investigating several parameters of the pituitary-testicular axis and correlating these to age. Illustrations revelant to the present discussion will be quoted here by permission of the authors.

Baker et al. (1976) found that from the age of 40 years there was a steady decline of plasma testosterone levels with advancing age (Fig. 1a). While only 5 of the 37 men over the age of 70 years had levels below the lowest seen in men aged 21–50 years, none had levels above 24 nmol/liter. The distribution of testosterone levels of adult men aged 21–70 years was also best approximated by a logarithmic normal distribution. Men over the age of 50 years had significantly lower levels of testosterone (mean 17.5 nmol/liter) than did the younger men (mean 22.0 nmol/liter; $P < 0.001$).

Kirschner and Coffman (1968) found significantly lower testosterone levels in six men aged 55–65 years compared with levels in men aged 18–38 years. Vermeulen et al. (1972) and Rubens et al. (1974) studied in detail age-related changes in testosterone secretion and metabolism and demonstrated a significant fall in plasma testosterone levels after the age of 60 years. The pattern seen was very similar to that shown in Fig. 1a, although a number of their old men had levels below 6–9 nmol/liter. Similar results have been reported by Nieschlag et al. (1973), Doerr and Pirke (1973), Stearns et al. (1974), Frick and Kinel (1969), Kirschner and Coffman (1968), and Vermeulen et al. (1972).

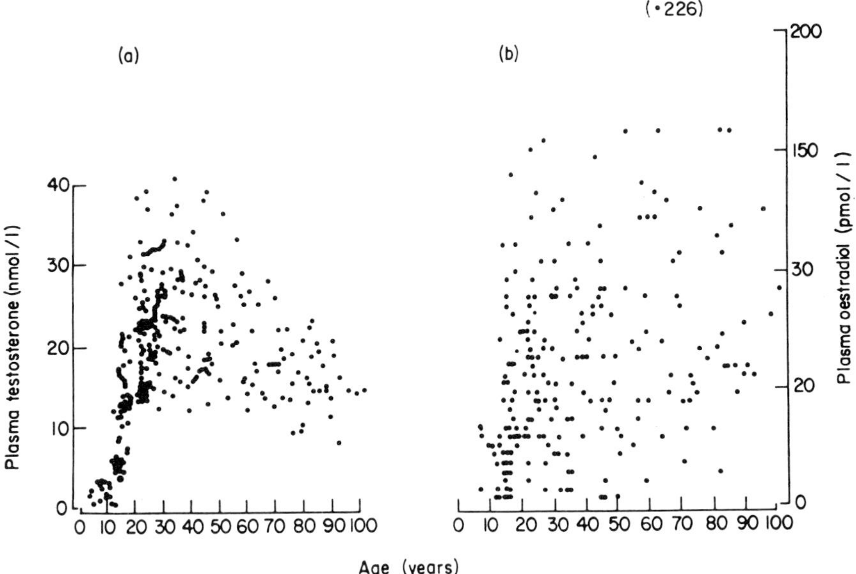

Fig. 1a, b. Testosterone (nmol/liter) (**a**) and estradiol (pmol/liter) (**b**) as functions of age in normal males. (BAKER et al., 1976)

Plasma estradiol (Fig. 1b) appeared to rise with advancing age, but the difference between the levels of young and old men was relatively small. The mean levels in the two groups were 59.2 and 77.8 pmol/liter ($P < 0.005$).

The results of BAKER et al. (1976) confirm the findings of DOERR and PIERKE (1973) and LONGCOPE (1973) who also found Estradiol (E_2) levels higher in older men. Closer inspection of Fig. 1b reveals a wide scatter of E_2 levels at all ages and also that a large group of men above the age of 50 years have E_2 levels below the mean level (59 pmol/liter) of the younger age group. The lack of uniformity of the E_2 pattern is only partially a reflection of testicular function since peripheral conversion is a main contributor to the levels found in plasma. The binding capacity of the sex hormone-binding globulin (SHBG) gradually increases with advancing age (VERMEULEN et al., 1972; DOERR and PIRKE, 1973; STEARNS et al., 1974; NIESCHLAG et al., 1973). This increase does not only occur in individuals with elevated estrogen levels (potent stimulator of SHBG) but also as a result of a decrease in the rate of metabolic disposal. The increased SHBG binding capacity leads to an increase in the portion of the bound steroids and a concomitant decrease in the available free testosterone. Indeed, BAKER et al. (1976) showed that free testosterone in adults after the age of 50 years was 1.1% and in the younger group 1.7%. This, in addition to the decreased production rate of testosterone, leads to a decrease of about one-half of the physiologically available testosterone; the mean free testosterone level above the age of 51 years was 0.19 nmol/liter whereas in the younger age group it was 0.38 nmol/liter.

Decreased levels of free sex hormones will evoke an elevation of the gonadotropin hormones. HENDERSON and ROWLANDS reported in 1938 that the pituitary content of gonadotropins increased in men with advancing age. ALBERT (1956)

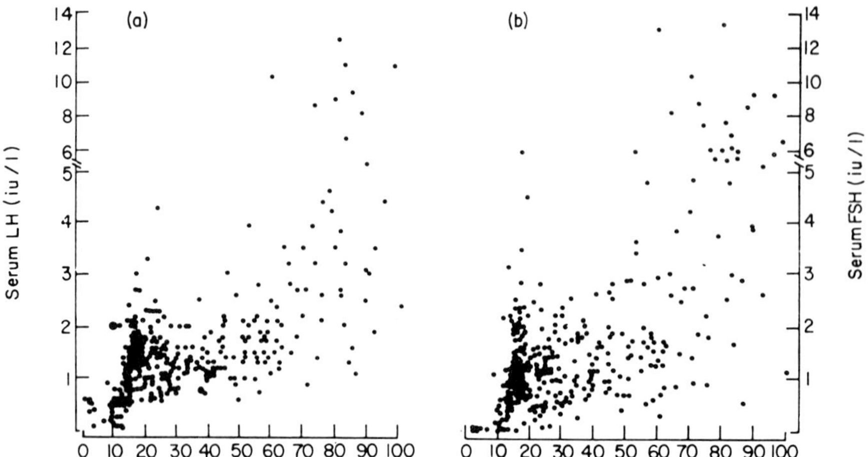

Fig. 2a, b. Serum LH (IU/liter) (**a**) and serum FSH (IU/liter) (**b**) as functions of age in normal males. (Baker et al., 1976)

demonstrated a progressive rise in urinary gonadotropins in men after the age of 40 years and a sharp rise after the age of 60 years. These findings were later confirmed by Johnsen (1959). Baker et al. (1976) described luteinizing hormone (LH) and follicle-stimulating hormone (FSH) levels in serum of men of different ages (Fig. 2a and 2b). Changes in levels of LH and FSH presented similar patterns with increasing age of the subjects. The mean LH and FSH levels in men over the age of 50 years (LH 3.04, FSH 7.27 IU/liter) were significantly higher than in men aged 21–50 years (LH 1.42, FSH 1.95 IU/liter) ($P < 0.001$). Of the 37 men over the age of 70 years, 22 had LH levels above the upper limit of the range for men aged 21–50 years, and 15 had levels within the normal range. FSH levels were elevated in 25 men over the age of 70 years. The gonadotropin levels exhibited a logarithmic normal distribution. Increased levels of gonadotropins concomitant with a decreased rate of androgen production are indicative of a reduced responsiveness of the steroidogenic target cells. This has been investigated by studying the effect of human chorionic gonadotropin (HCG) stimulation. Luisi et al. (1969) studied the effect of HCG on testosterone secretion in elderly men who had elevated levels of gonadotropins and in whom plasma and urinary testosterone levels and testosterone production rates were significantly lower than in younger persons. HCG stimulation (concomitant with dexamethasone suppression) resulted in a significant rise of both plasma and urinary testosterone (from 0.38 ± 11 to 0.62 ± 29 and from 41.6 ± 11.6 to 69 ± 27.1 µg/24 h, respectively). The testosterone production rate also significantly increased following HCG stimulation (3.1 ± 1.1 to 5.3 ± 2.6 µg/day). In the above-mentioned study it was also found that testosterone production rates in elderly subjects complaining of climacteric symptoms were similar to those of the symptom-free group and that the increase in the testosterone production rate was even greater (3.6 ± 1.13 to 7.5 ± 1.8 µg/day).

The data reported by Nieschlag et al. (1973), and Mazzi et al. (1974) confirm the above-mentioned results concerning plasma testosterone increase following HCG stimulation. However, NIESCHLAG et al. (1973) showed that in men between the ages of 20–60 years, the mean increase of plasma testosterone following HCG stimulation was 2.3 (± 0.05) fold, whereas in the age group of 61–90 years the stimulation coefficient was only 1.6 (± 0.1).

All the above-mentioned papers examined the effect of relative short-term HCG stimulation (1–3 days of stimulation) and thus investigated the capacity of the available Leydig cells to secrete testosterone upon HCG stimulation. MOTT (1919) and TILLINGER (1957) showed that the number of Leydig cells decreases with age. The decreased rise of testosterone upon short-term HCG stimulation might thus be due either to the reduced number of responsive cells, a reduced responsiveness of the target cells, or a combination of both.

All the above observations confirm that testicular function in general declines with age. However, when inspecting the individual values (Fig. 1), it becomes clear that this does not occur consistently or suddenly at a particular age. Furthermore, it can be speculated that the process leading to andropause occurs gradually and passes through several phases:
1. Decreased responsiveness of Leydig cells to LH stimulation
2. Decrease in testosterone levels
3. The weakened impulse toward the negative feedback system leads to an increase of LH and FSH
4. The elevated LH brings about a transient compensatory effect
5. As a result of the age-dependent decreased metabolic disposal of SHBG the portion of free testosterone is further reduced and andropause is established

The sequence is not necessarily initiated at the testicular level but could be started by the reduction of the metabolic disposal rate. Whatever the starting point, the end result will be similar.

B. Diagnosis and Management

As outlined in the introduction, the diagnosis of andropause can only be confirmed if clinical symptoms of the male climacteric are associated with decreased potency or libido and with laboratory parameters of decreased androgenicity. The laboratory investigation should include determination of serum levels of testosterone (preferably free testosterone) and LH. If testosterone levels (total) are 30% below the normal mean (with respect to the normal mean value of each particular center) or free testosterone is reduced by 50% and this is associated with a doubling of LH values (with respect to the normal mean value of each particular center), then the diagnosis of andropause is established. Despite the existence of testosterone deficiency, replacement therapy with androgens should not be initiated as long as Leydig cells have residual capacity to respond to stimulation. Testosterone administration in such cases will inhibit LH secretion, which will further diminish (possibly irreversibly) Leydig cell function.

To assess Leydig cell function, the responsiveness to HCG stimulation as reflected by testosterone secretion should be evaluated. Following the assessment of baseline testosterone levels, 5000 IU HCG is administered IM, and testosterone is again estimated 48–72 h later. The injections are repeated at 5-day intervals, and plasma testosterone is again estimated 48–72 h after the third injection. If a 50% increase in testosterone occurs, then periodical administration of HCG (5000 IU/week) is recommended.

A treatment course is continued for 6–12 weeks during and following which testosterone levels are measured and compared to baseline levels. If during the treatment course testosterone levels increase and remain elevated thereafter with concomitant increase of potency and amelioration of symptoms, HCG treatment is considered to be the treatment of choice. At the reoccurrence of the typical symptomatology, a reevaluation of the Leydig cell response to HCG is instituted as previously outlined, and the decision for further treatment is made accordingly.

When testosterone levels do not increase following HCG injections or increased levels cannot be maintained following cessation of HCG injections, an irreversible stage of andropause may be assumed, which should be treated by long-acting androgen preparations. If Leydig cells are responsive to HCG stimulation but testosterone levels are maintained for only short intervals following cessation of HCG injections (e.g., less than 3 months), one should consider long-acting androgen preparations as a better form of therapy.

References

Albert A (1956) Human urinary gonadotropin. In: Pincus G (ed) Recent progress in hormone research, vol 12. Academic Press, New York, pp 227–301

Baker HWG, Burger HG, de Kretser DM, Hudson B, O'Connor S, Wang C, Mirovics A, Court J, Dunlop M and Rennie GC (1976) Changes in the pituitary-testicular system with age. Clin Endocrinol 5:349–372

Doerr P, Pirke KM (1973) Influence of male senescence on plasma oestradiol, testosterone and binding capacity of testosterone-binding globulin (Abstract). Acta Endocrinol [Suppl] (Kbh) 177:123

Engle ET, Pincus G (1956) Hormones and the ageing process. Academic Press, New York, pp 1–20

Frick J, Kincl FA (1969) The measurement of plasma testosterone by competitive protein binding assay. Steroids 13:495–505

Henderson WR, Rowlands IW (1938) Gonadotropic activity of anterior pituitary gland in relation to increased intracranial pressure. Br Med J 1:1094–1097

Hollander N, Hollander VP (1958) The microdetermination of testosterone in human spermatic vein blood. J Clin Endocrinol Metab 18:966–971

Johnsen SG (1969) A clinical routine-method for the quantitative determination of gonadothrophins in 24 hour urine samples. II. Normal values for men and women at all age groups from puberty to senescence. Acta Endocrinol (Kbh) 34:209–227

Kies N (1974) Die klimakterische Symptomatologie aus klinischer-psychologischer Sicht. Med Welt 25:228

Kirschner MA, Coffman GD (1968) Measurement of plasma testosterone and Δ4-androstenedione using electron capture gas-liquid chromatography. J Clin Endocrinol Metab 28:1347–1355

Longcope C (1973) The effect of human chorionic gonadotropin in plasma steroid levels in young and old men. Steroids 21:583–590

Luisi M, Franchi F, Morescotti V, Fassorra C, Todescini C (1969) Effect of chorionic gonadotrophin administration on plasma levels, urinary excretion and production of testosterone in elderly subjects and in patients with climacteric syndrome. Acta Eur Fertil 1:617–632

Mazzi C, Riva LP, Bernasconi D (1974) Gonadotrophin and plasma testosterone in senescence. In: James VHT, Serio M, Martini L (eds) The endocrine function of the human testis. vol 2. Academic Press, New York, pp 51–66

Morer-Fargas F, Nowakosky H (1965) Die Testosteronausscheidung im Harn bei männlichen Individuen. Acta Endocrinol (Kbh) 49:443–452

Mott FW (1919) Normal and morbid conditions of the testis from birth to old age in one hundred asylum and hospital cases. Br Med J 2:655

Nieschlag E, Kley HK, Wiegelmann W, Solback HG, Krueskemper HL (1973) Lebensalter und endokrine Funktion der Testes des erwachsenen Mannes. Dtsch Med Wochenschr 98:1281

Rubens R, Dhont M, Vermeulen A (1974) Further studies on Leydig cell function in old age. J Clin Endocrinol Metab 39:40–45

Stearns EL, Macdonell JA, Kaufman BJ, Padua R, Lucman TS, Winter JSD, Faiman C (1974) Declining testicular function with age: Hormonal and clinical correlates. Am J Med 57:761–766

Tillinger KG (1957) Testicular morphology. Acta Endocrinol [Suppl] (Kbh) 30:1

Vermeulen A, Rubens R, Verdonck L (1972) Testosterone secretion and metabolism in male senescence. J Clin Endocrinol Metab 34:730–735

Werner AA (1939) The male climacteric. J Am Med Assoc 112:1441

Subject Index

Handbuch der Urologie/ Encyclopedia of Urology

Outline
Gesamtübersicht

Volume 1
Anatomie und Embryologie
Von K. Conrad, H. Ferner, A. Gisel, H. v. Hayek,
W. Krause, Ch. Zaki
1969. 363 Abbildungen, davon 46 farbig.
XI, 637 Seiten
Gebunden DM 360,–; approx. US $ 167.60
Subskriptionspreis
Gebunden DM 288,–; approx. US $ 134.10
ISBN 3-540-04534-1

Volume II
**Physiologie und pathologische Physiologie/
Physiology and Pathological Physiology/
Physiologie normale et pathologique**
By. B. Fey, F. Heni, A. Kuntz, D. F. McDonald,
L. Quénu, L. G. Wesson jr.,C. Wilson
1965. 169 figures. XX, 1009 pages
(273 pages in German, 60 pages in French)
Cloth DM 420,–; approx. US $ 195.60
Subscription price
Cloth DM 372,–; approx. US $ 173.20
ISBN 3-540-03315-7

Volume III
**Symptomatologie und Untersuchungen von Blut,
Harn und Genitalsekreten/ Symptomatology and
Examination of the Blood, Urine and Genital
Secretions**
Von K. Hinsberg, J. Kimmig, J. Meyer-Rohn,
R. H. Robinson, C. Schirren, R. Wehrmann
1960. 61 Abbildungen. XVI, 337 Seiten
(30 Seiten in Englisch)
Gebunden DM 210,–; approx. US $ 97.80
Subskriptionspreis
Gebunden DM 168,–; approx. US $ 78.30
ISBN 3-540-02550-2

Volume IV
L'insuffisance rénale
Par J. Hamburger, G. Richet, J. Crosnier,
J.-L. Funck-Brentano
1962. 151 figures. XXIV, 637 pages
Relié DM 320,–; approx. US $ 149.00
Prix de souscription
Relié DM 256,–; approx. US $ 119.20
ISBN 3-540-02845-5

Volume V/1
Diagnostic Radiology
By R. H. Flocks, G. Jönsson, K. Lindblom,
O. Olsson, R. Romanus, Ch. C. Winter
1962. 402 figures. XII, 533 pages
Cloth DM 320,–; approx. US $ 149.00
Subscription price
Cloth DM 256,–; approx. US $ 119.20
ISBN 3-540-02846-3

Volume V/2
Radiotherapy
In preparation

Volume VI
Endoscopy
By R. W. Barnes, R. Th. Bergman, H. L. Hadley
1959. 184 figures. XXIV, 282 pages
(5 pages in German)
Cloth DM 200,–; approx. US $ 93.10
Subscription price
Cloth DM 160,–; approx. US $ 74.50
ISBN 3-540-02419-0

Volume VII/1
Malformations
By A. D. Amar, O. S. Culp, F. Farman, J. A. Hutch,
H. W. Jones Jr., V. F. Marshall, J. W. McRoberts,
E. C. Muecke, J. J. Murphy, R. J. Prentiss,
Th. A. Tristan, K. Waterhouse
1968. 348 figures. XV, 479 pages
Cloth DM 220,–; approx. US $ 102.50
Subscription price
Cloth DM 176,–; approx. US $ 82.00
ISBN 3-540-04165-6

Volume VII/2
**Die urologische Begutachtung und Dokumen-
tation/The Urologist's Expert Opinion and
Documentation/ L'Expertise et Documentation en
Urologie**
Von F. Baumbusch, E. Schindler, Th. Schultheis,
W. Vahlensieck
1965. 10 Tabellen. XXIV, 648 Seiten
Gebunden DM 270,–; approx. US $ 125.70
Subskriptionspreis
Gebunden DM 216,–; approx. US $ 100.60
ISBN 3-540-03316-5

Volume VIII
Entleerungsstörungen
Von R. Chwalla, U. Comuzzi, F. de Gironcoli,
G. Hartmann, Z. Kairis, R. Übelhör
1962. 299 Abbildungen. XII, 706 Seiten
Gebunden DM 340,–; approx. US $ 158.30
Subskriptionspreis
Gebunden DM 272,–; approx. US $ 126.70
ISBN 3-540-02847-1

Springer-Verlag
Berlin Heidelberg New York